Inflammation and Allergy Drug Design

Inflammation and Allergy Drug Design

Edited by

Kenji Izuhara MD, PhD
Professor
Department of Biomolecular Sciences
Division of Medical Biochemistry
Saga Medical School
Nabeshima
Saga, Japan

Stephen T. Holgate MD, DSc, FMedSci
Professor
School of Medicine, Allergy and Inflammation Research
Southampton General Hospital
University Medicine
Southampton, UK

Marsha Wills-Karp PhD
Director
Division of Immunology
Cincinnati Children's Medical Center
Cincinnati, OH, USA

WILEY-BLACKWELL

A John Wiley & Sons, Ltd., Publication

This edition first published 2011, © 2011 by Blackwell Publishing Ltd

Blackwell Publishing was acquired by John Wiley & Sons in February 2007. Blackwell's publishing program has been merged with Wiley's global Scientific, Technical and Medical business to form Wiley-Blackwell.

Registered office: John Wiley & Sons, Ltd, The Atrium, Southern Gate, Chichester, West Sussex, PO19 8SQ, UK

Editorial offices: 9600 Garsington Road, Oxford, OX4 2DQ, UK
The Atrium, Southern Gate, Chichester, West Sussex, PO19 8SQ, UK
350 Main Street, Malden, MA 02148-5020, USA
111 River Street, Hoboken, NJ 07030-5774, USA

For details of our global editorial offices, for customer services and for information about how to apply for permission to reuse the copyright material in this book please see our website at www.wiley.com/wiley-blackwell

The right of the author to be identified as the author of this work has been asserted in accordance with the UK Copyright, Designs and Patents Act 1988.

Designations used by companies to distinguish their products are often claimed as trademarks. All brand names and product names used in this book are trade names, service marks, trademarks or registered trademarks of their respective owners. The publisher is not associated with any product or vendor mentioned in this book. This publication is designed to provide accurate and authoritative information in regard to the subject matter covered. It is sold on the understanding that the publisher is not engaged in rendering professional services. If professional advice or other expert assistance is required, the services of a competent professional should be sought.

The contents of this work are intended to further general scientific research, understanding, and discussion only and are not intended and should not be relied upon as recommending or promoting a specific method, diagnosis, or treatment by physicians for any particular patient. The publisher and the author make no representations or warranties with respect to the accuracy or completeness of the contents of this work and specifically disclaim all warranties, including without limitation any implied warranties of fitness for a particular purpose. In view of ongoing research, equipment modifications, changes in governmental regulations, and the constant flow of information relating to the use of medicines, equipment, and devices, the reader is urged to review and evaluate the information provided in the package insert or instructions for each medicine, equipment, or device for, among other things, any changes in the instructions or indication of usage and for added warnings and precautions. Readers should consult with a specialist where appropriate. The fact that an organization or Website is referred to in this work as a citation and/or a potential source of further information does not mean that the author or the publisher endorses the information the organization or Website may provide or recommendations it may make. Further, readers should be aware that Internet Websites listed in this work may have changed or disappeared between when this work was written and when it is read. No warranty may be created or extended by any promotional statements for this work. Neither the publisher nor the author shall be liable for any damages arising herefrom.

Library of Congress Cataloging-in-Publication Data

Inflammation and allergy drug design / edited by Kenji Izuhara, Stephen T. Holgate, Marsha Wills-Karp.
    p. ; cm.
  Includes bibliographical references and index.
  ISBN 978-1-4443-3014-4 (hardcover : alk. paper)
1. Antiallergic agents. 2. Allergy–Treatment. 3. Anti-inflammatory agents. 4. Drugs–Design. I. Izuhara, Kenji. II. Holgate, S. T. III. Wills-Karp, Marsha.
  [DNLM: 1. Anti-Allergic Agents. 2. Hypersensitivity–drug therapy. 3. Anti-Inflammatory Agents. 4. Drug Design. QV 157]
  RM666.A5I54 2011
  615'.7–dc22

                                    2010052266

A catalogue record for this book is available from the British Library.

This book is published in the following electronic formats: ePDF 978-1-4443-4666-4; Wiley Online Library 978-1-4443-4668-8; ePub 978-1-4443-4667-1.

Set in 9/11.5 pt Sabon by Toppan Best-set Premedia Limited
Printed and Bound in Singapore by Fabulous Printers Pte Ltd

01 2011

Contents

Contributors

Jessica L. Allen PhD
Division of Molecular Immunology
Cincinnati Children's Hospital Research Foundation
    and the University of Cincinnati College of
    Medicine
Cincinnati, OH, USA

Yassine Amrani MSc, PhD
Reader
Respiratory Immunology
Institute for Lung Health
University of Leicester School of Medicine
Leicester, UK

Kazuhiko Arima MD, PhD
Assistant Professor
Department of Biomolecular Sciences
Division of Medical Biochemistry
Saga Medical School
Nabeshima, Saga, Japan

Maria G. Belvisi PhD, FBPharmacolS
Head of Respiratory Pharmacology
Pharmacology and Toxicology Section
National Heart & Lung Institute
Imperial College London
London, UK

Neville Berkman MBBCh, FRCP
Director
Invasive Pulmonology
Institute of Pulmonology Medicine
Hadassah-Hebrew University Medical Center
Jerusalem, Israel

Larry Borish MD
Asthma and Allergic Disease Center
Carter Immunology Center
University of Virginia Health Systems
Charlottesville, VA, USA

Christopher Brightling MRCP PhD
Wellcome Senior Clinical Fellow
Honorary Consultant
Institute for Lung Health
Leicester, UK

Latifa Chachi MSc
University of Leicester School of Medicine
Leicester, UK

Deborah L. Clarke PhD
Research Fellow
Respiratory Pharmacology
Pharmacology and Toxicology Section
National Heart and Lung Institute
Imperial College London
London, UK

Chris Corrigan MD
Department of Asthma, Allergy & Respiratory
    Science
King's College London School of Medicine;
MRC and Asthma UK Centre for Allergic
    Mechanisms of Asthma
London, UK

Mark V. Dahl MD
Consultant
Department of Immunology, Dermatology, and
    Pathology
Professor of Dermatology
Mayo Clinic College of Medicine
Mayo Clinic Arizona
Scottsdale, AZ, USA

Dhan Desai MBBS
Clinical Fellow
Institute for Lung Health
Leicester, UK

Ramzi Fattouh PhD
Department of Pathology and Molecular Medicine
Centre for Gene Therapeutics
Division of Respiratory Diseases and Allergy
McMaster University
Hamilton, ON, Canada

Stephen J. Galli MD
Chair
Department of Pathology
Professor
Pathology and Microbiology and Immunology
Stanford University School of Medicine
Stanford, CA, USA

Yasuhiro Gon MD
Department of Internal Medicine
Division of General Medicine
Nihon University School of Medicine
Tokyo, Japan

Tillie-Louise Hackett PhD
Department of Anesthesiology, Pharmacology and
    Therapeutics
UBC James Hogg Research Centre
Providence Heart and Lung Institute
University of British Columbia
Vancouver, BC, Canada

Andrew J. Halayko PhD
Professor
Physiology, Internal Medicine and Pediatrics and
    Child Health
Canada Research Chair
Airway Cell and Molecular Biology
University of Manitoba;
Leader
Biology of Breathing Theme
Manitoba Institute of Child Health
Winnipeg, MB, Canada

Hamida Hammad PhD
Department of Respiratory Diseases
Laboratory of Immunoregulation and Mucosal
    Immunology
University Hospital Ghent
Ghent, Belgium

Mitchishige Harada PhD
Research Scientist
Laboratory for Immune Regulation
RIKEN Research Center for Allergy and
    Immunology
Yokohama, Kanagawa, Japan

Shu Hashimoto MD
Department of Internal Medicine
Division of Respiratory Medicine
Nihon University School of Medicine
Tokyo, Japan

Masashi Ikutani PhD
Assistant Professor
Department of Immunobiology and Pharmacological
    Genetics
Graduate School of Medicine and Pharmaceutical
    Science
University of Toyama
Toyama, Japan

Itsuo Iwamoto MD, PhD
Director
Research Center for Allergy and Clinical
    Immunology
Asahi General Hospital
Chiba, Japan

Elizabeth A. Jacobsen PhD
Research Associate
Division of Pulmonary Medicine
Assistant Professor
Department of Biochemistry and Molecular Biology
Mayo Clinic Arizona
Scottsdale, AZ, USA

Manel Jordana MD, PhD
Department of Pathology and Molecular Medicine
Centre for Gene Therapeutics
Division of Respiratory Diseases and Allergy
McMaster University
Hamilton, ON, Canada

Christopher L. Karp MD
Gunnar Esiason/Cincinnati Bell Chair
Director
Division of Molecular Immunology
Professor of Pediatrics
Cincinnati Children's Hospital Research Foundation
    and the University of Cincinnati College of
    Medicine
Cincinnati, OH, USA

Darryl Knight PhD
UBC James Hogg Research Centre
Providence Heart and Lung Institute
Department of Anesthesiology, Pharmacology and
    Therapeutics
University of British Columbia
Vancouver, BC, Canada

Bart N. Lambrecht MD, PhD
Department of Respiratory Diseases
Laboratory of Immunoregulation and Mucosal
    Immunology
University Hospital Ghent
Ghent, Belgium;
Department of Pulmonary Medicine
Erasmus University Medical Center
Rotterdam, Netherlands

Nancy A. Lee PhD
Consultant
Division of Hematology and Oncology
Associate Professor
Department of Biochemistry and Molecular Biology
Mayo Clinic Arizona
Scottsdale, AZ, USA

Francesca Levi-Schaffer PhD
Professor and Head
Immunopharmacology Laboratory for Allergy and
    Asthma Research
Isaac and Myrna Kaye Chair
Immunopharmacology
Institute for Drug Research
School of Pharmacy, Faculty of Medicine
The Hebrew University of Jerusalem
Jerusalem, Israel

Alba Llop-Guevara BSc
Department of Pathology and Molecular Medicine
Centre for Gene Therapeutics
Division of Respiratory Diseases and Allergy
McMaster University
Hamilton, ON, Canada

Yong-Jun Liu MD, PhD
Professor and Chair
Department of Immunology
Director
Center for Cancer Immunology Research
University of Texas, M.D. Anderson Cancer Center
Houston, TX, USA

Donald MacGlashan, Jr. MD
Johns Hopkins University
Baltimore, MD, USA

Sarah A. Maher PhD
Postdoctoral Research Associate
Respiratory Pharmacology
Pharmacology and Toxicology Section
National Heart and Lung Institute
Imperial College London
London, UK

Josip Marcinko BHSc
Department of Pathology and Molecular Medicine
Centre for Gene Therapeutics
Division of Respiratory Diseases and Allergy
McMaster University
Hamilton, ON, Canada

Yoshinori Nagai MD, PhD
Associate Professor
Department of Immunobiology and Pharmacological
  Genetics
Graduate School of Medicine and Pharmaceutical
  Science
University of Toyama
Toyama, Japan

Hiroshi Nakajima MD, PhD
Professor
Department of Molecular Genetics
Graduate School of Medicine
Chiba University
Chiba, Japan

Kenji Nakanishi MD, PhD
President and Professor
Department of Immunology and Medical Zoology
Hyogo College of Medicine
Nishinomiya, Hyogo, Japan

Keisuke Oboki PhD
Department of Allergy and Immunology
National Research Institute for Child Health and
  Development
Tokyo, Japan

Sergei I. Ochkur PhD
Senior Research Associate
Department of Biochemistry and Molecular Biology
Division of Pulmonary Medicine
Mayo Clinic Arizona
Scottsdale, AZ, USA

Shoichiro Ohta MD, PhD
Lecturer
Department of Laboratory Medicine
Saga Medical School
Saga, Japan

Katsuhide Okunishi MD, PhD
Postdoctoral Research Fellow
Division of Pulmonary and Critical Care Medicine
Department of Internal Medicine
University of Michigan Health System
Ann Arbor, MI, USA

Marc Peters-Golden MD
Professor
Internal Medicine
Division of Pulmonary and Critical Care Medicine
Department of Internal Medicine
University of Michigan Health System
Ann Arbor, MI, USA

Maud Plantinga MSc
Department of Respiratory Diseases
Laboratory of Immunoregulation and Mucosal
  Immunology
University Hospital Ghent
Ghent, Belgium

Kimuli Ryanna MD
Department of Asthma, Allergy and Respiratory
  Science
King's College London School of Medicine;
MRC and Asthma UK Centre for Allergic
  Mechanisms of Asthma
London, UK

Hirohisa Saito MD, PhD
Department of Allergy and Immunology
National Research Institute for Child Health and
  Development
Tokyo, Japan

Michael Schuliga PhD
Research Fellow
Department of Pharmacology
University of Melbourne
Parkville, VIC, Australia

Pawan Sharma MPharm
Department of Physiology
University of Manitoba
Biology of Breathing Group
Manitoba Institute of Child Health
Winnipeg, MB, Canada

Hiroshi Shiraishi PhD
Assistant Professor
Division of Medical Biochemistry
Department of Biomolecular Sciences
Saga Medical School
Saga, Japan

Lilian Soon PhD
Senior Lecturer
Australian Centre for Microscopy and
   Microanalysis
University of Sydney
Sydney, NSW, Australia

Dorota Stefanowicz BSc
UBC James Hogg Research Centre
Providence Heart and Lung Institute
Department of Medicine
University of British Columbia
Vancouver, BC, Canada

John W. Steinke PhD
Asthma and Allergic Disease Center
Carter Immunology Center
University of Virginia Health Systems
Charlottesville, VA, USA

Whitney W. Stevens PhD
Asthma and Allergic Disease Center
Carter Immunology Center
University of Virginia Health Systems
Charlottesville, VA, USA

Alastair G. Stewart PhD
Professor
Department of Pharmacology
University of Melbourne
Parkville, VIC, Australia

Shoichi Suzuki PhD
Assistant Professor
Division of Medical Biochemistry
Department of Biomolecular Sciences
Saga Medical School
Saga, Japan

Kiyoshi Takatsu PhD
Professor
Department of Immunobiology and Pharmacological
   Genetics
Graduate School of Medicine and Pharmaceutical
   Science
University of Toyama
Toyama, Japan

Masaru Taniguchi MD, PhD
Director
RIKEN Research Center for Allergy and
   Immunology
Yokohama, Kanagawa, Japan

Mayumi Tamari MD, PhD
Team Leader
Laboratory for Respiratory Diseases
RIKEN Center for Genome Medicine
Yokohama, Kanagawa, Japan

Luis M. Teran PhD
Head of Allergy and Clinical Immunology
National Institute of Respiratory Diseases
Mexico City, Mexico

Aurelien Trompette MS
University Hospital Center of Lausanne
Lausanne, Switzerland

Mindy Tsai DMSc
Senior Research Scientist
Department of Pathology
Stanford University School of Medicine
Stanford, CA, USA

Hiroka Tsutsui MD, PhD
Professor
Department of Microbiology
Hyogo College of Medicine
Nishinomiya, Hyogo, Japan

Juan R. Velazquez PhD
Immunology and Asthma Laboratory
National Institute of Respiratory Diseases
Mexico City, Mexico

Stephanie Warner BSc
UBC James Hogg Research Centre
Providence Heart and Lung Institute
Department of Medicine
University of British Columbia
Vancouver, BC, Canada

Hiroshi Watarai PhD
Senior Research Scientist
Laboratory for Immune Regulation
RIKEN Research Center for Allergy and
    Immunology
Yokohama, Kanagawa, Japan

Monique Willart MSc
Department of Respiratory Diseases
Laboratory of Immunoregulation and Mucosal
    Immunology
University Hospital Ghent
Ghent, Belgium

Tomohiro Yoshimoto MD, PhD
Director and Professor
Laboratory of Allergic Diseases
Institute for Advanced Medical Sciences
Hyogo College of Medicine
Nishinomiya, Hyogo, Japan

Preface

Our knowledge and understanding of allergic diseases of the respiratory tract, such as asthma and rhinoconjunctivitis, has improved to a point where new therapies are being developed for patient benefit. Part of the problem in developing therapies has been our rather simplistic view of the allergic cascade and its components, as well as the over-reliance of the pharmaceutical and biotechnology industries on simple animal models of antigen sensitization and subsequent challenge to screen for active compounds. Asthma is a chronic relapsing disorder that varies its natural history over the life course and in which many environmental factors play a role beyond allergen exposure. This does not mean that enormous progress is not being made in these diseases, but that our ability to model the differing manifestations of asthma and associated disorders is limited. In addition, new technologies have led to the discovery of new targets in the airways that help link immunologic and inflammatory features to those of altered airway structure and function. Even within these immunologic mechanisms, we are gaining a wider appreciation of the role of the innate as well as the adaptive response and the importance of the formed airway elements such as epithelial cells, smooth muscle, nerves, and blood vessels in contributing to and supporting ongoing inflammation and tissue injury.

To give greater consideration to these issues in *Inflammation and Allergy Drug Design*, we have asked world leaders in their respective fields to provide us with the most up-to-date knowledge of the biologic science that underpins the pathophysiology of asthma and related disorders. We have divided the book into three parts covering the cells involved, their cytokines, chemokines, and growth factors, and mediators. What is so different about this book is the authors' skills in embedding their field of interest in the concept of asthma being a chronic relapsing condition. While each chapter develops in some detail the cutting-edge developments in a particular field, it is also clear that important interconnections between the fields are providing a new framework for reviewing asthma, especially the interactions between environmental exposures and the subsequent development of different subphenotypes (stratified medicine).

We believe the book is state-of-the art in terms of providing the reader with a superb reference source and a global perspective of each field, which should be helpful for clinical and basic scientists interested in the mechanisms of these disorders, irrespective of their academic, clinical, or industrial affiliations. The three editors are indebted to the way the authors have responded to requests for chapters in their fields, covering the most exciting recent developments, and as a result the value of the book as a whole has greatly increased. The editors would also value readers' views on this publication and interactions that may flow from it.

Kenji Izuhara, Stephen T. Holgate,
and Marsha Wills-Karp
April 2011

Part I
Cells contributing to the pathogenesis of allergic diseases in the respiratory tract

1

Novel anti-inflammatory drugs based on targeting lung dendritic cells and airway epithelial cells

Bart N. Lambrecht,[1,2] *Maud Plantinga,*[1] *Monique Willart,*[1] *and Hamida Hammad*[1]

[1]Department of Respiratory Diseases, Laboratory of Immunoregulation and Mucosal Immunology, University Hospital Ghent, Ghent, Belgium
[2]Department of Pulmonary Medicine, Erasmus University Medical Center, Rotterdam, the Netherlands

General function of dendritic cells in the immune system: induction of immunity

Dendritic cells (DCs) were originally defined by their capacity both to efficiently process and present antigens and to prime naïve T cells [1]. Immature DCs are situated in the periphery at sites of antigen exposure. In the periphery, DCs are specialized in antigen recognition and uptake. Under homeostatic conditions and particularly upon recognition of pathogens, DCs migrate to the T-cell area of draining nodes, where they screen the repertoire of naïve T cells for antigen-specific T cells that can be directed against the pathogen. Upon cognate T-cell receptor (TCR)–major histocompatibility complex (MHC)–peptide interaction, DCs subsequently form more stable interactions, and optimally induce T-cell effector function by providing co-stimulatory molecules and T-cell stimulatory and survival cytokines. In homeostatic conditions, only harmless antigens or self antigens are presented to T cells. Owing to their lack of complete induction of co-stimulatory molecules and cytokines in DCs, these antigens induce only abortive T-cell proliferation and/or lead to a T-cell response in which regulatory T cells (Tregs) are induced. This system allows for dangerous antigens to be eliminated, while avoiding overt immune-mediated damage in response to harmless environmental antigens and self antigens.

The increasing complexity of lung dendritic cell subsets

It is now clear that at least five different subsets of DCs can be found in the lungs (Figure 1.1). These subsets vary in origin, anatomical location, expression of cell surface markers and endocytic receptors, responsiveness to chemokines, and migratory behavior. Most importantly, there is division of labor between these various lung DC subsets, which makes a closer distinction between subsets almost imperative if one is to understand the biology of lung DCs [2]. The mouse lung is grossly divided into large conducting airways and lung interstitium, which contains alveolar septa and capillaries where gas exchange takes place [3]. The conducting airways of all species studied are lined with an intraepithelial, highly dendritic network of MHCII[high] CD11c[chi] cells that are mostly CD11b[−] and, at least in the mouse and rat, express langerin and the mucosal integrin CD103 ($\alpha_E\beta_7$), and have the propensity to extend dendrites into the airway lumen by forming tight junctions with bronchial epithelial cells [4]. Immediately below the epithelium, the lamina propria of the conducting airways contains MHCII[high] CD11c[high] cells that are mostly CD11b and are a rich source of proinflammatory chemokines [5]. A similar broad division into CD11b[+] and CD11b[−] can also be applied to lung interstitial DCs [6,7]. As both CD11b[+] and CD11b[−] subsets express high levels of CD11c, they are best

Inflammation and Allergy Drug Design, First Edition. Edited by Kenji Izuhara, Stephen T. Holgate, Marsha Wills-Karp.
© 2011 Blackwell Publishing Ltd. Published 2011 by Blackwell Publishing Ltd.

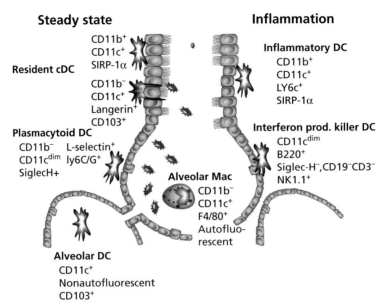

Steady state

Resident cDC
CD11b⁺
CD11c⁺
SIRP-1α

CD11b⁻
CD11c⁺
Langerin⁺
CD103⁺

Plasmacytoid DC
CD11b⁻ L-selectin⁺
CD11cᵈⁱᵐ ly6C/G⁺
SiglecH+

Alveolar Mac
CD11b⁻
CD11c⁺
F4/80⁺
Autofluo-
rescent

Alveolar DC
CD11c⁺
Nonautofluorescent
CD103⁺

Inflammation

Inflammatory DC
CD11b⁺
CD11c⁺
LY6c⁺
SIRP-1α

Interferon prod. killer DC
CD11cᵈⁱᵐ
B220⁺
Siglec-H⁻,CD19⁻CD3⁻
NK1.1⁺

Figure 1.1 Lung dendritic cell (DC) subsets. In steady-state conditions (depicted on the left) conventional DCs (subdivided into CD11b⁺ and CD11b⁻ subsets) line the conducting airways. They can also be found back in the deeper interstitial compartments, obtained by enzymatic digestion of peripheral lung. Plasmacytoid DCs (pDCs) are also found in both compartments with a slight preference for the interstitial compartment. Finally, the alveolar space contains DCs that can be easily confused with alveolar macrophages if one does not take autofluorescence of the latter into account. Under inflammatory conditions, there is recruitment of CD11b⁺ monocytes to the lungs and these rapidly become DCs. They can still express Ly6C as part of their monocytic descent. In viral infection as well as in some cancers there is also recruitment of interferon-producing killer DCs, a subset of natural killer (NK) cells that can be mistaken for pDCs in view of their intermediate expression of CD11c and expression of the B-cell marker B220. One way of discriminating these is via staining for NK1.1. cDC, conventional DC.

described as conventional DCs (cDCs) in order to differentiate them from another population of CD11cⁱⁿᵗ plasmacytoid DCs (pDCs) that express Siglec-H, the bone marrow stromal antigen 1, and the B-cell marker B220. Under inflammatory conditions, such as viral infection, allergen challenge, or lipopolysaccharide (LPS) administration, there is recruitment of additional subsets of CD11b⁺ monocyte-derived DCs that rapidly upregulate CD11c and retain expression of Ly6C as a remnant of their monocytic descent, and are easily confused with resident CD11b⁺ cDCs [7].

Function of lung dendritic cells: induction of tolerance in steady state and bridging innate and adaptive immunity

Airway DCs form a dense network in the lung that is ideally placed for sampling inhaled antigens by forming tight junctions with airway epithelial cells and extending their dendrites into the airway lumen, analogous to the situation in the gut. Following antigen uptake across the airway epithelial barrier, DCs migrate to draining mediastinal lymph nodes (LNs) in order to stimulate naïve T cells [8,9]. As most allergens are immunologically inert proteins, the usual outcome of their inhalation is tolerance and thus inflammation does not develop upon chronic exposure [10]. This is best displayed in the model antigen ovalbumin (OVA). When given to the airways of naïve mice, it induces tolerance to a subsequent immunization with OVA in adjuvant, and effectively inhibits the development of airway inflammation—a feature of true immunologic tolerance [10]. It was therefore long enigmatic how sensitization to natural allergens occurred. An important discovery was the fact that most clinically important allergens, such as the major house dust mite (HDM) allergen Der p 1, are proteolytic enzymes that can directly activate DCs or epithelial cells to break the process of tolerance and promote Th2 responses [11,12]. However, other allergens such as the experimental allergen OVA do not have any intrinsic activating properties. For these antigens, contaminating molecules or environmental exposures (respiratory viruses, air pollution) might initiate on DC activation [13]. Eisenbarth [14] showed that low-level Toll-like receptor (TLR) 4 agonists mixed with harmless OVA prime DCs to induce a Th2 response by inducing their full maturation, yet not their production of interleukin 12 (IL-12). This is clinically important information as most natural allergens such as HDM, cockroach, and animal dander contain endotoxin and undoubtedly other TLR agonists [15].

From the above, is seems that the decision between tolerance or immunity (in the lungs) is controlled by the degree of maturity of the myeloid DCs (mDCs) that interact with naïve T cells, a process that is driven by signals from the innate immune system [16]. Indeed, it has been shown that immature mDCs induce abortive proliferation in responding T cells and induce Tregs [17]. Another level of complexity arose when it was shown that (respiratory) tolerance might be a function of a subset of pDCs [10]. The removal of pDCs from mice using depleting antibodies led to a break in inhalational tolerance to OVA and to the development of asthmatic inflammation [10].

Sentinel function of lung dendritic cells requires instruction by epithelial cells

Most of the lung DC migration to the mediastinal lymph node results from some form of insult to the lung, be it microbial, physical, or toxic in nature. Based on the anatomical distribution of even the most exposed DCs, it is immediately clear that DCs are basically always covered by a layer of epithelial cells that seals off the inhaled air by the formation of tight junctions (Figure 1.2). It is therefore possible that in the absence of any TLRs or other activating signals, the DCs do not extend dendrites across this epithelial barrier. We recently hypothesized that airway epithelial cells might be instructive in causing

DC sentinel behavior and activation in the lungs [18]. Using a series of radiation chimeric mice in which either radioresistant stromal cells or radiosensitive hematopoietic cells were deficient in the LPS receptor TLR4, we demonstrated that the initial dynamic scanning behavior of lung DCs as well as their directed migration to the mediastinal nodes in response to LPS inhalation was largely dependent on TLR4 signaling on epithelial cells [19].

It is immediately clear from analysis of the common characteristics of clinically relevant allergens that most have the potential to modify epithelial barrier function and to activate airway epithelial cells or innate and adaptive immune cells, like DCs and basophils (see Chapter 21). For example, HDM (*Dermatophagoides pteronyssinus)* fecal pellets contain many allergens (Der p 1 to 9) that have either proteolytic activity or enhance TLR responsiveness, explaining why HDM acts as an allergen and a Th2 adjuvant. Der p 1 increases the permeability of the bronchial epithelium, as measured by a decrease in transepithelial electrical resistance by cleaving the tight junction proteins claudin and occludin, thus increasing access to the DC network [20]. In addition to these proteolytic effects of HDM, β-glucan-rich motifs of HDM were able to trigger human bronchial epithelial cells, most likely via the dectin-1 receptor, and downstream Syk signaling to produce CCL20, a major chemokine, thus causing attraction of lung DCs (see Figures 1.2 and 1.3) [21]. Along the same line, TLR4 signaling is also involved in the recognition of the HDM allergen [22]. In an elegant study, Trompette *et al.* [23] recently demonstrated that Der p 2 is a functional homolog of the adaptor MD-2 (also known as LY96), the LPS-binding component of the TLR4 signaling complex, thus stabilizing TLR4 expression on bronchial epithelial cells. In the same setting of TLR4 radiation chimerics, we have shown that it is mainly the epithelial TLR4-driven response that activates Th2 immunity to the HDM allergen by releasing innate pro-Th2 cytokines, like granulocyte–macrophage colony-stimulating factor (GM-CSF), thymic stromal lymphopoietin (TSLP), IL-33, and IL-25 (Figures 1.2 and 1.3) [19]. The TLR C-type lectin, or proteolytic-mediated activation of epithelial cells by HDM can lead to release of these innate cytokines or other mediators that subsequently program DCs to become Th2 inducers [19].

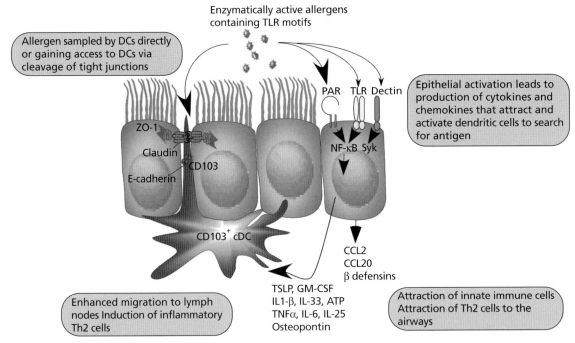

Enzymatically active allergens
containing TLR motifs

Allergen sampled by DCs directly
or gaining access to DCs via
cleavage of tight junctions

Epithelial activation leads to
production of cytokines and
chemokines that attract and
activate dendritic cells to search
for antigen

PAR TLR Dectin

ZO-1

Claudin

E-cadherin

CD103

NF-κB Syk

CD103⁺ cDC

CCL2
CCL20
β defensins

TSLP, GM-CSF
IL1-β, IL-33, ATP
TNFα, IL-6, IL-25
Osteopontin

Enhanced migration to lymph
nodes Induction of inflammatory
Th2 cells

Attraction of innate immune cells
Attraction of Th2 cells to the
airways

Figure 1.2 Interactions between epithelial cells and dendritic cells (DCs) in the airways. DCs sample the airway lumen by forming dendritic extensions in between epithelial cells. The cells form tight junctions with epithelial cells by expressing occludin and claudin family members as well as zona occludens 1. In addition, the cells attach to airway epithelial cells using E-cadherin and CD103 expressed by a subset of DCs that probes the airway lumen. Enzymatically active allergens can activate protease-activated receptors (PARs) expressed by epithelial cells followed by nuclear factor-κB (NF-κB) activation and the production of chemokines and cytokines by epithelial cells that attract and activate DCs. Allergens often contain Toll-like receptor (TLR) agonists and C-type lectin agonists; triggering through these also induces NF-κB activation and DC activation either directly or indirectly via effects on epithelial cells that also express TLRs and C-type lectin receptors.

Induction of Th2 responses: collaboration between DCs and innate immune cells

In the field of lung immunology, several groups have shown that either endogenous lung DCs [10,24,25] or adoptively transferred bone marrow-derived DCs [26] are sufficient to induce Th2 responses to inhaled antigens. Studies by Eisenbarth's group [24] have elegantly shown that triggering TLR4 on lung-derived DCs by administering low doses of LPS promotes Th2 cell development through a myeloid differentiation primary response gene 88 (MyD88)-dependent pathway. There is also evidence to suggest that CD11c⁺ DCs are necessary for Th2 responses. The Th2-inducing adjuvant alum is used by many groups to induce Th2 sensitization to inhaled OVA. However, these Th2 responses, as read out by induced T-cell proliferation, Th2 cytokine production, and IgG1 production, were eliminated when CD11c⁺ DCs were depleted when using diphtheria toxin treatment in CD11cDTR Tg mice [27,28]. Likewise, alum-exposed DCs clearly induced Th2 polarization from naïve TCR Tg T cells in a process requiring caspase-1 and IL-1β production. *In vitro* studies have also amply demonstrated that human DCs exposed to allergens like the HDM Der p 1 allergen [29] and pollen extracts (containing phytoprostanes and NADPH oxidases) [30] acquire Th2 polarizing capacity, even if IL-4 is not made by these exposed DCs. Several papers have recently demonstrated a crucial role for basophils in Th2 immunity [31–33], as they provide

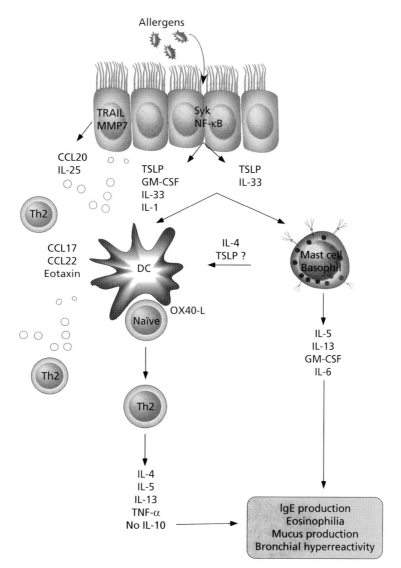

Figure 1.3 Early innate cytokine responses that promote allergic inflammation. Allergen triggering of protease-activated receptor 2 (PAR2) by C-type lectin receptors or by contaminating endotoxin acting on Toll-like receptors (TLRs) initiates the production of thymic stromal lymphopoeitin (TSLP), granulocyte–macrophage colony-stimulating factor (GM-CSF), and interleukin 33 (IL-33) by airway epithelial cells. These cytokines are known as DC-activating cytokines. For example, TSLP induces immediate innate immune functions in DCs leading to chemokine-driven recruitment of Th2 cells and eosinophils to the airways, possibly providing a source for polarizing Th2 cell-associated cytokines. Epithelial cells produce CCL20 in a process involving tumor necrosis factor alpha-related apoptosis-inducing ligand (TRAIL) and IL-25 in a process requiring matrix metalloproteinase 7 (MMP7). The effects of CCL20 and IL-25 are to further attract innate immune cells and Th2 cells to the lungs.

TSLP and IL-33 stimulate the functions of mast cells and basophils. In mast cells, there is immediate release of the Th2 effector cytokines that can attract and activate eosinophils in a T-cell-independent way. Following innate immune induction, TSLP (and IL-33) trigger the maturation of DCs so that they migrate to the mediastinal lymph nodes and induce the polarization of inflammatory Th2 cells in an OX40L-dependent fashion. In contrast to most other triggers that induce DC maturation, TSLP-induced maturation is not accompanied by the production of IL-12, thereby explaining Th2 cell polarization. Mast cells and basophils can also serve an important role for providing an early source of IL-4 for Th2 development. Basophils are recruited to draining lymph nodes in a process requiring TSLP. Together with mediators released by mast cells and basophils, effector Th2 cells control the salient features of asthma.

an important source of IL-4 early during an innate response to parasite infection and proteolytic allergens like HDM or papain, and at the same time also serve as bona fide antigen-presenting cells (APCs) that provide peptide-major histocompatibility complex (MHC), co-stimulatory molecules, and instructive Th polarizing signals. We foresee a scenario by which resident lymph node basophils collaborate with migratory DCs, providing an early source of IL-4 to promote or sustain Th2 immunity (Figure 1.3). In this regard, eosinophils, mast cells, and natural killer T (NKT) cells might be similar innate helpers for Th2 immunity driven by DCs [34,35].

Dendritic cells in established allergic airway inflammation

Not only do DCs play a role in the primary immune response to inhaled allergens, they are also crucial for the outcome of the effector phase in asthma. The number of mDCs is increased in the airways of sensitized and challenged mice during the acute phase of the response [36]. The mechanisms for this enhanced recruitment are that DC precursors, most likely at the monocyte stage of development, are attracted from the bone marrow via the bloodstream to the lung in a CCR2-dependent way [37]. However, during the chronic phase of the pulmonary response, induced by prolonged exposure to a large number of aerosols, respiratory tolerance develops through unclear mechanisms. During this regulatory phase, the number of mDCs in the lungs steadily decreased, and this was associated with a reduction of bronchial hyperreactivity (BHR). Inflammation, however, reappeared when mDCs were given [38]. The role of mDCs in the secondary immune response was further supported by the fact that their depletion at the time of allergen challenge abrogated all the features of asthma, including airway inflammation, goblet cell hyperplasia, and bronchial hyperresponsiveness [9,39]. antigenain the defect was restored by intratracheal injection of CD11b$^+$ inflammatory mDCs, but not by other APCs such as macrophages. It therefore seems that inflammatory mDCs are both necessary and sufficient for secondary immune responses to allergens.

In humans, allergen challenge leads to an accumulation of myeloid, but not plasmacytoid DCs to the airways of asthmatics, concomitantly with a reduc-

tion in circulating CD11c$^+$ cells, showing that these cells are recruited from the bloodstream in response to allergen challenge [40,41]. In stable asthma, the number of CD1a$^+$ DCs is increased in the airway epithelium and lamina propria, and these numbers are reduced by treatment with inhaled corticosteroids [42]. Based on the above argumentation in mice studies of asthma, it is very likely that part of the efficacy of inhaled steroids might be due to their effects in dampening airway DC function.

Novel targets for anti-inflammatory disease based on knowledge of DC-epithelial biology

Blocking innate pro-Th2 instructive cytokines

Thymic stromal lymphopoietin, a unique dendritic cell-instructive signal
Thymic stromal lymphopoietin is a 140 amino acid IL-7-like four-helix bundle cytokine that has potent DC-modulating capacities by binding its receptor complex, composed of the IL-7 receptor (IL-7R) and the TSLP receptor (TSLPR) [43]. TSLP can directly activate DCs to prime naïve CD4$^+$ T cells to differentiate into proinflammatory Th2 cells that secrete IL-4, IL-5, IL-13, and TNF-α, but not IL-10, and express the prostaglandin D$_2$ receptor CRTH2 (chemoattractant receptor-homologous molecule expressed on Th2 cells), a T-cell phenotype that is also found in asthmatic airways [44]. This pathway involves the induction of the Th2-prone co-stimulatory molecule OX40L and the production of the Th2-attractive chemokines CCL17 and CCL22 by DCs [44] (Figure 1.3). In addition to its effects on DCs, TSLP can also activate human mast cells to produce Th2-associated effector cytokines in the absence of T cells or IgE cross-linking [45] (Figure 1.3).

The most convincing evidence for a role for TSLP in DC-driven Th2 cell development came from studies in mice that conditionally overexpressed TSLP in the lungs. These mice mounted a vigorous DC-driven primary Th2 cell response to environmental antigens in the airways [46]. By contrast, *Tlspr*$^{-/-}$ mice fail to develop an antigen-specific Th2 cell inflammatory response in the airways unless they are supplemented with wild-type CD4$^+$ T cells [47]. Taken together, these data suggest that TSLP produced by the lung epithelium might represent a crucial factor that can initiate allergic responses at the epithelial-cell surface. Therefore, it will be very important to study how the production of TSLP by epithelial cells and other inflammatory cells is regulated.

IL-25, IL-33, and GM-CSF
The polarization of Th2 cells induced by TSLP-matured DCs is further enhanced by IL-25, which is produced by epithelial cells, basophils, and eosinophils [48]. Several reports showed that airway epithelial cells can produce IL-25 in response to an innate immune response to allergens, a process requiring epithelial cleaving of IL-25 by matrix metalloproteinase 7 (Figure 1.3) [19,49]. GM-CSF is released by bronchial epithelial cells in response to HDM exposure, as well as a number of environmental sensitizers like diesel exhaust particles and cigarette smoke. GM-CSF promotes DC maturation and breaks inhalation tolerance, and previous studies demonstrated that HDM-driven asthma is neutralized by blocking GM-CSF [50]. IL-33 is made by epithelial cells, boosts Th2-cytokine production, and promotes goblet cell hyperplasia. It was recently shown to also promote Th2 differentiation by programming the function of DCs [51]. Obviously, these cytokines could be high on the list for targeting inflammation in asthma, either individually or simultaneously, by blocking the innate receptors like TLR4, C-type lectin receptors, or protease-activated receptors that induce them [19,21,52].

Blocking endogenous DAMPs that contribute to DC activation in asthma

Dendritic cells express a plethora of receptors for endogenous danger-associated molecular patterns (DAMPs; Figure 1.4) that are released at sites of ongoing inflammation. For example, DCs express receptors (protease activated receptors [PARs]) that are activated by proteolytic proteins like tryptase and thrombin [29]. Shortly after insult to the vascular compartment or after pathogen entry in the mucosa, complement activation occurs. Lung DCs can sense this "acute alert" through expression of the C5a and C3a anaphylatoxin receptors [53]. DCs also express neuropeptide receptors, which can respond to the neurotransmitters that are released in response to axon reflexes or efferent neural responses, this is supported by the fact that lung DCs synapse

with unmyelinated nerve endings in and beneath the airway mucosa and produce neurotransmitters [54]. Lung DCs express receptors for prostaglandins and these acutely released inflammatory mediators can profoundly impact on the migration and maturation of the cell [55,56]. Endogenously released metabolites like extracellular adenosine triphosphate (ATP) trigger purinergic receptors on lung DCs, and in this way relay information about allergen-induced platelet aggregation or metabolic cell stress to the cells of the immune system through widely expressed purinergic receptors [57,58]. Eosinophil and mast cell degranulation can lead to the release of eosinophil-derived neurotoxin (EDN) and histamine that can feed back on DCs and promote further Th2 responses [59]. Clearly, much more effort is required before we can fully grasp the importance of these inflammatory mediators and DAMPs in explaining the chronicity of asthma [58]. These endogenous DAMPs are obvious targets for intervention, and blocking their production or neutralizing their effects has proven to be successful in intervening in mouse models of asthma.

Direct blocking of dendritic cell function

If DCs are so crucial in mounting and maintaining immune responses to inhaled allergens, then interfering directly with their function could constitute a novel form of treatment for allergic diseases. A strategy to eliminate DCs from the airways is probably not a valuable option, as local depletion of airway DCs was recently shown to lead to severe exacerbation of respiratory viral infections like influenza, whereby the virus failed to be cleared from the lungs and led to severe systemic illness [7]. Therefore, we are favoring the idea of targeting the fine-tuning mechanisms whereby DCs maintain allergic inflammation. Recently, several new molecules have been identified that may alter DC function in allergic inflammation and therefore could be possible therapeutic targets. Many of these compounds were first discovered by their potential to interfere with DC-driven Th2 cell sensitization. The sphingosine 1-phosphate receptor antagonist FTY720 is currently used in clinical trials for multiple sclerosis and transplant rejection. When given locally in the lungs of mice with established inflammation, it strongly reduced inflammation by suppressing the T-cell stimulatory capacity and migratory behavior of lung DCs without causing

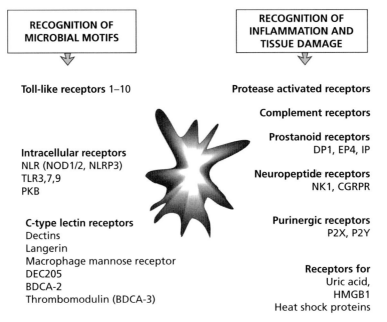

RECOGNITION OF MICROBIAL MOTIFS	RECOGNITION OF INFLAMMATION AND TISSUE DAMAGE

Toll-like receptors 1–10

Intracellular receptors
NLR (NOD1/2, NLRP3)
TLR3,7,9
PKB

C-type lectin receptors
Dectins
Langerin
Macrophage mannose receptor
DEC205
BDCA-2
Thrombomodulin (BDCA-3)

Protease activated receptors

Complement receptors

Prostanoid receptors
DP1, EP4, IP

Neuropeptide receptors
NK1, CGRPR

Purinergic receptors
P2X, P2Y

Receptors for
Uric acid,
HMGB1
Heat shock proteins

Figure 1.4 Dendritic cells (DCs) express extracellular and intracellular receptors that recognize pathogen-associated molecular patterns (PAMPs) that are found inside microbial motifs, as well as a wide variety of C-type lectin receptors that discriminate glycosylation patterns on self versus non-self proteins. What is less emphasized in the literature is that they also express receptors that recognize an ongoing inflammation response. Although PAMP receptors are mainly triggered by microbial motifs, it is possible that they are also activated by self ligands such as heat shock proteins. Tryptase, which is released by mast cells, and thrombin, which is released during the blood coagulation process, can trigger protease-activated receptors (PARs). Complement activation is an early innate immune reaction in response to allergen inhalation and can also lead to alterations in DC function. Inflammation often leads to the production of prostaglandins that can either stimulate (through the type 4 prostaglandin E_2 receptor, EP4) DC activation or dampen it (through the type 1 prostaglandin D_2 [DP1] and prostaglandin I_2 receptor [IP]). As airway DCs "live" in close proximity to unmyelinated nerve endings, the various neuropeptides that are released during neurogenic inflammation can also activate DCs by triggering neurokinin 1 (NK1) and the calcitonin gene-related protein receptor (CGRPR). Necrotic cell death leads to the release of damage-associated molecular patterns (DAMPs). Extracellular adenosine triphosphate (ATP) triggers a broad family of purinergic P2X and P2Y receptors. Uric acid is recognized by the NALP3 (NACHT-, LRR-, and pyrin-domain-containing protein) receptor. The chromatin-binding protein high-mobility group box 1 protein (HMGB1) is released by necrotic cells and triggers the receptor for advanced glycation end products (RAGE). (BDCA, blood dendritic cell antigen; TLR, Toll-like receptor; NLR, NOD-like receptor).

lymphopenia, which is caused when the drug is given orally [60]. FTY720 inhibited the potential of DCs to form stable synapses with naïve antigen-specific T cells as well as effector Th2 cells, providing a possible explanation as to how these drugs might work to inhibit allergic inflammation. The drugable spleen tyrosine kinase (Syk) pathway has been shown to be crucial for Th2 induction by airway DCs [61], and downstream of this pathway the signaling intermediate PI3Kδ might similarly be very drugable.

As the number and activation status of lung CD11b+ DCs during secondary challenge seems crucial for controlling allergic inflammation, studying the factors that control recruitment, survival, or egress of DCs from the lung during allergic inflammation will be important, as this might reveal new therapeutic targets [37]. Eicosanoid lipid mediators, such as prostaglandins and leukotrienes, can also influence the migration of lung DCs [56]. Selective agonists of particular receptors for members of the prostaglandin family might also suppress DC function. Prostaglandin D_2 has pleiotropic effects in the immune system owing to its activity on the DP1 and CRTH2 (also known as DP2) receptors, which are widely expressed on immune cells. The DP1 agonist BW245C strongly suppressed the spontaneous migration of lung DCs to the mediastinal lymph node [62]. More importantly, BW245C suppressed airway inflammation and bronchial hyperreactivity when given to allergic mice by inhibiting the maturation of lung DCs. More detailed information on the interactions between DCs, epithelial cells, basophils, and other inflammatory cells will undoubtedly lead to the discovery of more potentially interesting drugs. In this regard, blocking the interaction of TSLP and GM-CSF with their respective receptors with small molecule inhibitors or blocking antibodies might prove very useful. Downstream of these, blocking CCR4 or its ligands might prevent DC-driven recruitment of Th2 cells.

Disease modification based on interfering with DC function

Stimulation of the immunoregulatory properties of DCs might reset the balance of the allergic immune response in favor of the development of Tregs, and could lead to a more long-lasting effect on the natural course of allergic disease. One way of achieving this would be by using a combination of steroids and vitamin D analogs to impact DC function and stimulate Treg differentiation. Steroids are currently the cornerstone of anti-inflammatory treatment in allergic disease. Inhaled steroids reduce (but do not eliminate) the number and modulate the function of DCs in the lungs and noses of individuals with allergic asthma and allergic rhinitis [63]. Steroids also induce the activation of the IDO enzyme in pDCs in a glucocorticoid-induced TNF receptor-related protein ligand (GITRL)–dependent way, thereby broadly suppressing inflammatory responses [64]. Prostaglandins or their metabolites might have the same effect. In the presence of the DP1 agonist BW245C, DCs induced the formation of forkhead box P3 positive (FOXP3+) Tregs from FOXP3− antigen-specific T cells in a process requiring cyclic adenosine monophosphate (cAMP) and protein kinase A [56]. A very similar mechanism was described for inhaled iloprost, a prostacyclin analog that acts on the I prostanoid (IP) receptor expressed by lung DCs [55,65]. Downstream metabo-

lites of prostaglandins include agonists of the peroxisome proliferator-activated receptor γ (PPARγ) family. Pharmacologic PPARγ agonists like the antidiabetic drug rosiglitazone were able to modify lung DC function and stimulate the formation of IL-10-producing T cells, thus suppressing features of asthma [66]. Finally, the stimulation of the IgA-inducing capacities of lung DCs might be a possible strategy that could have prolonged effects in allergic disease akin to the effects of desensitization immunotherapy [67].

Concluding remarks

It is now clear that DCs and epithelial cells play crucial roles in the initiation and maintenance of allergic airway inflammation. Interfering with their function, either directly or indirectly via disruption of intercellular communication, promises to provide novel therapeutics for this disease.

References

1 Steinman RM, Cohn ZA. Identification of a novel cell type in peripheral lymphoid organs of mice. I. Morphology, quantitation, tissue distribution. *J Exp Med* 1973; **137**: 1142–62.

2 GeurtsvanKessel Ch, Lambrecht BN. Division of labor between dendritic cell subsets of the lung. *Mucosal Immunology* 2008; **1**: 442–50.

3 Wikstrom ME, Stumbles PA. Mouse respiratory tract dendritic cell subsets and the immunological fate of inhaled antigens. *Immunol Cell Biol* 2007; **85**: 182–8.

4 Holt PG, Schon-Hegrad MA, Phillips MJ, McMenamin PG. Ia-positive dendritic cells form a tightly meshed network within the human airway epithelium. *Clin Exp Allergy* 1989; **19**: 597.

5 Sung SS, Fu SM, Rose CE, Jr., Gaskin F, Ju ST, Beaty SR. A major lung CD103 (alphaE)-beta7 integrin-positive epithelial dendritic cell population expressing Langerin and tight junction proteins. *J Immunol* 2006; **176**: 2161–72.

6 von Garnier C, Filgueira L, Wikstrom M, *et al.* Anatomical location determines the distribution and function of dendritic cells and other APCs in the respiratory tract. *J Immunol* 2005; **175**: 1609–18.

7 GeurtsvanKessel Ch, Willart MA, van Rijt LS, *et al.* Clearance of influenza virus from the lung depends on migratory langerin+CD11b− but not plasmacytoid dendritic cells. *J Exp Med* 2008; **205**: 1621–34.

8 Vermaelen KY, Carro-Muino I, Lambrecht BN, Pauwels RA. Specific migratory dendritic cells rapidly transport antigen from the airways to the thoracic lymph nodes. *J Exp Med* 2001; **193**: 51–60.

9 Lambrecht BN, Salomon B, Klatzmann D, Pauwels RA. Dendritic cells are required for the development of chronic eosinophilic airway inflammation in response to inhaled antigen in sensitized mice. *J Immunol* 1998; **160**: 4090–7.

10 De Heer HJ, Hammad H, Soullie T, *et al.* Essential role of lung plasmacytoid dendritic cells in preventing asthmatic reactions to harmless inhaled antigen. *J Exp Med* 2004; **200**: 89–98.

11 Hammad H, Charbonnier AS, Duez C, *et al.* Th2 polarization by Der p 1—pulsed monocyte-derived dendritic cells is due to the allergic status of the donors. *Blood* 2001; **98**: 1135–41.

12 Kheradmand F, Kiss A, Xu J, Lee SH, Kolattukudy PE, Corry DB. A protease-activated pathway underlying Th cell type 2 activation and allergic lung disease. *J Immunol* 2002; **169**: 5904–11.

13 Dahl ME, Dabbagh K, Liggitt D, Kim S, Lewis DB. Viral-induced T helper type 1 responses enhance allergic disease by effects on lung dendritic cells. *Nat Immunol* 2004; **5**: 337–43.

14 Eisenbarth SC, Zhadkevich A, Ranney P, Herrick CA, Bottomly K. IL-4-dependent Th2 collateral priming to inhaled antigens independent of toll-like receptor 4 and myeloid differentiation factor 88. *J Immunol* 2004; **172**: 4527–34.

15 Braun-Fahrlander C, Riedler J, Herz U, *et al.* Environmental exposure to endotoxin and its relation to asthma in school-age children. *N Engl J Med* 2002; **347**: 869–77.

16 de Heer HJ, Hammad H, Kool M, Lambrecht BN. Dendritic cell subsets and immune regulation in the lung. *Semin Immunol* 2005; **17**: 295–303.

17 Akbari O, DeKruyff RH, Umetsu DT. Pulmonary dendritic cells producing IL-10 mediate tolerance induced by respiratory exposure to antigen. *Nat Immunol* 2001; **2**: 725–31.

18 Hammad H, Lambrecht BN. Dendritic cells and epithelial cells: linking innate and adaptive immunity in asthma. *Nat Rev Immunol* 2008; **8**: 193–204.

19 Hammad H, Chieppa M, Perros F, Willart MA, Germain RN, Lambrecht BN. House dust mite allergen induces asthma via Toll-like receptor 4 triggering of airway structural cells. *Nat Med* 2009; **15**: 410–16.

20 Wan H, Winton HL, Soeller C, *et al.* Der p 1 facilitates transepithelial allergen delivery by disruption of tight junctions. *J Clin Invest* 1999; **104**: 123–33.

21 Nathan AT, Peterson EA, Chakir J, Wills-Karp M. Innate immune responses of airway epithelium to house dust mite are mediated through beta-glucan-dependent pathways. *J Allergy Clin Immunol* 2009; **123**: 612–18.

22 Phipps S, Lam CE, Kaiko GE, *et al.* Toll/IL-1 signaling is critical for house dust mite-specific Th1 and Th2 responses. *Am J Respir Crit Care Med* 2009; **179**: 883–93.

23 Trompette A, Divanovic S, Visintin A, *et al.* Allergenicity resulting from functional mimicry of a Toll-like receptor complex protein. *Nature* 2009; **457**: 585–8.

24 Eisenbarth SC, Piggott DA, Huleatt JW, Visintin I, Herrick CA, Bottomly K. Lipopolysaccharide-enhanced, toll-like receptor 4-dependent T helper cell type 2 responses to inhaled antigen. *J Exp Med* 2002; **196**: 1645–51.

25 Krishnamoorthy N, Oriss TB, Paglia M, *et al.* Activation of c-Kit in dendritic cells regulates T helper cell differentiation and allergic asthma. *Nat Med* 2008; **14**: 565–73.

26 Lambrecht BN, De Veerman M, Coyle AJ, Gutierrez-Ramos JC, Thielemans K, Pauwels RA. Myeloid dendritic cells induce Th2 responses to inhaled antigen, leading to eosinophilic airway inflammation. *J Clin Invest* 2000; **106**: 551–9.

27 Kool M, Soullie T, van Nimwegen M, *et al.* Alum adjuvant boosts adaptive immunity by inducing uric acid and activating inflammatory dendritic cells. *J Exp Med* 2008; **205**: 869–82.

28 Kool M, Petrilli V, De Smedt T, *et al.* Cutting Edge: alum adjuvant stimulates inflammatory dendritic cells through activation of the NALP3 inflammasome. *J Immunol* 2008; **181**: 3755–9.

29 Hammad H, Charbonnier AS, Duez C, *et al.* Th2 polarization by Der p 1—pulsed monocyte-derived dendritic cells is due to the allergic status of the donors. *Blood* 2001; **98**: 1135–41.

30 Boldogh I, Bacsi A, Choudhury BK, *et al.* ROS generated by pollen NADPH oxidase provide a signal that augments antigen-induced allergic airway inflammation. *J Clin Invest* 2005; **115**: 2169–79.

31 Yoshimoto T, Yasuda K, Tanaka H, *et al.* Basophils contribute to T(H)2-IgE responses *in vivo* via IL-4 production and presentation of peptide-MHC class II complexes to CD4[+] T cells. *Nat Immunol* 2009; **10**: 706–12.

32 Sokol CL, Chu NQ, Yu S, Nish SA, Laufer TM, Medzhitov R. Basophils function as antigen-presenting cells for an allergen-induced T helper type 2 response. *Nat Immunol* 2009; **10**: 713–20.

33 Perrigoue JG, Saenz SA, Siracusa MC, *et al.* MHC class II-dependent basophil-CD4[+] T cell interactions promote T(H)2 cytokine-dependent *Immunity Nat Immunol* 2009; **10**: 697–705.

34 Shi HZ, Humbles A, Gerard C, Jin Z, Weller PF. Lymph node trafficking and antigen presentation by endobronchial eosinophils. *J Clin Invest* 2000; **105**: 945–53.

35 Suto H, Nakae S, Kakurai M, Sedgwick JD, Tsai M, Galli SJ. Mast cell-associated TNF promotes dendritic cell migration. *J Immunol* 2006; **176**: 4102–12.

36 van Rijt LS, Prins JB, deVries VC, *et al.* Allergen-induced accumulation of airway dendritic cells is supported by an increase in CD31[hi] Ly 6C[neg] hematopoietic precursors. *Blood* 2002; **100**: 3663–71.

37 Robays LJ, Maes T, Lebecque S, *et al.* Chemokine receptor CCR2 but not CCR5 or CCR6 mediates the increase in pulmonary dendritic cells during allergic airway inflammation. *J Immunol* 2007; **178**: 5305–11.

38 Koya T, Kodama T, Takeda K, *et al.* Importance of myeloid dendritic cells in persistent airway disease after repeated allergen exposure. *Am J Respir Crit Care Med* 2006; **173**: 42–55.

39 van Rijt LS, Jung S, Kleinjan A, *et al.* In vivo depletion of lung CD11c[+] dendritic cells during allergen challenge abrogates the characteristic features of asthma. *J Exp Med* 2005; **201**: 981–91.

40 Upham JW, Denburg JA, O'Byrne PM. Rapid response of circulating myeloid dendritic cells to inhaled allergen in asthmatic subjects. *Clin Exp Allergy* 2002; **32**: 818–23.

41 Jahnsen FL, Moloney ED, Hogan T, Upham JW, Burke CM, Holt PG. Rapid dendritic cell recruitment to the bronchial mucosa of patients with atopic asthma in response to local allergen challenge. *Thorax* 2001; **56**: 823–6.

42 Moller GM, Overbeek SE, Van Helden-Meeuwsen CG, *et al.* Increased numbers of dendritic cells in the bronchial mucosa of atopic asthmatic patients: downregulation by inhaled corticosteroids. *Clin Exp Allergy* 1996; **26**: 517–24.

43 Liu YJ, Soumelis V, Watanabe N, *et al.* TSLP: an epithelial cell cytokine that regulates T-cell differentiation by conditioning dendritic cell maturation. *Annu Rev Immunol* 2007; **25**: 193–219.

44 Ito T, Wang YH, Duramad O, *et al.* TSLP-activated dendritic cells induce an inflammatory T helper type 2 cell response through OX40 ligand. *J Exp Med* 2005; **202**: 1213–23.

45 Allakhverdi Z, Comeau MR, Jessup HK, *et al.* Thymic stromal lymphopoietin is released by human epithelial cells in response to microbes, trauma, or inflammation and potently activates mast cells. *J Exp Med* 2007; **204**: 253–8.

46 Zhou B, Comeau MR, De Smedt T, *et al.* Thymic stromal lymphopoietin as a key initiator of allergic airway inflammation in mice. *Nat Immunol* 2005; **6**: 1047–53.

47 Al-Shami A, Spolski R, Kelly J, Keane-Myers A, Leonard WJ. A role for TSLP in the development of inflammation in an asthma model. *J Exp Med* 2005; **202**: 829–39.

48 Wang YH, Angkasekwinai P, Lu N, *et al.* IL-25 augments type 2 immune responses by enhancing the expansion and functions of TSLP-DC-activated Th2 memory cells. *J Exp Med* 2007; **204**: 1837–47.

49 Goswami S, Angkasekwinai P, Shan M, *et al.* Divergent functions for airway epithelial matrix metalloproteinase 7 and retinoic acid in experimental asthma. *Nat Immunol* 2009; **10**: 496–503.

50 Stampfli MR, Wiley RE, Scott Neigh G, *et al.* GM-CSF, transgene expression in the airway allows aerosolized ovalbumin to induce allergic sensitization in mice. *J Clin Invest* 1998; **102**: 1704–14.

51 Rank MA, Kobayashi T, Kozaki H, Bartemes KR, Squillace DL, Kita H. IL-33-activated dendritic cells induce an atypical TH2-type response. *J Allergy Clin Immunol* 2009; **123**: 1047–54.

52 Knight DA, Lim S, Scaffidi AK, *et al.* Protease-activated receptors in human airways: upregulation of PAR-2 in respiratory epithelium from patients with asthma. *J Allergy Clin Immunol* 2001; **108**: 797–803.

53 Kohl J, Baelder R, Lewkowich IP, *et al.* A regulatory role for the C5a anaphylatoxin in type 2 immunity in asthma. *J Clin Invest* 2006; **116**: 783–96.

54 Lambrecht BN, Germonpre PR, Everaert EG, *et al.* Endogenously produced substance P contributes to lymphocyte proliferation induced by dendritic cells and direct TCR, ligation. *Eur J Immunol* 1999; **29**: 3815–25.

55 Idzko M, Hammad H, van Nimwegen M, *et al.* Inhaled iloprost suppresses the cardinal features of asthma via inhibition of airway dendritic cell function. *J Clin Invest* 2007; **117**: 464–72.

56 Hammad H, Kool M, Soullie T, Narumiya, *et al.* Activation of the D prostanoid 1 receptor suppresses asthma by modulation of lung dendritic cell function and induction of regulatory T cells. *J Exp Med* 2007; **204**: 357–67.

57 Idzko M, Hammad H, van Nimwegen M, *et al.* Extracellular ATP triggers and maintains asthmatic airway inflammation by activating dendritic cells. *Nat Med* 2007; **13**: 913–19.

58 Willart MA, Lambrecht BN. The danger within: endogenous danger signals, atopy and asthma. *Clin Exp Allergy* 2009; **39**: 12–19.

59 Yang D, Chen Q, Su SB, *et al.* Eosinophil-derived neurotoxin acts as an alarmin to activate the TLR2-MyD88 signal pathway in dendritic cells and enhances Th2 immune responses. *J Exp Med* 2008; **205**: 79–90.

60 Idzko M, Hammad H, van Nimwegen M, *et al.* Local application of FTY720 to the lung abrogates experimental asthma by altering dendritic cell function. *J Clin Invest* 2006; **116**: 2935–44.

61 Matsubara S, Koya T, Takeda K, *et al.* Syk activation in dendritic cells is essential for airway hyperresponsiveness and inflammation. *Am J Respir Cell Mol Biol* 2006; **34**: 426–33.

13

62 Hammad H, de Heer HJ, Souillie T, Hoogsteden HC, Trottein F, Lambrecht BN. Prostaglandin D2 modifies airway dendritic cell migration and function in steady-state conditions by selective activation of the DP-receptor. *J Immunol* 2003; **171**: 3936–40.

63 Hammad H, Lambrecht BN. Recent progress in the biology of airway dendritic cells and implications for understanding the regulation of asthmatic inflammation. *J Allergy Clin Immunol* 2006; **118**: 331–6.

64 Grohmann U, Volpi C, Fallarino F, *et al.* Reverse signaling through GITR ligand enables dexamethasone to activate IDO in allergy. *Nat Med* 2007; **13**: 579–86.

65 Zhou W, Hashimoto K, Goleniewska K, *et al.* Prostaglandin I2 analogs inhibit proinflammatory cytokine production and T cell stimulatory function of dendritic cells. *J Immunol* 2007; **178**: 702–10.

66 Hammad H, de Heer HJ, Souillie T, *et al.* Activation of peroxisome proliferator-activated receptor pathway in dendritic cells inhibits development of eosinophilic airway inflammation in a mouse model of asthma. *Am J Pathol* 2004; **164**: 263–71.

67 Smits HH, Gloudemans AK, van Nimwegen M, *et al.* Cholera toxin B suppresses allergic inflammation through induction of secretory IgA. *Mucosal Immunol* 2009; **2**: 331–9.

2

Role of Th2 cells in the allergic diathesis

Marsha Wills-Karp

Division of Immunobiology, Cincinnati Children's Hospital Medical Center, University of Cincinnati College of Medicine, Cincinnati, OH, USA

Introduction

Allergic diseases continue to plague modernized societies, with an estimated 20% of the world's population currently afflicted with one or more allergic diseases (i.e., atopic dermatitis, allergic rhinitis, allergic asthma, eosinophilia esophagitis). Allergy is thought to result from maladaptive immune responses to ubiquitous, otherwise innocuous, environmental proteins, referred to as allergens. The propensity for developing allergic reactions is referred to as atopy and is defined operationally by elevations in levels of serum immunoglobulin E (IgE) reactive with, or by skin test reactivity to, such allergens. The recognition in the late 1980s that a particular subset of CD4$^+$ T lymphocytes, namely the T helper 2 (Th2) subset, were important orchestrators of IgE-mediated inflammatory processes led to the hypothesis that Th2 cytokine-producing CD4$^+$ T cells play a pivotal role in the pathogenesis of allergic disorders. The goal of this review is to discuss our current understanding of the pathogenic role of CD4$^+$ Th2 cytokine-producing cells in allergy, the molecular mechanisms driving the differentiation of naïve CD4$^+$ T cells into the Th2 phenotype, and possible therapeutic approaches to preventing or reversing the development of pathogenic Th2-mediated immune responses.

Role of CD4$^+$ T cells in allergy

Several lines of evidence support a causal role for T lymphocytes in allergic disorders. Increased numbers of T lymphocytes are found in the bronchial mucosa, nasal mucosa, and skin of patients with allergic asthma, rhinitis, and dermatitis, respectively, when compared with nonatopic controls [1]. In asthma and allergic rhinitis, CD4$^+$ T cells predominate; however, CD8$^+$ T cells, γ/δ T cells [2], and natural killer (NK) T cells have also been found in the respiratory tissues of allergic individuals [3]. In atopic dermatitis, however, both excess CD4$^+$ and CD8$^+$ T populations are present in skin lesions [4]. Further, there is a generalized increase in T-cell activation in allergic individuals both at the site of disease and systemically. Experimental data support a generalized increase in T-cell activation in all disorders of the atopic triad, with increased expression of the interleukin 2 (IL-2) receptor, class II histocompatibility antigen (HLA) DR, and very late activation antigen 1 (VLA-1). These activated T cells have the capacity to rapidly expand in response to specific stimuli, and through the release of a variety of cytokines they recruit and activate other immune cells (B cells, CD8 T cells, macrophages, mast cells, neutrophils, eosinophils, basophils), thereby initiating a complex series of events resulting in the symptoms

Inflammation and Allergy Drug Design, First Edition. Edited by Kenji Izuhara, Stephen T. Holgate, Marsha Wills-Karp.
© 2011 Blackwell Publishing Ltd. Published 2011 by Blackwell Publishing Ltd.

of allergic diseases. Following initial activation, CD4+ T cells remain in lymphoid tissues as memory cells. These memory cells retain the ability to respond to specific antigens upon re-exposure throughout the lifetime of the individual.

The identification of functionally distinct subsets of CD4+ T cells provided considerable theoretical insight into the pathophysiology of allergic diseases in both mice and humans. These populations have been distinguished at both clonal and population levels by their unique functions, their unique pattern of cytokine secretion, and their specific transcription factors. Unfortunately, no cell surface markers have been consistently shown to identify these various subsets, likely reflecting their plasticity. To date, CD4+ T cells have been classified into four major subsets, Th1, Th2, Th17, and T regulatory (Treg) cells. Th1 cells producing tumor necrosis factor beta (TNF-β) and interferon gamma (IFN-γ) are critical in the development of cell-mediated immunity, macrophage activation, and the production of complement-fixing antibody isotypes. Th2 cells producing IL-4, IL-13, IL-5, and IL-9 are important in the stimulation of IgE production, mucosal mastocytosis, eosinophilia, and macrophage deactivation. Tregs have immunosuppressive functions and cytokine profiles which are distinct from either Th1 or Th2 cells (IL-10; transforming growth factor beta [TGF-β]). These cells are thought to play an important role in limiting immune responses to self or exogenous antigens by preventing the activation and function of other CD4+ T-cell subsets through cell–cell interactions or through elaboration of IL-10 and/or TGF-β. Th17 cells are a recently identified subset of CD4+ T cells that produce IL-17A, IL-21, IL-22, and have been shown to be important in regulating neutrophilic inflammation and autoimmune diseases.

Based on the theoretical construct that Th2 cells were the primary regulators of eosinophilia and humoral immunity, it was hypothesized that they would regulate the development of allergic diseases. Indeed a tremendous amount of experimental evidence gathered over the last 20 years supports a pivotal role of CD4+ T cells and Th2 cytokines in the pathogenesis of allergic disorders. Firstly, T cells at the site of disease (bronchoalveolar lavage, bronchial biopsies, nasal biopsies) in allergic individuals (allergic asthma, atopic rhinitis) express elevated levels of mRNA for IL-4, IL-13, and IL-5 [5]. In patients with atopic dermatitis, elevated Th2 cytokines and their receptors (IL-4R; IL-5R) are found in skin lesions in acute disease, while cytokine patterns in chronic lesions are mixed, with both Th2 cytokines (IL-5 and IL-13) and Th1 cytokines (IFN-γ) being expressed [4]. However, in some instances Th2 cytokines themselves have been difficult to measure, but the downstream gene signatures of IL-4 and IL-13 have been consistently observed in lung tissues obtained from severe asthmatics. The IL-4- and IL-13-inducible genes observed in asthmatic tissues include eotaxin-1 and -3 (CCL11 and CCL26) [6] and inducible nitric oxide synthase (iNOS) [7]. Secondly, it has been shown that successful therapeutic treatment of these disorders is associated with a reduction in the Th2 cytokine pattern. For example, both steroid treatment and immunotherapeutic regimes result in reductions in Th2 cytokine levels in the nasal mucosa4 and in the cells and tissues of patients with allergic asthma [8,9].

Although IFN-γ-producing Th1 cells have also been identified in the airways of asthmatics, broncho-provocation of allergic asthmatics with an allergen leads to an increase in Th2 cytokine-producing lymphocytes, not IFN-γ-producing cells [10]. These results indicate that the Th1 cells present in the airways of asthmatics are not allergen-specific and may be responding to other antigens such as bacterial and viral antigens. Alternatively, they may function in a counterregulatory fashion to inhibit Th2 cell-mediated pathology.

It is thought that the Th2 cytokine pattern is established in early childhood as Martinez and colleagues [11] demonstrated that the propensity to develop asthma is associated with low stimulated levels of IFN-γ in children at 9 months of age, which suggests that a type I response is a protective factor. This has been more recently supported by Holt and colleagues [12], who showed that although the levels of IgE vary considerably during early childhood, atopic subjects eventually lock into a stable pattern of increasing antibody production and Th2-polarized cellular immunity that is associated with stable expression of the IL-4 receptor in allergen-specific Th2 memory cells, which is absent during infancy.

Pathogenic role of Th2 cytokines in allergic disorders

Although descriptive evidence suggests a pathogenic role for Th2 cytokine-producing cells in allergic disorders, cause and effect has been difficult to establish in human disease. Consequently, experimental animal models have been extremely useful in delineation of the role of CD4+ T cells and Th2 cell-derived cytokines in the pathogenesis of allergic disorders. Mouse models of allergen-driven asthma have consistently shown an absolute requirement for CD4+ T cells in the development of the common symptoms of allergic airway disease (i.e., airway hyperresponsiveness [AHR], eosinophilic inflammation, elevations in IgE levels, and mucus hypersecretion) [1]. Similar roles for CD4+ T cells and Th2 cytokines have been demonstrated in experimental mouse models of each of the atopic disorders including atopic dermatitis [13], food allergy [14], atopic rhinitis [15], and experimental allergic encephalomyelitis (EAE) [16]. Moreover, studies have shown that the Th2 subset, not the Th1 subset, drives the allergic phenotype. Specifically, the adoptive transfer of TCR-transgenic Th2 cells derived from DO11.10 mice and subsequent ovalbumin (OVA) challenge of recipients induces eosinophilic airway inflammation and AHR [17]. In contrast, the transfer of Th1 cells resulted in a neutrophil-predominant inflammatory response without any of the characteristic features of asthma. The involvement of each of the specific Th2 cytokines in allergic airway responses has been demonstrated in studies in which IL-4, IL-5, IL-13, and IL-9 have been manipulated through either antibody blockade [18–21] or gene targeting [22–24].

The elaboration of the Th2 cytokines sets into motion a complex series of events leading to IgE production: the development, recruitment, and activation of effector cells such as mast cells, basophils, eosinophils and effector T cells; and a variety of downstream effector cascades. Specifically, Th2 cells regulate B cell class switching to IgE through their production of IL-4 and IL-13 in humans and IL-4 in mice. IgE immune complexes activate innate immune cells including basophils and mast cells, resulting in their degranulation by cross-linking high-affinity Fc receptors for IgE (FcεRI) on the surface of these cells. Activated basophils and mast cells secrete various products, including cytokines, chemokines, histamine, heparin, serotonin, and proteases, which result in smooth muscle constriction, vascular permeability, and inflammatory cell recruitment. IL-4, together with IL-9, also contributes to IgE-mediated processes through their ability to stimulate mastocytosis. IL-5

has been shown to play a pivotal role in eosinophil development, recruitment, and activation at the site of Th2-inflammatory responses. The importance of IL-5 in antigen-induced eosinophilia has been well established in mice with either a targeted deletion in IL-5 [19] or those overexpressing the IL-5 gene [25]. If taken at face value, this result would suggest that IL-5 alone is sufficient for tissue eosinophilia; however, it has been shown that overexpression of IL-5 in mice results in a marked elevation of circulating eosinophils, but that the tissue levels of eosinophils remain similar to their wild-type controls. These results suggest that other processes also contribute to the recruitment of eosinophils to sites of inflammation. Indeed, IL-4 and IL-13 synergize with IL-5 to promote eosinophil recruitment to the lungs through their ability to regulate vascular cell adhesion molecule 1 (VCAM-1) and the eosinophil-specific chemokine, eotaxin. This is evidenced by the ability of overexpression of both of these cytokines in the lungs to enhance eosinophil recruitment.

By directly acting on epithelial cells, smooth muscle cells, and fibroblasts, Th2 cells induce goblet cell metaplasia, mucus production, and fibrosis in mucosal tissues. Tissue fibrosis and AHR are primarily mediated through IL-13, as evidenced by the fact that administration of recombinant IL-13 (rIL-13) [20,21] or overexpression of the IL-13 gene [26] can induce AHR and subepithelial fibrosis, while overexpression of IL-4 in the lung does not induce these responses [27]. In regards to mucus cell metaplasia, the story is more complex. Several lines of evidence suggest that mucus cell metaplasia is an IL-13-, not IL-4-, dependent process. For example, transfer of Th2 cells devoid of IL-4 or IL-5 genes still induces extensive goblet cell metaplasia in the mouse lung [28]. However, a blockade of the IL-4R alpha (IL-4RA) chain [18] or a deficiency in STAT6 [29] prevents the development of mucus cell metaplasia following allergen challenge, suggesting that IL-13 may be the ligand for the type II IL-4R–STAT6 pathway regulation of mucus cell changes. Indeed, administration of the soluble form of the IL-13 binding protein, IL-13RA2, which does not bind IL-4, completely reversed the metaplastic response of goblet cells induced by allergen sensitization and challenge [20,21]. Administration of rIL-13 *in* vivo [20,21] or overexpression of the IL-13 gene recapitulates antigen effects on mucus production. [26] Conversely, allergen-induced goblet cell metaplasia is significantly reduced in IL-13-deficient mice [30]. This was not further reduced when IL-4 was blocked with neutralizing antibodies, suggesting that indeed IL-13 is the primary regulator of mucus cell hyperplasia *in vivo*. The exact reasons for the differences in the role of IL-4 and IL-13 are unknown, as they both signal through type II IL-4R composed of the IL-4RA and the IL-13RA1 chain. Several explanations for this paradox have been postulated, including the possibility that IL-4 production at the site of inflammation is short lived and that IL-13 may persist, giving the illusion that IL-13 is the more important mediator of the effector phase of the response. This hypothesis is not without merit, as IL-4 is difficult to measure at the site of inflammation and kinetic studies have shown sustained IL-13 production in the lungs of asthmatic patients. However, several *in vitro* studies have shown that these cytokines have unique functions in systems in which the level of cytokines is controlled. Another potential explanation is that IL-13 may act through an as yet unidentified receptor complex. In support of this hypothesis, a recent study [31] demonstrates that although AHR induced by adoptive transfer of IL-13-sufficient T cells is STAT6 dependent, these effects appear to occur independently of the IL-4RA chain. These studies suggest that an as yet unidentified IL-13 binding chain may exist or that different configurations of the existing chains may mediate distinct effects of IL-13 stimulation. It is possible that binding IL-13 to IL-13RA2 may alter the output of the functional receptor complex. Alternatively, it has recently been shown that IL-4 may induce inhibitory pathways through the type I IL-4R which limit its proallergic effects mediated through the type II IL-4R [32]. On the other hand, it has been shown that IL-13 induces a small set of epithelial-specific genes that are not upregulated by IL-4 *in vivo* [33]. This apparent IL-13 selectivity either occurs via IL-13 stimulation of a unique receptor complex or as a result of IL-4 inhibition of these putative pathways. Clearly, further studies are required to resolve this mystery. Thus, although much remains to be determined about the mechanisms by which Th2 cytokines elicit the distinct pathologic features of diverse allergic diseases, collectively the evidence suggests that the individual Th2 cytokines work in concert to induce a constellation of pathophysiologic changes that culminate in the symptoms associated with various allergic disorders.

Susceptibility to Th2-skewed immune responses

Another line of evidence supporting the importance of Th2 cytokines in the pathogenesis of allergic diseases is the association of polymorphisms in Th2 cytokine genes with allergic subphenotypes. Genetic studies have demonstrated that multiple genes are involved in asthma. Several genome-wide screens point to chromosome 5q31–33 as a major susceptibility locus for asthma and high IgE values [34]. This region includes a cluster of cytokine genes (IL-3, IL-4, IL-5, IL-9, IL-13, GM-CSF [granulocyte–macrophage colony-stimulating factor], IL-12RB2 [interleukin 12 receptor beta 2]). A specific polymorphism in the IL-4 gene itself has been shown to correlate with high serum IgE levels and enhanced IL-4 gene expression [35]. Likewise, polymorphisms in the *Il13* promoter (−1055 C/T and −1112 C/T) and coding regions (R110Q) are strongly associated with asthma susceptibility and various aspects of allergic disease [36]. Moreover, polymorphisms in genes important in IL-4 and IL-13 signaling, such as IL-4RA [37] and STAT6 [38], have also been shown to be associated with an increased prevalence of several atopic disorders (bronchial asthma, atopic dermatitis, food allergies). Taken together, these studies suggest that genetic differences in Th2 genes themselves and genes regulating their production or responsiveness may contribute to asthma susceptibility. Although it is not likely that polymorphisms in these genes alone confer susceptibility to atopy and asthma, considerable evidence is mounting to suggest that genetic differences in factors important in Th2 cell commitment and function may contribute to the risk of developing atopic disorders.

Regulation of Th2 cell differentiation

A variety of factors have been shown to influence Th cell differentiation including the nature of the peptide presented by antigen-presenting cells to T cells and the expression and activity of co-stimulatory molecules (CD40-CD40L, CD80/CD86–CTLA-4/CD28). However, one of the most important determinants of T-cell differentiation are the cytokines/mediators produced either by antigen-presenting cells such as dendritic cells, basophils, or

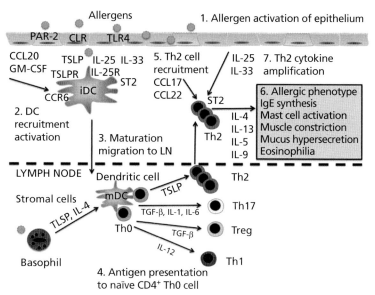

Figure 2.1 Initiation of Th2-mediated allergic responses. (1, 2) Upon encounter with allergen, epithelial cells of the respiratory tract, the intestinal tract, and the skin release mediators that recruit (CCL20), activate (granulocyte–macrophage colony-stimulating factor [GM-CSF]), and/or drive Th2 cell differentiation (thymic stromal lymphopoietin [TSLP], interleukin 25 [IL-25], IL-33). (3) Mature dendritic cells (DCs) then migrate to the draining lymph node to stimulate naïve T-cell differentiation and proliferation. (4) Allergens can also directly stimulate basophils to produce TSLP and IL-4 in the lymph nodes. Basophils and DCs drive Th2 cell differentiation under the influence of various cytokines such as TSLP, IL-4, and IL-25. (5) Activated Th2 cells in turn migrate back to the site of antigen stimulation under the influence of Th2 selective chemokines (CCL17, CCL12). (6) Once in the tissues, Th2 cells secrete a profile of Th2 cytokines (IL-4, IL-5, IL-13, IL-9), which initiate a cascade of downstream pathways that collectively lead to the development of the allergic phenotype. (7) Th2 responses may be further amplified by their ability to induce the release of Th2-selective chemokines (CCL17, CCL12), IL-25, and IL-33 from the epithelium, initiating a positive feedback loop. PAR, protease-activated receptor; CLR, C-type lectin receptor; TCR, T-cell receptor; iDC, immature dendritic cell; mDC, mature dendritic cell.

structural cells. Although the factors driving Th1 and Th17 responses have largely been identified, the elucidation of the factors driving Th2 differentiation has proven more challenging. Nonetheless, recent studies suggest a model in which allergens are sensed by pattern-recognition receptors such as Toll-like receptor 4 (TLR4), protease-activated receptor 2 (PAR-2), and C-type lectin receptors (CLRs) residing on epithelial surfaces and/or on DCs [39] (Figure 2.1). Stimulation of one or more of these receptors leads to the release of cytokines including thymic stromal lymphopoietin (TSLP), IL-25, and IL-33 from epithelial cells of the respiratory tract, the intestinal tract, and the skin that either activate DCs or drive Th2 cell differentiation. Each of these cytokines has been shown to be important in both driving and amplifying Th2 cell polarization and genetic variants in these genes have been associated with disease. Once DCs are activated, they migrate to the draining lymph node to stimulate T-cell differentiation and proliferation. Activated CD4+ T cells in turn differentiate and proliferate in the lymph nodes and migrate back to the site of antigen stimulation. Once in the tissues, Th2 cells produce Th2 cytokines and initiate a cascade of downstream pathways that lead to the development of the allergic phenotype. As the receptors for IL-25 and IL-33 are also found on Th2 cells, they induce additional Th2 cytokine production, thereby amplifying Th2 responses in the tissues.

19

Molecular mechanisms of Th2 cell differentiation

Although the exact molecular events that drive Th2 differentiation have not been fully elucidated, a picture is beginning to emerge (Figure 2.2) [40]. A model has been put forth in which, following the presentation of an antigen in the context of MHC II and TCR stimulation of naïve CD4+ T cells, a modest increase in the mRNA levels of the master regulator of Th2 differentiation, GATA-3, occurs, which steadily accumulates over the first 24 hours. Once produced, GATA-3 remodels chromatin (demethyla-

tion) around the Th2 cytokine locus, resulting in the opening of the Th2 locus and marked upregulation of IL-4 [41]. GATA-3 also enhances Th2 differentiation by inhibiting expression of the IL-12RB2 and the STAT4 genes, which are required for Th1 differentiation programming. In parallel, TCR stimulation induces IL-2 production [42], which in turn activates STAT5 [43]. TSLP and IL-7 may also contribute to STAT5 activation. The combination of STAT5 activation and GATA-3 induction stabilizes IL-4 expression in developing Th2 cells [44]. Another potential signal involved in early IL-4 production is the binding of jagged-1 on antigen-presenting cells (APCs) with

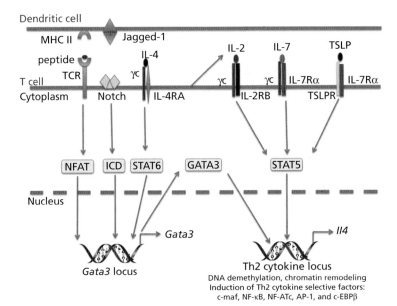

Figure 2.2 Molecular mechanisms of T helper 2 (Th2) differentiation. Following T-cell receptor (TCR) stimulation through engagement of MHCII and antigen, on naïve CD4+ T cells a modest increase in the mRNA levels of the master regulator of Th2 differentiation, GATA-3 occurs. Another potential signal involved in early interleukin (IL) 4 production is the binding of the Notch ligand, jagged-1, on antigen-presenting cells with Notch ICD expressed on naïve CD4 T cells that further induces GATA-3 expression. Once produced, GATA-3 remodels chromatin (demethylation) around the Th2 cytokine locus resulting in opening of the Th2 locus and marked upregulation of IL-4. In parallel, TCR stimulation induces IL-2 production, which in turn activates STAT5. TSLP and IL-7 may also contribute to STAT5 activation. The

combination of STAT5 activation and GATA-3 induction stabilizes Il4 expression in developing Th2 cells. Once the early IL-4 accumulates, it binds its receptor composed of the IL-4 receptor α and the g/c chain and activates STAT6, which further enhances GATA-3 and induces the expression of other Th2-specific factors such as c-maf, which together, in combination with continued STAT5 activation, results in further upregulation of IL-4, initiating a positive feedback loop that drives commitment to a Th2 phenotype. The expression of specific Th2 cytokine genes (IL-4, IL-5, IL-13, IL-9) is controlled by the synergistic actions of the GATA-3 and c-Maf, and by the more widely expressed and transiently induced transcription factors such as NF-ATc, NF-κB, AP-1, and c-EBPb.

Notch ICD, expressed on naïve CD4 T cells [45]. The induction of IL-4 by Notch is thought to be partially due to its ability to increase expression of GATA-3.

Once the early IL-4 accumulates it binds its receptor, which is composed of the IL-4RA and γ/c, and activates STAT6, which further enhances GATA-3 and induces the expression of other Th2-specific factors such as c-Maf, which, together in combination with continued STAT5 activation, results in further upregulation of IL-4 and initiates a positive feedback loop that drives commitment to a Th2 phenotype [46]. The expression of specific Th2 cytokine genes is controlled by the synergistic actions of GATA-3 and c-Maf, and by the more widely expressed and transiently induced transcription factors such as NF-ATc, NF-κB, AP-1, and c-EBPβ. NF-ATc, unlike GATA-3, has been shown to directly activate the IL-4 promoter [47]. In contrast, NF-κB appears to be more important for antigen-induced IL-5 gene expression than for IL-4 gene expression [48]. During subsequent antigenic stimulation of the effector/memory cells, which maintain an open chromatin structure with high levels of GATA-3 and c-Maf expression, they are able to rapidly induce Th2 cytokine gene expression. The differences in the combination of transcription factors required for specific Th2 cytokine expression might explain the differential expression of Th2 cytokines observed in atopic and nonatopic individuals. It is reasonable to speculate that once cells have been committed to the Th2 lineage, different microenvironmental factors might activate different sets of transcription factors, such as GATA-3, c-Maf, NF-AT, and NF-κB, to cause differential expression of cytokine genes.

Therapeutic targeting of Th2 immune responses in allergic diseases

As substantial evidence implicates Th2 cytokines in the pathogenesis of allergic disorders, it stands to reason that a rational strategy for the treatment of allergic diseases may be to target Th2 immune pathways. Suppression of Th2 cell activity can be achieved through several approaches, including the blockade of CD4+ Th2 cell differentiation, activation, and cytokine secretion, as well as the inhibition of the biologic functions on individual Th2 cytokines.

Blockade of CD4+ Th2 differentiation

Th2 differentiation may be inhibited by blockade of the production of or responsiveness to several factors, including TSLP, OX40L–OX40 pathways, GATA-3, IL-25, and IL-33. Although this approach is being investigated, there are clearly not sufficient data to determine whether it will be an effective method for suppressing allergic inflammation. An alternative method for reducing Th2 cell generation is to increase the levels of either Th1-promoting cytokines, such as IL-12 and IFN-γ, or Treg cytokines, such as IL-10, TGF-β, thus shifting the Th balance away from Th2. Several groups are developing approaches to stimulate Th1 responses. Specifically, immunostimulatory DNA sequences, which activate TLR9 and upregulate Th1 immune responses, are currently in clinical trials for asthma. This approach allows stimulation of Th1 immune responses in the absence of infection, thereby preventing the untoward effects of acute infection on the lung. Alternatively, agents that enhance Treg function such as vitamin D and probiotics may be beneficial in the treatment of allergy and asthma by increasing the induction of allergen-specific IL-10-secreting Treg cells, concomitant with a reduction in allergen-specific Th2 responses. As these broad modulators of the immune response have the potential to disturb the delicate balance between tolerance and immunity within the mucosal tissues and either lead to enhanced inflammatory responses to infections or to the development of autoimmune diseases, therapies aimed at altering T-cell subset balance need to be carefully tested in long-term studies before becoming mainstream therapies.

Blockade of downstream effects of Th2 cytokines

As there is strong evidence that IL-4 and IL-13 play essential roles in asthma pathogenesis, blocking the effects of these two cytokines at the target tissue is another potential strategy for reducing the pathogenic effects of Th2 cells. To date, several different approaches have been used to target the IL-4/IL-13 signaling pathway.

Early studies with a soluble IL-4R were initially promising [49], but did not meet expectations in subsequent trials [50]. Whether the failure of this soluble receptor to ameliorate disease was due to its inability to fully neutralize IL-4 or to the inability of IL-4 blockade alone to impact disease is not currently known.

Either way, attention turned toward the development of neutralizing IL-13 antibodies because compelling evidence from animal models has suggested that IL-13 may the dominant mediator of the functional aspects of asthma. To date, a number of IL-13-neutralizing antibodies have been developed and are in various phases of clinical testing. These include anrukinzumab, IMA-026, TNX650, QAX576, MILR1444, GSK-679586, and CAT-354 [51–53]. Each of these anti-IL-13 antibodies has been shown to have a good safety and tolerability profile. However, the early results have been mixed, with some studies reporting that anti-IL-13 blockade did not effectively inhibit the primary outcome measure of the study, while other early studies showed that it effectively blocked changes in pulmonary function following allergen provocation. Whether this variation in efficacy is due to the specific formulations being used, the differences in outcome variables being examined, or the small size of the studies is not currently known. Determination of whether blockade of IL-13 alone will be an effective approach to the treatment of asthma awaits the results of the many ongoing studies.

Several reagents that block both IL-4 and IL-13 are further along in development than the single IL-13 mAbs and have shown some promise. For example, pitrakinra (AER 001, Aerovant™), a recombinant IL-4 variant that competitively antagonizes the IL-4Rα, and therefore interferes with the function of both IL-4 and IL-13 at the IL-4Rα–IL-13Rα1 receptor complex, has shown encouraging results. Specifically, in a "proof of concept" phase IIa trial it reduced the severity of late airway responses following allergen provocation, concomitant with a reduction in exhaled nitric oxide levels [54]. In a recently completed phase IIb double-blind randomized placebo-controlled dose-ranging study of 534 patients, the authors reported that pitrakinra treatment significantly reduced the incidence of asthma exacerbations, the time to exacerbations, and asthma symptom scores in patients with eosinophilic asthma compared with placebo in the same patients . However, it did not show efficacy when the entire group of asthmatics were evaluated.

In another study, AMG 317, a fully human monoclonal antibody to IL-4Rα that blocks both IL-4 and IL-13 pathways, failed to show a significant benefit in the primary endpoint, which was a change from baseline at week 12 in Asthma Control Questionnaire (ACQ) symptom score across the overall group of patients [55]. However, clinically significant improvements were observed in several outcome measures in patients with higher baseline ACQ scores, suggesting that a subset group of patients may benefit from the treatment.

Another approach to blocking the IL-4/IL-13 pathway is through the use of antisense targeting the mRNA that encodes the IL-4R subunit (AIR645). In a phase 1 trial of AIR645, it was shown to reduce several biomarkers of allergic inflammation including reductions in serum total IgE, sputum eosinophils, and levels of 15-HETE in sputum [56]. A phase II trial of AIR645 in asthma is currently under way (Altair Therapeutics, Inc.). Lastly, although more work needs to be done to identify the pertinent targets, modulating the downstream effector molecules (i.e., arginase I, etc.) induced by Th2 cytokines may be the safest approach to targeting this pathway. Although these studies are promising, we await the results of the ongoing asthma clinical trials to determine with certainty the efficacy of therapies based on IL-4/IL-13 blockade.

An anti-IL-5 mAb (mepolizumab) has been developed and evaluated in the setting of several allergic disorders. It has been shown to be effective in inhibiting both blood and tissue eosinophils in patients with eosinophilic esophagitis [57]. Initial studies of the effects of the anti-IL-5 mAb in asthma showed that while it effectively reduced circulating eosinophils, it had no discernible effect on asthma outcomes [58]. However, it has recently been shown to have a significant effect on asthma exacerbations in two recent small clinical trials in severely asthmatic patients requiring high-dose inhaled and oral corticosteroids [59,60]. However, as reported previously, it had no effect on bronchial hyperresponsiveness or forced expiratory volume in 1 s [58]. Another approach to blocking IL-5 has recently been developed in which an antibody-dependent cell cytotoxic defucosylated IgG1 monoclonal antibody (MEDI-563) is directed against all cells expressing the IL-5Rα [61,62]. Initial results suggest that the antibody is well tolerated and induces prolonged depletion of blood eosinophils. It remains to be seen whether it will have appreciable effects on asthma outcomes.

Conclusions

The preponderance of evidence derived from a variety of studies suggests that the pathophysiology of allergic diseases is mediated by a loss of immune tolerance and the skewing of immune responses to inhaled environmental antigens toward pathways driven by Th2-type CD4[+] T cells through the elaboration of a repertoire of interleukins, including IL-4, IL-5, IL-9, and IL-13. Therefore, biologic modifiers of Th2 immune responses represent rational targets for developing new treatment strategies for asthma. As Th2 cytokines work in concert to elicit the pathophysiologic features of disease, it may be that blockade of individual Th2 cytokines may not be sufficient to ameliorate disease, suggesting that targeting molecules that regulate Th2 cell differentiation, recruitment, and/or activation may be more efficacious. Establishment of the efficacy and safety of biologic modifiers of Th2 immune pathways in the treatment of asthma awaits the results of ongoing clinical trials.

References

1 Wills-Karp M. Immunologic basis of antigen-induced airway hyperresponsiveness. *Annu Rev Immunol* 1999; **17**: 255–81.

2 Krug N, Erpenbeck VJ, Balke K, *et al.* Cytokine profile of bronchoalveolar lavage-derived CD4(+), CD8(+), and gamma delta T cells in people with asthma after segmental allergen challenge. *Am J Respir Cell Mol Biol* 2001; **25**: 125–31.

3 Akbari O, Faul JL, Hoyte EG, *et al.* CD4[+] invariant T-cell-receptor[+] natural killer T cells in bronchial asthma. *N Engl J Med* 2006; **354**: 1117–29.

4 Grewe M, Bruijnzeel-Koomen CA, Schopf E, *et al.* A role for Th1 and Th2 cells in the immunopathogenesis of atopic dermatitis. *Immunol Today* 1998; **19**: 359–61.

5 Robinson D, Hamid Q, Bentley A, Ying S, Kay AB, Durham SR. Activation of CD4[+] T cells, increased TH2-type cytokine mRNA expression, and eosinophil recruitment in bronchoalveolar lavage after allergen inhalation challenge in patients with atopic asthma. *J Allergy Clin Immunol* 1993; **92**: 313–24.

6 Lamkhioued B, Renzi PM, Abi-Younes S, *et al.* Increased expression of eotaxin in bronchoalveolar lavage and airways of asthmatics contributes to the chemotaxis of eosinophils to the site of inflammation. *J Immunol* 1997; **59**: 4593–601.

7 Chibana K, Trudeau JB, Mustovich AT, *et al.* IL-13 induced increases in nitrite levels are primarily driven by increases in inducible nitric oxide synthase as compared with effects on arginases in human primary bronchial epithelial cells. *Clin Exp Allergy* 2008; **38**: 936–46.

8 Fokkens WJ, T Godthelp, AF Holm, *et al.* Allergic rhinitis and inflammation: the effect of nasal corticosteroid therapy. *Allergy* 1997; **52**: 29–32.

9 Secrist H, Chelen CJ, Wen Y, *et al.* Allergen immunotherapy decreases interleukin 4 production in CD4[+] T cells from allergic individuals. *J Exp Med* 1993; **178**: 2123–30.

10 Kelly EA, Rodriguez RR, Busse WW, *et al.* The effect of segmental bronchoprovocation with allergen on airway lymphocyte function. *Am J Respir Crit Care Med* 1997; **156**: 1421–8.

11 Martinez FD, Stern DA, Wright AL, *et al.* Association of interleukin 2 and interferon-gamma production by blood mononuclear cells in infancy with parental allergy skin tests and with subsequent development of atopy. *J Allergy Clin Immunol* 1995; **96**: 652–60.

12 Holt PG, Rowe J, Kusel M, *et al.* Toward improved prediction of risk for atopy and asthma among preschoolers: a prospective cohort study. *J Allergy Clin Immunol* 2010; **125**: 653–9.

13 Spergel JM, Mizoguchi E, Oettgen H, *et al.* Roles of Th1 and Th2 cytokines in a murine model of allergic dermatitis. *J Clin Invest* 1999; **103**: 1103–11.

14 Prescott VE, Forbes E, Foster PS, *et al.* Mechanistic analysis of experimental food allergen-induced cutaneous reactions. *J Leukoc Biol* 2006; **80**: 258–66.

15 Ogasawara H, Asakura K, Saito H, *et al.* Role of CD4-positive T cells in the pathogenesis of nasal allergy in the murine model. *Int Arch Allergy Immunol* 1999; **118**: 37–43.

16 Mishra A, Schlotman J, Wang M, *et al.* Critical role for adaptive T cell immunity in experimental eosinophilic esophagitis in mice. *J Leukoc Biol* 2007; **81**: 916–24.

17 Cohn L, Tepper JS, Bottomly K, *et al.* IL-4-independent induction of airway hyperresponsiveness by Th2: but not Th1: cells. *J Immunol* 1998; **161**: 3813–16.

18 Gavett SH, O'Hearn DJ, Karp CL, *et al.* Interleukin 4 receptor blockade prevents airway responses induced by antigen challenge in mice. *Am J Physiol* 1997; **272**: L253–61.

19 Kung TT, Stelts DM, Zurcher JA, *et al.* Involvement of IL-5 in a murine model of allergic pulmonary inflammation: prophylactic and therapeutic effect of an anti-IL-5 antibody. *Am J Respir Cell Mol Biol* 1995; **13**: 360–5.

20 Wills-Karp M, Luyimbazi J, Xu X, *et al.* Interleukin 13: central mediator of allergic asthma. *Science* 1998; **282**: 2258–61.

21 Grunig G, Warnock M, Wakil AE, *et al.* Requirement for IL-13 independently of IL-4 in experimental asthma. *Science* 1998; **282**: 2261–3.

22 Brusselle G, Kips J, Joos G, *et al.* Allergen-induced airway inflammation and bronchial responsiveness in wild type and interleukin 4-deficient mice. *Am J Respir Cell Mol Biol* 1995; **12**: 254–9.

23 Foster PS, Hogan SP, Ramsay AJ, *et al*. Interleukin 5 deficiency abolishes eosinophilia, airways hyperreactivity, and lung damage in a mouse asthma model. *J Exp Med* 1996; **183**: 195–201.

24 Townsend JM, Fallon GP, Matthews JD, *et al*. IL-9-deficient mice establish fundamental roles for IL-9 in pulmonary mastocytosis and goblet cell hyperplasia but not T cell development. *Immunity* 2000; **13**: 573–83.

25 Lee JJ, McGarry MP, Farmer SC, *et al*. Interleukin 5 expression in the lung epithelium of transgenic mice leads to pulmonary changes pathognomonic of asthma. *J Exp Med* 1997; **185**: 2143–56.

26 Zhu Z, Homer RJ, Wang Z, *et al*. Pulmonary expression of interleukin 13 causes inflammation, mucus hypersecretion, subepithelial fibrosis, physiologic abnormalities, and eotaxin production. *J Clin Invest* 1999; **103**: 779–88.

27 Rankin JA, Picarella DE, Geba GP, *et al*. Phenotypic and physiologic characterization of transgenic mice expressing interleukin 4 in the lung: lymphocytic and eosinophilic inflammation without airway hyperreactivity. *Proc Natl Acad Sci USA* 1996; **93**: 7821–5.

28 Cohn L, Homer RJ, MacLeod H, Mohrs M, Brombacher F, Bottomly K. Th2-induced airway mucus production is dependent on IL-4Ralpha, but not on eosinophils. *J Immunol* 1999; **162**: 6178–83.

29 Kuperman D, Schofield B, Wills-Karp M, *et al*. Signal transducer and activator of transcription factor 6 (Stat6)-deficient mice are protected from antigen-induced airway hyperresponsiveness and mucus production. *J Exp Med* 1998; **87**: 939–48.

30 Webb DC, McKenzie AN, Koskinen AM, *et al*. Integrated signals between IL-13: IL-4: and IL-5 regulate airways hyperreactivity. *J Immunol* 2000; **165**: 108–13.

31 Mattes J, M Yang, A Siqueira, *et al*. IL-13 induces airways hyperreactivity independently of the IL-4R alpha chain in the allergic lung. *J Immunol* 2001; **167**: 1683–92.

32 Finkelman FD, Yang M, Perkins C, *et al*. Suppressive effect of IL-4 on IL-13-induced genes in mouse lung. *J Immunol* 2005; **174**: 4630–8.

33 Lewis CC, Aronow B, Hutton J, *et al*. Unique and overlapping gene expression patterns driven by IL-4 and IL-13 in the mouse lung. *J Allergy Clin Immunol* 2009; **123**: 795–804.

34 Ober C, Hoffjan S. Asthma genetics 2006: the long and winding road to gene discovery. *Genes Immun* 2006; **7**: 95–100.

35 Hook S, Cheng P, Holloway J, *et al*. Analysis of two IL-4 promoter polymorphisms in a cohort of atopic and asthmatic subjects. *Exp Clin Immunogenet* 1999; **16**: 33–5.

36 Graves PE, Kabesch M, Halonen M. A cluster of seven tightly linked polymorphisms in the IL-13 gene is associated with total serum IgE levels in three populations of white children. *Allergy Clin Immunol* 2000; **105**: 506–13.

37 Hershey GK, Friedrich MF, Esswein LA, *et al*. The association of atopy with a gain-of-function mutation in the alpha subunit of the interleukin 4 receptor. *N Engl J Med* 1997; **337**: 1720–5.

38 Tamura K, Arakawa H, Suzuki M, *et al*. Novel dinucleotide repeat polymorphism in the first exon of the STAT6 gene is associated with allergic diseases. *Clin Exp Allergy* 2001; **31**: 1509–14.

39 Wills-Karp M, Nathan A, Page K, *et al*. New insights into innate immune mechanisms underlying allergenicity. *Mucosal Immunol* 2010; **3**: 104–10.

40 Paul WE, Zhu J. How are Th2-type immune responses initiated and amplified? *Nature Rev Immunol* 2010; **10**: 225–35.

41 Zhang D-H, Cohn L, Ray P, *et al*. Transcription factor GATA-3 is differentially expressed in Th1 and Th2 cells and controls Th2-specific expression of the interleukin 5 gene. *J Biol Chem* 1997; **272**: 21597–603.

42 Cote-Sierra J, Foucras G, Guo L, *et al*. Interleukin 2 plays a central role in Th2 differentiation. *Proc Natl Acad Sci USA* 2004; **101**: 3880–5.

43 Kagami S, Nakajima H, Suto A, *et al*. STAT5a regulates T helper cell differentiation by several distinct mechanisms. *Blood* 2001; **97**: 2358–65.

44 Yamane H, Zhu J, Paul WE. Independent roles for IL-2 and GATA-3 in stimulating naïve CD4[+] T cells to generate a Th2-inducing cytokine environment. *J Exp Med* 2005; **202**: 793–804.

45 Amsen D, Antov A, Jankovic D, *et al*. Direct regulation of GATA-3 expression determines the T helper differentiation potential of Notch. *Immunity* 2007; **27**: 89–99.

46 Ho I-C, Hodge MR, Rooney JW, *et al*. The proto-oncogene c-maf is responsible for tissue-specific expression of interleukin 4. *Cell* 1996; **85**: 973–83.

47 Glimcher LH, Singh H. Transcription factors in lymphocyte development—T and B cells get together. *Cell* 1999; **96**: 13–23.

48 Yang L, Cohn L, Zhang DH, *et al*. Essential role of nuclear factor kB in the induction eosinophilia in allergic airway inflammation. *J Exp Med* 1998; **188**: 1739–50.

49 Borish LC, Nelson HS, Lanz MJ, *et al*. Interleukin 4 receptor in moderate atopic asthma. A phase I/II randomized, placebo controlled trial. *Am J Respir Crit Care Med* 1999; **160**: 1816–23.

50 Borish LC, Nelson HS, Corren J, *et al*. Efficacy of soluble IL-4 receptor for the treatment of adults with asthma. *J Allergy Clin Immunol* 2001; **107**: 963–70.

51 Kariyawasam HH, Nicholson GC, Tan AJ, *et al*. Effects of anti-IL-13 (Novartis QAX576) on inflammatory responses following nasal allergen challenge (NAC). *Am J Respir Crit Care Med* 2009; **179**: A3642.

52 Gauvreau GM, Boulet LP, Fitzgerald JM, *et al.* The effects of IMA-638 on allergen induced airway responses in subjects with mild atopic asthma. *Eur Respir J* 2008; **32** (Suppl 52): 827s.

53 Singh D, Kane B, Molfino NA, Faggioni R, Roskos L, Woodcock A. A phase 1 study evaluating the pharmacokinetics, safety and tolerability of repeat dosing with a human IL-13 antibody (CAT-354) in subjects with asthma. *BMC Pulm Med* 2010; **10**: 3–11.

54 Wenzel S, Wilbraham D, Fuller R, *et al.* Effect of an interleukin 4 variant on late phase asthmatic response to allergen challenge in asthmatic patients: results of two phase 2a studies. *Lancet* 2007; **370**: 1422–31.

55 Corren J, Busse W, Meltzer EO, *et al.* A randomized, controlled, phase 2 study of AMG 317: an IL-4Ralpha antagonist, in patients with asthma. *Am J Respir Crit Care Med* 2010; **181**: 788–96.

56 Hodges MR, Castelloe E, Chen A, *et al.* Randomized, double-blind, placebo controlled first in human study of inhaled AIR645: an IL-4Rα oligonucleotide in healthy volunteers. *Am J Respir Crit Care Med* 2009; **179**: A3640.

57 Stein ML, Collins MH, Villanueva JM, *et al.* Anti-IL-5 (mepolizumab) therapy for eosinophilic esophagitis. *J Allergy Clin Immunol* 2006; **118**: 1312–19.

58 Flood-Page P, Swenson C, Faiferman I, *et al.* A study to evaluate safety and efficacy of mepolizumab in patients with moderate persistent asthma. *Am J Respir Crit Care Med* 2007; **176**: 1062–71.

59 Nair P, Pizzichini MM, Kjarsgaard M, *et al.* Mepolizumab for prednisone-dependent asthma with sputum eosinophilia. *N Engl J Med* 2009; **360**: 985–93.

60 Haldar P, Brightling CE, Hargadon B, *et al.* Mepolizumab and exacerbations of refractory eosinophilic asthma. *N Engl J Med* 2009; **360**: 973–84.

61 Busse WW, Katial R, Gossage D, *et al.* Safety profile, pharmacokinetics, and biologic activity of MEDI-563: an anti-IL-5 receptor alpha antibody, in a phase I study of subjects with mild asthma. *J Allergy Clin Immunol* 2010; **125**: 1237–44.

62 Kolbeck R, Kozhich A, Koike M, *et al.* MEDI-563: a humanized anti-IL-5 receptor alpha mAb with enhanced antibody-dependent cell-mediated cytotoxicity function. *J Allergy Clin Immunol* 2010; **125**: 1344–53.

3

Importance of Th17- and Th1-associated responses for the development of asthma

Tomohiro Yoshimoto,[1] *Hiroko Tsutsui,*[2] *and Kenji Nakanishi*[3]

[1]Laboratory of Allergic Diseases, Institute for Advanced Medical Sciences, Hyogo College of Medicine, Nishinomiya, Hyogo, Japan
[2]Department of Microbiology, Hyogo College of Medicine, Nishinomiya, Hyogo, Japan
[3]Department of Immunology and Medical Zoology, Hyogo College of Medicine, Nishinomiya, Hyogo, Japan

Introduction

In 1986, Mosmann *et al.* [1] proposed the presence of two distinct T helper (Th) cell subsets, each expressing a definite cytokine profile. Th1 cells develop in the presence of interleukin 12 (IL-12), produce primarily interferon gamma (IFN-γ) and IL-2, and are involved in cell-mediated immunity. IFN-γ elicits delayed-type hypersensitivity response, activates macrophages, and is highly effective in the clearance of intracellular pathogens. Th2 cells differentiate in the presence of IL-4, produce IL-4, IL-5, IL-6, IL-9, and IL-13, and are critical for humoral immunity. These Th2 cytokines are important for the development of allergic diseases and the clearance of helminth infections by induction of immunoglobulin E (IgE) production, activation of mast cells and basophils, and eosinophilic inflammation. IFN-γ, IL-12, and T-bet control Th1 development, while IL-4 and GATA-3 control Th2 development (Figure 3.1). Thus, the concept of a Th1–Th2 balance provided the basis for understanding the molecular mechanisms of immune responses and/or diseases and has been widely accepted as a paradigm of the immune system for the past two decades.

However, this Th1–Th2 paradigm cannot necessarily explain onsets of autoimmune diseases. For example, IFN-γ/IFN-γ receptor (IFN-γR) deficiency or IFN-γ neutralization results in exacerbation of, rather than protection against, the development of autoimmune diseases such as experimental autoimmune encephalomyelitis (EAE) [2–4] and collagen-induced arthritis (CIA), both of which were classically considered to be mediated by Th1 responses. Thus, another Th cell subset different from the Th1 subset might participate in the induction of EAE, CIA, and perhaps other organ-specific autoimmune diseases. Recent studies strongly suggest that the Th17 cell subset is important for the development of autoimmune diseases and for the clearance of extracellular pathogens by producing IL-17 in large amounts (described below).

Seven functionally unique populations of Th cells are now known (Figure 3.1). The regulatory T (Treg) cell subset [5] is essential for the regulation of allergy and autoimmunity. Recently, Th9 cells that produce IL-9 in large quantities [6] are separated from Th2 cells. In the follicles there exist unique Th cells named T follicular helper (TFH) cells [7], which produce IL-21 and help B cells. Our study revealed that, in response to exogenous IL-18 together with their antigen, the established Th1 cells begin to produce Th2 cytokines as well as their proper Th1 cytokines [8]. They produce Th2 cytokines (IL-9, IL-13), granulocyte–macrophage colony-stimulating factor (GM-CSF), and various chemokines that can recruit granulocytes, macrophages, and lymphocytes. We designated these Th2 cytokine-producing Th1 cells as

Inflammation and Allergy Drug Design, First Edition. Edited by Kenji Izuhara, Stephen T. Holgate, Marsha Wills-Karp.
© 2011 Blackwell Publishing Ltd. Published 2011 by Blackwell Publishing Ltd.

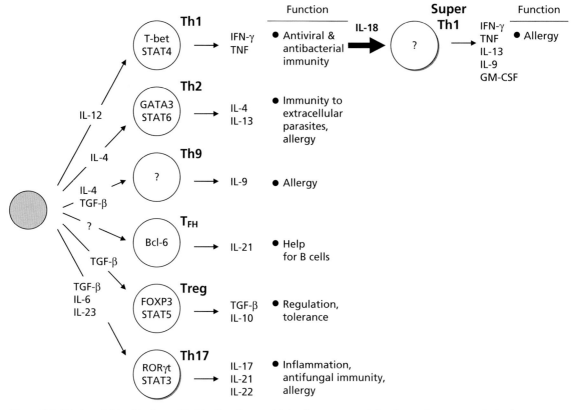

Figure 3.1 T helper (Th) cell subsets. Th17 cell and super Th1 cell responses might play an important role in the development of recurrent asthma and infectious type asthma.

"super Th1 cells." Among these Th cell subsets, Th2, Th9, Th17, and super Th1 cells are involved in the pathogenesis of allergic diseases. In this chapter, we will focus on the roles of Th17 and super Th1 cells.

Th17 cells

Th17 cell development

In mice, to develop into Th17 cells, naïve CD4+ cells have to be activated through the T-cell receptor (TCR) in the presence of both immunoregulatory cytokine TGF-β and proinflammatory cytokine IL-6, which lead to the expression of the transcription factor retinoic acid-related orphan receptor γt (RORγt) [9,10] (Figure 3.1).

In addition to IL-6 and TGF-β, IL-21 together with TGF-β or TGF-β plus IL-23 has been described as supporting Th17 polarization [11–13]. IL-21 pro-

duced by Th17 cells provides a positive feedback loop for the further expansion of differentiated Th17 cells [14]. However, the role of IL-21 in the differentiation of Th17 cells *in vivo* is questioned because Th17 cells and autoimmune diseases develop normally in the absence of IL-21 or IL-21 receptor (R) [15,16]. In the early studies on Th17 cells, IL-23 was proposed to initiate Th17 differentiation [17,18]. However, IL-23R expression is induced only on the activated memory Th cells or on the already differentiated Th17 cells [13], suggesting that IL-23 promotes the expansion and maintenance of IL-17-producing effector T cells [14].

In contrast to Th17 cells in mice, the conditions favoring the development of Th17 cells in humans are not yet fully elucidated. In particular, the role of TGF-β remains controversial [19,20]. However, recent studies confirmed that naïve human cord blood T cells differentiate into Th17 cells after being stimulated with TGF-β and a "proinflammatory" cytokine [21]. TGF-β plus IL-21, TGF-β plus a combination of IL-6 and IL-23, or IL-6 plus IL-21 [19] can induce the expression of RORc, the human counterpart of mouse RORγt.

IL-17 and IL-17R

Upon stimulation, Th17 cells produce various members of IL-17 family, which includes IL-17 (also called IL-17A), IL-17B, IL-17C, IL-17D, and IL-17F [14]. IL-17E, also called IL-25, is not produced by Th17 cells, but is produced by Th2 cells [22]. Mouse Th17 cells express the lineage-specific cytokines IL-17A, IL-17F, and IL-22, in addition to other inflammatory cytokines, such as IL-21, tumor necrosis factor (TNF) α, and GM-CSF [14]. Human Th17 cells also secrete the IL-22-related cytokine IL-26 [14]. IL-17A and IL-17F display high sequence homology and can be secreted as homodimers, as well as IL-17A/F heterodimers, by both mouse and human cells [23,24].

The cognate receptor for IL-17A is IL-17RA, which is expressed at high levels on hematopoietic cells and at lower levels on fibroblasts, endothelial cells, and epithelial cells. IL-17RA also binds IL-17F, albeit with a lower affinity. In mice, the cognate receptor for IL-17F is IL-17RC, and in humans IL-17RA and IL-17RC can form a heterodimer that is able to bind both IL-17A and IL-17F [14]. The receptor for IL-17E (IL-25) is IL-17RB, which also binds IL-17B with low affinity [14].

Biological functions of Th17-associated cytokines (IL-17A and IL-17F)

IL-17A and IL-17F are key cytokines for the recruitment, activation, and migration of neutrophils [14]. IL-17A and IL-17F have proinflammatory properties [25] and induce a wide range of cell types to secrete cytokines (TNF-α, IL-1β, IL-6, GM-CSF, granulocyte colony-stimulating factor [G-CSF]), chemokines (CXCL1, CXCL8, CXCL10), and metalloproteinases [14]. Focusing on the respiratory tracts, human bronchial fibroblast cells respond to stimulation with IL-17 *in vitro* by producing IL-6/IL-11, IL-8, and GRO-α [26]. IL-8 and GRO-α are known chemoattractants for neutrophils, and IL-6 is a neutrophil-activating cytokine [27]. Thus, the increased expression of IL-17

in the lung during bronchial asthma may explain the increased accumulation and activation of lung neutrophils. Similarly, cultured human airway smooth muscle cells produce IL-8 and IL-6 upon activation with IL-17, and the production is enhanced by IL-1β and TNF-α, respectively [28,29]. Likewise, eotaxin-1 (CCL11) was produced by human airway smooth muscle cells cultured with IL-17, which was upregulated by the addition of IL-1β [30]. IL-17 and TNF-α cooperatively stimulate human lung epithelial cells to produce IL-8 and IL-6 [31]. In addition to its local and systemic effects on neutrophils, IL-17, acting through stimulation of IL-6, is shown to induce gene expression of the mucins MUC5B and MUC5AC in human bronchial epithelial cells [32].

Th17 cells in allergic diseases in respiratory tract

Th17-associated cytokines in allergic asthma

Allergic asthma is a complex and chronic inflammatory airway disease characterized by airway hyper-responsiveness (AHR), airway inflammation and remodeling, and occasional high serum levels of IgE, in which many cells, such as mast cells, basophils, eosinophils, T lymphocytes, macrophages, neutrophils, and epithelial cells, play a role. The imbalance of Th1–Th2 immunity was believed to play an important role in the pathogenesis of allergic asthma. However, there is significant evidence to suggest that IL-17 plays an important role in the pathogenesis of bronchial asthma [26,33–37]. IL-17 mRNA and/or proteins are reported to be increased in the lungs, sputum, and bronchoalveolar lavage (BAL) fluids or sera from asthmatics [26,33–37], and the levels of IL-17 correlate with the degree of severity of airway hypersensitivity in individuals with asthma [33], implying a contribution of IL-17 to the development of asthma.

Very recently, Th17 immunity in patients with allergic asthma was reported [38]. The percentages of Th2 and Th17 cells as well as the concentrations of Th2- and Th17-related cytokines (IL-4, IL-17, IL-22, and IL-23) are higher in allergic asthmatics than in healthy controls, even though some patients received treatment with inhaled glucocorticoid [38]. The percentages of Th17 cells and the plasma concentrations of IL-17 and IL-22 tend to increase with the severity of the disease, while the IL-25 level is elevated in patients with mild asthma. Furthermore, a parallel elevation of IL-17 and IL-23 concentrations and an increase in RORγt level were found in allergic asthmatics [38]. Involvement of Th17 cells in asthma is verified in mice. Although adoptive transfer of ovalbumin (OVA)-specific Th17 cells alone cannot induce asthmatic changes in naïve mice, this treatment in collaboration with OVA-specific Th2 cells enhances Th2 cell-induced eosinophilic airway inflammation [39]. These results suggested the involvement of Th2 cells and Th17 cells in the pathogenesis of allergic asthma.

Th17-associated cytokines in severe asthma
Most studies have been conducted on patients with mild-to-moderate asthma who have an association with Th2 cell activation, peribronchial eosinophilic infiltration, mucous hypersecretion, and Th2 cytokine production. Usually, combination therapy with broad-spectrum anti-inflammatory agents (typically inhaled glucocorticoids) and long-acting β agonists can control the Th2 cytokine-induced eosinophilic inflammation and clinical features of the asthma [40]. However, 10% of the asthmatic population comprises patients with severe asthma who are unresponsive to treatment with glucocorticoids [41]. Thus, severe asthma has greater morbidity and mortality and uses a considerable amount of healthcare expenditures. Furthermore, the population of patients with severe asthma appears to manifest a different pattern of airway inflammation that is not associated with either classic Th1 or Th2 cells [41]. For example, IL-8 chemoattractant for neutrophils is prominently expressed in the airways of such patients [42]. These observations suggest the possibility of "non-Th2-type" asthma.

Based on the heterogeneity in the symptoms, asthma has been categorized into atopic and nonatopic type [43], or eosinophilic and noneosinophilic type [44,45]. Patients with atopic-type asthma show Th2-type airway inflammation with a numerical increase of cells expressing IL-4 and/or IL-5 and eosinophils in bronchial biopsies and are accompanied by increased serum IgE levels. Patients with nonatopic-type asthma exhibit non-Th2-type airway inflammation and a numerical increase of cells expressing IL-8 and neutrophils, and are characterized by the absence of elevation of serum IgE [43]. As mentioned above, individuals with mild and moderate asthma

have predominant airway inflammation with eosinophils, while severe asthmatics show predominant neutrophilic inflammation [45]. Importantly, the severity of asthma is well paralleled with the number of neutrophils [44–48].

Al-Ramli *et al.* [41] performed immunohistologic analysis for the expression of IL-17A and IL-17F in the lung biopsies sampled from patients with severe asthma, moderate asthma, mild asthma, and controls without asthma. IL-17A is expressed in all groups and is almost exclusively expressed in mononuclear cells present in the subepithelial region within clusters of inflammatory cells. Some IL-17A+ cells are observed within the epithelial layer and smooth muscle bundle. The number of IL-17A+ cells is significantly elevated in the patients with severe asthma than in other groups [41]. In contrast, IL-17F is expressed in both epithelial cells and inflammatory infiltrates. The number of IL-17F+ cells in the subepithelial compartment is increased only in individuals with severe asthma, whereas the number of IL-17F+ epithelial cells is elevated even in individuals with moderate asthma compared with healthy controls [41]. They did not perform the colocalization studies of IL-17A and IL-17F. Quantitative real-time polymerase chain reaction (RT-PCR) analysis confirms a significant increase of IL-17A and IL-17F in individuals with severe asthma.

Steroid unresponsiveness in those with severe asthma has been attributed to the presence of neutrophilic inflammation [40]. Activation of human bronchial fibroblasts with IL-17 induces chemoattractants (IL-8 and GRO-α) for neutrophils and activates cytokine (IL-6) of neutrophils [26,27]. McKinley *et al.* [49] have shown in a murine model that Th17 cells not only induce airway inflammation but also may induce steroid resistance. They demonstrated that *in vitro* polarized Th17 cells are nonresponsive to glucocorticoids. Adoptive transfer of these cells into a model of antigen-induced airway inflammation results in the pulmonary increase of KC (CXCL8) and G-CSF, both of which are associated with neutrophil influx. Treatment of Th17 cell-reconstituted mice with dexamethasone does not alter the airway inflammation, but it can attenuate Th2-mediated airway inflammation. Reconstitution of mice with either Th2 or Th17 cells resulted in increased AHR to methacholine challenge. However, dexamethasone treatment significantly reduces AHR in mice transferred with Th2 cells but not in Th17-reconstituted mice [49]. These data clearly demonstrated the significance of the contribution of Th17 cells to diseases in the respiratory tract and the association of Th17 cells in steroid-resistant asthma.

Super Th1 cells

Introduction of super Th1 cells

We previously demonstrated that stimulation of naïve CD4+ T cells or B cells with IL-12 induces the expression of IL-18R, and that these IL-18R-expressing cells produce IFN-γ in response to IL-18 [50]. Naïve CD4+ T cells, when stimulated with antigen and IL-12 or IL-4, develop into Th1 cells or Th2 cells, respectively. Then, we examined the expression of IL-18R on Th1 cells and Th2 cells. As expected, only Th1 cells express IL-18R and produce IFN-γ in response to antigen stimulation and further increase IFN-γ production in response to additional IL-18 stimulation [8,50]. Thus, IL-18 was initially regarded as the Th1 response-

enhancing cytokine. However, to our surprise Th1 cells simultaneously produced Th2 cytokines (e.g., IL-9 and IL-13), GM-CSF, and chemokines (e.g., regulated on activation, normal T cell-expressed, and secreted [RANTES] and macrophage inflammatory protein 1) [8]. We also demonstrated that human Th1 cells produce Th1 and Th2 cytokines and IL-8 in response to anti-CD3 plus IL-18 [51]. As a combination of IFN-γ and IL-13 induces severe bronchial asthma [52], we examined the capacity of Th1 cells to induce bronchial asthma after treatment with antigen, IL-2, and IL-18 in mice and found that Th1 cells become very pathologic and induce bronchial asthma by production of IL-13 and IFN-γ. We further demonstrated that Th1 cells also induce intrinsic atopic dermatitis by production of Th1 and Th2 cytokines and chemokines [53]. Thus, Th1 cells develop into the cells that produce both Th1 cytokines and Th2 cytokines and induce allergic inflammation. Based on this unique pathologic function, we proposed to designate antigen plus IL-18-stimulated Th1 cells as "super Th1 cells" [53] (Figure 3.2).

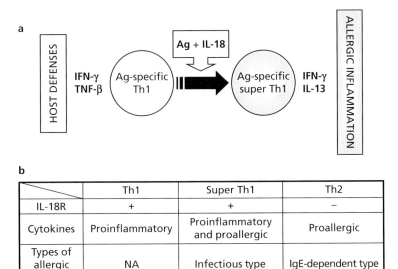

	Th1	Super Th1	Th2
IL-18R	+	+	−
Cytokines	Proinflammatory	Proinflammatory and proallergic	Proallergic
Types of allergic disorder	NA	Infectious type	IgE-dependent type

Figure 3.2 Super T helper 1 (Th1) cells. (a) When activated with antigen together with interleukin 18 (IL-18), Th1 cells begin to exert their actions as super Th1 cells by producing both Th1 and Th2 cytokines. Among the cytokines, interferon gamma (IFN-γ) and IL-13 are critical for the development of airway hyperresponsiveness (AHR) and airway fibrosis, respectively. (b) Th2 responses are essential for immunoglobulin E (IgE)-dependent type allergy principally by their production of proallergic cytokine IL-13, while super Th1 cells are critical for the development of infectious type allergy by producing both IFN-γ and IL-13.

Super Th1 cells and asthma

Bronchial asthma is characterized by AHR and reversible airflow obstruction. This syndrome is usually associated with airway inflammation and remodeling and occasional high serum levels of IgE [54–60]. Histologic examination reveals that there are infiltrates of eosinophils, subbasement membrane thickening, hyperplasia and hypertrophy of bronchial smooth muscle, and hyperplasia of airway goblet cells [54,55]. Th2 cells have been recognized as cells that induce bronchial asthma by producing Th2 cytokines [54–65]. Among these Th2 cytokines, IL-13 is suggested to play a critical role in induction of AHR, eosinophilic infiltration, goblet cell hyperplasia, and lung fibrosis [61,62,64–66]. In contrast, Th1 cells had been regarded as inhibiting bronchial asthma by producing IFN-γ [67–69]. However, several studies have revealed the incapability of Th1 cells to suppress Th2 cell-induced AHR [52,70–73]. On the contrary, a combination of Th1 cells and Th2 cells or their products rather augment each activity to induce airway inflammation and AHR [52,70,73]. Thus, it is very important to define the functions of Th1 cells in bronchial asthma.

We prepared monoclonal Th1 cells that express OVA-specific TCR and IL-18R by culturing naïve CD4$^+$ T cells derived from OVA-specific TCR-transgenic mice (DO11.10) under Th1 conditions. We wished to reveal the pathologic role of super Th1 cells *in vivo*. We simultaneously generated Th2 cells from OVA-specific naïve DO11.10 CD4$^+$ cells by *in vitro* incubation under Th2 conditions. As reported elsewhere, naïve mice transferred with OVA-specific Th2 cells, namely "passive Th2 mice," develop asthmatic responses upon intranasal OVA challenge [8]. They develop AHR, airway eosinophilic inflammation, and goblet cell metaplasia of airway epithelial cells. As we expected, an IL-13 blockade protected against the development of all of those manifestations. In contrast, "passive Th1 mice," which are generated by a similar protocol to passive Th2 mice except for the *in vitro* incubation of naïve OVA-specific CD4$^+$ cells under Th1 conditions, do not show any asthmatic signs and/or symptoms after intranasal challenge with OVA alone. However, whenever challenged with OVA together with IL-18, passive Th1 mice start to succumb to AHR, airway eosinophilia, and peribronchial fibrosis, suggesting the pathologic function of

super Th1 cells (Figure 3.2b). Thus, nasally administered OVA and IL-18 act on memory Th1 cells to induce AHR and eosinophilic inflammation. In contrast to Th2-type asthma observed in passive Th2 mice, IL-13 blockade prevents airway eosinophilic inflammation and peribronchial fibrosis partly and profoundly, but not AHR [74]. This AHR can be protected by IFN-γ blockade. Thus, super Th1 cells might be involved in the pathogenesis of certain types of allergic disorders by producing both IFN-γ and IL-13 (Figure 3.2a).

Infectious-type bronchial asthma

It is well documented that lower respiratory infection with rhinovirus, a common microbe relevant to colds, or with *Mycoplasma pneumoniae* and *Chlamydophila pneumoniae*, common bacterial causatives of pneumonia, frequently provokes or exacerbates bronchial asthma [75,76]. Epithelial cells are a major cell source of various proallergic cytokines such as IL-18, IL-25, thymic stromal lymphopoietin (TSLP), and IL-33 [77]. As they are accumulated preferentially in the inflammatory sites of patients with Th2-type allergic diseases, IL-25, TSLP, and IL-33 might be involved in the development of Th2-type allergy [56,78,79]. By contrast, epithelium-derived IL-18 might trigger infectious types of the allergic diseases as described above, although the mechanism for the secretion of IL-18 from the epithelial cells is still to be elucidated [80,81]. As microbial infection sometimes evokes IL-18 secretion [82,83], we may assume that microbial products might cause local release of IL-18, which in turn triggers bronchial asthma by activation of super Th1 cells. As expected, murine bronchial epithelial cells can respond to lipopolysaccharide (LPS) by releasing IL-18 [84]. We could demonstrate that passive Th1 mice or wild-type mice immunized with OVA in Th1 adjuvant ("active Th1 mice") show AHR and peribronchial eosinophilic inflammation upon intranasal OVA challenge in combination with LPS, a cell wall component of Gram-negative bacteria [74]. As IL-18 blockade can rescue active Th1 mice from these clinical manifestations after intranasal challenge with OVA and LPS, we concluded that LPS induces production of endogenous IL-18 [74]. Furthermore, IL-18$^{-/-}$ mice immunized with OVA in Th1 adjuvant can evade them after being similarly challenged [74]. Thus, endogenously produced IL-18 and exogenously

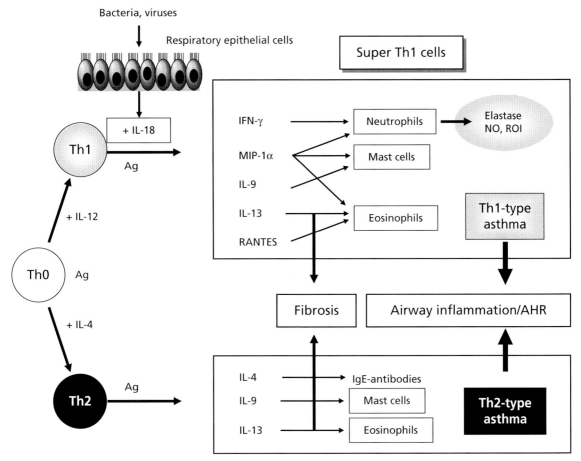

Figure 3.3 Mechanisms involved in super T helper 1 (Th1) asthma. In Th2-type asthma, interleukin 4 (IL-4) induces B-cell immunoglobulin E (IgE) production, IL-9 activates mast cells, and IL-13 induces eosinophilic inflammation, airway hyperresponsiveness (AHR), and pulmonary fibrosis. In Th1-type asthma, when pathogen-specific Th1 cells are activated with pathogen-derived antigen and IL-18 from epithelial cells infected with microbes, they exert their pathologic effects by producing Th1 cytokines, Th2 cytokines, and chemokines. Interferon gamma (IFN-γ) stimulates neutrophils to produce nitric oxide-producing hilic elastase and reactive oxygen intermediate (ROI), which in combination induce AHR. IL-13 induces airway eophinophilic inflammation and pulmonary fibrosis. IL-9 induces proliferation of mast cells. These changes are usually observed in the lung of Th2-type asthma. In addition, chemokines produced by super Th1 cells augment airway inflammation.

administered OVA both induce OVA-specific super Th1 cells, leading to the development of asthmatic manifestations in infectious types of asthma (Figure 3.3).

We further investigated whether IL-18 induces and/or exacerbates AHR and airway inflammation in mice immunized with bacterial products in the Th1 adjuvant, complete Freund adjuvant (CFA). Upon intranasal exposure to the protein A (SpA) derived from

Staphylococcus aureus that frequently colonizes in the human nasal tract, mice immunized with SpA/CFA developed asthma-like inflammation with AHR and airway eosinophilic inflammation [85]. Their CD4+ T cells in draining lymph nodes produced robust IFN-γ and IL-13. IL-18 blockade prevented airway inflammation by inhibiting this T-cell differentiation. Furthermore, naïve mice receiving CD4+ T cells from the draining lymph nodes of SpA-immunized mice developed airway inflammation as well. Importantly, immunodeficient mice transferred with SpA-stimulated human peripheral blood mononuclear cells (PBMCs) developed airway inflammation with a dense accumulation of human CD4[+] T cells after intranasal challenge with SpA. Neutralizing antihuman IL-18 could protect this airway inflammation [85]. These results suggest that animals immunized with bacterial products under Th1 cell-inducing conditions develop IL-18-dependent bronchial asthma upon challenge with the same product, indicating that IL-18 is a potent therapeutic target molecule for the treatment of Th1 cell-induced bronchial asthma.

Clinical evidence for IL-18

Accumulating evidence suggests a positive relationship between IL-18 levels in the lesion or circulation and allergic diseases, such as asthma, allergic rhinitis, and atopic dermatitis (AD) [81,86,87]. In particular, after an inhalatory challenge test with flour allergens, patients with occupational allergic asthma and/or rhinitis show a significant increase in IL-18 levels in nasal lavage fluid. Furthermore, the IL-18 polymorphism that ensures higher production of IL-18 upon appropriate stimuli is preferentially accumulated in patients with allergic disorders [88,89]. Further association studies using polymorphic markers of the IL-18 gene have been performed to discover genetic components in the pathogenesis of bronchial asthma [90–94]. We recently examined an association study in a Japanese population and discovered variants of IL-18 that might have an effect on asthma susceptibility and/or progression, and we conducted functional analyses of the related variants [95]. In this study, the IL-18 gene locus was resequenced in 48 human chromosomes. Asthma severity was determined according to the 2002 Global Initiative for Asthma (GINA) guidelines. Association and haplotype analyses were performed using 1172 individuals (including 453 adults with asthma). Although no polymorphisms differed significantly in frequency between the healthy control and adult asthma groups, rs5744247 C>G was significantly associated with the severity of adult asthma (steps 1 and 2 vs. steps 3 and 4; $P = 0.0034$) [95]. By in vitro functional analyses, the rs5744247 variant was found to increase enhancer-reporter activity of the IL-18 gene in bronchial epithelial cells. Expression levels of IL-18 in response to LPS stimulation in monocytes were significantly greater in individuals who are homozygous for the susceptibility G allele at rs5744247 C>G. This LPS-induced IL-18 mRNA expression was not affected by treatment with dexamethasone and salmeterol. Furthermore, we found a significant correlation between the serum IL-18 level and the genotype of rs5744247 ($P = 0.031$) [95].

Concluding remarks

Th17 cells seem to be critical mediators of steroid-resistant severe, recurrent asthma with neutrophilic inflammation. Recent reports suggest the importance of Th17 cells for the pathogenesis of AD [96]. Loss of function null mutation of filaggrin, which is important for the skin barrier, is a genetic risk factor of AD in humans [97]. Filaggrin-deficient mice develop Th17-dominated skin inflammation upon epicutaneous application with OVA concomitant with serum elevation of OVA-specific IgE [96]. Thus, Th17 cells seem to be important for Th2-type atopic diseases. However, there remain several issues to be elucidated. Is Th2 response preceded by Th17 response, or vice versa? How are Th17 cells differentiated in allergic diseases? Does Th17-type asthma preferentially develop after respiratory microbial infection? One may accept that super Th1 cells are activated upon microbial infection of allergic lesion. What is a super Th1 cell subset? Do super Th1 cells, like Th1 cells, require the proper epigenetic regulation? If so, what is a transcription factor essential for the differentiation into super Th1 cells, like T-bet/STAT4 for Th1 cells (Figure 3.1)?

Although we need further studies to settle those issues, targeting Th17/super Th1 cells and Th17/super Th1-associated cytokines might be of value in the therapy of severe recurrent asthma and perhaps of infectious-type allergic diseases. As IL-6 contributes to the Th17 cell differentiation, humanized anti-IL-6R mAb, which is now utilized as the potent therapeutic reagent for autoimmune diseases such as rheumatoid arthritis and Crohn disease [98,99], might be beneficial for the treatment of Th17-involved allergy. We have generated human antihuman IL-18 mAb by the gene-manipulating technique [100]. This human-derived mAb that targets human IL-18 might be highlighted as a therapeutic agent against infectious-type allergic diseases as well.

Acknowledgment

We thank Dr. Hayashi for the enthusiastic discussion.

References

1 Mosmann TR, Cherwinski H, Bond MW, Giedlin MA, Coffman RL. Two types of murine helper T cell clone. I. Definition according to profiles of lymphokine activities and secreted proteins. *J Immunol* 1986; **136**: 2348–57.

2 Ferber IA, Brocke S, Taylor-Edwards C, *et al.* Mice with a disrupted IFN-gamma gene are susceptible to the induction of experimental autoimmune encephalomyelitis (EAE). *J Immunol* 1996; **156**: 5–7.

3 Krakowski M, Owens T. Interferon-gamma confers resistance to experimental allergic encephalomyelitis. *Eur J Immunol* 1996; **26**: 1641–6.

4 Willenborg DO, Fordham S, Bernard CC, Cowden WB, Ramshaw IA. IFN-gamma plays a critical downregulatory role in the induction and effector phase of myelin oligodendrocyte glycoprotein-induced autoimmune encephalomyelitis. *J Immunol* 1996; **157**: 3223–7.

5 Miyara M, Wing K, Sakaguchi S. Therapeutic approaches to allergy and autoimmunity based on FoxP3+ regulatory T-cell activation and expansion. *J Allergy Clin Immunol* 2009; **123**: 749–55.

6 Soroosh P, Doherty TA. Th9 and allergic disease. *Immunology* 2009; **127**: 450–8.

7 King C, Tangye SG, Mackay CR. T follicular helper (TFH) cells in normal and dysregulated immune responses. *Annu Rev Immunol* 2008; **26**: 741–66.

8 Sugimoto T, Ishikawa Y, Yoshimoto T, Hayashi N, Fujimoto J, Nakanishi K. Interleukin 18 acts on memory T helper cells type 1 to induce airway inflammation and hyperresponsiveness in a naïve host mouse. *J Exp Med* 2004; **199**: 535–45.

9 Ivanov II, McKenzie BS, Zhou L, *et al.* The orphan nuclear receptor RORgammat directs the differentiation program of proinflammatory IL-17+ T helper cells. *Cell* 2006; **126**: 1121–33.

10 Ivanov II, Zhou L, Littman DR. Transcriptional regulation of Th17 cell differentiation. *Semin Immunol* 2007; **19**: 49–417.

11 Korn T, Bettelli E, Gao W, *et al.* IL-21 initiates an alternative pathway to induce proinflammatory T(H)17 cells. *Nature* 2007; **448**: 484–7.

12 Nurieva R, Yang XO, Martinez G, *et al.* Essential autocrine regulation by IL-21 in the generation of inflammatory T cells. *Nature* 2007; **448**: 480–3.

13 Zhou L, Ivanov II, Spolski R, *et al.* IL-6 programs T(H)–17 cell differentiation by promoting sequential engagement of the IL-21 and IL-23 pathways. *Nat Immunol* 2007; **8**: 967–74.

14 Korn T, Bettelli E, Oukka M, Kuchroo VK. IL-17 and Th17 cells. *Annu Rev Immunol* 2009; **27**: 485–517.

15 Coquet JM, Chakravarti S, Smyth MJ, Godfrey DI. Cutting edge: IL-21 is not essential for Th17 differentiation or experimental autoimmune encephalomyelitis. *J Immunol* 2008; **180**: 7097–101.

16 Sonderegger I, Kisielow J, Meier R, King C, Kopf M. IL-21 and IL-21R are not required for development of Th17 cells and autoimmunity *in vivo*. *Eur J Immunol* 2008; **38**: 1833–8.

17 Harrington LE, Hatton RD, Mangan PR, *et al.* Interleukin 17-producing CD4+ effector T cells develop via a lineage distinct from the T helper type 1 and 2 lineages. *Nat Immunol* 2005; **6**: 1123–32.

18 Langrish CL, Chen Y, Blumenschein WM, *et al.* IL-23 drives a pathogenic T cell population that induces autoimmune inflammation. *J Exp Med* 2005; **201**: 233–40.

19 Manel N, Unutmaz D, Littman DR. The differentiation of human T(H)–17 cells requires transforming growth factor-beta and induction of the nuclear receptor RORgammat. *Nat Immunol* 2008; **9**: 641–9.

20 Volpe E, Servant N, Zollinger R, *et al.* A critical function for transforming growth factor-beta, interleukin 23 and proinflammatory cytokines in driving and modulating human T(H)–17 responses. *Nat Immunol* 2008; **9**: 650–7.

21 Yang L, Anderson DE, Baecher-Allan C, *et al.* IL-21 and TGF-beta are required for differentiation of human T(H)17 cells. *Nature* 2008; **454**: 350–2.

22 Fort MM, Cheung J, Yen D, *et al.* IL-25 induces IL-4: IL-5: and IL-13 and Th2-associated pathologies *in vivo*. *Immunity* 2001; **15**: 985–95.

23 Liang SC, Long AJ, Bennett F, *et al.* An IL–17F/A heterodimer protein is produced by mouse Th17 cells and induces airway neutrophil recruitment. *J Immunol* 2007; **179**: 7791–9.

24 Wright JF, Guo Y, Quazi A, *et al.* Identification of an interleukin 17F/17A heterodimer in activated human CD4+ T cells. *J Biol Chem* 2007; **282**: 13447–55.

25 Kolls JK, Linden A. Interleukin-17 family members and inflammation. *Immunity* 2004; **21**: 467–76.

26 Molet S, Hamid Q, Davoine F, *et al.* IL-17 is increased in asthmatic airways and induces human bronchial fibroblasts to produce cytokines. *J Allergy Clin Immunol* 2001; **108**: 430–8.

27 Linden A. Role of interleukin-17 and the neutrophil in asthma. *Int Arch Allergy Immunol* 2001; **126**: 179–84.

28 Dragon S, Rahman MS, Yang J, Unruh H, Halayko AJ, Gounni AS. IL-17 enhances IL-1beta-mediated CXCL-8 release from human airway smooth muscle cells. *Am J Physiol Lung Cell Mol Physiol* 2007; **292**: L1023–9.

29 Henness S, Johnson CK, Ge Q, Armour CL, Hughes JM, Ammit AJ. IL-17A augments TNF-alpha-induced IL-6 expression in airway smooth muscle by enhancing mRNA stability. *J Allergy Clin Immunol* 2004; **114**: 958–64.

30 Rahman MS, Yamasaki A, Yang J, Shan L, Halayko AJ, Gounni AS. IL-17A induces eotaxin-1/CC chemokine ligand 11 expression in human airway smooth muscle cells: role of MAPK (Erk1/2: JNK and p38) pathways. *J Immunol* 2006; **177**: 4064–71.

31 van den Berg A, Kuiper M, Snoek M, *et al.* Interleukin-17 induces hyperresponsive interleukin-8 and interleukin-6 production to tumor necrosis factor-alpha in structural lung cells. *Am J Respir Cell Mol Biol* 2005; **33**: 97–104.

32 Chen Y, Thai P, Zhao YH, Ho YS, DeSouza MM, Wu R. Stimulation of airway mucin gene expression by interleukin (IL)–17 through IL-6 paracrine/autocrine loop. *J Biol Chem* 2003; **278**: 17036–43.

33 Barczyk A, Pierzchala W, Sozanska E. Interleukin-17 in sputum correlates with airway hyperresponsiveness to methacholine. *Respir Med* 2003; **97**: 726–33.

34 Chakir J, Shannon J, Molet S, *et al.* Airway remodeling-associated mediators in moderate to severe asthma: effect of steroids on TGF-beta, IL-11: IL-17: and type I and type III collagen expression. *J Allergy Clin Immunol* 2003; **111**: 1293–8.

35 Laan M, Palmberg L, Larsson K, Linden A. Free, soluble interleukin-17 protein during severe inflammation in human airways. *Eur Respir J* 2002; **19**: 534–7.

36 Sun YC, Zhou QT, Yao WZ. Sputum interleukin-17 is increased and associated with airway neutrophilia in patients with severe asthma. *Chin Med J (Engl)* 2005; **118**: 953–6.

37 Wong CK, Ho CY, Ko FW, Chan Ch, Ho AS, Hui DS, Lam CW. Proinflammatory cytokines (IL-17: IL-6: IL-18 and IL-12) and Th cytokines (IFN-gamma, IL-4: IL-10 and IL-13) in patients with allergic asthma. *Clin Exp Immunol* 2001; **125**: 177–83.

38 Zhao Y, Yang J, Gao YD, Guo W. Th17 Immunity in patients with allergic asthma. *Int Arch Allergy Immunol* 2009; **151**: 297–307.

39 Wakashin H, Hirose K, Maezawa Y, *et al.* IL-23 and Th17 cells enhance Th2 cell-mediated eosinophilic airway inflammation in mice. *Am J Repir Crit Care Med* 2008; **178**: 1023–32.

40 Gold DR, Fuhlbrigge AL. Inhaled corticosteroids for young children with wheezing. *N Engl J Med* 2006; **354**: 2058–60.

41 Al-Ramli W, Prefontaine D, Chouiali F, *et al.* T(H)17-associated cytokines (IL-17A and IL-17F) in severe asthma. *J Allergy Clin Immunol* 2009; **123**: 1185–7.

42 Shannon J, Ernst P, Yamauchi Y, *et al.* Differences in airway cytokine profile in severe asthma compared to moderate asthma. *Chest* 2008; **133**: 420–6.

43 Amin K, Ludviksdottir D, Janson C, *et al.* Inflammation and structural changes in the airways of patients with atopic and nonatopic asthma. BHR Group. *Am J Respir Crit Care Med* 2000; **162**: 2295–301.

44 Gibson PG, Simpson JL, Saltos N. Heterogeneity of airway inflammation in persistent asthma: evidence of neutrophilic inflammation and increased sputum interleukin-8. *Chest* 2001; **119**: 1329–36.

45 Wenzel SE, Schwartz LB, Langmack EL, *et al.* Evidence that severe asthma can be divided pathologically into two inflammatory subtypes with distinct physiologic and clinical characteristics. *Am J Respir Crit Care Med* 1999; **160**: 1001–8.

46 Fahy JV, Kim KW, Liu J, Boushey HA. Prominent neutrophilic inflammation in sputum from subjects with asthma exacerbation. *J Allergy Clin Immunol* 1995; **95**: 843–52.

47 Jatakanon A, Uasuf C, Maziak W, Lim S, Chung KF, Barnes PJ. Neutrophilic inflammation in severe persistent asthma. *Am J Respir Crit Care Med* 1999; **160**: 1532–9.

48 Ordonez CL, Shaughnessy TE, Matthay MA, Fahy JV. Increased neutrophil numbers and IL-8 levels in airway secretions in acute severe asthma: Clinical and biologic significance. *Am J Respir Crit Care Med* 2000; **161**: 1185–90.

49 McKinley L, Alcorn JF, Peterson A, *et al.* TH17 cells mediate steroid-resistant airway inflammation and airway hyperresponsiveness in mice. *J Immunol* 2008; **181**: 4089–97.

50 Yoshimoto T, Takeda K, Tanaka TK, *et al.* IL-12 upregulates IL-18 receptor expression on T cells, Th1 cells, and B cells: synergism with IL-18 for IFN-gamma production. *J Immunol* 1998; **161**: 3400–7.

51 Hata H, Yoshimoto T, Hayashi N, Hada T, Nakanishi K. IL-18 together with anti-CD3 antibody induces human Th1 cells to produce Th1- and Th2-cytokines and IL-8. *Int Immunol* 2004; **16**: 1733–9.

52 Ford JG, Rennick D, Donaldson DD, *et al.* IL-13 and IFN-gamma: interactions in lung inflammation. *J Immunol* 2001; **167**: 1769–77.

53 Terada M, Tsutsui H, Imai Y, *et al.* Contribution of IL-18 to atopic-dermatitis-like skin inflammation induced by *Staphylococcus aureus* product in mice. *Proc Natl Acad Sci USA* 2006; **103**: 8816–21.

54 Bochner BS, Undem BJ, Lichtenstein LM. Immunological aspects of allergic asthma. *Annu Rev Immunol* 1994; **12**: 295–335.

55 Busse WW, Lemanske RF, Jr. Asthma. *N Engl J Med* 2001; **344**: 350–62.

56 Cohn L, Elias JA, Chupp GL. Asthma: mechanisms of disease persistence and progression. *Annu Rev Immunol* 2004; **22**: 789–815.

57 Davies DE, Wicks J, Powell RM, Puddicombe SM, Holgate ST. Airway remodeling in asthma: new insights. *J Allergy Clin Immunol* 2003; **111**: 215–25.

58 Elias JA, Lee CG, Zheng T, Ma B, Homer RJ, Zhu Z. New insights into the pathogenesis of asthma. *J Clin Invest* 2003; **111**: 291–7.

59 Umetsu DT, McIntire JJ, Akbari O, Macaubas C, DeKruyff RH. Asthma: an epidemic of dysregulated immunity. *Nat Immunol* 2002; **3**: 715–20.

60 Wills-Karp M. Immunologic basis of antigen-induced airway hyperresponsiveness. *Annu Rev Immunol* 1999; **17**: 255–81.

61 Grunig G, Warnock M, Wakil AE, *et al.* Requirement for IL-13 independently of IL-4 in experimental asthma. *Science* 1998; **282**: 2261–3.

62 Kuperman DA, Huang X, Koth LL, *et al.* Direct effects of interleukin-13 on epithelial cells cause airway hyperreactivity and mucus overproduction in asthma. *Nat Med* 2002; **8**: 885–9.

63 Nakamura Y, Ghaffar O, Olivenstein R, *et al.* Gene expression of the GATA-3 transcription factor is increased in atopic asthma. *J Allergy Clin Immunol* 1999; **103**: 215–22.

64 Wills-Karp M, Luyimbazi J, Xu X, *et al.* Interleukin-13: central mediator of allergic asthma. *Science* 1998; **282**: 2258–61.

65 Zhu Z, Homer RJ, Wang Z, *et al.* Pulmonary expression of interleukin-13 causes inflammation, mucus hypersecretion, subepithelial fibrosis, physiologic abnormalities, and eotaxin production. *J Clin Invest* 1999; **103**: 779–88.

66 Wynn TA. IL-13 effector functions. *Annu Rev Immunol* 2003; **21**: 425–56.

67 Cohn L, Homer RJ, Niu N, Bottomly K. T helper 1 cells and interferon gamma regulate allergic airway inflammation and mucus production. *J Exp Med* 1999; **190**: 1309–18.

68 Huang TJ, MacAry PA, Eynott P, *et al.* Allergen-specific Th1 cells counteract efferent Th2 cell-dependent bronchial hyperresponsiveness and eosinophilic inflammation partly via IFN-gamma. *J Immunol* 2001; **166**: 207–17.

69 Iwamoto I, Nakajima H, Endo H, Yoshida S. Interferon gamma regulates antigen-induced eosinophil recruitment into the mouse airways by inhibiting the infiltration of CD4$^+$ T cells. *J Exp Med* 1993; **177**: 573–6.

70 Hansen G, Berry G, DeKruyff RH, Umetsu DT. Allergen-specific Th1 cells fail to counterbalance Th2 cell-induced airway hyperreactivity but cause severe airway inflammation. *J Clin Invest* 1999; **103**: 175–83.

71 Li L, Xia Y, Nguyen A, Feng L, Lo D. Th2-induced eotaxin expression and eosinophilia coexist with Th1 responses at the effector stage of lung inflammation. *J Immunol* 1998; **161**: 3128–35.

72 Randolph DA, Carruthers CJ, Szabo SJ, Murphy KM, Chaplin DD. Modulation of airway inflammation by passive transfer of allergen-specific Th1 and Th2 cells in a mouse model of asthma. *J Immunol* 1999; **162**: 2375–83.

73 Randolph DA, Stephens R, Carruthers CJ, Chaplin DD. Cooperation between Th1 and Th2 cells in a murine model of eosinophilic airway inflammation. *J Clin Invest* 1999; **104**: 1021–9.

74 Hayashi N, Yoshimoto T, Izuhara K, Matsui K, Tanaka T, Nakanishi K. T helper 1 cells stimulated with ovalbumin and IL-18 induce airway hyperresponsiveness and lung fibrosis by IFN-γ and IL-13 production. *Proc Natl Acad Sci USA* 2007; **104**: 14765–70.

75 Gern JE. Rhinovirus and the initiation of asthma. *Curr Opin Allergy Clin Immunol* 2009; **9**: 73–8.

76 Rand Sutherland E, Martin RJ. Asthma and atypical bacterial infection. *Chest* 2007; **132**: 1962–6.

77 Bulek K, Swaidani S, Aronica M, Li X. Epithelium: the interplay between innate and Th2 immunity. *Immunol Cell Biol* 2010; **88**: 257–68.

78 Liu Y-J, Soumelis V, Watanabe N, *et al.* TSLP: An epithelial cell cytokine that regulates T-cell differentiation by conditioning dendritic cell maturation. *Annu Rev Immunol* 2007; **25**: 193–219.

79 Saenz SA, Taylor BC, Artis D. Welcome to the neighborhood: epithelial cell-derived cytokines license innate and adaptive immune responses at mucosal sites. *Immunol Rev* 2008; **226**: 172–90.

80 Nakano H, Tsutsui H, Terada M, *et al.* Persistent secretion of IL-18 in the skin contributes to IgE response in mice. *Int Immunol* 2003; **15**: 611–21.

81 Wong CK, Ho CY, Ko FW, *et al.* Proinflammatory cytokines (IL-17: IL-6: IL-18 and IL-12) and Th cytokines (IFN-g, IL-4: IL-10 and IL-13) in patients with allergic asthma. *Clin Exp Immunol* 2001; **125**: 177–83.

82 Nakanishi K, Yoshimoto T, Tsutsui H, Okamura H. Interleukin-18 regulates both Th1 and Th2 responses. *Annu Rev Immunol* 2001; **19**: 423–74.

83 Tsutsui H, Yoshimoto T, Hayashi N, Mizutani H, Nakanishi K. Induction of allergic inflammation by interleukin-18 in experimental animal models. *Immunol Rev* 2004; **202**: 115–38.

84 Cameron LA, Taha RA, Tsicopoulos A, *et al.* Airway epithelium expresses interleukin-18. *Eur Respir J* 1999; **14**: 553–9.

85 Kuroda-Morimoto M, Tanaka H, Hayashi N, *et al.* Contribution of IL-18 to eosinophilic airway inflammation induced by immunization and challenge with Staphylococcus aureus proteins. *Int Immunol* 2010; **22**: 561–70.

86 Tanaka T, Tsutsui H, Yoshimoto T, *et al.* Interleukin-18 is elevated in the sera from patients with atopic

dermatitis and from atopic dermatitis model mice, NC/Nga. *Int Arch Allergy Immunol* 2001; **125**: 236–40.

87 Krakowiak A, Walusiak J, Krawczyk P, *et al*. IL-18 levels in nasal lavage after inhalatory challenge test with flour in bakers diagnosed with occupational asthma. *Int J Occup Med Environ Health* 2008; **21**: 165–72.

88 Novak N, Kruse S, Potreck J, *et al*. Single nucleotide polymorphisms of the IL-18 gene are associated with atopic eczema. *J Allergy Clin Immunol* 2005;**115**: 828–33.

89 Sebeloba S, Izakovicova-Holla L, Stejskalova A, Schüller M, Znojil V, Vasku A. Interleukin-18 and its three gene polymorphisms relating to allergic rhinitis. *J Hum Genet* 2007; **52**: 152–158.

90 Heinzmann A, Gerhold K, Ganter K, *et al*. Association study of polymorphisms within interleukin-18 in juvenile idiopathic arthritis and bronchial asthma. *Allergy* 2004; **59**: 845–9.

91 Higa S, Hirano T, Mayumi M, *et al*. Association between interleukin-18 gene polymorphism 105A/C and asthma. *Clin Exp Allergy* 2003; **33**: 1097–102.

92 Imboden M, Nicod L, Nieters A, *et al*. The common G-allele of interleukin-18 single nucleotide polymorphism is a genetic risk factor for atopic asthma. The SAPALDIA Cohort Study. *Clin Exp Allergy* 2006; **36**: 211–18.

93 Reijmerink NE, Postma DS, Bruinenberg M, *et al*. Association of IL-1RL1: IL-18R1: and IL-18RAP gene cluster polymorphisms with asthma and atopy. *J Allergy Clin Immunol* 2008; **122**: 651–4 e658.

94 Shin HD, Kim LH, Park BL, *et al*. Association of interleukin 18 (IL-18) polymorphisms with specific IgE levels to mite allergens among asthmatic patients. *Allergy* 2005; **60**: 900–6.

95 Harada M, Obara K, Hirota T, *et al*. A functional polymorphism in IL-18 is associated with severity of bronchial asthma. *Am J Respir Crit Care Med* 2009; **180**: 1048–55.

96 Gao PS, Rafaels NM, Hand T, *et al*. Filaggrin mutations that confer risk of atopic dermatitis confer greater risk for eczema herpeticum. *J Allergy Clin Immunol* 2009; **124**: 507–13.

97 Oyoshi MK, Murphy GS, Geha RS. Filaggrin-deficient mice exhibit Th17-dominated skin inflammation and permissiveness to epicutaneous sensitization with protein antigen. *J Allergy Clin Immunol* 2009; **124**: 485–93.

98 Kimura A, Kishimoto T. IL-6: Regulator of Treg/Th17 balance. *Eur J Immunol* 2010; **40**: 1830–5.

99 Kishimoto T. IL-6: from its discovery to clinical applications. *Int Immunol* 2010; **22**: 347–52.

100 Hamasaki T, Hashiguchi S, Ito Y, *et al*. Human anti-human IL-18 antibody recognizing the IL-18-binding site 3 with IL-18 signaling blocking activity. *J Biochem* 2005; **138**: 433–42.

4 Regulatory T cells

Chris Corrigan and Kimuli Ryanna
Department of Asthma, Allergy & Respiratory Science, King's College London
School of Medicine, and MRC and Asthma UK Centre for Allergic Mechanisms of
Asthma, London, UK

Introduction

Early-developing T cells in the thymus express both CD4 and CD8, and their epitope specificity is determined by random association of their T-cell antigen receptor genes. During thymic development, T cells, the receptors of which happen by chance to recognize peptides derived from "self" antigens, must be silenced or eliminated, otherwise they would attack the host. The fact that autoimmune diseases do exist demonstrates that this silencing system, while ingenious and very efficient, is not perfect. Developing T cells in the thymic epithelium that happen to bind self peptide/major histocompatibility complex (MHC) class I or II complexes presented by thymic cortical epithelial cells proliferate: this process is called primary positive selection. The remainder of the cells, which have no affinity for self antigens at all, die by neglect. Surviving T cells migrate on to the thymic medulla. T cells with a very high affinity for self antigens begin to proliferate but, in the absence of co-stimulatory signals provided by dendritic cells, undergo activation-induced apoptotic cell death. This is reflected by surface expression of Fas (CD95) and its ligand (CD95L), which interact and activate caspase enzymes that direct cell death. Mutations in Fas, its ligand, and caspase genes result in autoimmune lymphoproliferative syndrome (ALS) in humans [1]. Although this process, called negative selection, is a major one for establishment of self-tolerance,

many T cells with a medium/high affinity for self antigens do not die but rather undergo a process called nondeletional central tolerance, or secondary positive selection, in which they give rise to immunosuppressive CD4+ T cells, now known as naturally occurring T regulatory cells [2]. These cells are characterized by expression of CD25 and of forkhead box P3 (FOXP3), one of the fork head family of DNA-binding transcription factors. This factor likely plays a critical role in the development of naturally occurring T regulatory cells, since congenital mutations of the FOXP3 gene result in major disruption of immune regulation, in particular the IPEX (immune dysregulation, polyendocrinopathy, enteropathy X-linked) syndrome in humans (see account below). T cells with low-affinity receptors for self antigens escape all these processes completely and enter the periphery as conventional naïve T cells. Only about 3% of all T-cell precursors entering the thymus survive selection, migrate to the periphery, and colonize secondary lymphoid organs such as the spleen and lymph nodes. They bind self antigenic peptides with low avidity, yet constitute the population of T cells that will deal with foreign peptides presented by dendritic cells in the binding grooves of MHC molecules.

The removal by these mechanisms of T cells with a high affinity for self antigenic peptides, occurring as it does solely in the thymus gland, is a remarkable feat. Several mechanisms have been proposed to explain how this phenomenon occurs. There is

Inflammation and Allergy Drug Design, First Edition. Edited by Kenji Izuhara, Stephen T. Holgate, Marsha Wills-Karp.
© 2011 Blackwell Publishing Ltd. Published 2011 by Blackwell Publishing Ltd.

evidence, for example, for promiscuous expression of a huge variety of self antigens from outside the thymus in thymic medullary epithelial cells, so that T cells can be exposed to the entire repertoire of self antigenic peptides. This is in part regulated by a gene called "autoimmune regulator" or AIRE [3]. Mutations in AIRE result in immune polyendocrinopathy syndrome type I [4]. This mechanism may be principally involved in the removal of self-reactive T cells by negative selection (again by antigen presentation by dendritic cells in the absence of co-stimulation), since in mice AIRE deficiency results in compromised negative selection of T cells that recognize self antigenic peptides, but does not compromise the development of $CD4^+CD25^+FOXP3^+$ T regulatory cells [5]. Another process that may be important in self-tolerance involves the IL-7-like cytokine thymic stromal lymphopoietin (TSLP), which, as its name suggests, is produced by stromal cells such as epithelial and endothelial cells as well as inflammatory leukocytes. Recent studies show that TSLP is selectively expressed in the Hassall corpuscles in the thymic medulla in association with an activated subpopulation of myeloid dendritic cells [6]. Upon activation by TSLP, these dendritic cells have the capacity to induce the production of T regulatory cells in the thymus, since they have the capability to express the T-cell co-stimulatory molecules CD80 and CD86, ligands for CD28, on the T-cell surface. Development of T regulatory cells in the thymus depends on CD28 signaling [6]. There is evidence that these dendritic cells migrate into the thymus from the periphery [7] and could sample peripheral self antigens and present them to developing T cells within the thymus, resulting in self tolerance.

Thus, while many T cells that recognize self antigenic peptides are eliminated in the thymus, others acquire a T regulatory phenotype and actively suppress antiself responses. Reversal of this phenotype in particular circumstances may give rise to autoimmune disease; there is also some evidence to suggest that gaps in the repertoire of naturally occurring T regulatory cells may also cause exaggerated responses to external antigens, including allergens (see below). T cells in human neonates developing *in utero* and soon after birth are almost certainly exposed to external antigens, including allergens, at the time that the natural T regulatory cell repertoire evolves, providing a mechanistic rationale for the influence of early life exposure to allergens in regulating subsequent immune effector responses.

Although T helper (Th) 1 and Th2 T cells are mutually inhibitory, it has long been apparent that simple, mutually antagonistic interactions between these cells cannot explain the regulation of Th2 activity in humans. For example, in animal models of asthma, allergen-specific Th1 cells have in some cases been reported to augment allergic inflammation [8]. Helminthic infections, which promote Th2 responses, do not appear to be associated with increased risk of allergy and asthma, but rather, in some studies, appear to be protective [9]. Finally, epidemiologic data in the last 40 years have shown a parallel rise in the prevalence of "Th1-type" diseases such as diabetes and "Th2-type" diseases such as asthma [10], an observation that, although not necessarily reflecting direct mutual Th1/Th2 antagonism, certainly does not support it. It is in this setting that T regulatory cells have come to the fore as being capable of suppressing Th1 and Th2 T cells independently. Environmental influences altering the function of T regulatory cells seem a more likely candidate to explain the aforementioned data, rather than mutual antagonism of Th1 and Th2 responses within individuals.

T regulatory cells may be "natural" (that is, arising in course of normal development of the immune system) or "adaptive" (arising because of immune encounters). As described above, natural T regulatory cells arise largely to promote tolerance to self antigens (Figure 4.1). They constitute 5–10% of circulating $CD4^+$ T cells [11], and there is some evidence that they recognize self antigens, but with broad specificity [12]. They are characterized by high expression of CD25 (which confounds their identification since this is also an activation marker of effector T cells). They proliferate poorly *in vitro* in response to conventional T-cell activation stimuli. Adaptive T regulatory cells arise generally in the periphery from naïve T cells on encounter with antigens presented by tolerogenic dendritic cells. Tolerogenic dendritic cells are generally semimature cells with increased expression of MHC class II molecules and CD86, but low expression of CD40 and low secretion of proinflammatory cytokines such as IL-6 and TNF-α [13]. Repetitive stimulation of T cells with such dendritic cells generates IL-10-producing Tr1-adaptive T regulatory cells [14]. Similarly, inhibition of dendritic cell maturation by inhibiting NF-κB activation

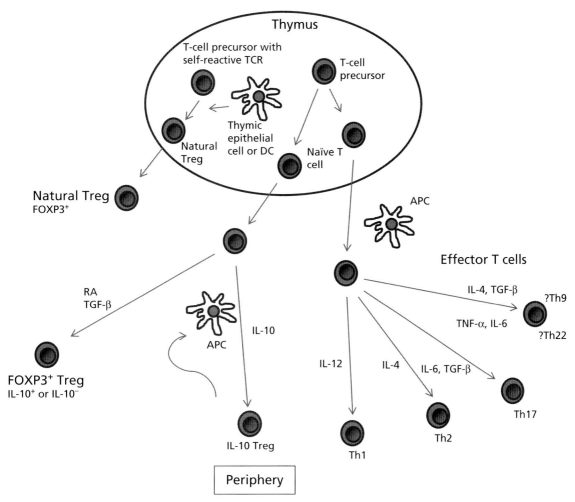

Figure 4.1 Development of regulatory CD4+ T cells. T-cell precursors in the thymus have T-cell receptors (TCRs) with varying antigen specificity. Natural regulatory T cells (Tregs) are derived from some precursors bearing TCRs with a medium/high affinity for self antigen (following contact with thymic epithelial cells or dendritic cells [DCs]). These cells will be CD4+CD25+FOXP3+. Other Tregs will be derived from the periphery. Naïve T cells may differentiate into FOXP3+ Tregs or interleukin 10 (IL-10) Tregs depending on antigen stimulus/contact with antigen-presenting cells and the cytokine environment in which they develop (IL-10, retinoic acid, or transforming growth factor (TGF) β). IL-10 Tregs comprise a distinct subset of Tregs, although some FOXP3+ Tregs may be IL-10+. TNF-α, tumor necrosis factor alpha.

with 1,25-dihydroxyvitamin D3, glucocorticoids, or mycophenolate mofetil induces development of Tr1 T regulatory cells; this may also occur directly in the presence of such drugs by activating naïve CD4+ T cells in the absence of dendritic cells [15]. Again, the mechanism is not completely understood but appears to depend on secretion of IL-10 (Tr1) or transforming growth factor (TGF) β (Tr3) by immature dendritic cells. Tolerance induced to mucosally applied antigens also appears to induce tolerogenic dendritic cells producing IL-10 or TGF-β [16].

The mechanisms of action of T regulatory cells are not well understood. One mechanism of action is through contact with effector T cells when they synapse with dendritic cells during activation. The precise mechanisms are unclear, but signaling through surface molecules such as CTLA-4, Notch 3, and LAG-3 has been implicated. Ligation of CTLA-4 on dendritic cells induces the enzyme indoleamine-2,3-dioxygenase (IDO), which starves T cells of tryptophan [17]. Other studies suggest that they exert their suppressive functions on potential effector T cells through membrane-bound TGF-β and its receptor CD152 [18]. However, other studies suggest that these cells can interfere with the direct contact of naïve T cells with dendritic cells, thus preventing their activation [19,20]. Finally, some of their suppressive activity may be caused by the secretion of inhibitory cytokines such as IL-10 and TGF-β [21].

In summary, T regulatory cells limit the generation of immune responses to self antigens and innocuous environmental antigens. They also likely limit immune responses to pathogens, preventing excessive tissue damage following pathogen clearance. While the majority of published studies have described the regulatory functions of CD4$^+$ T lymphocytes, it is clear that natural killer (NK) and NKT cells, CD8 T cells, λδ T cells, B cells, and even mast cells may in certain circumstances possess important regulatory activities. Indeed, any cell with the capacity to secrete inhibitory cytokines has regulatory potential. CD4$^+$ T regulatory cells are arguably of greatest interest, however, given the possibility of generating or expanding cells with unique and disease-relevant antigen specificity.

Biomarkers of T regulatory cells

The investigation of regulatory T cells *in vivo* is hampered by the lack of specific markers. For example, constitutive expression of CD25, the IL-2 receptor α chain, is commonly used to identify CD4$^+$ T regulatory cells, although CD25 is also expressed transiently by all T cells upon activation, resulting in confusion in *in vivo* studies addressing T regulatory function in conditions characterized by inappropriate immune activation. Additional described biomarkers of T regulatory cells include CD38, CD45RO, CD62L, CTLA-4, the glucocorticoid-induced tumor necrosis factor receptor gene GITR [22], neurophilin-1, and the folic acid receptor [21], but again most of these are also expressed, at least transiently, by activated effector T cells. As mentioned above, the transcriptional FOXP3 is overexpressed in natural T regulatory cells compared with resting and conventionally

activated T cells. However, this is troublesome as an identification marker for these cells since FOXP3 is not a surface marker, and again its expression is not entirely limited to T regulatory cells and may be expressed, at least transiently, upon activation of effector T cells. The precise actions of FOXP3 are not clear, but retroviral transfer of FOXP3 is sufficient to confer regulatory T-cell function [23]. Furthermore, whereas natural thymus-derived T regulatory cells are typically CD4$^+$CD25$^+$FOXP3$^+$, adaptive antigen-induced CD4$^+$ T regulatory cells comprise both FOXP3$^+$ and FOXP3$^-$ populations [24,25]. In practice, many investigators consider T cells that express high FOXP3 and CD25 but low CD127 to be the majority population of T regulatory cells. More specific, robust markers would be highly desirable.

Other influences on the development and function of adaptive T regulatory cells

Adaptive T regulatory cells develop outside the thymus (Figure 4.1), and this development is likely contingent upon the local environment. For example, organ-specific structural cells likely also play an active role in mediating immune responses to inhaled or ingested allergens at mucosal surfaces. In the murine respiratory tract, alveolar epithelial cells can present antigens and promote development of FOXP3$^+$ cells using a TGF-β-dependent mechanism [26]. Further, airways epithelial cells are able to initiate specific tolerogenic mechanisms on exposure to allergens with proteinase activity. In mice, retinal dehydrogenase 1 (RALDH-1), an enzyme involved in the production of retinoic acid, is induced under these circumstances and promotes the development of T regulatory cells [27]. This enzyme is in turn downregulated *in vivo* by epithelial-derived matrix metalloproteinase (MMP) 7, so that MMP-7 deficiency results in further enhancement of T regulatory cell activity. Again in the respiratory tract, alveolar macrophages have long been described as suppressing immune responses in the lung [28]. Although as yet there is scant direct evidence that they operate through the induction of T regulatory cells, there is some *in vitro* evidence that suggests that they can tolerize CD4$^+$ T cells in an antigen-specific manner [29]. Resident dendritic cells also seem to be vital in regulating mucosal immune responses. For example, in mice plasmacytoid dendritic cells appear to limit immune responses to harmless inhaled allergens [30], and again this may involve induction of T regulatory cells.

The external environment may also influence the development of adaptive (and conceivably natural) T regulatory cells. For example, in mice, delivery of Toll-like receptor (TLR) ligands to the airways along with an antigen can enhance both Th2 and Th1 effector T-cell responses depending on the relative concentrations of the TLR ligand and antigen [31]. Conversely, TLR signaling may impair, directly or indirectly, T regulatory cell function, a phenomenon which has been postulated to facilitate the clearance of pathogens [32,33]. Such data suggest that, in humans, environmental pathogens, pollutants, and allergens may interact in particular combinations, variably and on multiple occasions, to regulate allergen-specific T-cell responses.

The appropriate localization of regulatory T cells is potentially important for their function because they may exert their suppressive activity by direct cell contact as well as by the secretion of cytokines. Studies on T-cell homing *in vivo* suggest that the CC chemokine receptor CCR4 is required for the recruitment of CD4$^+$FOXP3$^+$ regulatory cells [34]. Moreover, mice with a complete loss of CCR4 in the T regulatory cell compartment develop lymphocytic infiltration and severe inflammatory disease of the airways [35]. This finding is intriguing because CCR4 is also one of the key chemokine receptors thought to be responsible for the recruitment of allergen-specific Th2 effector T cells to the lung. CD4$^+$CD25$^+$ T regulatory cells from human donors have been shown preferentially to express CCR4 and migrate in response to the CCR4 ligands CCL17 and CCL22 [36]. Adoptive transfer studies in mice have also highlighted a role for these ligands in the recruitment and retention of CD4$^+$CD25$^+$ T regulatory cells in the lung during repeated allergen challenge [37].

There is also some evidence from animal models to suggest that the retention of regulatory T cells at mucosal surfaces is dependent upon continued antigen exposure. In one study involving chronic antigen challenge [38], interruption of exposure resulted in a reduction in T regulatory cell activity concomitant with a resurgence of Th2-type inflammation. There is a parallel in humans, with beekeepers who are tolerant of bee venom allergen showing an *in vivo* switch of venom-specific T cells to an IL-10-secreting phenotype during the beekeeping season, which wanes during periods of nonexposure [39]. These observations cast some doubt upon the maxim that allergen avoidance is always the best way to prevent or turn off allergic responses. Finally, recent evidence suggests that effector and regulatory T cells may mutually regulate their accumulation at sites of inflammation. Paradoxically, in animal models the absence of T regulatory cells during mucosal viral infections results in uncontrolled inflammation and early death resulting from delayed migration of effector T cells to the site [40]. These data allow the possibility that T regulatory cells control inflammation partly by regulating the recruitment of antigen-specific effector T cells; thus, they may be important not only for the resolution but also for the initiation of immune responses. Although these phenomena may reflect the functional interaction of different populations of fully differentiated T cells, another possibility is that there is much more functional plasticity between effector and regulatory T cells than is currently recognized. For example, in mice, expression of interferon regulatory factor 4 (IRF-4), a transcription factor essential for Th2 effector cell differentiation, is dependent on FOXP3 expression. Ablation of a conditional IRF-4 allele in T regulatory cells resulted in selective dysregulation of Th2 cell responses [41], suggesting either that expression of IRF-4 somehow endows T regulatory cells with the capacity to inhibit Th2 cell responses or that one is observing different functional facets of the same cell. Other studies suggest that Th2 effector cells may be converted into alternate phenotypes expressing IL-9 and IL-10, depending on the cytokine milieu [42,43]. This flexibility in T-cell differentiation may explain the reduction of Th2 cytokine production *in vivo*, but it remains to be seen whether these changes are transient or represent more fundamental "reprogramming" of the cells' genetic machinery.

In summary, we have yet a great deal to learn about the mechanisms of immune regulation. Data to date emphasize that the local environment of T regulatory cells may greatly influence their function, that there may be competition for or ordered progression of recruitment of T cells with different functional properties to inflammatory sites, and that the functional phenotypes of T cells themselves may be more plastic than is currently understood. This is not to mention the potential regulatory properties of other leukocytes such as IL-10-secreting NK cells [44], CD8+ T cells, and γδ cells. At present, the relative importance of natural and adaptive T regulatory cells in regulating allergic inflammation and asthma is unclear and difficult to ascertain. Peripheral induction may represent an important mechanism for broadening the T-regulatory antigenic repertoire [45] or to maintain immune regulation with age [46]. The mechanisms of action of T regulatory cells may vary according to the situation in the target organ in which they were induced. In animals, data from antigenic stimulation regimens developed to promote the generation of adaptive T regulatory cells that secrete a range of inhibitory cytokines [24] suggest that IL-10-secreting adaptive T regulatory cells are likely relevant to immune homoeostasis in the respiratory tract, whereas T regulatory cells secreting TGF-β may be more relevant in the gut [47,48].

The role of T regulatory cells in allergy and asthma: evidence from animal models

It has long been known that particular regimens of exposure of animals to antigens can result in a state of subsequent immunologic tolerance. There is accumulating evidence that this phenomenon involves, at least in part, the generation of adaptive T regulatory cells. The use of these "models" to mimic tolerance induction and the role of regulatory T cells and their possible relevance to human disease have been widely reviewed [49–52] and in general they support the paradigm that a failure of tolerance plays a prominent role in the development of allergic disease. For example, repeated exposure of mice to inhaled antigens results in the development of T regulatory cell populations characterized by the production of TGF-β and FOXP3 (low inhaled concentrations) or IL-10 (higher inhaled concentrations), both of which inhibit sensitization in naïve animals following adoptive transfer [53,54]. In the latter case, IL-10-producing pulmonary dendritic cells induced T regulatory cell differentiation and tolerance could be transferred with these cells as well.

Moving on from these early experiments, adoptive transfer of CD4+CD25+ T regulatory cells induced by an antigen inhalation regimen was found to suppress airways inflammation and hyperreactivity in an IL-10-dependent fashion not only before induction of the inflammation but also after its inception [37,55]. On the other hand, intratracheal but not intravenous administration of naïve lung CD4+CD25+ T cells prior to antigen challenge of sensitized mice resulted in reduced airways responsiveness and inflammation [56], but with this regimen both IL-10 and TGF-β appeared to be necessary for the suppressive function of these cells. Yet further studies have not suggested an obligatory role for IL-10 [57]. Conversely, depletion of CD4+CD25+ T regulatory cells before inhaled antigen sensitization enhanced the severity of the associated inflammation and airways hyperresponsiveness [58], although this effect was dependent upon the strain of mouse employed, being clearly evident only in the "allergy-resistant" C3H strain. Depletion of CD25+ T cells also resulted in increased numbers of airway dendritic cells, with higher expression of activation markers and an enhanced potential to promote effector T cell proliferation.

Other themes have emerged from these animal experiments. Two studies [37,38] have suggested that maintenance of T regulatory cell activity after antigen inhalation is dependent on the continuing presence of allergen stimulation, which may in turn reflect a requirement for ongoing recruitment to and/ or retention of these cells in the respiratory mucosa. A second theme, as mentioned above, is that regulatory mechanisms appear to depend on the concentration and route of administration of the tolerizing antigens. Generally speaking, TGF-β-dependent mechanisms are more evident with low tolerizing concentrations of inhaled antigens [53,59] whereas IL-10-dependent mechanisms are more evident when higher tolerizing concentrations are employed [54,60]. Oral antigen administration has also been shown to reduce lung inflammation following subsequent inhaled challenge by a mechanism dependent on TGF-β [61]. Furthermore, such antigens may appear in breast milk and in animals have been shown [62] to induce tolerance to the same inhaled antigen in neonate offspring in a TGF-β-dependent fashion, in line with a significant body of earlier data highlighting the role of this cytokine in the induction of oral tolerance [63].

A final theme from these studies is that T regulatory cells that protect against the inflammatory effects of inhaled antigens need not be induced by the antigen itself or indeed through the respiratory tract. For example, regulatory cells induced by mycobacterial antigens or helminths can protect against antigen challenge of the respiratory tract [64–67]. The effects of therapeutic maneuvers thought to be important in conferring reduced reactivity to allergens in humans, such as allergen immunotherapy, have also been modeled in animals [68].

In summary, while these phenomena in animals provide clear "proof of principle" that antigen-specific and nonspecific T regulatory cells may play a role in modifying the development and natural history of allergic diseases, precise conclusions about mechanisms must be very guarded since these appear to depend very much on the experimental regimen, the concentration and route of administration of antigen, and the strain of animal. Furthermore, in the main they involve short-term sensitization of previously naïve animals in otherwise sterile conditions, which does not reflect a lifetime of exposure to protean environmental influences as occurs in humans. At the very least, these experiments provide a loose mechanistic framework for understanding how T regulatory cells might mediate some of the effects of the environment on the development of allergic disease, how maternal exposure to allergens may be significant and that allergen avoidance may not always be the best way to promote allergen tolerance.

T regulatory cell products: possible roles of IL-10

IL-10 is a potent anti-inflammatory cytokine produced by a wide range of leukocytes including B cells, macrophages, dendritic cells, mast cells, and eosinophils [69]. Many T-cell subsets synthesize IL-10, including CD8+ T cells, CD25+FOXP3+ T regulatory cells, and effector CD4+ T-cell populations including Th1 cells, Th2 cells, and Th17 cells. Even effector Th2 T cells have been subdivided into high IL-10-producing regulatory Th2 cells and high TNF-α-producing inflammatory Th2 cells [70]. IL-10 production by effector T cells is likely to be important in limiting their inflammatory potential. IL-10 has broad immunosuppressive and anti-inflammatory actions relevant to the inhibition of allergic inflammation and asthma pathology [69]. It inhibits proinflammatory cytokine production by T cells and also acts on antigen-presenting cells, attenuating T-cell activation. It inhibits a wide range of effector leuko-

cytes involved in allergic inflammation such as mast cells and eosinophils. IL-10 promotes the production of IgG4 by activated B cells, an immunoglobulin isotype generally believed to be protective in the context of allergic responses and induced following allergen immunotherapy [71]. At least in mice, IL-10 is absolutely required for immune homoeostasis at mucosal surfaces, since mice with a targeted deletion of IL-10 in regulatory (FOXP3+) cells develop spontaneous colitis and show exaggerated pulmonary inflammation following sensitization to inhaled antigens [72]. A series of studies suggest that IL-10 is implicated in limiting respiratory mucosal inflammation following "allergic" sensitization [55–57] or infection with respiratory tract pathogens [73,74]. Concomitant intranasal instillation of recombinant IL-10 during antigen sensitization of the airways [75] and IL-10 gene delivery to the lung suppressed subsequent airways inflammation [76,77]. In other mouse inhalative sensitization studies, adoptive transfer of IL-10-secreting T regulatory cells inhibited Th2-specific responses in vivo [78], and CD4+ T cells engineered to express IL-10 limited the ensuing airways hyperactivity and inflammation [79]. Some, but not all, animal studies employing inhalative regimens that induce tolerance also support a mechanistic role for IL-10 in this process [60,80].

Circumstantial evidence implicates IL-10 in reducing asthmatic and allergic inflammation in humans. Patients with asthma compared with controls were reported to express less IL-10 mRNA and protein but elevated proinflammatory cytokines in bronchoalveolar lavage fluid and alveolar macrophages [81]. A polymorphism in the IL-10 gene promoter resulting in reduced IL-10 expression was associated with an elevated risk of severe asthma [82]. Allergen-specific blood T cells from nonatopic individuals were more likely to express IL-10 than those from sensitized atopic individuals [83]. Natural immune tolerance to bee venom in beekeepers, who are frequently exposed to venom allergen when stung, was associated with increased venom allergen-specific IL-10+ CD4+ T cells [39]. Rhinoviral infection, one of the commonest causes of asthma exacerbation, was associated with reduced IL-10 production and augmented Th2 T cell-mediated immunity [84]. Overall, these and more generalized epidemiologic studies [85] suggest a role for IL-10 in preventing or curtailing allergic and asthmatic inflammation in humans, although they do not set the importance of IL-10 against other mechanisms and do not address the fundamental question of why some individuals develop these diseases whereas others do not. Finally, as discussed more fully below, therapies associated with amelioration of disease, including glucocorticoid therapy and allergen immunotherapy, are associated with the induction of IL-10 synthesis by T cells [86–88].

T regulatory cell products: possible roles of TGF-β

TGF-β is a pleiotropic cytokine which regulates lymphocyte homoeostasis, inhibits Th2- and Th1-cell responses, and has important influences on T-cell differentiation (see below). It also inhibits immunoglobulin E (Ig-E) but promotes IgA switching by activated B cells [47]. TGF-β induces expression of FOXP3 in peripheral naïve T cells, which as described above appears to be central to the function of natural and some adaptive T regulatory cells [89]. Homozygous TGF-β gene-deleted mice die early from multiorgan inflammation [90], suggesting a critical although as yet uncharacterized role for this cytokine in self tolerance in the periphery. Following airways antigen sensitization and challenge, heterozygous mice show exaggerated airways inflammation compared with wild-type animals, again suggesting a role for endogenous TGF-β in suppressing the development of allergic responses to antigens encountered in the respiratory tract [91]. As with similar animal experiments involving IL-10 described above, intratracheal delivery of TGF-β suppressed airways inflammation following inhaled antigen sensitization and challenge [56]. CD4+ T cells engineered to secrete latent TGF-β showed a similar effect [92]. Conversely, blocking TGF-β signaling specifically in T cells resulted in enhancement of airways hyperresponsiveness, inflammation, and Th2 cytokine production [93]. These data are consistent with the hypothesis that, at least in mice, TGF-β plays some part in regulating the immune response to novel antigens presented to the respiratory tract. The apparent relative roles of TGF-β and IL-10 in these acute sensitization models depend very much on the experimental regimen, although at least two studies [53,56] suggest an obligatory role for TGF-β. The effects of each cytokine may be partly complementary. This contrasts with the situation in

the gut, where naturally occurring TGF-β-secreting T regulatory cells appear to play a more critical, nonredundant role in maintaining immune homoeostasis [94]. One might speculate that this reflects the fundamentally different environments of the normally sterile respiratory tract and the gut, which is normally colonized with a wide variety of microorganisms, not to mention food-derived antigens.

TGF-β can exert important influences on the lineage specificity of T-cell subsets. It activates the retinoic acid-related orphan receptor (ROR) γT-dependent differentiation pathway in CD4+ T cells, resulting in the development either of Th17 or of T regulatory cells depending on the concurrent presence of maturation and polarization factors such as IL-6, IL-21, retinoic acid, IL-23, and IL-10. TGF-β has also been shown to have the potential to reprogram apparently differentiated T helper cells to form another functional subset that produces IL-9 [42,43]. Thus, mucosal effector T cells may exhibit a degree of plasticity over which TGF-β has some influence, which might be exploitable in therapeutic strategies. Allergen immunotherapy has been reported to induce TGF-β as well as IL-10 in allergen-specific T cells in various studies [95,96] but it is still not clear if and how these cytokines contribute to the clinical benefit of immunotherapy.

The potentially beneficial effects of TGF-β on airways diseases such as asthma cannot be described without also pointing out that it has also been implicated in contributing to a range of changes in the chronically inflamed airways of asthmatics collectively described as remodeling. Thus, TGF-β has been shown to promote proliferation and differentiation of fibroblasts into myofibroblasts capable of secreting extracellular matrix proteins such as collagen [97], apoptosis of airways epithelial cells, and possible denudation of intercellular adhesion, which may cause sloughing [98], goblet cell hyperplasia and increased mucus secretion [97,99], and airways smooth muscle hyperplasia [97], although the precise pathophysiologic consequences of many of these changes are still unclear. Some studies have shown elevated expression of TGF-β in the bronchial mucosa and airways of asthmatics compared with controls, with correlation in some cross-sectional studies with the extent of subepithelial fibrosis [100]. An increase in TGF-β2 has been associated with airways remodeling following acute allergen challenge of atopic asthmatics [101]. TGF-β was also reported to be increased following experimental infection of bronchial epithelial cells with rhinovirus, an important respiratory pathogen responsible for many asthma exacerbations [102].

In short, the relative benefits and drawbacks of increasing TGF-β production therapeutically, especially in the context of asthma as opposed to other allergic diseases that do not involve the lower airways, are currently very difficult to assess. Typically, animal modeling has not clarified the issue, with one study in which animals were sensitized by intraperitoneal injection of antigen and then challenged with inhaled antigen suggesting that TGF-β neutralization reduced remodeling [99], and another in which naïve mice repeatedly (and possibly more physiologically) inhaled house dust mite allergen [103] suggesting that TGF-β neutralization did not affect remodeling but did augment airways inflammation.

Finally, and to add further to the complexity, TGF-β exists in three isoforms and is also a member of a complex superfamily that includes the bone morphogenic proteins and activins. Other members of this family might have similar influences on immune homoeostasis and airways structural changes. Activin A appears to be acutely increased in the airways following allergen bronchial challenge of atopic asthmatics [104], and in an animal model of inhaled antigen sensitization it suppressed antigen-specific Th2 cell responses and protected against airways hyperresponsiveness and inflammation through induction of antigen-specific T regulatory cells, which suppressed effector responses *in vitro* and on adoptive transfer *in vivo* [105]. The receptor for bone morphogenic protein has been described in the asthmatic bronchial mucosa, although its function if any is not yet clear [106].

Evidence for a role for T regulatory cells in human allergic disease

"Experiments of nature" involving mutations of the T regulatory cell transcriptional regulatory protein FOXP3 provide perhaps the most convincing evidence to date for involvement of T regulatory cells in the prevention of allergic disease in early life in humans. As described above, FOXP3 expression is characteristic of natural T regulatory cells developing in the thymus before birth and some adaptive T regulatory cells. In many young males the IPEX (immune dysregulation, polyendocrinopathy, enteropathy X-linked) syndrome is caused by a variety of mutations in FOXP3 [107–109]. They have absent, reduced, or nonfunctional CD4+CD25high T regulatory cells. IPEX presents perinatally as a syndrome of autoimmune disease, allergy, and failure to thrive. It is generally rapidly fatal without allogeneic stem cell transplantation or profound immunosuppression [109,110]. Successful transplantation may be curative and restores CD4+CD25highCD127low FOXP3-expressing cells of donor origin [111,112]. These boys suffer from all diseases of the "atopic march" including severe eczema, elevated allergen-specific IgE, food allergy, and asthma [110]. These studies suggest that FOXP3+ CD25+high natural T regulatory cells play a prominent role in the prevention of allergic sensitization in early life. The scurfy mouse is the natural murine equivalent of IPEX [108,109], but mice with targeted loss-of-function mutations of FOXP3 similarly develop multiorgan inflammation including Th2-type airways inflammation, elevated IgE, and deregulated Th1 and Th2 cytokine production [113]. A significant proportion of patients with IPEX seem to have mutations of CD25, the IL-2 receptor α-chain, rather than FOXP3 [25,114,115]. A comparison of two patients with FOXP3 or CD25 deficiency [115] showed normal and deficient IL-10 production respectively by peripheral blood CD4+ T cells, suggesting that natural and adaptive T regulatory cells may play separate, nonredundant roles in the prevention of allergic disease.

As has been discussed, the role of T regulatory cells in controlling the development and expression of allergic diseases in asthma is only beginning to be explored [116]. Whether or not these cells play an important role in sensitization to allergens in intrauterine or early life is not yet clear, although phenomena such as the IPEX syndrome strongly suggest that they may be. In individuals with established allergy, evidence of deficiency of allergen-specific natural T regulatory cells has been reported in some [117] but not all [118] studies. The former study suggested that allergen-specific T regulatory cell activity was reduced compared with nondiseased controls in subjects with allergic rhinitis during the pollen season when they have symptoms, rather than outside it, suggesting that deficient T regulatory cell activity may somehow be involved with the clinical expression of allergic disease, although these experiments do not make it clear if clinical disease is caused by reduced natural T regulatory cell activity or is a consequence of it. What these studies do show for certain is that external allergens seem to be included in the antigenic repertoire of natural T regulatory cells. A further study [119] showed increased numbers of CD4$^+$ CD25$^+$ β-lactoglobulin-specific T cells in the blood of children who had grown out of cow's milk allergy compared with others who had not. The inhibitory effect of these cells appeared to depend on cell contact, implying a role for natural T regulatory cells. There are similar data suggesting deficiency of allergen-specific, IL-10-producing Tr1-adaptive T regulatory cells in patients who develop sensitization and symptoms in response to aeroallergens compared with those who do not [83].

Many of the studies addressing a possible role for T regulatory cells in limiting asthma are difficult to interpret because of the use of CD25 as a phenotypic marker. As discussed, this may be expressed on activated effector T cells as well as natural and adaptive T regulatory cells. Furthermore, these studies have typically been performed using peripheral blood T cells, whereas it has been emphasized that the precise situational environment of T regulatory cells may influence their function. Finally, they have tended to compare numbers of cells rather than address their functions. One study in children [120] showed reduced numbers of CD4$^+$CD25high$^+$ T cells in the airways lumen, but not the peripheral blood of asthmatics compared with controls: this imbalance was restored in association with glucocorticoid therapy. In a second study in children [121] a slight deficiency of these cells was noted in the peripheral blood of those with asthma and allergic rhinitis compared with controls. Both studies reported reduced FOXP3 mRNA expression in the peripheral blood, although protein was not measured. Other observational studies have reported elevated [122,123] or similar [124] numbers of CD4$^+$CD25$^+$ T cells in the peripheral blood of asthmatics compared with controls, but the precise functional phenotype(s) of these cells is unknown. Some of these studies have suggested that the putative T regulatory cells express elevated CTLA-4, GITR, and latency-associated peptide (LAP) but reduced CD127 [118,124,125]. So far there are few descriptions of putative T regulatory cells within the mucosa of the respiratory tract. A

biopsy study of the proximal airways of infants with symptoms suggestive of reversible airways obstruction [126] showed CD3$^+$FOXP3$^+$ cells in the mucosa, but there was no association with lung function or atopic status.

Functional studies of putative T regulatory cells in asthma have so far been limited. Bronchial allergen challenge of atopic asthmatics was associated with greater depletion of blood T cells with a regulatory phenotype in those failing to show a late phase bronchoconstrictor response compared with those who did [125]. Several studies [117,118,127] purporting to demonstrate impaired suppressor activity of blood CD4$^+$CD25$^+$ cells in patients with atopic disease or asthma compared with controls did not differentiate regulatory and effector activity of these cells. In the study on asthmatic children referred to above [120], a reduction in the numbers of CD4$^+$CD25$^+$ T cells in the airways lumen compared with controls was accompanied by impaired suppressive activity of these cells *in vitro*; both were reversed in association with inhaled corticosteroid therapy. In a second study [123], the suppressive activity of CD4$^+$CD25hi FOXP3 expressing blood T cells, as well as the expression of FOXP3 itself, was reduced in child atopic asthmatics sensitized to house dust mite compared with controls; both were enhanced following allergen-specific immunotherapy. In addition, incubation of T cells from the asthmatics with recombinant tumor necrosis factor (TNF) α further reduced FOXP3 expression and suppressor activity of these cells, whereas incubation with the TNF-α antagonist etanercept restored both. This might be relevant to the reported clinical benefits of TNF-α antagonists in severe asthma [128,129], although subsequent studies have not looked so promising.

In conclusion, these studies provide some indirect evidence for a functional role for T regulatory cells in limiting and reversing allergic disease and asthma, but confusion arises from the problems with identifying these cells accurately *in vivo*. Further, examination of the function of cells within their natural inflammatory environment presents a formidable challenge, whereas it is clear from animal experiments that global blockade of cytokines such as TNF-α and IL-6 [130] can lead to expansion of putative T regulatory cell populations within the airways mucosa, suggesting that local influences on T regulatory cell development may be even more significant in this regard.

Experimental and therapeutic influences on T regulatory cell development and function in allergic diseases

Typically, although not invariably, allergic diseases including asthma develop at an early age, implying that in many cases early life events are critical for the development of protective regulatory mechanisms within the immune system. Indeed, evidence exists that T regulatory cells are already impaired in the cord blood of neonates at hereditary risk of allergy [131,132]. Epidemiologic evidence about the influence of environmental factors on the risk of development of allergic disease, which could be used to frame hypotheses about the influence of these factors on the early development of the immune system, remains somewhat confusing. The "hygiene hypothesis" proposes that early childhood infections and exposure to microbial products inhibit the tendency to develop allergic disease. Epidemiologic evidence seems to support this in the sense that living in a developing country, having several older siblings, mixing with other children early at day care, and exposure to livestock have been associated with a lower incidence of allergic disease. This in turn has been linked with the development of regulatory pathways [133]. On the other hand, some viral infections in childhood, for example with respiratory syncitial virus, seem to increase the risk of subsequent asthma at least in a proportion of infected children [134–136]. Environmental factors may influence the development of the neonatal immune system before birth and even before conception, because prenatal exposure to a farming environment influences innate immune patterning. Maternal exposure during pregnancy to an environment rich in microbial compounds was associated with higher expression of Toll-like receptors 2 and 4 CD14 on peripheral blood cells, implying that exposure might prevent sensitization of the children [137]. More directly, farm exposure during pregnancy has been associated with enhanced numbers and functional activity of regulatory T cells within cord blood as well as reduced Th2 cytokine production and lymphocyte proliferation after innate restimulation [138]. Studies in mice have shown that exposure of pregnant females to endotoxin inhibits subsequent antigen-induced airways sensitization and inflammation in the offspring [139]. Further, immunologic tolerance can be transferred from parent to offspring if the parent is tolerized before pregnancy, implying that even before conception the immune status of the mother is critical in defining the immune response of the offspring to allergens [140]. In addition to infection and exposure to aeroallergens, environmental pollution and diet [141–143] have recently been proposed to influence the development of allergic disease in early life. Reduced maternal intake of vitamins D and E and zinc during pregnancy has been associated with increased risk of asthma in children [143,144]. Vitamin D in particular has been implicated in the development or maintenance of both natural and adaptive FOXP3[+] and IL-10[+] T regulatory cells in humans and mice [33,145,146] (Figure 4.2). There is also some evidence, at least from animal studies, to suggest that diet may modify the risk of allergic diseases through epigenetic mechanisms [141]. Mice given a diet rich in methyl donors such as folate or vitamin B12 gave rise to offspring who showed enhanced allergic airways inflammation after sensitization: the phenomenon was heritable over multiple generations. This was hypothesized to reflect increased DNA methylation, reducing the transcriptional rate of inhibitory genes. A similar scenario may apply in humans [142]. Intriguing as these studies are, they have provided little direct evidence for a role for specific regulatory T-cell populations. A more direct animal study showed that exposure of lactating mice to an airborne antigen protected their progeny from airways sensitization on exposure to the same antigen [62]. This protection depended upon transference of the inhaled antigen to the breast milk and the presence of TGF-β originating from regulatory CD4[+] T cells. Food allergens have long been known to appear in human breast milk, but whether and in what circumstances they might induce tolerance is not clear.

A role for T regulatory cells has been suggested in the mechanisms of the therapeutic interventions that ameliorate allergic diseases and asthma. Perhaps the best studied is allergen immunotherapy, the only therapeutic intervention which has been suggested to alter the natural history of allergic disease [147]. Immunotherapy reduces and skews allergen-specific Th2 cell responses and promotes development of IL-10-secreting T regulatory cells. This is observable quite quickly after initiation of immunotherapy and is followed by an increase in circulating allergen-specific IgG$_4$, an isotype known to be regulated by

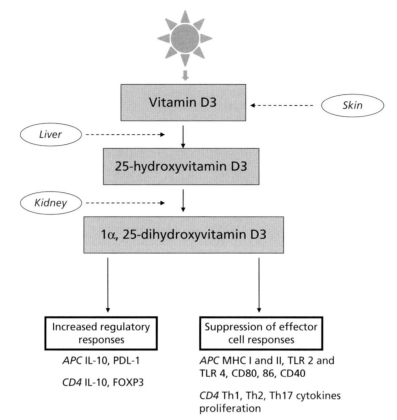

Figure 4.2 Vitamin D. Exposure to sunlight in the skin converts 7-dehydrocholesterol to vitamin D3. Vitamin D3 is then metabolized in the liver to 25-hydroxyvitamin D3, the main circulating form of the vitamin. 25 hydroxyvitamin D3 undergoes further conversion in the kidney to the active metabolite 1α,25-dihydroxyvitamin D3. Vitamin D has widespread immunoregulatory effects, leading to suppression of effector responses in antigen-presenting cells (APCs) and CD4 T cells, and induction of regulatory responses. MHC, major histocompatibility complex.

IL-10 and postulated to play a role in reducing clinical responses to subsequent allergen exposure, for example by inhibiting IgE-mediated allergen capture and presentation by antigen-presenting cells [71,148]. This high IL-10 phenotype is characteristic of the allergen-specific T-cell response of nonatopic donors [83] and those who develop natural tolerance of allergens despite repeated exposure [39]. There is direct evidence that allergen immunotherapy induces T regulatory cells. In one study [149], rush venom immunotherapy was associated with a progressive increase in $CD4^+CD25^{+high}FOXP3^+$ allergen-specific T cells, the numbers of which correlated with serum venom-specific IgG_4/IgE ratios. Grass pollen immunotherapy of individuals with hay fever was associated with elevated numbers of $FOXP3^+CD25^+CD3^+$ cells in the target nasal mucosa, some of which co-expressed IL-10 [150]. Other studies have reported elevated allergen-induced T-cell TGF-β production in association with immunotherapy, implying that not all of the immunomodulatory effects of immunotherapy operate through IL-10 [148].

Several lines of evidence, some briefly referred to above, suggest that corticosteroids, the mainstay of asthma therapy, act at least partly by enhancing IL-10 production and T regulatory cell numbers and function. IL-10 is the only cytokine whose expression is increased rather than decreased by corticosteroids. Thus, corticosteroids may assert their immunomodulatory effects through activities on both effector and T regulatory cells. IL-10 production has been reported to be increased in the serum and airways and in putative T regulatory cells in both the blood and the airways following corticosteroid therapy [81,120,151,152]. Furthermore, corticosteroid-induced IL-10 production was reduced in peripheral blood T cells of patients with clinically corticosteroid refractory asthma [86]. This deficiency was reversible by $1\alpha,25$-dihydroxyvitamin D3 (calcitriol), not only *in vitro* but also *in vivo* after the patients ingested vitamin D3 at standard dosages for just a few days [33,87]. Long-acting β_2-agonist was also reported to synergize with corticosteroids to promote the development of allergen-specific T regulatory cells [153].

This observation returns us full circle to the importance of environment and diet on the development of allergic diseases. There is a growing awareness of the prevalence of vitamin D insufficiency and its association with respiratory diseases including asthma as well as allergy worldwide [143,154]. This has focused attention on the possible importance of vitamin D in maintaining and possibly programming T regulatory cell populations that are important for immune homoeostasis (Figure 4.2). *In vitro*, vitamin D induces a tolerogenic dendritic cell phenotype characterized by elevated production of IL-10, which promotes the development of FOXP3+ T regulatory cells [145] and also acts directly on human CD4+ T cells to induce IL-10+ T regulatory cells [33]. These phenomena suggest the possibility that vitamin D may be important for the induction of T regulatory cell populations, which could for example limit immune responsiveness to inhaled aeroallergens. This, coupled with the capacity of vitamin D to enhance antimicrobial defense, might suggest an important role for vitamin D in immune homoeostasis in the respiratory tract [155]. Further, they suggest that agents such as vitamin D may enhance T regulatory cell production in situations where these cells are already known to be produced, such as with corticosteroid therapy or allergen immunotherapy. While these observations offer promise for the future, it is salutary to remember that not all T regulatory cells seem to operate through the production of IL-10, and that *in vitro* experiments may not paint a true picture of the functions of these cells when out of contact with other cells in the environment of the mucosal surface.

Finally, a return to the hygiene hypothesis, which in essence suggests that lack of exposure to environmental infectious agents is one factor responsible for the increasing prevalence of allergy in the past 30 or 40 years. As originally formulated, it cannot now apply to the concept of directing a battle between Th1 and Th2 T-cell supremacy. Environmental influences on the development and persistence of allergic disease, if they truly exist, must now be examined in light of their possible influences on T regulatory cells. Interestingly, pathogen-specific Tr1-adaptive T regulatory cells are induced in the course of infections with many viruses, bacteria, and parasites [156]. In some cases this results in incomplete elimination of the pathogen, which could theoretically result in "bystander" suppression of allergic responses by both natural and adaptive T regulatory cells. Such findings may necessitate investigation of the hygiene hypothesis in the context of a much broader range infectious agents, not only pathogens but also commensal bacteria such as the intestinal flora [157].

References

1 Worth A, Thrasher AJ, Gaspar B. Autoimmune lymphoproliferative syndrome: molecular basis of disease and clinical phenotype. *Br J Haematol* 2006; **133**: 124–40.

2 Sakaguchi S. Naturally arising CD4+ regulatory T cells for immunologic self-tolerance and negative control of immune responses. *Annu Rev Immunol* 2004; **14**: 73–99.

3 Su M, Anderson MS. AIRE: an update. *Curr Opin Immunol* 2004; **16**: 748–52.

4 Peterson P, Peltonen L. Autoimmune polyendocrinopathy syndrome type 1 (APS1) and the AIRE gene: new views on the molecular basis of auto. *J Autoimmunity* 2005; **25**: 49–55.

5 Anderson MS, Venanzi ES, Klein L, *et al.* Projection of an immunological self shadow within the thymus by the Aire protein. *Science* 2002; **298**: 1395–401.

6 Watanabe N, Wang YH, Lee HK, Ito T, Cao W, Liu YJ. Hassall's corpuscles instruct dendritic cells to induce CD4+ CD25+ regulatory T cells in human thymus. *Nature* 2005; **436**: 1181–5.

7 Donskoy E, Goldenschneider I. Two developmentally distinct populations of dendritic cells inhabit the adult mouse thymus: demonstration by differential importation of haematogenous precursors under steady-state conditions. *J Immunol* 2003; **170**: 3514–21.

8 Hansen G, Berry G, Dekruyff RH, Umetsu DT. Allergen-specific Th1 cells fail to counterbalance Th2 cell-induced airway hyperactivity but cause severe airway inflammation. *J Clin Invest* 1999; **103**: 175–83.

9 Yazdanbakhsh M, Kremsner PG, van Ree R. Allergy, parasites, and the hygiene hypothesis. *Science* 2002; **296**: 490–4.

10 Sheikh A, Smeeth L, Hubbard R. There is no evidence of an inverse relationship between TH2-mediated atopy and TH1-mediated autoimmune disorders: lack of support for the hygiene hypothesis. *J Allergy Clin Immunol* 2003; **111**: 131–5.

11 Fehervari Z, Sakaguchi S. Development and function of CD25⁺CD4⁺ regulatory T cells. *Curr Opin Immunol* 2004; **16**: 203–8.

12 Hsieh CS, Liang Y, Tyznik AJ, Self SG, Liggitt D, Rudensky AY. Recognition of the peripheral self by naturally arising CD25⁺CD4⁺ T cell receptors. *Immunity* 2004; **21**: 267–77.

13 Lutz MB, Schuler G. Immature, semi-mature and fully mature dendritic cells which signals induce intolerance or immunity? *Trends Immunol* 2002; **23**: 445–9.

14 Jonuleit H, Schmitt E, Steinbrink K, Enk AH. Dendritic cells as a tool to induce anergic and regulatory T cells. *Trends Immunol* 2001; **22**: 394–400.

15 Barrat FJ, Cua DJ, Boonstra A, *et al. In vitro* generation of interleukin 10-producing regulatory CD4⁺ T cells is induced by immunosuppressive drugs and inhibited by T helper type 1 (Th1)- and Th2-inducing cytokines. *J Exp Med* 2002; **195**: 603–16.

16 Weiner HL. The mucosal milieu creates tolerogenic dendritic cells and Tr1 and Tr3 regulatory cells. *Nat Immunol* 2001; **2**: 671–2.

17 Mellor AL, Munn DH. IDO expression by dendritic cells: tolerance and tryptophan catabolism. *Nat Rev Immunol* 2004; **4**: 762–74.

18 Nakamura K, Kitani A, Strober W. Cell contact-dependent immunosuppression by CD4⁺CD25⁺ regulatory T cells is mediated by surface-bound transforming growth factor β. *J Exp Med* 2001; **194**: 629–44.

19 Bluestone JA, Tang Q. How do CD4⁺CD25⁺ regulatory T cells control autoimmunity? *Curr Opin Immunol* 2005; **17**: 638–42.

20 Tadokoro CE, Shakhar G, Shen S, *et al.* Regulatory T cells inhibit stable contacts between CD4⁺ T cells and dendritic cells. *J Exp Med* 2006; **203**: 505–11.

21 Vignali DA, Collison LW, Workman CJ. How regulatory T cells work. *Nat Rev Immunol* 2008; **8**: 523–32.

22 Yi H, Zhen Y, Jiang L, Zheng J, Zhao Y. The phenotypic characterization of naturally occurring regulatory CD4⁺ CD25⁺ T cells. *Cell Mol Immunol* 2006; **3**: 189–95.

23 Yagi H, Nomura T, Nakamura K, *et al.* Crucial role of FoxP3 in the development and function of human CD25⁺CD4⁺ regulatory T cells. *Int Immunol* 2004; **16**: 1643–56.

24 Hawrylowicz CM, O'Garra A. Potential role of interleukin-10-secreting regulatory T cells in allergy and asthma. *Nat Rev Immunol* 2005; **5**: 271–83.

25 Roncarolo MG, Gregori S, Battaglia M, Bacchetta R, Fleischhauer K, Levings MK. Interleukin-10-secreting type 1 regulatory T cells in rodents and humans. *Immunol Rev* 2006; **212**: 28–50.

26 Gereke M, Jung S, Buer J, Bruder D. Alveolar type II epithelial cells present antigen to CD4(⁺) T cells and induce Foxp3(⁺) regulatory T cells. *Am J Respir Crit Care Med* 2009; **179**: 344–55.

27 Goswami S, Angkasekwinai P, Shan M, *et al.* Divergent functions for airway epithelial matrix metalloproteinase 7 and retinoic acid in experimental asthma. *Nat Immunol* 2009; **10**: 496–503.

28 Holt PG, Strickland DH, Wikstrom ME, Jahnsen FL. Regulation of immunological homeostasis in the respiratory tract. *Nat Rev Immunol* 2008; **8**: 142–52.

29 Blumenthal RL, Campbell DE, Hwang P, DeKruyff RH, Frankel LR, Umetsu DT. Human alveolar macrophages induce functional inactivation in antigen-specific CD4 T cells. *J Allergy Clin Immunol* 2001; **107**: 258–64.

30 Lambrecht BN. Biology of lung dendritic cell subsets at the origin of asthma. *Immunity* 2009; **31**: 412–24.

31 Eisenbarth SC, Piggott DA, Huleatt JW, Visintin I, Herrick CA, Bottomly K. Lipopolysaccharide-enhanced, toll-like receptor 4-dependent T helper cell type 2 responses to inhaled antigen. *J Exp Med* 2002; **196**: 1645–51.

32 Sutmuller RP, Morgan ME, Netea MG, Grauer O, Adema GJ. Toll-like receptors on regulatory T cells: expanding immune regulation. *Trends Immunol* 2006; **27**: 387–93.

33 Urry Z, Xystrakis E, Richards D, *et al.* Ligation of TLR9 induced on human IL-10-secreting Tregs by 1a,25-dihydroxyvitamin D3 abrogates regulatory function. *J Clin Invest* 2009; **119**: 387–98.

34 Sather BD, Treuting P, Perdue N, *et al.* Altering the distribution of Foxp3(⁺) regulatory T cells results in tissue-specific inflammatory disease. *J Exp Med* 2007; **204**: 1335–47.

35 Lloyd CM, Delaney T, Nguyen T, *et al.* CC chemokine receptor (CCR)3/eotaxin is followed by CCR4/monocyte-derived chemokine in mediating pulmonary T helper lymphocyte type 2 recruitment after serial antigen challenge *in vivo. J Exp Med* 2000; **191**: 265–74.

36 Iellem A, Mariani M, Lang R, *et al.* Unique chemotactic response profile and specific expression of chemokine receptors CCR4 and CCR8 by CD4(⁺)CD25(⁺) regulatory T cells. *J Exp Med* 2001; **194**: 847–53.

37 Kearley J, Robinson DS, Lloyd CM. CD4⁺CD25⁺ regulatory T cells reverse established allergic airway inflammation and prevent airway remodelling. *J Allergy Clin Immunol* 2008; **122**: 617–24.

38 Strickland DH, Stumbles PA, Zosky GR, *et al.* Reversal of airway hyperresponsiveness by induction of airway mucosal CD4⁺CD25⁺ regulatory T cells. *J Exp Med* 2006; **203**: 2649–60.

39 Meiler F, Zumkehr J, Klunker S, Ruckert B, Akdis CA, Akdis M. *In vivo* switch to IL-10-secreting T regulatory cells in high dose allergen exposure. *J Exp Med* 2008; **205**: 2887–98.

40 Lund JM, Hsing L, Pham TT, Rudensky AY. Coordination of early protective immunity to viral infection by regulatory T cells. *Science* 2008; **320**: 1220–4.

41 Zheng Y, Chaudhry A, Kas A, *et al.* Regulatory T-cell suppressor program co-opts transcription factor IRF4 to control T(H)2 responses. *Nature* 2009; **458**: 351–6.

42 Dardalhon V, Awasthi A, Kwon H, *et al.* IL-4 inhibits TGF-beta-induced Foxp3⁺ T cells and, together with TGF-beta, generates IL-9⁺ IL-10⁺ Foxp3(-) effector T cells. *Nat Immunol* 2008; **9**: 1347–55.

43 Veldhoen M, Uyttenhove C, van Snick J, *et al.* Transforming growth factor-beta 'reprograms' the differentiation of T helper 2 cells and promotes an interleukin 9-producing subset. *Nat Immunol* 2008; **9**: 1341–6.

44 Deniz G, Erten G, Kucuksezer UC, *et al.* Regulatory NK cells suppress antigen specific T-cell responses. *J Immunol* 2008; **180**: 850–7.

45 Curotto de Lafaille MA, Kutchukhidze N, Shen S, Ding Y, Yee H, Lafaille JJ. Adaptive Foxp3⁺ regulatory T cell-dependent and -independent control of allergic inflammation. *Immunity* 2008; **29**: 114–26.

46 Akbar AN, Vukmanovic-Stejic M, Taams LS, Macallan DC. The dynamic co-evolution of memory and regulatory CD4⁺ T cells in the periphery. *Nat Rev Immunol* 2007; **7**: 231–7.

47 Li MO, Wan YY, Sanjabi S, Robertson AK, Flavell RA. Transforming growth factor-beta regulation of immune responses. *Annu Rev Immunol* 2006; **24**: 99–146.

48 Faria AM, Weiner HL. Oral tolerance and TGF-beta-producing cells. *Inflamm Allergy Drug Targets* 2006; **5**: 179–90.

49 Hawrylowicz CM. Regulatory T cells and IL-10 in allergic inflammation. *J Exp Med* 2005; **202**: 1459–63.

50 Boyce JA, Austen KF. No audible wheezing: nuggets and conundrums from mouse asthma models. *J Exp Med* 2005; **201**: 1869–73.

51 Tournoy KG, Hove C, Grooten J, Moerloose K, Brusselle GG, Joos GF. Animal models of allergen-induced tolerance in asthma: are T-regulatory-1 cells (Tr-1) the solution for T-helper-2 cells (Th-2) in asthma? *Clin Exp Allergy* 2006; **36**: 8–20.

52 Lloyd CM. Building better mouse models of asthma. *Curr Allergy Asthma Rep* 2007; **7**: 231–6.

53 Ostroukhova M, Seguin-Devaux C, Oriss TB, *et al.* Tolerance induced by inhaled antigen involves CD4(⁺) T cells expressing membrane-bound TGF-beta and FOXP3. *J Clin Invest* 2004; **114**: 28–38.

54 Akbari O, Freeman GJ, Meyer EH, *et al.* Antigen-specific regulatory T cells develop via the ICOS-ICOS-ligand pathway and inhibit allergen-induced airway hyperreactivity. *Nat Med* 2002; **8**: 1024–32.

55 Kearley J, Barker JE, Robinson DS, Lloyd CM. Resolution of airway inflammation and hyperreactivity after *in vivo* transfer of CD4⁺CD25⁺ regulatory T cells is interleukin 10 dependent. *J Exp Med* 2005; **202**: 1539–47.

56 Joetham A, Takada K, Taube C, *et al.* Naturally occurring lung CD4⁺CD25⁺ T cell regulation of airway allergic responses depends on IL-10 induction of TGF-beta. *J Immunol* 2007; **178**: 1433–42.

57 Leech MD, Benson RA, De Vries A, Fitch PM, Howie SE. Resolution of Der p1-induced allergic airway inflammation is dependent on CD4⁺CD25⁺Foxp3⁺ regulatory cells. *J Immunol* 2007; **179**: 7050–8.

58 Lewkowich IP, Herman NS, Schleifer KW, *et al.* CD4⁺CD25⁺ T cells protect against experimentally induced asthma and alter pulmonary dendritic cell phenotype and function. *J Exp Med* 2005; **202**: 1549–61.

59 Van Hove CL, Maes T, Joos GF, Tournoy KG. Prolonged inhaled allergen exposure can induce persistent tolerance. *Am J Respir Cell Mol Biol* 2007; **36**: 573–84.

60 Akbari O, DeKruyff RH, Umetsu DT. Pulmonary dendritic cells producing IL-10 mediate tolerance induced by respiratory exposure to antigen. *Nat Immunol* 2001; **2**: 725–31.

61 Mucida D, Kutchukhidze N, Erazo A, Russo M, Lafaille JJ, Curotto de Lafaille MA. Oral tolerance in the absence of naturally occurring Tregs. *J Clin Invest* 2005; **115**: 1923–33.

62 Verhasselt V, Milcent V, Cazareth J, *et al.* Breast milk-mediated transfer of an antigen induces tolerance and protection from allergic asthma. *Nat Med* 2008; **14**: 170–5.

63 Faria AM, Weiner HL. Oral tolerance and TGF-beta-producing cells. *Inflamm Allergy Drug Targets* 2006; **5**: 179–90.

64 Zuany-Amorim C, Sawicka E, Manlius C, *et al.* Suppression of airway eosinophilia by killed *Mycobacterium vaccae*-induced allergen-specific regulatory T-cells. *Nat Med* 2002; **8**: 625–9.

65 Wilson MS, Taylor MD, Balic A, Finney CA, Lamb JR, Maizels RM. Suppression of allergic airway inflammation by helminth-induced regulatory T cells. *J Exp Med* 2005; **202**: 1199–212.

66 Yang J, Zhao J, Yang Y, *et al.* *Schistosoma japonicum* egg antigens stimulate CD4 CD25 T cells and modulate airway inflammation in a murine model of asthma. *Immunology* 2007; **120**: 8–18.

67 Wilson MS, Maizels RM. Regulation of allergy and autoimmunity in helminth infection. *Clin Rev Allergy Immunol* 2004; **26**: 35–50.

68 Taher YA, van Esch BC, Hofman GA, Henricks PA, van Oosterhout AJ. 1Alpha,25-dihydroxyvitamin D3 potentiates the beneficial effects of allergen immunotherapy in a mouse model of allergic asthma: role for IL-10 and TGF-beta. *J Immunol* 2008; **180**: 5211–21.

69 O'Garra A, Barrat FJ, Castro AG, Vicari A, Hawrylowicz C. Strategies for use of IL-10 or its antagonists in human disease. *Immunol Rev* 2008; **223**: 114–31.

70 Ito T, Wang YH, Duramad O, *et al.* TSLP-activated dendritic cells induce an inflammatory T helper type 2 response through OX40 ligand. *J Exp Med* 2005; **20**: 1213–23.

71 Till SJ, Francis JN, Nouri-Aria K, Durham SR. Mechanisms of immunotherapy. *J Allergy Clin Immunol* 2004; **113**: 1025–34.

72 Rubtsov YP, Rasmussen JP, Chi EY, *et al.* Regulatory T cell-derived interleukin-10 limits inflammation at environmental interfaces. *Immunity* 2008; **28**: 546–58.

73 Higgins SC, Lavelle EC, McCann C, *et al.* Toll-like receptor 4-mediated innate IL-10 activates antigen-specific regulatory T cells and confers resistance to *Bordetella pertussis* by inhibiting inflammatory pathology. *J Immunol* 2003; **171**: 3119–27.

74 Sun J, Madan R, Karp CL, Braciale TJ. Effector T cells control lung inflammation during acute influenza virus infection by producing IL-10. *Nat Med* 2009; **15**: 277–84.

75 Zuany-Amorim C, Haile S, Leduc D, *et al.* Interleukin-10 inhibits antigen induced cellular recruitment into the airways of sensitized mice. *J Clin Invest* 1995; **95**: 2644–51.

76 Stampfli MR, Cwiartka M, Gajewska BU, *et al.* Interleukin-10 gene transfer to the airway regulates allergic mucosal sensitization in mice. *Am J Respir Cell Mol Biol* 1999; **21**: 586–96.

77 Nakagome K, Dohi M, Okunishi K, *et al.* In vivo IL-10 gene delivery suppresses airway eosinophilia and hyperreactivity by downregulating APC functions and migration without impairing the antigen-specific systemic immune response in a mouse model of allergic airway inflammation. *J Immunol* 2005; **174**: 6955–66.

78 Cottrez F, Hurst SD, Coffman RL, Groux H. T regulatory cells 1 inhibit a Th2-specific response *in vivo*. *J Immunol* 2000; **165**: 4848–53.

79 Oh JW, Seroogy CM, Meyer EH, *et al.* CD4 T-helper cells engineered to produce IL-10 prevent allergen-induced airway hyperreactivity and inflammation. *J Allergy Clin Immunol* 2002; **110**: 460–8.

80 Akbari O, Freeman GJ, Meyer EH, *et al.* Antigen-specific regulatory T cells develop via the ICOS-ICOS-ligand pathway and inhibit allergen-induced airway hyperreactivity. *Nat Med* 2008; **8**: 1024–32.

81 John M, Lim S, Seybold J, *et al.* Inhaled corticosteroids increase interleukin-10 but reduce macrophage inflammatory protein-1alpha, granulocyte–macrophage colony-stimulating factor, and interferon-gamma release from alveolar macrophages in asthma. *Am J Respir Crit Care Med* 1998; **157**: 256–62.

82 Lim S, Crawley E, Woo P, Barnes PJ. Haplotype associated with low interleukin-10 production in patients with severe asthma. *Lancet* 1998; **352**: 113.

83 Akdis M, Verhagen J, Taylor A, *et al.* Immune responses in healthy and allergic individuals are characterized by a fine balance between allergen-specific T regulatory 1 and T helper 2 cells. *J Exp Med* 2004; **199**: 1567–75.

84 Message SD, Laza-Stanca V, Mallia P, *et al.* Rhinovirus induced lower respiratory illness is increased in asthma and related to virus load and Th1/2 cytokine and IL-10 production. *Proc Natl Acad Sci USA* 2008; **105**: 13562–7.

85 Heaton T, Rowe J, Turner S, *et al.* An immunoepidemiological approach to asthma: identification of in-vitro T-cell response patterns associated with different wheezing phenotypes in children. *Lancet* 2005; **365**: 142–9.

86 Hawrylowicz C, Richards D, Loke TK, Corrigan C, Lee T. A defect in corticosteroid-induced IL-10 production in T lymphocytes from corticosteroid-resistant asthmatic patients. *J Allergy Clin Immunol* 2002; **109**: 369–70.

87 Xystrakis E, Kusumakar S, Boswell S, *et al.* Reversing the defective induction of IL-10-secreting regulatory T cells in glucocorticoid resistant asthma patients. *J Clin Invest* 2006; **116**: 146–55.

88 Akdis CA, Blesken T, Akdis M, Wuthrich B, Blaser K. Role of interleukin 10 in specific immunotherapy. *J Clin Invest* 1998; **102**: 98–106.

89 Chen W, Jin W, Hardegen N, *et al.* Conversion of peripheral CD4⁺CD25- naïve T cells to CD4⁺CD25⁺ regulatory T cells by TGF-beta induction of transcription factor Foxp3. *J Exp Med* 2003; **198**: 1875–86.

90 Shull MM, Ormsby I, Kier AB, *et al.* Targeted disruption of the mouse transforming growth factor-beta 1 gene results in multifocal inflammatory disease. *Nature* 1992; **359**: 693–9.

91 Scherf W, Burdach S, Hansen G. Reduced expression of transforming growth factor beta 1 exacerbates pathology in an experimental asthma model. *Eur J Immunol* 2005; **35**: 198–206.

92 Hansen G, McIntire JJ, Yeung VP, *et al.* CD4(⁺) T helper cells engineered to produce latent TGF-beta1 reverse allergen-induced airway hyperreactivity and inflammation. *J Clin Invest* 2000; **105**: 61–70.

93 Nakao A, Miike S, Hatano M, *et al.* Blockade of transforming growth factor beta/Smad signalling in T cells by overexpression of Smad7 enhances antigen-induced airway inflammation and airway reactivity. *J Exp Med* 2000; **192**: 151–8.

94 Barnes MJ, Powrie F. Regulatory T cells reinforce intestinal homeostasis. *Immunity* 2009; **31**: 401–11.

95 Jutel M, Akdis M, Budak F, *et al.* IL-10 and TGF-beta cooperate in the regulatory T-cell response to mucosal allergens in normal immunity and specific immunotherapy. *Eur J Immunol* 2003; **33**: 1205–14.

96 Larche M, Akdis CA, Valenta R. Immunological mechanisms of allergen-specific immunotherapy. *Nat Rev Immunol* 2006; **6**: 761–71.

97 Makinde T, Murphy RF, antigenrawal DK. The regulatory role of TGF-beta in airway remodelling in asthma. *Immunol Cell Biol* 2007; **85**: 348–56.

98 Szefler SJ. Airway remodelling: therapeutic target or not? *Am J Respir Crit Care Med* 2005; **171**: 672–3.

99 McMillan SJ, Xanthou G, Lloyd CM. Manipulation of allergen-induced airway remodelling by treatment with anti-TGF-β antibody: effect on the Smad signalling pathway. *J Immunol* 2005; **174**: 5774–80.

100 Doherty T, Broide D. Cytokines and growth factors in airway remodelling in asthma. *Curr Opin Immunol* 2007; **19**: 676–80.

101 Torrego A, Hew M, Oates T, Sukkar M, Fan Chung K. Expression and activation of TGF-beta isoforms in acute allergen-induced remodelling in asthma. *Thorax* 2007; **62**: 307–13.

102 Xatzipsalti M, Psarros F, Konstantinou G, *et al.* Modulation of the epithelial inflammatory response to rhinovirus in an atopic environment. *Clin. Exp. Allergy* 2008; **38**: 466–72.

103 Fattouh R, Midence NG, Arias K, *et al.* Transforming growth factor-beta regulates house dust mite-induced allergic airway inflammation but not airway remodelling. *Am J Respir Crit Care Med* 2008; **177**: 593–603.

104 Karagiannidis C, Hense G, Martin C, *et al.* Activin A is an acute allergen-responsive cytokine and provides a link to TGF-beta-mediated airway remodelling in asthma. *J Allergy Clin Immunol* 2006; **117**: 111–18.

105 Semitekolou M, Alissafi T, antigengelakopoulou M, *et al.* Activin-A induces regulatory T cells that suppress T helper cell immune responses and protect from allergic airway disease. *J Exp Med* 2009; **206**: 1769–85.

106 Kariyawasam HH, Xanthou G, Barkans J, Aizen M, Kay AB, Robinson DS. Basal expression of bone morphogenetic protein receptor is reduced in mild asthma. *Am J Respir Crit Care Med* 2008; **177**: 1074–81.

107 Bacchetta R, Passerini L, Gambineri E, *et al.* Defective regulatory and effector T cell functions in patients with FOXP3 mutations. *J Clin Invest* 2006; **116**: 1713–22.

108 Zheng Y, Rudensky AY. Foxp3 in control of the regulatory T cell lineage. *Nat Immunol* 2007; **8**: 457–62.

109 Torgerson TR, Ochs HD. Immune dysregulation, polyendocrinopathy, enteropathy, X-linked: forkhead box protein 3 mutations and lack of regulatory T cells. *J Allergy Clin Immunol* 2007; **120**: 744–50.

110 Chatila TA, Blaeser F, Ho N, *et al.* JM2: encoding a fork head-related protein, is mutated in X-linked autoimmunity-allergic dysregulation syndrome. *J Clin Invest* 2000; **106**: R75–R81.

111 Rao A, Kamani N, Filipovich A, *et al.* Successful bone marrow transplantation for IPEX syndrome after reduced-intensity conditioning. *Blood* 2007; **109**: 383–5.

112 Seidel MG, Fritsch G, Lion T, *et al.* Selective engraftment of donor CD4+25high FOXP3-positive T cells in IPEX syndrome after nonmyeloablative hematopoietic stem cell transplantation. *Blood* 2009; **113**: 5689–91.

113 Lin W, Truong N, Grossman WJ, *et al.* Allergic dysregulation and hyperimmunoglobulinemia E in Foxp3 mutant mice. *J Allergy Clin Immunol* 2005; **116**: 1106–15.

114 Gambineri E, Torgerson TR, Ochs HD. Immune dysregulation, polyendocrinopathy, enteropathy, and X-linked inheritance (IPEX), a syndrome of systemic autoimmunity caused by mutations of FOXP3: a critical regulator of T-cell homeostasis. *Curr Opin Rheumatol* 2003; **15**: 430–5.

115 Caudy AA, Reddy ST, Chatila T, Atkinson JP, Verbsky JW. CD25 deficiency causes an immune dysregulation, polyendocrinopathy, enteropathy, X-linked-like syndrome, and defective IL-10 expression from CD4 lymphocytes. *J Allergy Clin Immunol* 2007; **119**: 482–7.

116 Akdis M, Blaser K, Akdis CA. T regulatory cells in allergy: novel concepts in the pathogenesis, prevention, and treatment of allergic diseases. *J Allergy Clin Immunol* 2005; **116**: 961–8.

117 Ling EM, Smith T, Nguyen XD, *et al.* Relation of CD4+CD25+ regulatory T-cell suppression of allergen-driven T-cell activation to atopic status and expression of allergic disease. *Lancet* 2004; **363**: 608–15.

118 Bellinghausen I, Klostermann B, Knop J, Saloga J. Human CD4CD25 T cells derived from the majority of atopic donors are able to suppress Th1 and Th2 cytokine production. *J Allergy Clin Immunol* 2003; **111**: 862–8.

119 Karlsson MR, Rugtveit J, Brandtzaeg P. Allergen-responsive CD4+CD25+ regulatory T cells in children who have outgrown cow's milk allergy. *J Exp Med* 2004; **199**: 1679–88.

120 Hartl D, Koller B, Mehlhorn AT, *et al.* Quantitative and functional impairment of pulmonary CD4+CD25hi regulatory T cells in paediatric asthma. *J Allergy Clin Immunol* 2007; **119**: 1258–66.

121 Lee JH, Yu HH, Wang LC, Yang YH, Lin YT, Chiang BL. The levels of CD4$^+$CD25$^+$ regulatory T cells in paediatric patients with allergic rhinitis and bronchial asthma. *Clin. Exp. Immunol* 2007; **148**: 53–63.

122 Shi HZ, Li S, Xie ZF, Qin XJ, Qin X, Zhong XN. Regulatory CD4$^+$CD25$^+$ T lymphocytes in peripheral blood from patients with atopic asthma. *Clin Immunol* 2004; **113**: 172–8.

123 Lin YL, Shieh CC, Wang JY. The functional insufficiency of human CD4$^+$CD25 high T-regulatory cells in allergic asthma is subject to TNF-alpha modulation. *Allergy* 2008; **63**: 67–74.

124 Zhang Q, Qian FH, Liu H, *et al*. Expression of surface markers on peripheral CD4$^+$CD25high T cells in patients with atopic asthma: role of inhaled corticosteroid. *Chin Med J (Engl)* 2008; **121**: 205–12.

125 Moniuszko M, Kowal K, Zukowski S, Dabrowska M, Bodzenta-Lukaszyk A. Frequencies of circulating CD4$^+$CD25$^+$CD127 low cells in atopics are altered by bronchial allergen challenge. *Eur. J Clin Invest* 2008; **38**: 201–4.

126 Heier I, Malmstrom K, Pelkonen AS, *et al*. Bronchial response pattern of antigen presenting cells and regulatory T cells in children less than 2 years of age. *Thorax* 2008; **63**: 703–9.

127 Grindebacke H, Wing K, Andersson AC, Suri-Payer E, Rak S, Rudin A. Defective suppression of Th2 cytokines by CD4CD25 regulatory T cells in birch allergics during birch pollen season. *Clin Exp Allergy* 2004; **34**: 1364–72.

128 Berry MA, Hargadon B, Shelley M, *et al*. Evidence of a role of tumour necrosis factor alpha in refractory asthma. *N Engl J Med* 2006; **354**: 697–708.

129 Morjaria JB, Chauhan AJ, Babu KS, Polosa R, Davies DE, Holgate ST. The role of a soluble TNF alpha receptor fusion protein (etanercept) in corticosteroid refractory asthma: a double blind, randomised, placebo controlled trial. *Thorax* 2008; **63**: 584–91.

130 Doganci A, Eigenbrod T, Krug N, *et al*. The IL-6R alpha chain controls lung CD4$^+$CD25$^+$ Treg development and function during allergic airway inflammation *in vivo*. *J Clin Invest* 2005; **115**: 313–25.

131 Haddeland U, Karstensen AB, Farkas L, *et al*. Putative regulatory T cells are impaired in cord blood from neonates with hereditary allergy risk. *Pediatr Allergy Immunol* 2005; **16**: 104–12.

132 Smith M, Tourigny MR, Noakes P, Thornton CA, Tulic MK, Prescott SL. Children with egg allergy have evidence of reduced neonatal CD4($^+$)CD25($^+$)CD127(lo/$^-$) regulatory T cell function. *J Allergy Clin Immunol* 2008; **121**: 1460–6.

133 Bach JF. The effect of infections on susceptibility to autoimmune and allergic diseases. *N Engl J Med* 2002; **347**: 911–20.

134 Martinez FD, Wright AL, Taussig LM, Holberg CJ, Halonen M, Morgan WJ. Asthma and wheezing in the first six years of life. The Group Health Medical Associates. *N Engl J Med* 1995; **332**: 133–8.

135 Sly PD, Boner AL, Bjorksten B, *et al*. Early identification of atopy in the prediction of persistent asthma in children. *Lancet* 2008; **372**: 1100–6.

136 Morgan WJ, Stern DA, Sherrill DL, *et al*. Outcome of asthma and wheezing in the first 6 years of life: follow-up through adolescence. *Am J Respir Crit Care Med* 2005; **172**: 1253–8.

137 Ege MJ, Bieli C, Frei R, *et al*. Prenatal farm exposure is related to the expression of receptors of the innate immunity and to atopic sensitization in school-age children. *J Allergy Clin Immunol* 2006; **117**: 817–23.

138 Schaub B, Liu J, Hoppler S, *et al*. Impairment of T-regulatory cells in cord blood of atopic mothers. *J Allergy Clin Immunol* 2008; **121**: 1491–9.

139 Gerhold K, Avagyan A, Seib C, *et al*. Prenatal initiation of endotoxin airway exposure prevents subsequent allergen-induced sensitization and airway inflammation in mice. *J Allergy Clin Immunol* 2006; **118**: 666–73.

140 Polte T, Hennig C, Hansen G. Allergy prevention starts before conception: maternofoetal transfer of tolerance protects against the development of asthma. *J Allergy Clin Immunol* 2008; **122**: 1022–30.

141 Hollingsworth JW, Maruoka S, Boon K, *et al*. In utero supplementation with methyl donors enhances allergic airway disease in mice. *J Clin Invest* 2008; **118**: 3462–9.

142 Miller RL. Prenatal maternal diet affects asthma risk in offspring. *J Clin Invest* 2008; **118**: 3265–8.

143 Litonjua AA, Weiss ST. Is vitamin D deficiency to blame for the asthma epidemic? *J Allergy Clin Immunol* 2007; **120**: 1031–5.

144 Willers SM, Wijga AH, Brunekreef B, *et al*. Maternal food consumption during pregnancy and the longitudinal development of childhood asthma. *Am J Respir Crit Care Med* 2008; **178**: 124–31.

145 Penna G, Roncari A, Amuchastegui S, *et al*. Expression of the inhibitory receptor ILT3 on dendritic cells is dispensable for induction of CD4$^+$Foxp3$^+$ regulatory T cells by 1,25-dihydroxyvitamin D3. *Blood* 2005; **106**: 3490–7.

146 Adorini L, Penna G. Control of autoimmune diseases by the vitamin D endocrine system. *Nat Clin Pract Rheumatol* 2008; **4**: 404–12.

147 Moller C, Dreborg S, Ferdousi HA, *et al*. Pollen immunotherapy reduces the development of asthma in children with seasonal rhinoconjunctivitis (the PAT-study). *J Allergy Clin Immunol* 2002; **109**: 251–6.

148 Akdis M, Akdis CA. Mechanisms of allergen-specific immunotherapy. *J Allergy Clin Immunol* 2007; **119**: 780–91.

149 Pereira-Santos MC, Baptista AP, Melo A, *et al.* Expansion of circulating Foxp(3+)D25bright CD4+ T cells during specific venom immunotherapy. *Clin Exp Allergy* **38**: 291–7.

150 Radulovic S, Jacobson MR, Durham SR, Nouri-Aria KT. Grass pollen immunotherapy induces Foxp3-expressing CD4+ CD25+ cells in the nasal mucosa. *J Allergy Clin Immunol* 2008; **121**: 146772.

151 Stelmach I, Jerzynska J, Kuna P. A randomized, double-blind trial of the effect of glucocorticoid, antileukotriene and beta-agonist treatment on IL-10 serum levels in children with asthma. *Clin Exp Allergy* 2002; **32**: 264–9.

152 Karagiannidis C, Akdis M, Holopainen P, *et al.* Glucocorticoids upregulate FOXP3 expression and regulatory T cells in asthma. *J Allergy Clin Immunol* 2004; **114**: 1425–33.

153 Peek EJ, Richards DF, Faith A, *et al.* Interleukin-10-secreting "regulatory" T cells induced by glucocorticoids and beta2-agonists. *Am J Respir Cell Mol Biol* 2005; **33**: 105–11.

154 Holick MF. Vitamin D deficiency. *N Engl J Med* 2007; **357**: 266–81.

155 Adams JS, Hewison M. Unexpected actions of vitamin D: new perspectives on the regulation of innate and adaptive *Immunity Nat Clin Pract Endocrinol Metab* 2008; **4**: 80–90.

156 Mills KH. Regulatory T cells: friend or foe in immunity to infection? *Nat Rev Immunol* 2004; **4**: 841–55.

157 Kalliomaki M, Isolauri E. Role of intestinal flora in the development of allergy. *Curr Opin Allergy Clin Immunol* 2003; **3**: 15–20.

5

A role for natural killer T-cell subsets in the pathogenesis of various allergic disorders

Hiroshi Watarai,[1] *Michishige Harada,*[1,2] *Mayumi Tamari,*[2] *and Masaru Taniguchi*[1]

[1]RIKEN Research Center for Allergy and Immunology, Suehiro-cho, Tsurumi-ku, Yokohama, Kanagawa, Japan

[2]Center for Genome Medicine, Suehiro-cho, Tsurumi-ku, Yokohama, Kanagawa, Japan

Introduction

NKT cell function bridging innate and acquired immunity

Natural killer T (NKT) cells are characterized by a highly conserved single variant T-cell receptor (TCR) α chain that consists of Vα14Jα18 in mice [1] and Vα24Jα18 in humans [2,3], and is associated with a restricted set of Vβ chains (Vβ8, Vβ7, and Vβ2 in mice and Vβ11 in humans). In addition, NKT cells appear to be autoreactive and, as a result, are persistently activated by endogenous glycolipid ligands presented by the monomorphic major histocompatibility complex (MHC) class I-like molecule, CD1d [4]. Another characteristic feature of NKT cells is their promiscuous production of T helper cell (Th)1, Th2, and Th17 cytokines [5–7]. Their recognition of self ligands leads to the accumulation of cytokine mRNAs and upregulation of activation markers, indicating that NKT cells in steady-state are already primed and ready to quickly mediate their effector functions to serve as a bridge between innate and acquired immunity [1]. However, their recognition of endogenous ligands does not elicit any cytokine production, only transcript accumulation, because NKT cells require additional signals to produce cytokines mediating their functions.

The second signal is the key event that determines NKT cell function. A single *in vivo* injection of α-galactosylceramide (α-GalCer), a synthetic exogenous glycolipid ligand for NKT cells presented by CD1d [8], induces a burst of interleukin 12 (IL-12) production by dendiritic cells (DCs) followed by Th1 cytokine interferon gamma (IFN-γ) production by NKT cells [9,10]. The NKT cells together with IL-12 from DCs mediate strong adjuvant effects on innate and acquired immunity through the NKT cell production of IFN-γ [11], leading to the subsequent activation and expansion of NK cells, neutrophils, DCs, and macrophages in the innate system, and CD4[+] Th1 or CD8[+] T cells in the acquired immune system.

In contrast to the IL-12-initiated NKT cell-mediated protective function, NKT cells can also become regulatory-type cells producing IL-10, which mediates regulatory responses. This occurs in the absence of IL-12 when the NKT cells interact with marginal zone B220[+] B cells or regulatory DCs (DCregs), both of which mainly produce IL-10 but no IL-12 [12]. These regulatory NKT cells then induce naïve DCs to become DCregs characterized by the production of IL-10, which in turn induces antigen-specific IL-10 producing regulatory CD4[+] T cells (Tr1) in the presence of antigen, thereby suppressing antigen-specific immune responses.

Inflammation and Allergy Drug Design, First Edition. Edited by Kenji Izuhara, Stephen T. Holgate, Marsha Wills-Karp.
© 2011 Blackwell Publishing Ltd. Published 2011 by Blackwell Publishing Ltd.

Newly identified NKT cell subsets associated with various disease conditions

Various pathologic conditions are controlled by NKT cells, including asthma [13]. Numerous studies have been performed to identify distinct functional subsets of NKT cells, and three such subsets have now been proposed in relation to disease pathogenesis: (i) IL-17 receptor B-positive (IL-17RB$^+$) NKT cell subset producing mainly IL-13 in response to IL-25, which has a crucial role in the pathogenesis of airway hypersensitivity reaction (AHR) or asthma [14,15]; (ii) retinoic acid receptor-related orphan receptor (ROR)γt$^+$ NKT cells within the NK1.1$^-$ CD4$^-$ subset that induce autoimmune disorders by their production of IL-17 and IL-22 [7,16]; and (iii) CD4$^-$ NKT cells which are involved in chronic obstructive pulmonary disease (COPD) after respiratory viral infection [17]. It should be noted that distinct subsets of NKT cells are involved in different pathogenic conditions in the presence and absence of acquired immunity (see below).

IL-17RB$^+$ NKT cells

IL-17RB$^+$ NKT cells induce AHR in response to IL-25

Although NKT cells were shown to be divided into CD4$^+$ and CD4$^-$CD8$^-$ double negative (DN) populations, the former produce larger amounts of Th2 cytokines such as IL-4 and IL-13, and the latter predominantly mediate antitumor immunity by their production of cytotoxic molecules, such as killer receptors, perforin, and granzyme. CD4$^+$ NKT cells in mainly Balb/c mice were further divided into two groups based on their expression of IL-17RB [14]. It is interesting to note that IL-17RB expression was detected only on a fraction (~approximately one-third) of CD4$^+$ NKT cells in the lung, spleen, and thymus, but not on other cell types including B cells, $\alpha\beta$ T cells, $\gamma\delta$ T cells, DCs, mast cells, eosinophils, or neutrophils. The IL-17RB$^+$ NKT cells expressed lower levels of Th1-related transcripts, such as IFN-γ, T-bet, STAT4, IL-12RB2 and IL-18RB, while expressing higher levels of Th2-related transcripts such as IL-4 and CCR4. These cells also lacked the transcripts

that encode cytotoxicity molecules such as granzyme, perforin, and killer receptors [14]. Furthermore, the levels of IL-17A and RORγt transcripts in IL-17RB$^+$ NKT cells were lower than in the DN NKT cell subset [14]. These results clearly indicate that IL-17RB$^+$ NKT cells are Th2-type NKT cells, but are distinct from other NKT subtypes. In fact, in response to IL-25 (also known as IL-17E), a ligand for IL-17RB, IL-17RB$^+$ NKT, but not other NKT subtypes, are activated to produce mainly IL-13 and modest amounts of IL-4, and barely produce IFN-γ and IL-17A. They do not produce other cytokines, such as IL-5 and IL-10, but produce Th2 chemokines (CCL17, CCL22) for recruitment of Th2 cells, chitinases that are important for eosinophil recruitment [14].

IL-25, a member of the IL-17 cytokine family, has recently been reported to be expressed in activated lung epithelial cells and to induce Th2-type immune responses, including increased serum immunoglobulin E (IgE) levels, blood eosinophilia, and pathologic changes in the lung and other tissues [18–20], thus demonstrating a pivotal role of IL-25 as a mediator of Th2 responses [18,21]. Consistent with the existence of IL-17RB$^+$ NKT cells in a higher proportion among the total NKT cells in the lung, IL-17RB$^+$ NKT cells are required for the development of AHR induced by IL-25 and a suboptimal dose of ovalbumin (OVA) antigen [14]. This was clearly shown in the studies using NKT cell-deficient Jα18$^{-/-}$ mice, which, unlike control Balb/c mice, failed to develop significant AHR, eosinophil infiltration, and histologic changes in the lung, even after treatment with IL-25.

Significantly large amounts of IL-13 and IL-5 were detected in the bronchoalveolar (BAL) fluid of IL-25-treated wild-type, but not of Jα18$^{-/-}$, mice and controls [14]. The locally produced IL-13 plays a crucial role, not only in the recruitment and activation of macrophages but also in airway remodeling by direct activation of smooth muscle cells. Even though IL-17RB$^+$ NKT cells did not produce IL-5 upon IL-25 stimulation *in vitro*, they produced a set of chitinases important for recruitment of eosinophils, which do produce IL-5. These results strongly suggest that IL-25 directly acts on IL-17RB$^+$ NKT cells, recruits effector cell types, and induces AHR.

In addition, the transfer of IL-17RB$^+$ NKT cells, but not IL-17RB$^-$ NKT cells, into Jα18$^{-/-}$ mice restored AHR induced by OVA/IL-25, and the severity of the AHR depended on the number of IL-17RB+ NKT cells transferred. Together, these findings indicate that IL-17RB+ NKT cells have a crucial role in the development of IL-25-dependent AHR, which is mainly mediated by IL-13 and IL-5 [14].

IL-17RB+ NKT cells as a potential target for allergy and asthma therapy

Although antigen-specific Th2 cells and eosinophils are believed to have a central role in many of the pathologic features of allergic asthma [22,23], they are not always essential [24]. Elimination of Th2 cells, eosinophils, and their cytokines, for example by treatment with anti-IL-4, anti-IL-5 antibodies, or IL-13/IL-4 antagonists, has not reduced AHR in numerous clinical trials for asthma [25,26], suggesting that other immunologic factors may critically regulate asthma symptoms.

In one model of allergic asthma, IL-25-induced allergic airway inflammation as well as AHR [21,27] and, conversely, administration of an IL-25-blocking antibody [28] or use of IL-25-deficient mice [29] eliminated these Th2 responses. IL-25 has also been detected in lung biopsy samples from patients with asthma and reported to induce inflammatory cytokine and chemokine production by human lung fibroblasts as well as extracellular matrix components by airway smooth muscle cells [30]. Taken together, these observations suggest that IL-17RB+ NKT cells are the target of IL-25 in the development of AHR or asthma. The efficacy with which IL-17RB antibodies prevent AHR and reduce Th2 cytokine-induced inflammation *in vivo* suggests that IL-25 and IL-17RB are ideal therapeutic targets for asthma.

IL-17RB polymorphisms are associated with corticosteroid-resistance in childhood asthma

Based on our finding that IL-17RB+ NKT cells respond to IL-25 and contribute to AHR [14] and that IL-25 and IL-17RB transcripts have been shown to be elevated in asthmatic lung tissues [30], we conducted an association study of human IL-17RB as a candidate gene for bronchial asthma. Linkage disequilibrium (LD) was measured by coefficient r^2 among the 16 single nucleotide polymorphisms (SNPs) with a minor allele frequency greater than 10% (Figure 5.1A). Eight SNPs were finally selected as tag SNPs

representing each haplotype, and patients and controls were genotyped for association studies. We found no significant association between childhood asthma susceptibility and IL-17RB polymorphisms (Figure 5.1A).

We further compared allele frequencies of the eight SNPs among patients who had received inhaled corticosteroids in patients with childhood asthma. We divided the subjects into two groups based on the therapeutic dose of inhaled corticosteroid, beclomethasone dipropionate (BDP) ≤ 600 mg/day versus ≥ 800 mg/day. We found a strong association between the rs3017 (C > T) genotype and the therapeutic dose of inhaled corticosteroid in patients with childhood asthma (Figure 5.1B). The rs3017T allele was more frequent in patients with childhood asthma who required a high dose of inhaled corticosteroid (BDP ≥ 800 mg/day) to control their symptoms (dominant model: $P = 0.00060$, odds ratio 3.66; 95% confidence interval 1.71–7.84; allelic model: $P = 0.00015$, odds ratio 2.47, 95% confidence interval 1.54–3.94). Analysis using TRANSFAC® Professional 10.3 (BIOBASE, GmbH, Germany: http://www.biobase-international.com/) allowed us to predict a potential allelic difference in *cis*-acting transcriptional regulatory function (Figure 5.1C). The putative binding site of the transcription factor peroxisome proliferator-activated receptor (PPAR), which is known to be a target for chronic inflammatory lung diseases [31], is present in the 3′UTR SNP (rs3017) of the IL-17RB gene. The affinity of PPARs may differ between rs3017T and the related variant rs3017C; the rs3017T allele potentially decreases the binding affinity for PPARs. Since the activation of PPARs downregulates proinflammatory gene expression and inflammatory cell functions [31], the high-affinity binding of PPARs to the putative binding site in the 3′UTR of IL-17RB gene might lead to the downmodulation of IL-17RB transcription in the protective C allele. Mechanisms of corticosteroid-resistant (CR) asthma remain unclear, but this is an intriguing clue. Although replication of this finding in other larger samples is needed, these preliminary data indicate that IL-17RB may be involved in the chronic inflammatory lung diseases, including steroid resistance of childhood asthma through genetic polymorphisms altering the affinity for PPARs. Thus, the IL-17RB signaling pathway may play a key role in some forms of childhood asthma.

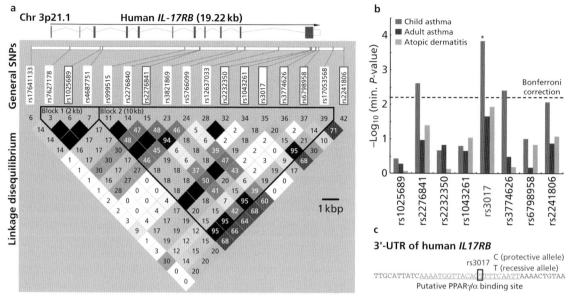

Figure 5.1 Association of IL-17RB polymorphisms with corticosteroid resistance in childhood asthma. (A) Pairwise linkage disequilibrium map of the human IL-17RB region. Linkage disequilibrium (LD) between 16 single nucleotide polymorphisms (SNPs) as measured by R^2 by using the Haploview 4.1 program (Massachusetts Institute of Technology, Cambridge, MA: http://www.broad.mit.edu/mpg/haploview/). The eight boxed polymorphisms were selected as tag SNPs among 16 SNPs in this study. The coefficient R^2 is calculated by the following formula; $R^2 = (PacPbd – PadPbc)2/PaPbPcPd$. (B) The association study of the *IL-17RB* gene with corticoid resistance in childhood asthma. SNPs in the red box in (A) were further analyzed. Differences in genotype frequencies of the polymorphisms between case and control subjects were compared by the Cochran–Armitage trend test. We applied the Bonferroni corrections, which is a statistical analysis for the multiple comparisons to adjust the P-values by the numbers (8) of tag SNPs. Dotted bars indicate statistically significant P-values after Bonferroni adjustment. The asterisk (*) indicates a significant difference. (C) Prediction of a potential allelic difference in cis-acting transcriptional regulatory function in rs3017C/T allele. TRANSFAC® Professional 10.3 was used for analysis. The putative PPARγ/α binding site in the 3′ untranslated region (UTR) of human *IL-17RB* gene was underlined.

Involvement of other NKT cell subsets in disease pathogenesis

IL-17A-producing NKT cells induce airway neutropilia

A requirement for IL-17A-producing NKT cells has also been shown in a model of asthma induced by ozone, a major component of air pollution. Mice repeatedly exposed to ozone developed severe AHR and airway inflammation accompanied by infiltration of neutrophils and macrophages [32]. Importantly, both Jα18$^{-/-}$ and IL-17A$^{-/-}$ mice, but not conventional CD4$^+$ T-cell-deficient MHC class II$^{-/-}$ mice, failed to develop ozone-induced AHR, indicating that IL-17A-producing NKT cells rather than Th17 cells are required for the development of this disease [32].

Ozone-induced, but not allergen-induced, AHR requires IL-17A produced from NKT cells [32]. This dichotomy suggests that ozone-induced or allergen-induced AHR requires distinct subsets of NKT cells that produce different sets of cytokines, which may account for the different inflammatory cell types recruited. Indeed, ozone-induced AHR is associated with neutrophils and IL-17A, whereas allergen-induced AHR is associated with eosinophils and primarily with IL-13 and IL-4, but not IL-17A. Of note, further studies are required to elucidate whether IL-17RB$^+$ NKT cells are also involved in the IL-17A production and play a crucial role in the AHR, which is independent of or in complete absence of Th2 cells and adaptive immunity. Nevertheless, IL-17A inhalation resulted in the induction of neutrophilia rather than eosinophilia in the lungs [33,34] and thus represents a unique target for effective asthma therapy.

NKT cell-macrophage immune axis in the chronic phase after viral infection

Acute infections with viruses, such as respiratory syncytial virus, Sendai virus, metapneumovirus, and parainfluenza virus, precipitate chronic pulmonary diseases that lead to asthma [35–37]. These viruses cause childhood asthma and COPD-like symptoms, which include AHR, airway inflammation, and mucus hypersecretion. However, it has long been difficult to understand how such symptoms develop even after the apparent clearance of viruses. Kim *et al.* [17] developed a mouse model of infection with parainfluenza virus or Sendai virus, in which chronic viral inflammation developed airway hypersensitivity reaction resembling human asthma and COPD. Surprisingly, the chronic pulmonary symptoms evolved independently of CD4 T cells but required CD4$^-$ NKT cells and did not occur in CD1d$^{-/-}$ and Jα18$^{-/-}$ mice. In this model, the NKT cells alternatively activated macrophages, which produced IL-13, which in turn drove increased mucus production and AHR. As the virus-induced AHR response occurred in MHC class II$^{-/-}$ mice, CD4 T cells are not required for the development of this type of AHR. These findings provide new insight into the pathogenesis of virus-induced inflammatory airways diseases and demonstrate the requirement for a novel subset of IL-13-producing CD4$^-$ NKT cells that drive chronic inflammatory lung disease by inducing alternatively activated IL-13-producing macrophages in the lung. Ultimately, it will be important to define how additional immune pathways respond to viral infection and how they interact with the NKT–macrophage pathway to provide a comprehensive model for chronic inflammatory disease after infection in order to be able to correct these abnormalities. It is possible to define the CD4$^-$ NKT cells in the chronic phase as functionally equivalent to the IL-17RB$^+$ NKT cells in the steady-state or acute phase based on their similarity of robust IL-13 production. However, the precursor pool of IL-13-producing CD4$^-$ NKT cells in the chronic phase remaining to be further characterized.

Our new understanding of the pathogenic role of NKT cells in chronic respiratory diseases [17] leads to a model distinct from previous models for the immunopathology of asthma and COPD. It is now clear that NKT cells are involved not only in the acute phase of respiratory viral infection by bridging innate and acquired immunity, but also in the chronic phase by producing IL-13 to stimulate macrophages. IL-13 drives a positive feedback loop to amplify IL-13 production from alternatively activated macrophages, resulting in sustained inflammation, stimulation of goblet cell metaplasia, and activation of mucus-producing cells.

Other cytokines as a second signal that activate NKT cells

The innate immune system is characterized by its ability to recognize pathogen products from bacteria, viruses, and fungi using a group of pattern recognition receptors (PRRs) such as Toll-like receptors (TLRs) [38] and Nod-like receptors (NLRs) [39], which trigger the first line of host defense. The pathogens are detected by PRRs and activate DCs and epithelial cells, leading to the production of cytokines such as IL-12 (DCs) and IL-25 (epithelial cells). Because NKT cells, but not T or NK cells, are continuously activated by endogenous ligands, they do express IL-12R or IL-17RB, even under normal physiologic conditions. Therefore, these cytokines initially produced by DCs or epithelial cells primarily act on NKT cells, such as IL-12 to enhance NKT cell production of IFN-γ [40], and IL-25 for NKT cell production of IL-13 and IL-4 [14], thereby eliciting effective NKT cell-mediated immunity.

IL-33, a new IL-1 family member, is constitutively expressed by epithelial cells and endothelial cells and is also reported to affect NKT cells [41,42]. The receptor for IL-33, ST2, is expressed on NKT cells and Th2 cells [43,44]. Although NKT cells do not directly respond to IL-33 alone, the cells produce both Th1 and Th2 cytokines upon stimulation with IL-33 synergized with α-GalCer or IL-12 *in vitro* [43]. Although intranasal administration of IL-33 into mice induces AHR and goblet cell hyperplasia [45], the precise mechanism of NKT cell involvement is totally unclear, particularly because this response could occur even in the absence of T, B, and NKT cells (i.e., RAG$^{-/-}$ mice) and may involve the direct activation of basophils and mast cells [43,45].

Thymic stromal lymphopoietin (TSLP) is an epithelial cell-derived cytokine that can strongly activate DCs [46], providing important evidence that the epithelial barrier can trigger allergic diseases by the induction and maintenance of Th2 responses [47]. In fact, TSLP transgenic mice developed massive infiltration of leukocytes, goblet cell hyperplasia, and subepithelial fibrosis [48]. NKT cells also express the TSLP receptor and respond to TSLP by preferentially increasing the production of IL-13 but not IFN-γ or IL-4 [49]. TSLP transgenic mice that lack NKT cells fail to develop AHR, supporting the notion that TSLP promotes AHR development through NKT-cell activation [49].

Future prospects

The studies described above indicate that AHR can be induced by allergens, air pollution (ozone), and viral infection, suggesting that NKT cells may provide a common disease mechanism for many different forms of airway inflammation, occurring even in the absence of acquired immune system. Moreover, these studies indicate that distinct subsets of NKT cells are involved in different forms of asthma. Although CD4$^+$ IL-17RB$^+$ NKT cells in concert with antigen-specific Th2 cells are crucial for allergen-induced AHR CD4$^-$ IL-17-producing NKT cells have a major role in ozone-induced AHR and CD4$^-$ NKT cells are involved in respiratory virus-induced AHR. It still remains to be elucidated how various NKT cell subtypes develop and are regulated, and how pulmonary NKT cells are activated and exert their functions.

Acknowledgment

We thank Professor Peter Burrows, University of Alabama at Birmingham, Alabama, USA, for his critical reading and editing of this manuscript.

References

1 Taniguchi M, Harada M, Kojo S, *et al.* The regulatory role of Valpha14 NKT cells in innate and acquired immune response. *Annu Rev Immunol* 2003; **21**: 483–513.

2 Lantz O, Bendelac A. An invariant T cell receptor alpha chain is used by a unique subset of major histocompatibility complex class I-specific CD4$^+$ and CD4–8$^-$ T cells in mice and humans. *J Exp Med* 1994; **180**: 1097–106.

3 Exley M, Garcia J, Balk SP, *et al.* Requirements for CD1d recognition by human invariant Va24$^+$CD4$^-$CD8$^-$ T cells. *J Exp Med* 1997; **186**: 109–20.

4 Bendelac A, Lantz O, Quimby ME, *et al.* CD1 recognition by mouse NK1$^+$ T lymphocytes. *Science* 1995; **268**: 863–5.

5 Bendelac A, Savage PB, Teyton L. The biology of NKT cells. *Annu Rev Immunol* 2007; **25**: 297–336.

6 Taniguchi M, Seino K, Nakayama T. The NKT cell system: bridging innate and acquired *Immunity Nat Immunol* 2003; **4**: 1164–5.

7 Michel ML, Keller AC, Paget C, *et al.* Identification of an IL-17-producing NK1.1^{neg} iNKT cell population involved in airway neutrophilia. *J Exp Med* 2007; **204**: 995–1001.

8 Kawano T, Cui J, Koezuka Y, *et al.* Requirement for Valpha14 NKT cells in IL-12-mediated rejection of tumors. *Science* 1997; **278**: 1626–9.

9 Tomura M, Yu WG, Ahn HJ, *et al.* A novel function of Vα14$^+$CD4$^+$ NKT cells: stimulation of IL-12 production by antigen-presenting cells in the innate immune system. *J Immunol* 1999; **163**: 93–101.

10 Kitamura H, Iwakabe K, Yahata T, *et al.* The natural killer T (NKT) cell ligand alpha-galactosylceramide demonstrates its immunopotentiating effect by inducing interleukin (IL)–12 production by dendritic cells and IL-12 receptor expression on NKT cells. *J Exp Med* 1999; **189**: 1121–8.

11 Fujii S, Shimizu K, Hemmi H, *et al.* Innate Vα14$^+$ natural killer T cells mature dendritic cells, leading to strong adaptive *Immunity Immunol Rev* 2007; **220**: 183–98.

12 Kojo S, Seino K, Harada M, *et al.* Induction of regulatory properties in dendritic cells by Vα14 NKT cells. *J Immunol* 2005;**175**: 3648–55.

13 Umetsu DT, DeKruyff RH. A role for natural killer T cells in asthma. *Nat Rev Immunol* 2006; **6**: 953–8.

14 Terashima A, Watarai H, Inoue S, *et al.* A novel subset of mouse NKT cells bearing the IL-17 receptor B responds to IL-25 and contributes to airway hyperreactivity. *J Exp Med* 2008; **205**: 2727–33.

15 Stock P, Lombardi V, Kohlrautz V, *et al.* Induction of airway hyperreactivity by IL-25 is dependent on a subset of invariant NKT cells expressing IL-17RB. *J Immunol* 2009; **182**: 5116–22.

16 Coquet JM, Chakravarti S, Kyparissoudis K, *et al.* Diverse cytokine production by NKT cell subsets and identification of an IL-17-producing CD4$^-$NK1.1$^-$ NKT cell population. *Proc Natl Acad Sci USA* 2008; **105**: 11287–92.

17 Kim EY, Battaile JT, Patel AC, et al. Persistent activation of an innate immune response translates respiratory viral infection into chronic lung disease. Nat Med 2008; 14: 633–40.

18 Fort MM, Cheung J, Yen D, et al. IL-25 induces IL-4: IL-5: and IL-13 and Th2-associated pathologies in vivo. Immunity 2001; 15: 985–95.

19 Pan G, French D, Mao W, et al. Forced expression of murine IL-17E induces growth retardation, jaundice, a Th2-biased response, and multiorgan inflammation in mice. J Immunol 2001; 167: 6559–67.

20 Kim MR, Manoukian R, Yeh R, et al. Transgenic overexpression of human IL-17E results in eosinophilia, B-lymphocyte hyperplasia, and altered antibody production. Blood 2002; 100: 2330–40.

21 Tamachi T, Maezawa Y, Ikeda K, et al. IL-25 enhances allergic airway inflammation by amplifying a Th2 cell-dependent pathway in mice. J Allergy Clin Immunol 2006; 118: 606–14.

22 Robinson DS, Hamid Q, Ying S, et al. Predominant TH2-like bronchoalveolar T-lymphocyte population in atopic asthma. N Engl J Med 1992; 326: 298–304.

23 Cohn L, Elias JA, Chupp GL. Asthma: mechanisms of disease persistence and progression. Annu Rev Immunol 2004; 22: 789–815.

24 Anderson GP. Endotyping asthma: new insights into key pathogenic mechanisms in a complex, heterogeneous disease. Lancet 2008; 372: 1107–19.

25 Leckie MJ, ten Brinke A, Khan J, et al. Effects of an interleukin-5 blocking monoclonal antibody on eosinophils, airway hyperresponsiveness, and the late asthmatic response. Lancet 2000;356: 2144–8.

26 Wenzel S, Wilbraham D, Fuller R, et al. Effect of an interleukin-4 variant on late phase asthmatic response to allergen challenge in asthmatic patients: results of two phase 2a studies. Lancet 2007; 370: 1422–31.

27 Angkasekwinai P, Park H, Wang YH, et al. Interleukin 25 promotes the initiation of proallergic type 2 responses. J Exp Med 2007; 204: 1509–17.

28 Ballantyne SJ, Barlow JL, Jolin HE, et al. Blocking IL-25 prevents airway hyperresponsiveness in allergic asthma. J Allergy Clin Immunol 2007; 120: 1324–31.

29 Fallon PG, Ballantyne SJ, Mangan NE, et al. Identification of an interleukin (IL)–25-dependent cell population that provides IL-4: IL-5: and IL-13 at the onset of helminth expulsion. J Exp Med 2006; 203: 1105–16.

30 Létuvé S, Lajoie-Kadoch S, Audusseau S, et al. IL-17E upregulates the expression of proinflammatory cytokines in lung fibroblasts. J Allergy Clin Immunol 2006; 117: 590–6.

31 Belvisi MG, Mitchell JA. Targeting PPAR receptors in the airway for the treatment of inflammatory lung disease. Br J Pharmacol 2009; 158: 994–1003.

32 Pichavant M, Goya S, Meyer EH, et al. Ozone exposure in a mouse model induces airway hyperreactivity that requires the presence of natural killer T cells and IL-17. J Exp Med 2008; 205: 385–93.

33 Hoshino H, Lotvall J, Skoogh BE, et al. Neutrophil recruitment by interleukin-17 into rat airways in vivo. Role of tachykinins. Am J Respir Crit Care Med 1999; 159: 1423–8.

34 Laan M, Cui ZH, Hoshino H, et al. Neutrophil recruitment by human IL-17 via C-X-C chemokine release in the airways. J Immunol 1999; 162: 2347–52.

35 Gern JE, Busse WW. The role of viral infections in the natural history of asthma. J Allergy Clin Immunol 2000; 106: 201–12.

36 Sigurs N, Gustafsson PM, Bjarnason R, et al. Severe respiratory syncytial virus bronchiolitis in infancy and asthma and allergy at age 13. Am J Respir Crit Care Med 2005; 171: 137–41.

37 Hamelin ME, Prince GA, Gomez AM, et al. Human metapneumovirus infection induces long-term pulmonary inflammation associated with airway obstruction and hyperresponsiveness in mice. J Infect Dis 2006; 193: 1634–42.

38 Takeda K, Kaisho T, Akira S. Toll-like receptors. Annu Rev Immunol. 2003; 21: 335–76.

39 Martinon F, Tschopp J. NLRs join TLRs as innate sensors of pathogens. Trends Immunol 2005; 26: 447–54.

40 Brigl M, Bry L, Kent SC, et al. Mechanism of CD1d-restricted natural killer T-cell activation during microbial infection. Nat Immunol 2003; 4: 1230–7.

41 Schmitz J, Owyang A, Oldham E, et al. IL-33: an interleukin-1-like cytokine that signals via the IL-1 receptor-related protein ST2 and induces T helper type 2-associated cytokines. Immunity 2005; 23: 479–90.

42 Moussion C, Ortega N, Girard JP. The IL-1-like cytokine IL-33 is constitutively expressed in the nucleus of endothelial cells and epithelial cells in vivo: a novel "alarmin"? PLoS One 2008; 3: e3331.

43 Smithgall MD, Comeau MR, Yoon BR, et al. IL-33 amplifies both Th1- and Th2-type responses through its activity on human basophils, allergen-reactive Th2 cells, iNKT, and NK cells. Int Immunol 2008; 20: 1019–30.

44 Bourgeois E, Van LP, Samson M, et al. The pro-Th2 cytokine IL-33 directly interacts with invariant NKT and NK cells to induce IFN-gamma production. Eur J Immunol 2009; 39: 1046–55.

45 Kondo Y, Yoshimoto T, Yasuda K, et al. Administration of IL-33 induces airway hyperresponsiveness and goblet cell hyperplasia in the lungs in the absence of adaptive immune system. Int Immunol 2008; 20: 791–800.

46 Liu YJ. TSLP in epithelial cell and dendritic cell cross talk. Adv Immunol 2009; 101: 1–25.

47 Liu YJ, Soumelis V, Watanabe N, *et al*. TSLP: an epithelial cell cytokine that regulates T-cell differentiation by conditioning dendritic cell maturation. *Annu Rev Immunol* 2007; **25**: 193–219.

48 Zhou B, Comeau MR, De Smedt T, *et al*. Thymic stromal lymphopoietin as a key initiator of allergic airway inflammation in mice. *Nat Immunol* 2005; **6**: 1047–53.

49 Nagata Y, Kamijuku H, Taniguchi M, *et al*. Differential role of thymic stromal lymphopoietin in the induction of airway hyperreactivity and Th2 immune response in antigen-induced asthma with respect to natural killer T cell function. *Int Arch Allergy Immunol* 2007; **144**: 305–14.

6

Regulatory roles of B cells in allergy and inflammation

Kiyoshi Takatsu,[1,2] *Masashi Ikutani,*[1] *and Yoshinori Nagai*[1]

[1]Department of Immunobiology and Genetic Pharmacology, Graduate School of Medicine and Pharmaceutical Science, University of Toyama, Sugitani, Toyama City, Toyama, Japan

[2]Toyama Prefectural Institute for Pharmaceutical Research, Naka-Taikouyama, Imizu-shi, Toyama, Japan

Introduction

Immune systems fall into at least two categories, innate and acquired immunity. Innate immune responses operate in all animals and are responsible for the first line of defense against common microorganisms or tissue injury [1–3]. These responses are mediated by macrophages and dendritic cells (DCs), natural killer T (NKT) cells, NK cells, B-1 cells, and certain leukocytes including eosinophils, neutrophils, basophils, and mast cells that recognize pathogen-associated molecular patterns (PAMPs) through germline-encoded pattern recognition receptors, the Toll-like receptor (TLR) family, or the Nod-like receptor (NLR) family [3–5]. TLRs, expressed on a variety of cells and tissues, recognize PAMPs that are derived from various classes of pathogens, including Gram-positive and -negative bacteria, DNA and RNA, viruses, fungi, and protozoa [3–6]. Ligand recognition induces a well-conserved host defense program, which includes production of inflammatory cytokines such as interleukin 6 (IL-6) and tumor necrosis factor alpha (TNF-α), upregulation of major histocompatibility complex (MHC) class II, and co-stimulatory molecules. TLR7 and TLR9 can recognize nucleic acids and trigger signaling cascades that activate plasmacytoid DCs (pDCs) to produce interferon alpha (IFN-α) [6–8]. NLR family proteins are activated by various crystals, adenosine triphosphate (ATP), amyloid-β, and PAMPs [9–11].

Acquired immune responses are involved in the late phase of infection and the generation of immunologic memory. The acquired immune response is regulated by a series of interactions among T cells, B cells, and antigen-presenting cells (APCs) such as macrophages and DCs [12]. Both T and B cells recognize antigens or individual peptides via cell surface antigen receptors. T helper (Th) cells recognize antigenic peptides in the context of MHC class II molecules on APCs and B cells and secrete cytokines upon re-stimulation with the same antigen as that seen during the primary stimulus. Th cells responding to and specific for the same antigen regulate the B-cell response to an antigen. During this process, B cells proliferate and differentiate into plasma cells that produce antibodies against distinct antigenic determinants [12,13]. The antibodies thus produced play a key role in the humoral immune response against invading microorganisms and exogenous antigens. Cytokines and chemokines secreted by T cells and inflammatory cells activate the phagocytosis of the innate cells and augment protection against pathogens [14]. Activation of DCs by TLR ligands plays a critical role in their maturation and consequent ability to initiate and activate acquired immune responses.

Inflammation is a series of reactions that bring cells and molecules of the innate immune response into the sites of infection or tissue damage where they then engulf and kill the pathogen. The main cell types seen in the initial phase of an inflammatory

Inflammation and Allergy Drug Design, First Edition. Edited by Kenji Izuhara, Stephen T. Holgate, Marsha Wills-Karp.
© 2011 Blackwell Publishing Ltd. Published 2011 by Blackwell Publishing Ltd.

response are phagocytic cells such as macrophages and neutrophils, both of which express PAMPs. Various cytokines and chemokines also potentiate the process of allergic inflammation. In addition, allergic inflammation enhances the flow of APCs to lymphoid tissues, where they are able to activate lymphocytes and initiate the acquired immune response efficiently.

The hallmark of the allergic response is the result of sensitization of mast cells and basophils in local tissues by immunoglobulin E (Ig-E) antibodies. Reducing IgE concentrations dampens allergic responses, such as those observed in asthma, anaphylaxis, and hyper-IgE disorders. There are at least four different events that are required in B cells for IgE production; namely cognate interaction of antigen-specific B cells with antigen-specific Th2 cells, B-cell division in the germinal center, IgE class switch recombination (CSR), and differentiation into memory B cells and IgE-secreting plasma cells. Regarding B-cell stimulatory signals, IL-4, IL-13, and CD40 ligand are indispensable for induction of germline ε (GLε) transcription and activation-induced cytidine deaminase (AID) that initiates IgE CSR by promoting double-strand breaks in switch region of ε gene. Transcriptional factors such as STAT6, NF-κB, NFIL-3, BCL6, and Id2 are implicated in regulation of IgE production.

B-cell subsets that regulate innate and acquired immune response

Mature B cells expressing surface IgM are divided into B-1 and conventional B (B-2) cells, which regulate the innate and acquired immune responses, respectively. B-1 cells can be distinguished from B-2 cells by their expression of CD5 and have numerous noteworthy characteristics, such as their self-replenishing ability and tissue distribution, Vh gene usage of IgM, and production of autoantibodies [15].

B-1 cells constitutively express three different markers, namely Mac-1, CD43, and IL-5Rα, and lack CD23 and CD21 expression [16]. B-1 cells produce natural antibodies in the IgM, IgG3, and IgA classes that can be included in the innate immune system by their preformed reactivity to various pathogens. In addition, natural antibodies are indispensable for the effective induction of acquired immune responses. As autoimmune-prone mice contain a higher number of B-1 cells and autoantibodies in serum than wild-type

mice, B-1 cells are thought to play important roles in the development and the pathogenesis of autoimmune diseases [17].

Despite their importance in innate and acquired immunity, the developmental pathway of B-1 cells is poorly understood. There are two hypothesis regarding B-1 cell development. One hypothesis is that B-1 cells are an activated form of B-2 cells through B-cell receptors (BCRs) with an autoantigen such as phosphatidylcholine. This hypothesis is supported by the observation that in the transgenic mice of BCR cloned from B-1 cell, all the B cells show a B-1 phenotype. Another hypothesis is that B-1 cells arise from progenitors other than B-2 cell progenitors. This idea stems from studies showing that transfer of adult bone marrow cells into irradiated recipient mice results in repopulation of B-2 cells but not of B-1 cells, whereas fetal liver cells give rise to both B-1 and B-2 cells in the same conditions. Consistent with the latter hypothesis, B-1 lineage-committed progenitors are recently identified as CD19$^+$ B220$^-$ cells in fetal and juvenile mouse bone marrow [18]. Accumulative evidence support the involvement of IL-5- and Btk-dependent signaling pathways in B-1 cell development and differentiation [19].

Mature B-2 cells recognize protein antigens and interact with Th cells that express a particular T-cell receptor (TCR), which leads to their proliferation and differentiation into antibody-secreting plasma cells (ASCs). The activated Th cells transiently express CD40 ligand (CD40L) and interact with B cells through CD40 and LMP-1 [20]. The activated Th cells produce a defined set of cytokines that support proliferation and differentiation of activated B-2 cells into ASCs [21–23].

Stimulation of the activated B-2 cells with antigen and cytokines induces genetic events in their IgH gene loci that are essential for the generation of effector function of the Ig and efficient antigen elimination. CSR replaces the heavy chain constant region (Ch) from Cμ to other Ch regions, and its process is highly regulated by cytokines and B-cell activators [24]. In the mouse, IL-4 is a survival factor for B-2 cells and an inducer of CSR, primarily to IgG1 and IgE. IL-5, IFN-γ, and transforming growth factor (TGF)-β are CSR-inducing cytokines for IgG1, IgG2a, IgG2b, and IgA, respectively [25–27]. The efficiency of antigen elimination is also augmented by affinity maturation, which is accomplished by excessive point mutations in the V-region gene by somatic hypermutation (SHM). AID is the essential and sole B cell-specific factor required for both CSR and SHM [28–31]. Finally, the switched B-cell genetic programs to high-level antibody secretion is regulated by transcriptional regulators, including Blimp-1, Bach 2, Bcl6, IRF-4, Xbp-1, and Pax5 [32–35]. Among these transcriptional regulators, Blimp-1, a transcriptional repressor, is essential for the terminal differentiation of ASCs [36].

Regulation of IgE production by B cells in local tissues

Immediate hypersensitivity is the consequence of sensitization of mast cells and basophils in tissues by IgE antibodies. Thus, IgE antibody plays a central role in allergic responses and is essential for host defense against pathogens in mucosal tissues [37]. IgE binds to high-affinity Fc-ε receptor, FcεRI, on mast cells and basophils, and cross-linking of IgE/FcεRI complexes by allergen causes the release of inflammatory mediators for immediate hypersensitivity and results in more prolonged allergic inflammation. Reducing IgE concentrations dampens allergic responses [38,39].

antigen-specific IgE synthesis is initiated by the interaction between DCs and Th2 cells in local lymph nodes. These Th2 cells, in turn, interact with allergen specific B cells, which divide and form germinal centers. B-cell division in the germinal center is associated with antibody affinity maturation, clonal expansion, CSR, and differentiation into memory B cells and ASCs. Plasma cells continue to secrete IgE antibodies that exert effector functions in the periphery.

In general, CSR requires transcription through switch regions upstream of the new constant region of the Ig heavy chain, DNA cleavage of single-stranded DNA at the site of transcription, and DNA repair to recombine the VDJ (variable, diverse, joining) domain with the new Ch domain. CSR replaces the Cμ constant region exons with one of several sets of downstream IgH constant region exons (e.g., Cγ, Cε, or Cα), which affects switching from IgM to another IgH class (e.g., IgG, IgE, or IgA). Cytokine stimulation of B cells in the germinal center can induce CSR [24]. For example, IL-4 and CD40 (or lipopolysaccharide [LPS]) stimulation induces GLε transcription from the Iε promoter. The production of GLε is essential for

CSR Cμ to Cε and IgE production [40]. AID initiates CSR by promoting DNA double-strand breaks (DSBs) within switch (S) regions flanking the donor Cμ (Sμ) and a downstream acceptor Ch (e.g., Sγ, Sε, Sα) [28–30] that are then joined to complete CSR.

Activation of the allergen-specific Th2 cells results in expression of IL-4, IL-13, and CD40 ligand and in induction of B-cell differentiation into IgE-secreting plasma cells [41]. The CSR from IgM to IgE requires two signals. Signal 1 is provided by IL-4 or IL-13 in B cells through its specific receptors and activates signal transducer and activator of transcription 6 (STAT6), which triggers transcription at Sε switch region. Signal 2 is provided by CD40L on T cells acting through CD40 on B cells, which activates DNA switch recombination. IL-4 and CD40L also induce expression of AID in B cells, leading to CSR. Patients with mutations in the genes encoding CD40, CD40L, and AID have been shown to exhibit defective CSR with hyper-IgM syndrome [30,41].

At the initiation of IgE CSR, T cells are the major source of both signals 1 and 2. However, basophils have been shown to express high levels of IL-4, IL-13, and CD40L, and it has been suggested that they play a pivotal role in polyclonal amplification of IgE production through the induction of Th2 cell differentiation [42,43]. The important roles of basophils in innate allergic responses are also described [44,45].

The CSR from IgM to IgE occurs in the respiratory mucosa of patients with allergic rhinitis and atopic asthma [45]. Kleinjan et al. [46] provided the first direct evidence for this local IgE synthesis. The CD40 stimulation of germinal center B cells through CD40 ligand and IL-4 induces GLε and ε-chain mRNA expression. In mucosal B cells, GLε, and ε-chain mRNA expressions are induced upon local allergen provocation of patients with allergic rhinitis [47].

Several transcription factors, including STAT6 and NF-κB, positively regulate Iε promoter activity. On the other hand, transcriptional repressors, such as Bcl-6 and Id2, are implicated in negative regulation of the promoter [48,49]. The balance of positive and negative transcriptional regulation is important for the control of IgE production. A transcription factor, Nfil3, is identified as a gene induced by IL-4 stimulation in B cells. Interestingly, NFIL-3 deficiency does not affect IgG1 CSR in vivo and has a small effect in vitro. Kashiwade et al. [50] reported that the induction of GLε transcripts after LPS and

IL-4 stimulation is significantly reduced in NFIL-3-deficient B cells leading to impaired IgE CSR. NFIL-3 is identified to be as a key regulator of IL-4-induced GLε transcription in response to IL-4 and subsequent IgE CSR.

B cells in innate immunity

The duration of the survival of the invading organism depends on the strength of the innate immune response that can quickly recognize and respond to microbial and viral products for eradication. TLRs sense well-conserved microbial and viral components [1–3]. For example, TLR4 recognizes LPS in combination with MD-2 [51,52]. Pathogen-derived nucleic acids and their analogs are also recognized via intracellular TLRs such as TLR9 and TLR7. TLR9 recognizes bacterial CpG DNA [53], while TLR7 recognizes viral RNA and antiviral compounds such as imidazoquinolines, imiquimod, and R-848 [54]. TLR7 also recognize guanosine analogs such as 7-allyl-8-oxoguanosine [55]. TLRs require intracellular adaptor proteins for transducing signals into nuclei. All TLRs except for TLR3 share MyD88 as an adaptor protein and induce the production of inflammatory cytokines [3]. There is a MyD88-independent pathway in TLR3 and TLR4 signaling. In this case Toll-like receptor domain-containing adapter-inducing interferon-β (TRIF, also known as TICAM-1) plays a role in place of MyD88 and induces type I interferon gene expression [56,57].

Mature B cells express both germline-encoded TLRs and the rearranged gene-encoded BCR. Thus, B cells contribute to both innate and acquired immunity by secreting antibodies against microbial glycolipids and peptides [58]. We recently identified a novel TLR7 ligand 8-deoxyguanosine whose stimulation of naïve B-2 cells induces NF-κB activation and the expression of GLγ1 transcription [59]. TLR stimulation also activates B cells to induce CSR and Ig production. For instance, LPS stimulation augments IgE and IgG1 production in B-2 cells together with IL-4. TLR9 ligand induces IgG2a, IgG2b, and IgG3 production in mouse B-2 cells activated by CD40 ligand and IL-4 and in human B cells in concert with BCR stimulation[60,61]. The B cells activated with CD38 or BCR undertake μ to γ1 CSR upon stimulation with TLR7 ligand and IL-5 [62].

Marginal zone B and B-1 cells respond to pathogen products

Mature splenic B-2 cells are divided into two subpopulations, marginal zone (MZ) and follicular (FO) B cells, based on a distinct phenotypic gene expression and functional features [63]. MZ B cells are IgM^{high}, CD21^{high}, CD1d^{high}, IgD^{low}, and CD23^{low}, while the FO B cells are IgM^{int}, IgD^{high}, CD21^{int}, CD23^{high}, and CD1d^{low}. The MZ B cells are located in a region at the border of the splenic white pulp and red pulp, and the FO B cells reside in the follicles of the splenic white pulp. This architectural structure contributes to the unique function of the MZ B cells to mount a rapid immune response to blood-borne antigens. The MZ B cells have a lower threshold for antigen activation than FO B cells and exhibit a potent response to TLR ligands. In contrast, the FO B cells respond to T-cell dependent (TD) antigens [64] and exhibit a delayed and weak response to LPS stimulation [65]. Furthermore, MZ B cells express high densities of radioprotective 105 (RP105)/MD-1, another TLR receptor for LPS that is involved in the potent LPS response [66].

As described, B-1 cells produce "natural antibodies" that cross-react with self antigens as well as bacterial pathogens, providing the first line of defense against pathogens. B-1 cells express TLR4, TLR7, and TLR9, and are more prone to differentiate into AFCs than B-2 cells upon TLR stimulation [67]. Furthermore, B-1 cell-mediated autoantibody production is enhanced upon stimulation with various TLR ligands [68,69].

LPS sensors in B cells: TLR4/MD-2 and RP105/MD-1

Lipopolysaccharide, a major Gram-negative bacterial component, is recognized by the TLR4/MD-2 complex (expressed by mature B cells) that activates B cells. Although the expression level of TLR4/MD-2 on B cells is relatively low, TLR4/MD-2 plays indispensable roles for the B-cell response to LPS [52,70].

Mouse B cells express RP105 that is identified as a mouse homolog of *Drosophila* Toll protein [71]. RP105 is a typeI transmembrane protein that forms a complex with MD-1, a homolog of MD-2 [72]. RP105-deficient B cells show little proliferation to LPS [73] and are hyporesponsive to TLR2 ligands, Pam$_3$CSK$_4$, and MALP-2, suggesting that RP105/

MD-1 functionally couples with TLR4/MD-2 and TLR2 [52]. As LPS interacts solely with MD-2 and TLR4/MD-2 associates with RP105/MD-1 [74,75], LPS-induced TLR4 oligomerization may induce RP105/MD-1 coclustering with TLR4/MD-2 that induces signal transduction. Divanovic *et al.* [76] reported that RP105-deficient DCs/macrophages are hyperresponsive to LPS, suggesting that RP105/MD-1 is a negative regulator for LPS responses. However, another report claimed that hyperresponsiveness to LPS was not observed in RP105-deficient DCs/macrophages [52]. Thus, the functional role of RP105 in DCs and macrophages still remains controversial.

RP105 stimulation of mouse B cells by anti-RP105 mAbs can transmit signals for survival and proliferation [71]. As MyD88- and TRIF-deficient B cells normally respond to RP105 cross-linking [77], RP105-mediated B-cell responses are independent on MyD88- and TRIF-mediated signaling. RP105 ligation leads to activation of ERK, JNK, and p38 [78]. Interestingly, B cells deficient in PKCβ or from Btk mutant X-linked immunodeficient mice respond poorly to RP105 ligation [74]. RP105-mediated B-cell activation may require Btk and PKCβ activation, which is distinct from TLR4 signaling pathway.

Innate activation of B cells in autoimmunity

Self-reactive B cells play a central role in the pathogenesis of SLE and other autoimmune diseases. The importance of B cells in these diseases is highlighted by the effectiveness of B cell depletion therapies. Increasing evidence suggest that autoreactive B cells promote autoimmune diseases not only by the production of autoantibody, but also by serving antigen as APCs for autoreactive T cells. Circumstantial evidence supports the notion that not only the onset and recurrence of systemic disease links to various types of infection, but also innate immunity or TLR signaling is critical for the onset and maintenance of autoimmune diseases.

TLR7, TLR8, and TLR9 are identified as receptors for viral RNA and bacterial DNA, and have the sensing ability of host RNA and DNA. A functional link between TLR9 signals and autoreactive B-cell activation was first described using the AM14 transgenic B cells that express mouse BCR specific for self IgG, thereby producing a rheumatoid factor (RF) upon activation [79]. These RF+ B cells are triggered in response to DNA- or RNA-containing immune complexes. Proliferative response of AM14 B cells to chromatin–IgG complexes is abolished in the absence of MyD88, TLR7, or TLR9 [80,81]. The analyses of TLR7- and TLR9-deficient autoimmune prone mice reveal that the various models of spontaneous lupus are differentially regulated by TLR7 and TLR9 [82–84].

The role of B-1 and regulatory B cells in contact sensitivity

Characterization of B-1 cell

Although B cells are key players in acquired immunity because of the high specificity of antibodies to immunized antigens and their long-lasting immunologic memory, particular subsets of B cells participate in innate immunity. Interestingly, antibodies are not always produced in response to pathogen or antigen, they are already prepared even in animals that have not experienced infection or grown in germ-free condition. These antibodies are termed as natural antibodies. These natural antibodies are represented by mainly IgM, but IgA and IgG3 are also included. With their circulation in the bloodstream and their ability to recognize a variety of antigens including LPS, phosphorylcoline, *Salmonella* spp., and phosphatidylcoline [15], they can eliminate pathogens immediately after they invade the host. This also augments the antigen-specific acquired immune response with affinity maturation. These natural antibodies are mainly produced by a unique subset of B cells called the B-1 cell.

B-1 cells can be distinguished from conventional B-2 cells by their location, self-replenishing activity, and expression pattern of cell surface antigens [15]. B-1 cells are exclusively located in the peritoneal and pleural cavities and virtually absent from the lymph nodes, Peyer patches, and peripheral blood where B-2 cells are abundantly observed. B-1 cells express CD19, surface IgM, CD11b (Mac-1), CD43, and IL-5Rα, and lack CD23 (FcεRII) expression. The B-1 cell homeostasis is severely impaired in IL-5 and IL-5Rα deficient mice [85]. B-1 cells can further be divided into CD5+ B-1a and CD5− B-1b cells. In general, B-1a cells produce natural antibodies, while B-1b cells produce IgM antibodies in response to infection by bacteria [86,87]. There are several observations describing increased number of B-1 cells in mice developing spontaneous autoimmune diseases and allergic disorders such as contact sensitivity (CS).

B-1 cell as an initiator of contact sensitivity

Contact hypersensitivity is a typical example of delayed-type hypersensitivity mediated by effector T cells. Contact skin sensitization with hapten–antigen induces migration of antigen-presenting Langerhans cells into lymph node, resulting in a generation of CS effector T cells within 3–4 days [88]. Subsequent separate local skin challenge with the same antigen recruits these effector T cells into the local tissue, initiating antigen-specific inflammation. Interestingly, B-cell deficient mice show apparently no signs of CS [89]. Furthermore, recruitment of CS effector T cells into the site of inflammation requires antigen-specific IgM antibodies produced by B-1 cells. Moreover, activated antigen-specific B-1 cells are detected in the spleen isolated from day 1 post-immunization mice, and these B-1 cells are able to reconstitute the CS response in B-cell deficient mice [89], strongly indicating the involvement of antigen-specific IgM antibodies derived from B-1 cells in the initiation of CS. Recently, the CD19$^+$CD5$^+$Thy1^{int}IgM^{high}IgD^{high} B-cell population, named initiator B cell, is identified in the spleen isolated from hapten-sensitized mice [90]. These initiator B cells reside in the peritoneal cavity without antigen-sensitization and migrate to the spleen in response to antigen-sensitization within 1 day. As AID-deficient mice are unable to initiate CS response, somatic hypermutation may be required for CS initiation. Selective depletion of the initiator B cell may be applicable to suppress CS initiation.

Regulatory B cells in contact sensitivity

In contrast to the roles of B-1 and B-1-like cells in initiating CS, there are B-cell populations responsible for negative regulation of CS. This negative regulation is partly attributed by B-cell-derived IL-10 [91]. It is reported that IL-10 inhibits differentiation of Th1 cells and production of Th2 cytokines and proinflammatory cytokines [92]. Furthermore, IL-10 is required to maintain the function of CD4$^+$CD25$^+$ regulatory T cells by stabilizing forkhead box P3 (FOXP3) expression [93]. These results support the notion that IL-10-producing B cells play a role to maintain the function of regulatory T cells. Interestingly, B-cell deficiency

results in a delay of emergence of CD4$^+$CD25$^+$ regulatory T cells in experimental autoimmune encephalomyelitis (EAE) [94]. IL-10-producing B cells appears to play a role in chronic collagen-induced arthritis and inflammatory bowel disease [95,96].

Although treatment of mice with recombinant IL-10 before the sensitization phase does not affect CS response, the IL-10 treatment of antigen-sensitized and challenged mice suppresses CS response [97]. Furthermore, the IL-10 neutralization at the challenging phase prolongs CS response. Thus, IL-10 production by B cells is important to regulate CS. The IL-10-producing B cells in the spleen were identified as CD1d^{high}CD5$^+$ B cells, termed B10 cells [91]. In addition to B10 cells, LPS-stimulated B cells also produce TGF-β that can induce apoptosis of pathogenic Th1 cells [98]. Control of these B cells may have great potential to manipulate allergic disorders.

Drug design

Enormous efforts to reveal the mechanisms underlying allergies have identified the importance of at least two types of important B-cell subsets, the initiator B cells and regulatory B cells. As both subsets of B cells function in an antigen-dependent manner [90,91], the depletion of initiator B cells before CS response in the local tissue or the activation of regulatory B cells after establishment of CS may suppress CS response.

Depletion of B cells in humans with anti-CD20 mAb (rituximab) was initially designed to deplete B cells in B-cell lymphoma and has been applied to target autoreactive B cells, resulting in clinical success in some cases including rheumatoid arthritis (RA) [99] and systemic lupus erythematosus (SLE) [100]. To avoid unwanted outcomes from B-cell depletion therapy, it may be necessary to target only the B-cell types responsible for the initiation of CS. Another threat possibly induced by the B-cell depletion is breakdown of the balance between Th1 and Th2 development. Several reports have demonstrated that Th1 development was dominant in the absence of B cells [101–103], suggesting that B-cell depletion leads to skewing toward a Th1 response and possibly induction of autoimmune diseases.

In addition to depleting initiator B cells, the activation of regulatory B cells to suppress allergic response might also induce unexpected results such as tumor development because tumor development is significantly reduced in B-cell-deficient mice [104] and anti-tumor cytoxic T lymphocyte generation mediated by Th1 cells is modulated by B-cell deficiency [101]. As regulatory T cells also repress tumor development together with IL-10 [105], total B-cell deletion including IL-10-producing regulatory B cells may result in a loss of the regulatory T-cell function.

Depletion of most of B cells is a double-edged sword, removing both malignant B cells and regulatory B cells. Instead of depleting B cells, targeting cytokines such as IL-5 may be applicable for therapies for CS. Anti-IL-5 mAbs have been used in clinical trials in asthma and hypereosinophilia to deplete eosinophils [106]. Although antigen-specific CS initiator B cells are identified in the spleen of antigen-sensitized mice [90], their origin is suggested to be B-1 (like) cells localized in the peritoneal cavity [89,90]. Furthermore, we reported that oxazolone-sensitized IL-5Rα KO mice showed impaired CS response following oxazolonechallenge, including poor ear swelling and significantly reduced eosinophil infiltration into the site of inflammation [107]. Since oxazolone-specific IgM-producing B cells were significantly reduced in IL-5Rα KO mice, we proposed that IL-5 plays a role in B-1 cell-mediated eosinophil infiltration as well as direct effect on eosinophil development and differentiation. Anti-IL-5RαmAb is a useful therapeutic to deplete eosinophils by antibody-dependent cell-mediated cytotoxicity (ADCC) [108]. Therefore, it is worthwhile to test whether these mAbs will be effective for CS treatment by depleting B-1 cells as well as eosinophils.

Conclusion

We have introduced evidence to suggest that B cells play a key role in allergic inflammation. IgE production by B cells requires a series of signals provided by other cell types. In particular, cytokine (IL-4, IL-13) stimulation and co-stimulatory molecules (CD40 ligand) provided by Th2 cells (possibly provided also by basophils) play a critical role in the induction of Gε transcription and AID, which initiates IgE CSR by promoting double-strand breaks in switch region of ε gene. Transcription factors such as NFIL-3 are also key regulator(s) of IL-4-induced IgE CSR and IgE production and may become target molecules to regulate allergic diseases.

In contrast to the positive defensive roles of B-1 cells, B cells appear also to be involved in development of allergy. There is a body of evidence showing the involvement of antigen-specific IgM antibodies secreted from B-1 cells in the initiation of CS. However, the potential role of B-1 cells in the allergic response and its mechanisms, particularly in CS, still remains elusive. Regarding regulatory B cells, they represent a relatively small population of entire B cells whose protective role from allergy should carefully be re-evaluated in various animal models.

Acknowledgment

We thank all of the collaborators for their tremendous contribution, sharing of data, and helpful discussion. Our project was supported in part by a Grant-in-Aid for Scientific Research and for Special Project Research, Cancer Bioscience from the Ministry of Education, Science, Sports, and Culture (MEXT); by a Grant-in-Aid for Scientific Research (S) and (B) from Japan Society for a Promotion of Science; and by Research Funds of Hokuriku Innovation Cluster for Health Science from MEXT Knowledge Custer Initiative Toyama/Ishikawa Region. The Department of Immunobiology and Genetic Pharmacology, Graduate School of Medicine and Pharmaceutical Science, University of Toyama is supported by Toyama Prefecture and Toyama Pharmaceutical Association.

References

1 Medzhitov R. Toll-like receptors and innate immunity. *Nat Rev Immunol* 2001; **1**: 135–45.

2 Janeway CA, Jr., Medzhitov R. Innate immune recognition. *Annu Rev Immunol* 2002; **20**: 197–216.

3 Akira S, Uematsu S, Takeuchi O, Pathogen recognition and innate immunity. *Cell* 2006; **124**: 783–801.

4 Takeda K, Kaisho T, Akira S. Toll-like receptors. *Annu Rev Immunol* 2003; **21**: 335–76.

5 Takeda K, Akira S. Toll-like receptors in innate immunity. *Int Immunol* 2005; **17**: 1–14.

6 Lund JM, Alexopoulou L, Sato A, *et al.* Recognition of single-stranded RNA viruses by Toll-like receptor 7. *Proc Natl Acad Sci USA* 2004; **101**: 5598–603.

7 Kaisho T. Type I interferon production by nucleic acid-stimulated dendritic cells. *Front Biosci* 2008; **13**: 6034–42.

8 Tanaka T, Grusby MJ, Kaisho T. PDLIM2-mediated termination of transcription factor NF-kappaB activation by intranuclear sequestration and degradation of the p65 subunit. *Nat Immunol* 2007; **8**: 584–91.

9 Eisenbarth SC, Colegio OR, O'Connor W, Jr., Sutterwale FS, Flavell RA. Crucial role for the Nalp3 inflammasome in the immunostimulatory properties of aluminium adjuvants. *Nature* 2008; **453**: 1122–6.

10 Hornung V, BauernFeind F, Halle A, *et al.* Silica crystals and aluminum salts activate the NALP3 inflammasome through phagosomal destabilization. *Nat Immunol* 2008; **9**: 847–56.

11 Atarashi K, Nishimura J, Shima T, *et al.* ATP drives lamina propria T(H)17 cell differentiation. *Nature* 2008; **455**: 808–12.

12 Paul WE (ed). *Fundamental Immunology*, 5th ed. Lippincott Williams & Wilkins: New York, 2003.

13 Takatsu K. Interleukin 5 and B cell differentiation. *Cytokines Growth Factor Rev* 1998; **9**: 25–35.

14 Pasare C, Medzhitov R. Control of B-cell responses by Toll-like receptors. *Nature* 2005; **438**: 364–8.

15 Hardy RR, Hayakawa K. B cell developmental pathway. *Annu Rev Immunol* 2001; **19**: 595–621.

16 Hitoshi Y, Yamaguchi N, Mita S, *et al.* Distribution of IL-5 receptor-positive B cells. Expression of IL-5 receptor on Ly 1(CD5)⁺ B cells. *J Immunol* 1990; **144** 4218–25.

17 Berland R, Wortis HH. Origins and functions of B-1 cells with notes on the role of CD5. *Annu Rev Immunol* 2002; **20**: 253–300.

18 Montecino-Rodriguez E, Leathers H, Dorshkind K. Identification of a B-1 B cell-specified progenitor. *Nat Immunol* 2006; **7**: 293–301.

19 Kouro T, Masashi Ikutani M, Kariyone A, Takatsu K. Expression of IL-5Rα on B-1 cell progenitors in mouse fetal liver and involvement of Bruton's tyrosine kinase in their development. *Immunol Lett* 2009; **123**: 169–78.

20 Rastelli J, Hömig-Hölzel C, Seagal J, *et al.* LMP1 signaling can replace CD40 signaling in B cells *in vivo* and has unique features of inducing class-switch recombination to IgG1. *Blood* 2008; **111**: 1448–55.

21 Hasbold J, Hong JS, Kehry MR, Hodgkin PD. Integrating signals from IFN-γ and IL-4 by B cells: positive and negative effects on CD40 ligand-induced proliferation, survival, and division-linked isotype switching to IgG1: IgE and IgG2a. *J Immunol* 1999; **163**: 4175–81.

22 Emslie D, D'Costa K, Hasbold J, *et al.* Oct2 enhances antibody-secreting cell differentiation through regulation of IL-5 receptor alpha chain expression on activated B cells. *J Exp Med* 2008; **205**: 409–21.

23 Horikawa K, Takatsu K. Interleukin-5 regulates genes involved in B-cell terminal maturation. *Immunology* 2006; **118**: 497–508.

24 Stavnezer J, Guikema JE, Schrader CE. Mechanism and regulation of class switch recombination. *Annu Rev Immunol* 2008; **26**: 261–92.

25 Sonoda E, Matsumoto R, Hitoshi Y, *et al.* Transforming growth factor β and interleukin 5 acts additively for IgA production. *J Exp Med* 1989; **170**: 1415–20.

26 Mizoguchi C, Uehara S, Akira S, Takatsu K. IL-5 induces IgG1 isotype switch recombination in mouse CD38-activated sIgD-positive B lymphocytes. *J Immunol* 1999; **162**: 2812–19.

27 Horikawa K, Kaku H, Nakajima H, *et al.* Essential role of STAT5 for IL-5-dependent IgH switch recombination in mouse B cells. *J Immunol* 2001; **167**: 5018–26.

28 Muramatsu M, Kinoshita K, Fagarasan S, Yamada S, Shinkai Y, Honjo T. Class switch recombination and hypermutation require activation-induced cytidine deaminase (AID), a potential RNA editing enzyme. *Cell* 2000; **102**: 553–63.

29 Muramatsu M, Nagaoka H, Shinkura R, Begum NA, Honjo T. Discovery of activation-induced cytidine deaminase, the engraver of antibody memory. *Adv Immunol* 2007; **94**: 1–36.

30 Revy P, Muto T, Levy Y, *et al.* Activation-induced cytidine deaminase (AID) deficiency causes the autosomal recessive form of the Hyper-IgM syndrome (HIGM2). *Cell* 2000; **102**: 565–75.

31 Kinoshita K, Honjo T. Linking class-switch recombination with somatic hypermutation. *Nat Rev Mol Cell Biol* 2001; **2**: 493–503.

32 Turner CA, Jr., Mack DH, Davis MM. Blimp-1: a novel zinc finger-containing protein that can drive the maturation of B lymphocytes into immunoglobulin-secreting cells. *Cell* 1994; **77**: 297–306.

33 Mittrucker HW, Matsuyama T, Grossman A, *et al.* Requirement for the transcription factor LSIRF/IRF4 for mature B and T lymphocyte function. *Science* 1997; **275**: 540–3.

34 Shaffer AL, Yu X, He Y, Boldrick J, Chan EP, Staudt LM. BCL-6 represses genes that function in lymphocyte differentiation, inflammation, and cell cycle control. *Immunity* 2000; **13**: 199–212.

35 Nera KP, Kohonen P, Narvi E, *et al.* Loss of Pax5 promotes plasma cell differentiation. *Immunity* 2006; **24**: 283–93.

36 Calame K. Transcription factors that regulate memory in humoral responses. *Immunol Rev* 2006; **211**: 269–79.

37 Gould HJ, Sutton BJ. IgE in allergy and asthma today. *Nat Rev Immunol* 2008; **8**: 205–17.

38 Geha RS, Jabara HH, Brodeur SR. The regulation of immunoglobulin E class switch recombination. *Nat Rev Immunol* 2003; **3**: 721–32.

39 Corry DB, Kheradmand F. Induction and regulation of the IgE response. *Nature* 1999; **402** (Suppl): B18–B23.

40 Snapper CM, Finkelman FD, Stefany D, Conrad DH, Paul WE. IL-4 induces coexpression of intrinsic membrane IgG1 and IgE by murine B cells stimulated with lipopolysaccharide. *J Immunol* 1988; **141**: 489–98.

41 Stone KD, Prussin C, Metcalfe DD. IgE, mast cells, basophils, and eosinophils. *J Allergy Clin Immunol* 2010; **125**: S73–80.

42 Yoshimoto T, Yasuda K, Tanaka H, et al. Basophils contribute to TH2-IgE responses *in vivo* via IL-4 production and presentation of peptide–MHC class II complexes to CD4[+] T cells. *Nat Rev Immunol* 2010; **7**: 706–10.

43 Sokol CL, Chu NQ, Yu S, Nish SA, Laufer TM, Medzhitov R. Basophils function as antigen-presenting cells for an allergen-induced T helper type 2 responses. *Nat Immunol* 2009; **10**: 713–20.

44 Karasuyama HK, Mukai K, Tsujimura Y, Obata K. Newly discovered roles for basophils: a neglected minority gains new respect. *Nat Rev Immunol* 2009; **9**: 9–13

45 Barrett NA, Austen KF. Innate cells and T helper 2 cell immunity in airway inflammation. *Immunity* 2009; **31**: 425–37.

46 KleinJan A, Vinke JG, Severijen LW, Fokkens WJ. Local production and detection of (specific) IgE in nasal B-cells and plasma cells of allergic rhinitis patients. *Eur Respir J* 2000; **15**: 491–7.

47 Cameron LA, Durham SR, Jacobson MR, et al. Expression of IL-4: Cε RNA and Iε RNA in the nasal mucosa of patients with seasonal rhinitis: effect of topical corticosteroids. *J Allergy Clin Immunol* 1998; **101**: 330–6.

48 Harris MB, Chang CC, Berton MT, et al. Transcriptional repression of Stat6-dependent interleukin-4-induced genes by BCL-6: Specific regulation of Iε transcription and immunoglobulin E switching. *Mol Cell Biol* 1999; **19**: 7264–75.

49 Sugai M, Gonda W, Kusunoki T, Katakai T, Yokota Y, Shimizu A. Essential role of Id2 in negative regulation of IgE class switching. *Nat Immunol* 2003; **4**: 25–30.

50 Kashiwada M, Levy DM, McKeag L, et al. IL-4-induced transcription factor NFIL-3/E4BP4 controls IgE class switching. *Proc Natl Acad Sci USA* 2010; **107**: 821–6.

51 Shimazu R, Akashi S, Ogata H, et al. MD-2: a molecule that confers lipopolysaccharide responsiveness on Toll-like receptor 4. *J Exp Med* 1999; **189**: 1777–82.

52 Nagai Y, Akashi S, Nagafuku M, et al. Essential role of MD-2 in LPS responsiveness and TLR4 distribution. *Nat Immunol* 2002; **3**: 667–72.

53 Hemmi H, Takeuchi O, Kawai T, et al. A Toll-like receptor recognizes bacterial DNA. *Nature* 2000; **408**: 740–5.

54 Hemmi H, Kaisho T, Takeuchi O, et al. Small antiviral compounds activate immune cells via the TLR7 MyD88-dependent signaling pathway. *Nat Immunol* 2002; **3**: 196–200.

55 Lee J, Chuang TH, Redecke V, et al. Molecular basis for the immunostimulatory activity of guanine nucleoside analogs: activation of Toll-like receptor 7. *Proc Natl Acad Sci USA* 2003; **100**: 6646–51.

56 Yamamoto M, Sato S, Hemmi H, et al. Role of adaptor TRIF in the MyD88-independent toll-like receptor signaling pathway. *Science* 2003; **301**: 640–3.

57 Oshiumi H, Matsumoto M, Funami K, Akazawa T, Seya T. TICAM-1: an adaptor molecule that participates in Toll-like receptor 3-mediated interferon-β induction. *Nat Immunol* 2003; **4**: 161–7.

58 Iwasaki A, Medzhitov R. Toll-like receptor control of the adaptive immune responses. *Nat Immunol* 2004; **5**: 987–95.

59 Tsukamoto Y, Uehara S, Mizoguchi C, Sato A, Horikawa K, Takatsu K. Requirement of 8-mercaptoguanosine as a costimulus for IL-4-dependent μ to γ1 class switch recombination in CD38-activated B cells. *Biochem Biophys Res Commun* 2005; **336**: 625–33.

60 Lin L, Gerth AJ, Peng SL. CpG DNA redirects class-switching towards "Th1-like" Ig isotype production via TLR9 and MyD88. *Eur J Immunol* 2004; **34**: 1483–7.

61 Fischer A. Human primary immunodeficiency diseases: a perspective. *Nat Immunol* 2004; **5**: 23–30.

62 Tsukamoto Y, Nagai Y, Kariyone A, et al. Toll-like receptor 7 cooperates with antigen receptors and CD38 for induction of class switch recombination and terminal B cell maturation. *Mol Immunol* 2009; **46**: 1278–88.

63 Martin F, Kearney JF. B-cell subsets and the mature preimmune repertoire: marginal zone and B1 B cells as part of a "natural immune memory." *Immunol Rev* 2000; **175**: 70–79.

64 Bendelac A, Bonneville M, Kearney JF. Autoreactivity by design: innate B and T lymphocytes. *Nat Rev Immunol* 2001; **1**: 177–86.

65 Oliver AM, Martin F, Kearney JF. IgMhigh CD21high lymphocytes enriched in the splenic marginal zone generate effector cells more rapidly than the bulk of follicular B cells. *J Immunol* 1999; **162**: 7198–207.

66 Nagai Y, Kobayashi T, Motoi Y, et al. The radioprotective 105/MD-1 complex links TLR2 and TLR4/MD-2 in antibody response to microbial membranes. *J Immunol* 2005; **174**: 7043–9.

67 Gururajan M, Jacob J, Pulendran B. Toll-like receptor expression and responsiveness of distinct murine splenic and mucosal B-cell subsets. *PLoS One* 2007; **2**: e863.

68 Baumgarth N, Tung JW, Herzenberg LA. B-1 B cells: development, selection, natural autoantibody and

leukemia. *Springer Semin Immunopathol* 2005; **26**: 347–62.

69 Carroll MC, Holers VM. Innate autoimmunity. *Adv Immunol* 2005; **86**: 137–57.

70 Hoshino K, Takeuchi O, Kawai T, *et al*. Cutting edge: Toll-like receptor 4 (TLR4)-deficient mice are hyporesponsive to lipopolysaccharide: evidence for TLR4 as the Lps gene product. *J Immunol* 1999; **162**: 3749–52.

71 Miyake K, Yamashita Y, Hitoshi Y, Takatsu K, Kimoto M. Murine B cell proliferation and protection from apoptosis with an antibody against a 105-kD molecule: unresponsiveness of X-linked immunodeficient B cells. *J Exp Med* 1994; **180**: 1217–24.

72 Miyake, K, Shimazu, R, Kondo, J, *et al*. Mouse MD-1: a molecule that is physically associated with RP105 and positively regulates its expression. *J Immunol* 1998; **161**: 1348–53.

73 Ogata H, Su I-h, Miyake K, *et al*. The Toll-like receptor protein RP105 regulates lipopolysaccharide signaling in B cells. *J Exp Med* 2000; **192**: 23–9.

74 Akashi S, Saitoh S-I, Wakabayshi Y, *et al*. Lipopolysaccharide interaction with cell surface Toll-like receptor 4-MD-2: higher affinity than that with MD-2 or CD14. *J Exp Med* 2003; **198**: 1035–42.

75 Tsuneyoshi N, Fukudome K, Kohara J, *et al*. The functional and structural properties of MD-2 required for lipopolysaccharide binding are absent in MD-1. *J Immunol* 2005; **174**: 340–4.

76 Divanovic S, Trompette A, Atabani SF, *et al*. Negative regulation for Toll-like receptor 4 signaling by the Toll-like receptor homolog RP105. *Nat Immunol* 2005; **6**: 571–8.

77 Yazawa N, Fujimoto M, Sato S, *et al*. CD19 regulates innate immunity by the toll-like receptor RP105 signaling in B lymphocytes. *Blood* 2003; **102**: 1374–80.

78 Chan VW, Mecklenbrauker I, Su I, *et al*. The molecular mechanism of B cell activation by toll-like receptor protein RP-105. *J Exp Med* 1998; **188**: 93–101.

79 Leadbetter EA, Rifkin IR, Hohlbaum AM, Beaudette BC, Shlomchik MJ, Marshak-Rothstein A. Chromatin–IgG complexes activate B cells by dual engagement of IgM and Toll-like receptors. *Nature* 2002; **416**: 603–7.

80 Viglianti GA, Lau CM, Hanley TM, Miko BA, Shlomchik MJ, Marshak-Rothstein A. Activation of autoreactive B cells by CpG-dsDNA. *Immunity* 2003; **19**: 837–47.

81 Lau CM, Broughton C, Tabor AS, *et al*. RNA-associated autoantigens activate B cells by combined B cell antigen receptor/Toll-like receptor 7 engagement. *J Exp Med* 2005; **202**: 1171–7.

82 Christensen SR, Kashgarian M, Alexopoulou L, Flavell RA, Akira S, Shlomchik MJ. Toll-like receptor 9 controls anti-DNA autoantibody production in murine lupus. *J Exp Med* 2005; **202**: 312–31.

83 Christensen SR, Shupe J, Nickerson K, Kashgarian M, Flavell RA, Shlomchik MJ. TLR7 and TLR9 dictate autoantibody specificity and have opposing inflammatory and regulatory roles in a murine model of lupus. *Immunity* 2006; **25**: 417–28.

84 Lartigue A, Courville P, Auquit I, *et al*. Role of TLR9 in antinucleosome and anti-DNA antibody production in lpr mutation-induced murine lupus. *J Immunol* 2006; **177**: 1349–54.

85 Yoshida T, Ikuta K, Sugaya H, *et al*. Defective B-1 cell development and impaired immunity against *Angiostrongylus cantonensis* in IL-5R alpha-deficient mice. *Immunity* 1996; **4**: 483–94.

86 Alugupalli KR, Leong JM, Woodland RT, Muramatsu M, Honjo T, Gerstein RM. B1b lymphocytes confer T cell-independent long-lasting immunity. *Immunity* 2004; **21**: 379–90.

87 Haas KM, Poe JC, Steeber DA, Tedder TF. B-1a and B-1b cells exhibit distinct developmental requirements and have unique functional roles in innate and adaptive immunity to *S. pneumoniae*. *Immunity* 2005; **23**: 7–18.

88 Kripke ML, Munn CG, Jeevan A, Tang JM, Bucana C. Evidence that cutaneous antigen-presenting cells migrate to regional lymph nodes during contact sensitization. *J Immunol* 1990; **145**: 2833–8.

89 Tsuji RF, Szczepanik M, Kawikova I, *et al*. B cell-dependent T-cell responses: IgM antibodies are required to elicit contact sensitivity. *J Exp Med* 2002; **196**: 1277–90.

90 Kerfoot SM, Szczepanik M, Tung JW, Askenase PW. Identification of initiator B cells, a novel subset of activation-induced deaminase-dependent B-1-like cells that mediate initiation of contact sensitivity. *J Immunol* 2008; **181**: 1717–27.

91 Yanaba K, Bouaziz JD, Haas KM, Poe JC, Fujimoto M, Tedder TF. A regulatory B cell subset with a unique CD1d^{hi}CD5^{+} phenotype controls T cell-dependent inflammatory responses. *Immunity* 2008; **28**: 639–50.

92 Fiorentino DF, Zlotnik A, Mosmann TR, Howard M, O'Garra A. IL-10 inhibits cytokine production by activated macrophages. *J Immunol* 1991; **147**: 3815–22.

93 Murai M, Turovskaya O, Kim G, *et al*. Interleukin 10 acts on regulatory T cells to maintain expression of the transcription factor Foxp3 and suppressive function in mice with colitis. *Nat Immunol* 2009; **10**: 1178–84.

94 Mann MK, Maresz K, Shriver LP, Tan Y, Dittel BN. B cell regulation of CD4^{+}CD25^{+} T regulatory cells and IL-10 via B7 is essential for recovery from experimental autoimmune encephalomyelitis. *J Immunol* 2007; **178**: 3447–56.

95 Mauri C, Gray D, Mushtaq N, Londei M. Prevention of arthritis by interleukin 10-producing B cells. *J Exp Med* 2003; **197**: 489–501.

96 Mizoguchi A, Mizoguchi E, Takedatsu H, Blumberg RS, Bhan AK. Chronic intestinal inflammatory condition generates IL-10-producing regulatory B cell subset characterized by CD1d upregulation. *Immunity* 2002; **16**: 219–30.

97 Ferguson TA, Dube P, Griffith TS. Regulation of contact hypersensitivity by interleukin 10. *J Exp Med* 1994; **179**: 1597–604.

98 Tian J, Zekzer D, Hanssen L, Lu Y, Olcott A, Kaufman DL. Lipopolysaccharide-activated B cells downregulate Th1 immunity and prevent autoimmune diabetes in nonobese diabetic mice. *J Immunol* 2001; **167**: 1081–9.

99 Edwards JC, Szczepanski L, Szechinski J, *et al.* Efficacy of B-cell-targeted therapy with rituximab in patients with rheumatoid arthritis. *N Engl J Med* 2004; **350**: 2572–81.

100 Cambridge G, Leandro MJ, Teodorescu M, *et al.* B cell depletion therapy in systemic lupus erythematosus: effect on autoantibody and antimicrobial antibody profiles. *Arthritis Rheum* 2006; **54**: 3612–22.

101 Harris DP, Haynes L, Sayles PC, *et al.* Reciprocal regulation of polarized cytokine production by effector B and T cells. *Nat Immunol* 2000; **1**: 475–82.

102 Bradley LM, Harbertson J, Biederman E, Zhang Y, Bradley SM, Linton PJ. Availability of antigen-presenting cells can determine the extent of CD4

103 Moulin V, Andris F, Thielemans K, Maliszewski C, Urbain J, Moser M. B lymphocytes regulate dendritic cell (DC) function *in vivo*: increased interleukin 12 production by DCs from B cell-deficient mice results in T helper cell type 1 deviation. *J Exp Med* 2000; **192**: 475–82.

104 Qin Z, Richter G, Schüler T, Ibe S, Cao X, Blankenstein T. B cells inhibit induction of T cell-dependent tumor *Immunity Nat Med* 1988; **4**: 627–30.

105 Jones E, Dahm-Vicker M, Simon AK, *et al.* Depletion of CD25[+] regulatory cells results in suppression of melanoma growth and induction of autoreactivity in mice. *Cancer Immun* 2002; **2**: 1.

106 Takatsu K, Nakajima H. IL-5 and eosinophilia. *Curr Opin Immunol* 2008; **20**: 288–94.

107 Itakura A, Kikuchi Y, Kouro T, *et al.* Interleukin 5 plays an essential role in elicitation of contact sensitivity through dual effects on eosinophils and B-1 cells. *Int Arch Allergy Immunol* 2006; **140** (Suppl. 1): 8–16.

108 Shinkawa T, Nakamura K, Yamane N, *et al.* The absence of fucose but not the presence of galactose or bisecting N-acetylglucosamine of human IgG1 complex-type oligosaccharides shows the critical role of enhancing antibody-dependent cellular cytotoxicity. *J Biol Chem* 2003; **278**: 3466–73.

effector expansion and priming for secretion of Th2 cytokines *in vivo*. *Eur J Immunol* 2002; **32**: 2338–46.

7 Mast cells

Mindy Tsai and Stephen J. Galli
Department of Pathology, Stanford University School of Medicine, Stanford, CA, USA

The basic biology of mast cells

Origin and tissue distribution

Mast cells are widely distributed throughout vascularized tissues in humans, mice, and other vertebrates. Relatively high numbers of mast cells occur near body surfaces, including the skin, airways, and gastrointestinal tract [1–4]. Accordingly, mast cells, together with dendritic cells (DCs), represent one of the first immune cells to interact with environmental antigens/allergens, invading pathogens, or external toxins.

Mast cells are derived from hematopoietic stem cells. Unlike granulocytes, only a small number of mast cells reside in the marrow and mature mast cells do not ordinarily circulate in the blood; instead, circulating mast cell precursors migrate to the peripheral tissues where they complete their differentiation and maturation and take up residence [1–4]. Mast cell numbers can be increased in a many human diseases, including asthma and atopic dermatitis, inflammatory bowel disease, rheumatoid arthritis, scleroderma, certain neoplasms, and other chronic diseases, such as osteoporosis, chronic liver disease, and chronic renal disease [2,5–8]. Mast cells can be long-life cells that can re-enter the cell cycle and proliferate following appropriate stimulation; increased recruitment and/or retention of mast cell progenitors, followed by their local maturation, also can contribute to the expansion of mast cell populations in the tissues [1–4].

Studies in mice have established that striking increases in the number of mast cells, as well as local changes in their tissue distribution and/or phenotypic characteristics, can occur during T helper 2 (Th2) cell-associated responses (e.g., as induced by certain parasites), and that increases in numbers of mast cells also can occur in settings of persistent inflammation and/or tissue remodeling [1–4]. The main survival and developmental factor for mast cells is stem cell factor (SCF; also known as Kit ligand), but many growth factors, cytokines, and chemokines can influence the number and phenotype of mast cells, including interleukin 3 (IL-3), Th2 cell-associated cytokines (such as IL-4 and IL-9), IL-10 [9], and transforming growth factor β1 (TGF-β1) [1–4,10,11]. Notably, certain cytokines such as TGF-β1 [12–14] and IL-4 [15,16] can negatively influence mast cell proliferation or survival, at least under certain circumstances.

In a study of airway biopsies from patients with asthma, Brightling *et al.* [17] showed that the numbers of mast cells in the airway submucosa were little different from those in control biopsies of normal individuals or subjects with eosinophilic bronchitis. By contrast, numbers of mast cells in the airway smooth muscle (ASM) were substantially and significantly elevated in the subjects with asthma compared with levels in either of the two control groups [17]. This is an intriguing finding because it suggests that changes in the anatomical distribution of mast cells in patients

Inflammation and Allergy Drug Design, First Edition. Edited by Kenji Izuhara, Stephen T. Holgate, Marsha Wills-Karp.
© 2011 Blackwell Publishing Ltd. Published 2011 by Blackwell Publishing Ltd.

with asthma can render such individuals particularly susceptible to the consequences of mast cell activation on ASM function. The mechanisms that explain the appearance of large numbers of mast cells in the ASM remain to be determined, but these may include changes in the production (by ASM cells and other cell types) of factors that influence the migration of mast cells or their precursors, or factors that influence the survival, maturation, phenotype, and/or functional properties of these cells [18–22].

Mast cell activation

Mast cell activation via the cross-linking of the high affinity immunoglobulin E (Ig-E) receptor, FcεRI, is the best studied mechanism by which mast cells express immunologically specific function, and IgE-dependent mast cell activation has been extensively studied [23–27; Table 7.1]. Recent work indicates that the binding of IgE itself in the absence of known encounters with antigens recognized by such IgE can also regulate mast cell function and survival. Exposure of human and mouse mast cells to IgE increases surface expression of FcεRI, which in turn enhances the sensitivity of mast cells to FcεRI cross-linking [47,48]. Moreover, some types of monomeric IgE can induce cytokine release by mast cells, in many cases without detectable degranulation or release of lipid mediators (e.g., leukotriene C_4 [LTC_4]) [49–51]. Certain IgE antibodies also can promote mast cell survival upon growth factor withdrawal *in vitro* [49,50,52,53]. Human mast cells primed with interferon gamma (IFN-γ) *in vitro* can be activated via FcγRI upon the binding of IgG1 immune complexes [54; Table 7.1]. However, the clinical relevance of IgG-dependent activation of human mast cells remains to be determined.

In addition to activation through Ig receptors, human mast cells express pathogen-associated molecular pattern (PAMP) receptors, including Toll-like receptors (TLRs; including TLR1, TLR2, TLR3, TLR4, TLR6, TLR7, and TLR9), which enable mast cells to react to pathogens or pathogen-derived products [28; Table 7.1]. Different mast cell populations exhibit different patterns of expression of TLRs [28,55,56], and activation of mast cells via different TLRs can induce these cells to secrete distinct patterns of cytokines or chemokines [28,55,56]. NOD2, an intracellular sensor of bacteria-derived muramyl dipeptide (MDP),

has recently been identified in human intestine and lung mast cells and in peripheral blood progenitor cell-derived human mast cells [57]. The expression of NOD2 in human mast cells is upregulated by IFN-γ, and stimulation of human mast cells with MDP pretreated with IFN-γ induces expression of CXCL10, urokinase type plasminogen activation (uPA), intercellular adhesion molecule (ICAM) 1, vascular cell adhesion molecule (VCAM) 1, and other products [57]. Mast cells also can be activated by many other stimuli, including products of complement activation (e.g., C3a, C5a), cytokines (e.g., SCF, tumor necrosis factor [TNF], IL-1, IL-12, thymic stromal lymphopoietin [TSLP], IL-33), neuropeptides (e.g., nerve growth factor [NGF], substance P, vasoactive intestinal peptide [VIP], somatostatin), proteases (tryptase), inflammatory mediators (adenosine, sphingosine-1-phospate [S1P], endothelin-1 [ET-1], neurotensin), as well as exogenous agents such as insect or reptile venoms and bacterial toxins (Table 7.1) [58].

Upon appropriate stimulation, mast cells can release a wide variety of biologically active products, many of which can potentially mediate proinflammatory, anti-inflammatory, and/or immunosuppressive functions; others can influence processes which participate in tissue remodeling [4,27,58–61]. Furthermore, mast cells can participate in multiple cycles of activation for mediator release and can be differentially activated to release distinct patterns of mediators or cytokines, depending on the type and strength of the activating stimuli [11,23,62–64]. While FcεRI-dependent activation induces degranulation with *de novo* synthesis and release of cytokines, chemokines, and lipid mediators, mast cells can be activated by other stimuli to release certain cytokines and mediators without degranulation. For example, IL-1 [65], SCF [66], and lipopolysaccharide (LPS) [67] can induce mast cell IL-6 release without degranulation or histamine release. Human mast cells can produce TNF, IL-5, IL-10, and IL-13 in response to TLR4 (LPS) or TLR2 (peptidoglycan [PGN]) agonists [68]; however, PGN, but not LPS, induces human mast cells to release histamine [69], GM-CSF, IL-1β, and LTC_4 [56]. Human mast cells produce type I IFNs, but not TNF, IL-1 β, IL-5, or granulocyte–macrophage colony-stimulating factor (GM-CSF), after exposure to the TLR3 agonist poly I:C (a synthetic mimic of viral double stranded RNA) [69].

Table 7.1 Mechanisms by which mast cells can be activated [23,24,28,31].

Via immune receptors	
IgE	By FcεRI; IgE can also bind to IgG receptors (FcγRII, and FcγRIII), and to galectin-3, which are expressed on some mast cell-populations
IgG$_1$	Mouse: FcγRIII, human: FcγRI, after treatment with IFN-γ
Ig-binding superantigens	Endogenous (e.g., protein Fv [in HBV & HCV infections]), bacterial (e.g., *S. aureus* Protein A, *P. magnus* protein L) or viral (e.g., HIV gp120)
Products of complement activation	
C3a, C5a, C3b, C4b	By their receptors: C3aR, C5aR, CR3, CR4
Ligands of Toll-like receptors	
Peptidoglycan	TLR2
ds viral RNA, polyI:C	TLR3
LPS	TLR4/CD14
Flagellin	TLR5 (human mast cells)
ss viral RNA	TLR7
CpG-DNA	TLR9
Bacteria and their products	
E. coli FimH	CD48
Pseudomonas aeruginosa	Human mast cells
Virulence factors/toxins	For example, *C. difficile* toxin A, cholera toxin, VacA (cytotoxin of *H. pylori*), streptolysin O
Viruses	
Respiratory syncytial virus, influenza virus, Dengue virus, Sendai virus	By TLR, and possibly by other mechanisms
Parasites	
Schistosoma mansoni	Activation by cercariae
Leishmania major	Activation by living promastigotes
Cytokines and inflammatory mediators	
Tryptase	Functional PAR2 has been shown in human skin mast cells and HMC-1 [32]
SCF	By c-Kit
IL-1, IL-12	Secretion of selective mediators (in human mast cells)
TNF	In human mast cells
PGE$_2$	Secretion of selective mediators (in human mast cells, via EP$_2$) or potentiation of IgE/antigen-induced mediator release (in mouse, via EP$_1$/EP$_3$)

(Continued)

Table 7.1 (*Continued*)

LIGHT	Activation via LTβR in the presence of ionomycin or activated T cells [33]
CD30	Reverse signaling via CD30L induces selective secretion of chemokines [34]
Adenosine	Increase of IgE/antigen-induced degranulation via A_3R
TSLP	TSLP, in synergy with IL-1 and TNF, stimulates human mast cells to produce high levels of Th2 cytokines [22,35]
IL-33	IL-33 promotes human mast cell survival, adhesion to fibronectin [29], and production of inflammatory cytokines and chemokines, but not lipid mediators (PGD_2) or histamine [29,30]. Maturation of human mast cell progenitors is markedly enhanced by IL-33 and TSLP [30]
Endogenous peptides	
Nerve growth factor, Substance P, CGRP, and other neuropeptides,	Via respective G protein-coupled or other receptors on mast cells
Endothelin-1	Via $ET_A > ET_B$
Neurotensin	Histamine release from rat peritoneal mast cells [36]
Antimicrobial peptides	e.g., β-defensin 2 and LL-37
Venoms or venom components	
Sarafotoxin 6b	Component of *Atractaspis engaddensis* venom, via ET_A [37]
Phospholipase A_2	Component of many different animal venoms [38]
Mast cell-degranulating peptide	And other components of honeybee venom [39]
Numerous venoms or venom components	e.g., from scorpions, the platypus [40], frogs [41], ants [42], sea urchins [43], Portuguese man-of-war [44], etc.
Physical stimuli	
UV, light, cold, heat, pressure, vibration	Possibly through direct and indirect effects on mast cells [45,46]

Modified from Metz *et al.* (2007).

IgG, immunoglobulin G; IFN, interferon; PAR, proteinase-activated receptor; LIGHT, lymphotoxin-like, exhibits inducible expression, and competes with herpes simplex virus glycoprotein D(gD) for herpesvirus entry mediator, a receptor expressed by T lymphocytes; TNF, tumor necrosis factor; SCF, stem cell factor; TSLP, thymic stromal lymphopoietin; IL, interleukin; CGRP, calcitonin gene-related peptide; UV, ultraviolet.

[a]Receptors other than the ones mentioned also may be involved in some cases, and, in some cases, the biological significance *in vivo* of mast cell activation via the listed receptors is not yet clear.

"Tuning" of mast cell phenotype and activation

The regulation of mast cell survival and proliferation and the modulation of important phenotypic characteristics of mast cells—including their susceptibility to activation by various stimuli during innate or adaptive immune responses, their ability to store and/or produce various secreted products, and the magnitude and nature of the secretory response of mast cells to specific activation stimuli—can be finely controlled or "tuned" by genetic and microenvironmental factors that affect the expression pattern or functional properties of the surface receptors or signaling molecules that contribute to such responses [23,27, 62]. For example, bone marrow-derived culture mast cells (BMCMCs) deficient in the expression of the src homology 2-containing inositol phosphatase (SHIP) exhibit enhanced degranulation upon FcεRI aggregation [70]; BMCMCs deficient in RabGEF1, another negative regulator of mast cell activation, exhibit delayed receptor internalization, elevated and prolonged intracellular signaling events, and enhanced cytokine and mediator release in response to FcεRI- or Kit-dependent activation [71–73]; and Syk-deficient human basophils and lung mast cells exhibit impaired responses to FcεRI-IgE-mediated stimulation [74,75].

In addition to the potential for exhibiting genetically determined variation in response to agonists of activation, the functional repertoire of mast cells also can vary based on anatomical location and/or their exposure to microenvironmental factors. Human mast cells isolated from different anatomic sites (lung, skin, and heart) have been shown to respond to different stimuli (e.g., FcεRI cross-linking, C5a anaphylatoxin, protamine, compound 48/80, substance P, morphine, and contrast media) by releasing distinct patterns of mediators [76,77]. In the mouse, incubation of BMCMCs with IL-4 *in vitro* leads to upregulation of FcγRIII, enhanced TNF, and IL-10 release after aggregation of FcγRIII [78,79]. Grimbaldeston *et al.* [79] reported that mast cells and mast cell-derived IL-10 can limit the magnitude of and promote the resolution of contact hypersensitivity (CHS) responses induced in response to the hapten DNFB (2,4-dinitro-1-fluorobenzene) or to urushiol, which is the hapten-containing sap of poison ivy (*Toxicodendron radicans*) or poison oak (*Toxicodendron diversilobum*); in these CHS responses, skin mast cell expression of FcRγ is required for the optimal production of IL-10 and contributes significantly to the ability of mast cells to suppress the responses [79]. As noted above, human mast cells can be activated by IgG1-dependent signaling after IFN-γ exposure. Human skin mast cells in patients with psoriasis, which contain high levels of IFN-γ, were found to express high affinity receptors for IgG (FcγRI), but FcγRI expression was not detectable in normal skin mast cells [80].

There is now substantial evidence that mast cells can have negative as well as positive effects on the development or intensity of innate or acquired immune responses [4,79,81–86]. Taken together with the evidence that mast cell functions (including their pattern of cytokine release) can be influenced by cytokines and other microenvironmental factors, which may vary at different stages of inflammatory or immune responses, this evidence raises the possibility that, in addition to their well-established roles as initiators and amplifiers of acquired immune responses (the most striking example of which is anaphylaxis), in some settings mast cells may be able both to enhance and later to limit certain innate or adaptive immune responses [4,27].

Approaches to analyze mast cell function

In vitro analyses

Mast cell development and function have been investigated by experiments using freshly isolated tissue mast cells or *in vitro*-derived cultured mast cells. Although the numbers of tissue mast cells that can be purified from dispersed human or mouse materials are limited, such freshly purified mast cells probably bear the most resemblance to tissue mast cells *in situ*. Some populations of purified human mast cells can also be maintained in long-term culture; while these cells can continue to express certain features of the corresponding mast cell population *in situ*, it is unlikely that such cells are (or could be rendered) fully identical to the original population of mast cells *in vivo* [87].

Mast cell development and function can also be analyzed using primary populations of mast cells generated from hematopoietic tissues *in vitro*. Human mast cells can be generated from progenitors present in bone marrow, cord blood, or peripheral blood [88–90]. Mouse mast cells have been generated from progenitors present in the bone marrow, fetal liver, or skin, and from embryonic stem cells [2,23,58,91]. Transformed human mast cell lines that are either growth factor-dependent (leukocyte adhesion deficiency type 1 [LAD-1] and LAD-2 [92]) or independent (human mast cell-1 [HMC-1] [93]) have been established from patients with mast cell leukemia (HMC-1) or other disorders affecting mast cells (LAD-1 and LAD-2).

In vivo analyses

Several approaches have been used to investigate mast cells *in vivo*. Histochemical and immunohistochemical staining can be used to assess the numbers, distribution, and mediator/protein expression of tissue mast cells, and *in situ* hybridization can be employed to analyze gene expression in these cells [94–97]. The potential involvement of mast cells in local or systemic disorders or adaptive immune responses can be assessed by measuring mast cell mediators in body fluids, e.g., bronchoalveolar lavage (BAL) fluid, urine, plasma, peritoneal fluid (in rats, mice), etc., or by using pharmacologic agents to attempt to interfere with mast cell activation or the actions of mast cell products.

Pharmacologic approaches, or using antibodies to deplete mast cells or to neutralize their products, may provide interesting information but are limited by the specificity of the drug or antibodies chosen. Some agents (such as antihistamines) obviously will block mediators derived from other cell types as well as mast cells. Antibodies that neutralize SCF [98] or block c-Kit [99,100] can result in the depletion of mast cells *in vivo*, but may also influence other cell types that express c-Kit.

Drugs (or antibodies) that interfere solely with mast cell activation would be highly desirable for experimental studies and possibly for evaluation as therapeutic agents. One drug, disodium cromoglycate, is often referred to as a "mast cell stabilizer" (i.e., an agent that blocks the release of mediators after mast cell activation) and is used to treat some patients with allergic disorders [101]. Sometimes this drug is used to suppress mouse mast cell function *in vivo* [102,103]. While the molecular targets and mechanism of action of disodium cromoglycate are not fully defined, some of the molecular targets of this drug are not restricted to mast cells [104] and this agent also influences the function of other cell types, including granulocytes and B cells [105].

Given the current limitations of using pharmacologic or antibody-based approaches either to eliminate mast cells or specifically to block their functional activation, we think that genetic approaches in mice, including those employing mast cell knock-in mice, mice deficient in specific mast cell-associated mediators, and, when they have been fully validated, approaches that can genetically delete specific media-

tors selectively in mast cells, are the most definitive ways to identify and characterize mast cell functions *in vivo*.

Mast cell knock-in mice and other mouse models

Although mice that specifically lack only mast cells have not been reported, *c-kit* mutant mice, which are deficient in mast cells and have several other phenotypic abnormalities, are available for analyzing the *in vivo* functions of mast cells [1,23,58,60,91,106]. The most commonly used animals for such studies are the WBB6F$_1$-*Kit*^{W}/*Kit*$^{W-v}$ mice and the more recently characterized C57BL/6-*Kit*$^{W-sh}$/*Kit*$^{W-sh}$ mice [23,58,60,91,106,107]. *Kit*^{W} is a point mutation that produces a truncated c-Kit, lacking the transmembrane domain, that is not expressed on the cell surface; *Kit*$^{W-v}$ is a (Thr^{660}→Met) mutation at the *c-kit* tyrosine kinase domain that substantially reduces the kinase activity of the receptor; and *Kit*$^{W-sh}$ is an inversion mutation of the transcriptional regulatory elements upstream of the *c-kit* transcription start site on mouse chromosome 5 (reviewed in references 23, 91,109).

Adult WBB6F$_1$-*Kit*^{W}/*Kit*$^{W-v}$ mice and C57BL/6-*Kit*$^{W-sh}$/*Kit*$^{W-sh}$ mice are profoundly deficient in mast cells and melanocytes [1,23,106]. WBB6F$_1$-*Kit*^{W}/*Kit*$^{W-v}$ mice also exhibit several other phenotypic abnormalities, such as macrocytic anemia, reductions in numbers of bone-marrow and blood neutrophils, sterility, and an almost complete lack of interstitial cells of Cajal [1,23,106–108]. By contrast, C57BL/6-*Kit*$^{W-sh}$/*Kit*$^{W-sh}$ mice are neither anemic nor sterile, but have increased numbers of neutrophils, basophils, and platelets [106,107,109,110]. However, because the *c-kit*-related phenotypic abnormalities that affect lineages other than mast cells are generally milder in C57BL/6-*Kit*$^{W-sh}$/*Kit*$^{W-sh}$ mice than in WBB6F$_1$-*Kit*^{W}/*Kit*$^{W-v}$ mice, and because C57BL/6-*Kit*$^{W-sh}$/*Kit*$^{W-sh}$ mice are fertile and (like many other mutant mice to which they might be bred) are fully on the C57BL/6 background, they are becoming increasingly popular for studies to elucidate the roles of mast cells *in vivo*.

Differences in the biologic responses in *c-kit* mutant mice compared with wild-type mice may be due to any one of the abnormalities that result from the *c-kit* mutations in these animals and not necessarily from their profound deficiency in mast cells. However, the lack of mast cells in *c-kit* mutant mice can be selectively repaired by the adoptive transfer of genetically compatible, *in vitro*-derived wild-type or mutant mast cells [1,23,58,60,91,106]. Such *in vitro*-derived mast cells, for example BMCMCs, can be administrated intravenously, intraperitoneally, or intradermally, or directly injected into the anterior wall of the stomach of *c-kit* mutant mice to create so-called "mast cell knock-in mice." These mast cell knock-in mice can then be used to assess the extent to which differences from wild-type mice in the expression of biologic responses observed in *c-kit* mutant mast cell-deficient mice reflect their lack of mast cells.

It is possible to investigate the role of specific mast cell-associated mediators *in vivo* by testing animals in which that mediator has been knocked out. If that mediator is selectively expressed by mast cells, and if its deletion does not significantly influence the expression of other mast cell products, then it is possible to draw conclusions about the role of that mast cell product *in vivo* [111–113]. For example, in mice that lack mouse mast cell carboxypeptidase A (mMC-CPA; a highly conserved secretory granule protease), the expression of mouse mast cell protease 5 (mMCP-5) is also reduced because it requires mMC-CPA for proper packaging in the cytoplasmic granules [112]. This problem can be circumvented by using mice in which mMC-CPA has been mutated specifically to eliminate its catalytic activity, a change that preserves mMC-CPA's ability to ensure proper packaging of mMCP-5 in the mast cell granule [112].

Other promising genetic approaches to investigate the specific functions of mast cells and their products are currently in development, such as "mast cell-specific Cre" mice that can be crossed with other strains in which genes of interest are "floxed" [114]. Cre recombinase recognizes the loxP consensus sequence and catalyzes the recombination of DNA sequences flanked (i.e., "floxed") by two loxP sites. When a gene sequence is flanked by loxP sites, Cre recombinase can then excise that specific segment from the gene sequence.

Mast cells and allergic inflammation

IgE-dependent mast cell activation

Mast cells are widely recognized as important effector cells in the pathophysiology of bronchial asthma and other allergic disorders [20,115–118]. Mast cells in sensitized individuals have allergen-specific IgE antibodies bound to their surface, high-affinity IgE receptors (FcεRI), and, upon cross-linking of adjacent IgE molecules by bi- or multivalent allergen, aggregation of the FcεRI triggers a complex intracellular signaling process that results in the secretion of three classes of biologically active products, those stored in the cytoplasmic granules, lipid-derived mediators, and newly synthesized cytokines, chemokines, and growth factors [23–26].

Mediators stored in the mast cells' cytoplasmic granules include biogenic amines (in humans, histamine with little or no serotonin; in murine rodents, both histamine and serotonin [23,24]), serglycin proteoglycans (such as heparin and chondroitin sulfate), serine proteases (such as tryptases, chymases, and carboxypeptidases) [119–121], as well as various other enzymes and certain cytokines and growth factors that may be associated with the granules, such as TNF, vascular endothelial growth factor A/vascular permeability factor (VEGF-A/VPF), TGF-β, etc. [23,24,122,123]. Mast cells activated via aggregation of FcεRI also metabolize arachidonic acid through the cyclooxegenase and lipoxegenase pathways, resulting in the release of prostaglandins (particularly prostaglandin D_2 [PGD_2], leukotriene B_4 [LTB_4], and cysteinyl leukotrienes [cys-LTs], particularly leukotriene C_4 [LTC_4]) [124]. Mast cells responding to IgE and specific allergen also release, with kinetics slower than those for the preformed mediators, a broad spectrum of newly synthesized cytokines, chemokines, and growth factors [23–26].

The release of preformed and lipid-derived mediators contributes to the acute signs and symptoms associated with early phase reactions (or type I immediate hypersensitivity reactions) of allergic inflammation (Figure 7.1a) [118]. Many of the clinically significant consequences of IgE-associated antigen-dependent reactions in the respiratory tract, skin, and other sites are now thought to depend critically on the actions of leukocytes recruited to these sites during late-phase responses (LPRs) rather than on the direct effects of the mediators released by mast cells at early intervals after antigen challenge [125,126]. LPRs can be defined as the recurrence, at a few to several hours after initial antigen challenge in sensitized hosts, of signs and symptoms of inflammation at the site of antigen challenge. In many but not all cases, such LPRs are preceded by

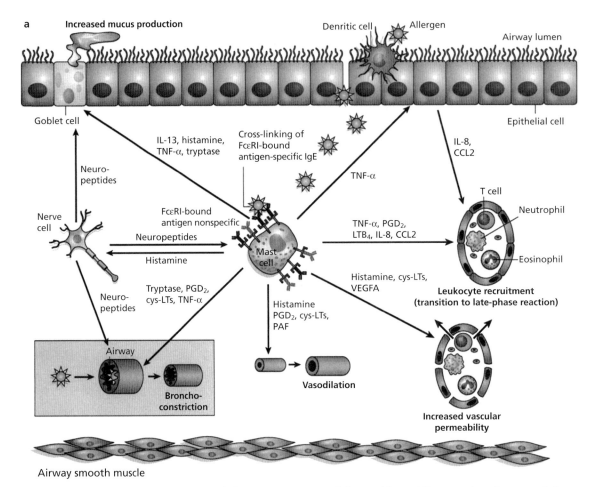

Figure 7.1 Early (a) and chronic (b) stages of allergen-induced airway inflammation. (a) Early-phase response to immunoglobulin E (IgE) and specific antigen in the airway of a subject without airway remodeling related to chronic allergic inflammation. The individual IgE molecules that are bound to the FcεRI molecules on a single mast cell can be specific for different antigens. The recognition of a particular allergen by FcεRI-bound IgE specific for antigen derived from that allergen (antigen-specific IgE) induces FcεRI aggregation, which activates mast cells to secrete preformed mediators and lipid-derived mediators and to increase the synthesis of many cytokines, chemokines, and growth factors. The rapidly secreted mediators result in bronchoconstriction (lower left), vasodilation, increased vascular permeability, and increased mucus production. Mast cells also contribute to the transition to the late-phase reaction by promoting an influx of inflammatory leukocytes, both by upregulating adhesion molecules on vascular endothelial cells (for example, through tumor necrosis factor [TNF]) and by secreting chemotactic mediators (such as LTB4 and PGD$_2$) and chemokines (such as interleukin 8 [IL-8] and CC-chemokine ligand 2 [CCL2]).

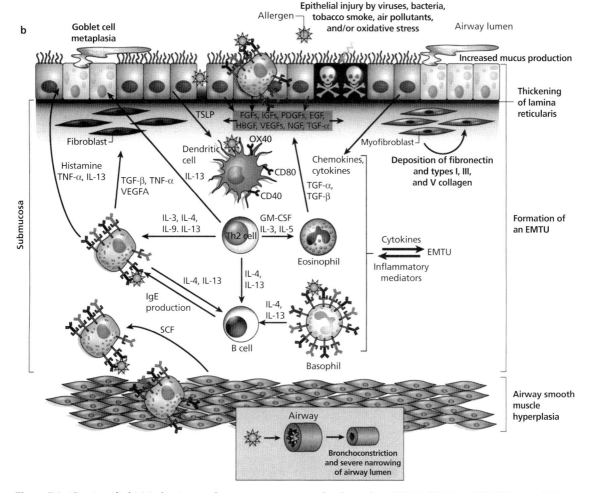

Figure 7.1 (*Continued*) (b) Mechanisms and consequences of chronic allergic inflammation in a subject with asthma and airway remodeling associated with repetitive or persistent exposure to allergens. Innate immune cells (including eosinophils, basophils, neutrophils, and monocyte–macrophage lineage cells) and adaptive immune cells (including T helper [Th] 2 cells, other types of T cells, and B cells) take up residence in the tissues. In addition, more mast cells develop in the tissue, and these cells display large amounts of IgE bound to FcεRI and have an altered anatomical distribution. Last, complex interactions are initiated between recruited and tissue-resident innate and adaptive immune cells, epithelial cells, and structural cells (such as fibroblasts, myofibroblasts, and airway smooth muscle cells), blood and lymphatic vessels, and nerves (not shown). Repetitive epithelial injury due to chronic allergic inflammation can be exacerbated by exposure to pathogens or environmental factors, and the consequent repair response results in an epithelial–mesenchymal trophic unit (EMTU) being established. This unit is thought to sustain Th2 cell-associated inflammation, to promote sensitization to additional allergens or allergen epitopes (for example, epithelial cell-derived thymic stromal lymphopoietin [TSLP] can upregulate the expression of co-stimulatory molecules such as OX40, CD40, and CD80 by dendritic cells), and to regulate the airway remodeling process. These processes result in many functionally important changes in the structure of the affected tissue. These changes include substantial thickening of the airway walls (including the epithelium, lamina reticularis, submucosa, and smooth muscle), increased deposition of extracellular-matrix proteins (such as fibronectin, and type I, III, and V collagen), and hyperplasia of goblet cells, which is associated with increased mucus production. In individuals who have such thickened airway walls, bronchoconstriction can result in more severe narrowing of the airway lumen than occurs in airways with normal wall thickness. In some individuals, especially those with severe asthma, Th17 cells (which secrete IL-17) may also contribute to the recruitment of neutrophils to sites of inflammation (not shown). EGF, epidermal growth factor; FGF, fibroblast growth factor; HBEGF, heparin-binding EGF-like growth factor; IGF, insulin-like growth factor; NGF, nerve growth factor; PDGF, platelet-derived growth factor; SCF, stem cell factor (also known as KIT ligand); TGF, transforming growth factor; GM-CSF, granulocyte–macrophage colony-stimulating factor; VEGF, vascular endothelial growth factor. Modified from Galli *et al.* (2008).

evidence of an acute allergic reaction at the same site [125,126].

Several lines of evidence, drawn from human experiments and mouse studies (including work in mast cell knock-in mice), indicate that IgE-dependent activation of mast cells can contribute importantly to the development of LPRs [2,91,125,127–129]; there is evidence that activation of effector T cells by antigenic peptides also can contribute to the development of LPRs [126,130]. The relative contribution of mast cells, T cells, and mast cell–T cell interactions in the development of LPRs in individual patients may differ, depending on the characteristics of the allergic disorder in that individual.

Mast cells in chronic allergic inflammation

When allergen exposure is continuous or repetitive, chronic inflammation can occur with many innate and immune cells found in the tissues at sites of allergen challenge (Figures 7.1b and 7.2). This persistent inflammation is associated with changes in structural cells at the affected sites, and in many cases with markedly altered function of the affected organs. For example, in chronic asthma, inflammation can involve all the layers of the airway wall and is typically associated with changes in the epithelium, including increased numbers of mucus-producing goblet cells; increased production of cytokines and chemokines by epithelial cells, as well as areas of epithelial injury and repair; substantial inflamma-

tion of the submucosa, including the development of increased deposition of extracellular matrix molecules in the lamina reticularis (beneath the epithelial basement membrane); changes in fibroblasts; increased development of myofibroblasts and increased vascularity; and increased thickness of the muscular layer of the airways, with increased size, numbers, and function of smooth muscle cells [118,131–134].

Extensive histologic and immunohistologic analyses of airway biopsies of subjects with chronic asthma, when taken together with emerging information from *in vitro* studies about possible mediators and cell–cell interactions that might contribute to tissue remodeling, have suggested that mast cells might play a variety of roles in regulating multiple features of the pathology of chronic asthma [20,135]. For the reasons already described, it can be difficult to prove that mast cells have such roles in human asthma. However, mast cells are clearly required for the full expression of multiple features of chronic allergic inflammation, and the accompanying tissue remodeling, in a mouse model of chronic asthma induced in animals sensitized to ovalbumin (OVA) without alum or other artificial adjuvants and then challenged weekly with OVA intranasally for 9 weeks [136]. The features of this model that required mast cells for optimal expression included enhanced airway responses to methacholine or specific antigen, chronic inflammation of the airways with infiltration of eosinophils and lymphocytes, airway epithelial

---

Figure 7.2 Chronic allergic inflammation and tissue remodeling in asthma. Tissue sections from the airway of an individual without asthma (a–c) and a patient with severe asthma (d–f) are shown. Specimens taken from lung resections (carried out for other indications) were fixed in 10% neutral buffered formalin and processed routinely; sections 5-μm thick, from the same area of tissue, were stained with hematoxylin and eosin (a and d), periodic acid–Schiff with diastase (to stain mucus red [shown here as dark gray; b and e], or pinacyanol erythrosinate to stain mast cells purple [shown here as dark gray or black]; c and f). (a–c) A normal small bronchus. There are few goblet cells (black arrows in insets) in the epithelium. The basement membrane and underlying lamina reticularis (at asterisk in a, hardly visible at this magnification) are normal. The submucosa (the length of the double-headed arrows in a contains few leukocytes and the occasional

mast cell (black arrowheads in c), and the bronchial smooth muscle (SM), the luminal surface of which is indicated by a dashed line, has few adjacent mast cells (white arrowhead in c). (d–f) A small bronchus from a patient with a history of severe asthma. Mucus (M) fills the airway lumen (d and e). There are many goblet cells (black arrows in insets) and the occasional intraepithelial mast cell (black arrows in f). The lamina reticularis (asterisk in inset in d) is markedly thickened. The submucosa (double-headed arrows in d) contains many eosinophils (inset in d) and other leukocytes, as well as mast cells (black arrowheads in f). There is more bronchial SM, the luminal surface of which is indicated by a dashed line, than in a–c, and there are many mast cells (white arrowheads in f) among bundles of SM cells. (Figure courtesy of GJ Berry, Stanford University, California). Modified from Galli *et al.* (2008).

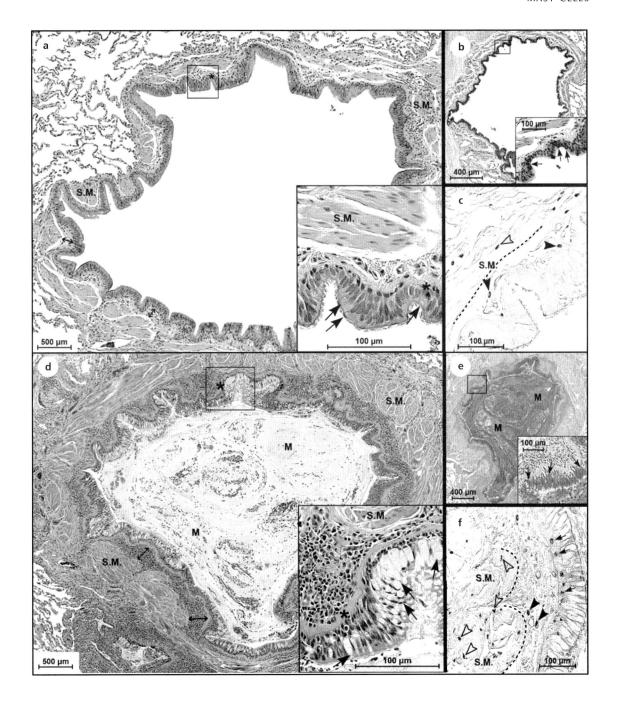

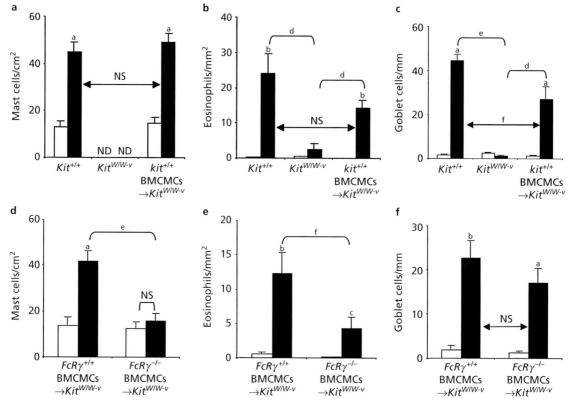

Figure 7.3 Signaling via FcRγ in mast cells contributes to different features of a chronic asthma model in mice. Wild type (Kit[+/+]) mice, genetically mast cell-deficient Kit[W/W-v] mice, and Kit[W/W-v] mice engrafted with wild-type mast cells (Kit[+/+] bone marrow-derived culture mast cells (BMCMCs) → Kit[W/W-v] or FcRγ[+/+] BMCMCs → Kit[W/W-v]) or mast cells lacking FcRγ (FcRγ[−/−] BMCMCs → Kit[W/W-v]) were immunized by three intraperitoneal injections of 50 μg ovalbumin (OVA) in 0.1 mL of phosphate buffered saline (PBS) on days 1, 4, and 7. Starting on day 12, mice were challenged intranasally with 20 μg OVA in 30 μL of PBS weekly for 9 weeks; control mice received intraperitoneal injections and intranasal challenges with PBS on the same schedule. Features observed in this model of chronic allergic inflammation were assessed 24 h after the ninth OVA or PBS challenge. (a, d) Numbers of lung mast cells, (b, e) eosinophils, and (c, f) goblet cells. White bars, PBS-treated group; black bars: OVA-sensitized/challenged group. [a]$P < 0.001$, [b]$P < 0.01$, or [c]$P < 0.05$ or versus corresponding PBS controls; [e]$P < 0.001$, [d]$P < 0.01$, or [f]$P < 0.05$ versus group indicated. ND, not detected; NS, not significant. Modified from Yu *et al.* (2006).

goblet cell hyperplasia, enhanced expression of mucin genes, and increased levels of lung collagen [136] (Figure 7.3a–c).

This study also demonstrated that both FcRγ-dependent and FcRγ-independent pathways of mast cell activation can contribute to the development of multiple features of chronic asthma in mice [136]. For example, much of the increase in lung mast cell numbers and eosinophil infiltration that is associated with this model required that mast cells be able to respond to IgE and/or IgG1 immune complexes (via the FcRγ chain that is shared by FcεRI and FcγRIII) [136] (Figure 7.3d,e). By contrast, the striking mast cell-dependent increase in numbers of airway goblet cells in this model occurred in mice whose mast cells lacked the FcRγ chain (Figure 7.3c,f), strongly suggesting that while this change was mast cell-dependent, it occurred as a result of the effects of mast cells that were mediated independently of antibody-dependent mast cell activation [136].

The mediators by which mast cells influence airway remodeling in the model of chronic allergic inflammation described in Yu *et al.* [136], and the relevance of these findings to human asthma, remain to be determined. However, there is a very long list of candidate mast cell-derived products that can directly or indirectly influence the biology of structural cells, including vascular endothelial cells, epithelial cells, fibroblasts, and smooth muscle or nerve cells [20,131,137]. In the mouse, data derived from studies of mast cell knock-in mice *in vivo* [138] and *in vitro* co-culture systems using mouse mast cells and fibroblasts [139] suggest that mast cell-derived TNF and TGF-β may influence fibroblast proliferation and function in chronic allergic inflammation.

Potential effects of mast cells on the development of acquired immune responses

In addition to contributing to the features of allergic inflammation, the ongoing release of cytokines, chemokines, and other mediators by mast cells that have been activated by IgE-dependent and other mechanisms at sites of antigen challenge can have additional effects. These include actions that have the potential to influence the development of acquired immune responses in such settings. For example, histamine derived from IgE- and antigen-stimulated skin mast cells can promote the migration of Langerhans cells (LCs) to draining lymph nodes (LNs) via H2 receptors [140]. This finding raises the possibility that, in individuals who already have developed IgE specific for particular epitopes of an environmental antigen, subsequent challenge with that antigen (alone, or in the presence of additional antigens) may result in IgE- and mast cell-dependent effects on local DCs, which in turn may function to increase the spectrum of epitopes of the original antigen (or of the additional antigens encountered at the same time) against which that individual develops sensitivity. As proposed in Jawdat *et al.* [140], should this mechanism actually occur in naturally acquired allergic disorders, it would have the potential to increase the severity of that individual's chronic allergic disease.

Mast cells have the potential to influence many aspects of the sensitization and effector phases of allergic responses [2,4,23,60,63,91,141]. Some mast cell products (such as histamine, leukotriene B$_4$ [LTB$_4$], and TNF) can promote the migration, recruitment, maturation, and activation of DCs and/or lymphocytes, whereas mast cell-derived histamine or IL-10 can have negative immunomodulatory effects [79,81]. Mast cell-derived factors (for example, PGD$_2$) [142] can influence the ability of DCs to polarize naïve T cells toward Th2 cells, can directly modulate cytokine production by CD4$^+$ T cells (for example, PGD$_2$ can enhance cytokine production by Th2 cells [143]), and, in the case of histamine, can promote Th1-cell activation through H1 receptors but suppress both Th1- and Th2 cell activation through H2 receptors [144]. Mast cells also can produce IL-2, IL-4, IL-6, IL-10, IL-12, IL-13, TNF, and TGF-β. These cytokines can influence the polarization of naïve T cells toward Th1, Th2, Th17, and T regulatory (Treg) cells [63] and/or can modulate the function of distinct T-cell subsets.

The expression of various co-stimulatory molecules by mast cells is further evidence that these cells can have immunomodulatory roles. Co-stimulatory molecules expressed by mouse and/or human mast cells include members of the B7 family inducible T-cell co-stimulator ligand (ICOSL), programmed cell death-1 ligand-1 (PD-L1), PD-L2, CD80 (also known as B7.1), and CD86 (also known as B7.2); members of TNF–TNF receptor families—OX40, CD153, CD95, 4-1BB, and glucocorticoid-induced TNF receptor-related protein (GITR); and CD28 and CD40 ligand (CD40L) [63,145]. Although the importance of mast cell co-stimulatory molecule expression *in vivo* has yet to be determined, *in vitro* evidence suggests that engagement of OX40L, expressed by mast cells, and OX40, expressed by T cells, is required for optimal mast cell-dependent enhancement of T-cell activation [145,146]. Moreover, certain mast cell mediators may exert autocrine or paracrine effects on mast cell expression of co-stimulatory molecules. For example, in co-culture experiments, mast cell-derived TNF increased the surface expression of OX40, ICOS, programmed cell death-1 (PD-1), and other co-stimulatory molecules on CD3$^+$ T, in addition to promoting T-cell proliferation and cytokine production [146].

While mast cell–T cell interactions represent a complex area of study that is beyond the scope of this chapter, *in vitro* experiments showed that Treg cells can directly inhibit FcεRI-dependent mast cell degranulation (but not mast cell production of IL-6 or TNF) through cell–cell contact involving interactions between OX40 expressed on Treg cells and OX40 ligand expressed by mast cells [147]. This study defined a novel Treg-dependent mechanism, which can suppress mast cell degranulation and which could serve to limit mast cell effector function.

Several mast cells products, including IL-4, IL-5, IL-6, IL-13, CD40L, and rat mast cell protease I, can influence B-cell development and function, including IgE production [91]. However, the relevance of these observations *in vivo* largely remains to be determined. For example, it has been reported that mast cell-deficient mice exhibit normal levels of antibodies at baseline and after antigen sensitization in several different experimental settings [91]. As discussed above, although mast cell effector functions in allergic inflammation are primary initiated by IgE-dependent mechanisms, mast cells express a wide spectrum of receptors that equip these cells to respond to other exogenous and endogenous stimuli, some of which can directly activate mast cells and others of which can modulate the cells' response to IgE and specific antigen. For example, in a mouse model of asthma, the administration of low dose LPS can enhance the levels of OVA-induced eosinophilic airway inflammation [148,149]. Using mast cell-deficient mice that had been acutely engrafted with wild-type or TLR4–/– mast cells, Nigo *et al.* [149] provided evidence that TLR4-dependent mast cell activation can enhance allergen sensitization in a mouse model of allergic inflammation [149]. However, because the mast cells had been injected intravenously into mast cell-deficient mice shortly before exposing the mice to antigen (and therefore these animals probably would have large numbers of phenotypically immature *in vitro*-derived mast cells in the lung), it will be of interest to repeat such studies with mice that had undergone long-term mast cell engraftment.

Mast cells are required for the optimal development of acquired immune responses in certain mouse models of contact hypersensitivity (CHS) [150]. Bryce *et al.* [150] reported that both mast cells and physiologic concentrations of antigen-nonspecific IgE are required for optimal sensitization to oxazolone (Ox) (and certain other haptens) and can enhance the emigration of skin LCs from the epidermis of naïve mice in response to epicutaneous application of Ox in ethanol. The binding of IgE to FcεRI on dermal mast cells, even in the absence of antigen known to be recognized by that IgE, enhanced levels of mRNA for certain mast cell-associated products that were

detected in the skin 1 h after the first epicutaneous application of the hapten. In addition, several products that might be secreted by such mast cells (e.g., TNF, IL-6, and monocyte chemoattractant protein-1 [MCP-1]) can influence the biology of DCs.

These findings represent the strongest evidence currently available that the effects of IgE on mast cells that can be detected in the absence of specific antigen known to be recognized by such IgE can be important in modulating mast cell function *in vivo*. As noted above, the clinical relevance of these findings, and other evidence that IgE can induce effects on mast cells in the absence of the cells' exposure to antigen recognized by such IgE, is not yet clear. However, Gould and colleagues [151] identified evidence of the local production of IgE in the affected airways of subjects with allergic rhinitis [152,153] or asthma [154,155], and suggested that, at least in some instances, such local IgE production might contribute to the pathology of asthma even in individuals with low circulating levels of IgE and in whom it has not been possible to identify an antigen to which they exhibit reactivity [151,156].

Recent work has suggested that mast cells might function as adjuvants during certain models of antigen sensitization or immunization. McLachlan *et al.* [157] showed that the subcutaneous or nasal administration of small-molecule mast cell activators together with vaccine antigens enhanced antigen-specific serum Ig responses and increased DC and lymphocyte recruitment to draining lymph nodes [157]. In another study, mast cell-deficient mice exhibited a markedly impaired peptide-specific cytotoxic T-lymphocyte response following transcutaneous immunization employing the synthetic TLR7 ligand, imiquimod, as an adjuvant. By using the mast cell knock-in approach in $Kit^{W-sh/W-sh}$ mice, this study provided evidence that IL-1β produced by TLR7-activated mouse skin mast cells can promote the emigration of LCs that is essential to initiate the development of the peptide-specific cytotoxic T-lymphocyte response in this setting [158]. The importance of mast cells as "endogenous adjuvants," or as targets of known exogenous adjuvants, may depend importantly on the details of the experimental model investigated. For example, aluminum hydroxide (alum) can induce mouse mast cell activation *in vivo*, but experiments in $Kit^{W/W-v}$ mast cell-deficient mice showed that, under the conditions tested, mast cells were not required to observe the efficacy of alum in the development of antigen-specific antibody and a Th2 cell-biased immune response, or in the enhancement of endogenous antigen-specific CD4 and CD8 T-cell responses [159].

The airway

In addition to IgE and specific antigen and TLR ligands, many mediators that are present in high levels in the airway of asthmatic patients can also stimulate lung mast cells to release products that may influence acute airway responses and/or allergic airway inflammation. Many of these mediators, including ET-1, S-1-P, adenosine, and products of complement activation, activate lung mast cells by binding to G protein-coupled receptors [160]. Adenosine, a metabolic by-product of adenosine triphosphate (ATP), binds to P1 purinoceptors and P1 purinoceptor subtypes A1, A2a, A2b, and A3. Adenosine receptors have been identified in human (A2b) and mouse (A3) mast cells. Adenosine stimulation directly activates human mast cells via A2b to produce chemokines and cytokines [161,162] and can also promote IgE synthesis by B lymphocytes [162]. Airway challenge with adenosine in asthmatics induced mast cell activation and acute release of mast cell-associated mediators, including PGD_2, histamine, and tryptase [163,164], which may contribute to adenosine-induced airway responses [163,165]. The effects of adenosine on IgE-dependent activation of human lung mast cells are rather complex. Adenosine was reported to potentiate IgE-dependent mast cell degranulation at low concentrations, while high concentrations of adenosine inhibited mast cell activation (as reviewed in Okayama *et al.* [160]). Mouse mast cells express A2a, A2b, and A3 receptors and release histamine in response to adenosine via A3 receptors [166]. In mice, adenosine induces airway inflammation and hyperresponsiveness through activation of A3 receptors on mast cells [167,168].

In the asthmatic airway, mast cells are found in close association with the bronchial epithelium (and some mast cells can infiltrate the epithelium itself [Figure 7.2]) [20], mucus glands [169], smooth muscle [17,170], and in the bronchoalveolar space [171]. Epithelial dysfunction is now recognized as a critical underlying mechanism in the pathogenesis of allergic disorders [132]. Mast cell infiltration into the bronchial epithelium may influence aspects of allergic airway inflammation. Asthmatic epithelial cells are a major source of TSLP, which in conjunction with inflammatory cytokines (e.g., TNF and IL-1) can promote Th2 cytokine production in human mast cells in an IgE-independent manner [22]. Mast cell upregulation of epithelial TSLP production contributes importantly to the development of a mouse model of allergic rhinitis [172]. Although mast cell products that upregulate TSLP production in the mouse model of allergic rhinitis have not been identified, mast cell tryptase has been shown to stimulate the release of IL-8 and the proliferation in bronchial epithelial cells [173]. Amphiregulin produced by FcεRI-activated human mast cells has also been shown to upregulate mucin gene expression in epithelial cells, and this mechanism has been hypothesized to promote goblet cell hyperplasia in bronchial asthma [174].

In individuals with asthma, infections with common respiratory viruses such as rhinoviruses, influenza viruses, and respiratory syncytial virus can produce marked exacerbation of the signs and symptoms of asthma [175]. While the mechanisms that account for this striking clinical observation are not fully understood, it is thought that effects of viruses on the function of bronchial epithelial cells may be involved [175]. Mast cells appear in the airway epithelium in asthma [20] and can be activated by viral products via TLRs [28]. However, the role of mast cells (if any) in viral exacerbations of asthma remains to be determined.

As mentioned above, mast cell infiltration of airway smooth muscle (ASM) represents a characteristic pathologic feature of human asthma, while few mast cells were found in the ASM of normal individuals or individuals with eosinophilic bronchitis, a disorder that shares several pathologic features with asthma [17]. Mast cells in the ASM of asthmatic individuals are of tryptase-positive–chymase-positive phenotype and can constitutively express IL-4, IL-13, and TNF [97,176]. Such mast cell derived-mediators and cytokines (and perhaps others) are thought to contribute to ASM hypertrophy, hyperplasia, and hyperreactivity [20,177]. For example, mast cell derived β-tryptase was shown to enhance ASM differentiation and contractibility, at least in part by upregulation of TGF-β secretion in ASM [178]. Tryptase, perhaps via the binding of protease activated receptor 2 (PAR2) on ASM, has also been shown to stimulate the proliferation of ASM *in vitro* [179,180]. ASM activated by mast cells can also secrete products that can promote mast cell recruitment, survival, and function [20]. Tryptase-stimulated ASM can induce mast cell chemotaxis via the production of TGF-β and SCF [18]. Other ASM-derived chemokines, such as CXCL-9, CXCL-10, and CXCL-11, also exhibit mast cell chemotactic activities that can recruit CXCR3+ mast cells into the ASM bundles [19]. TNF derived from IgE/anti-IgE-activated umbilical cord blood-derived mast cells induced TSLP release by ASM cells [22], and exposure to TNF and IL-1 together with ASM-derived TSLP in turn activated mast cells to produce Th2 cytokines [22]. These findings support the hypothesis that the intimate physical association between ASM and lung mast cells in asthma has functional consequences. The proximity of ASM and mast cells may also contribute to the development of nonspecific airway hyperreactivity to agonists such as histamine, cys-LTs, and methacholine [181].

In contrast to the reports by Brightling *et al.* [17] and Carroll *et al.* [169], Wenzel's group [164] did not find differences in the numbers of smooth muscle-associated mast cells in the airways of asthmatics versus control individuals, nor did they document a significant correlation between lung function and mast cell numbers/distribution/phenotype in the large airways of their patients [182]. However, they found that increases in the numbers of chymase-positive mast cells in the small airways were significantly correlated with improved lung function in severe asthma [183]. While it is not clear to what extent the differences in these findings from those of Brightling *et al.* [17] and Carroll *et al.* [170] reflect differences in the patient populations analyzed or other factors, such discrepancies highlight the challenges of using clinical material in efforts to understand the potentially complex roles of mast cells in asthma.

IL-33 is a tissue-derived cytokine involved in allergic inflammation and asthma [184]. Human mast cells constitutively express ST2, the receptor for IL-33, and produce inflammatory cytokines and chemokines, but not lipid mediators (e.g., PGD_2) or histamine, in response to IL-33 stimulation [29,30]. TSLP [30] or IgE cross-linking [29] can synergize with IL-33 to activate mast cells. Mouse mast cells are also responsive to direct activation by IL-33 [185,186]. ST2 is expressed at several stages during the development of the mast cell lineage in the mouse [187] and human

[30], and the maturation of human CD34+ mast cell progenitors is markedly enhanced by IL-33 and TSLP [30]. Furthermore, IL-33 promotes human mast cell survival and adhesion to fibronectin [29]. Therefore, in human asthma, IL-33 released from smooth muscle or other tissue cells could potentially enhance activation and tissue adherence of airway mast cells, as well as promote maturation of recruited mast cell progenitors.

The skin

Mast cells are thought to contribute to IgE-associated allergic inflammation in the skin, but their precise role in the pathogenesis of atopic dermatitis (AD) is uncertain [188,189,190]. Numbers of mast cells can be markedly increased in the involved skin in chronic AD and in mouse models of this disorder [188–191]. In acute lesions in human AD, mast cells are not increased in number, but show signs of degranulation [188]. Mast cells migrate into the epidermis in lesions of AD [192] where mast cells and mast cell products may directly influence keratinocytes, as well as influence local inflammation.

Mast cells are a major source of histamine in the skin. Histamine has been shown to induce keratinocytes to express chemokines (e.g., IL-8, CCL5), cytokines (e.g., IL-6), growth factors (e.g., NGF, GM-CSF), cell-surface molecules (e.g., ICAM-1, human leukocyte antigen (HLA) DR, major histocompatibility complex [MHC] 1) [193–195], and matrix metallopeptidase 9 (MMP-9) [196], a molecule involved in tissue remodeling. Mast cell chymase is increased in chronic atopic dermatitis and may contribute to the epithelial barrier defect which has been identified in this disorder, resulting in enhanced skin permeability to allergens and microbes, and thus aggravation of inflammation [197]. Variants of the mast cell chymase gene located on chromosome 14q11.2 [198,199], as well as mast cell chymase gene 1 (CMA1) promoter polymorphism (rs1800875) [200], have been linked to AD. Polymorphisms in the beta subunit of the high affinity IgE receptor are also strongly associated with AD [201]. These genetic studies are consistent with a role for mast cells in AD.

In AD lesions, the close physical association between mast cells and nerve fibers suggests a role for mast cells in the induction of neurogenic inflammation [202]. Human skin mast cells can be induced to degranulate and release histamine by substance P and VIP, somatostatin, or calcitonin gene-related peptide (CGRP) *in vitro* [203,204] or *in vivo* [205]. Several neuropeptides, including substance P and VIP, have been shown to activate mast cells to release TNF and certain chemokines, which in turn can promote inflammation [206,207]. Tryptase is increased in patients with AD and the activation of skin sensory nerve-associated PAR-2 by tryptase may contribute to pruritus, a clinical hallmark of AD [208].

The potential role of mast cells in mouse models of AD has been investigated in mast cell-deficient mice. In a mouse model of AD, elicited by epicutaneous sensitization with OVA, mast cells appear to be dispensable for the development of skin inflammation, although higher levels of IFNγ mRNA were detected in the sensitized skin in mast cell-deficient $Kit^{W/W-v}$ mice than in wild-type mice [209]. While both FcεRI and FcγRIII/CD16 contribute to the expression of the skin disease in the OVA-induced AD model [210], the cell type responsible for mediating the FcγR-dependent responses has yet to be identified. In another AD model, mast cell-deficient $Kit^{W/W-v}$ or $Kitl^{Sl/Sl-d}$ mice develop markedly reduced skin inflammation elicited by epicutaneous application of cedar pollen [211]. In the cedar pollen dermatitis model, mast cells are likely to be activated by an IgE-independent mechanism since cedar pollen-induced dermatitis was independent of STAT6 and IgE but required the expression of CRTH2, a PGD_2 receptor [211]. These studies indicate that the importance of mast cells in mouse models of AD depends on the experimental conditions. Incongruent results have also been reported in the studies that investigated the roles of mast cells in mouse models of CHS, allergic asthma, and autoimmune arthritis, indicating that mast cells can make significant contribution to certain models of such disorders, but may not detectably contribute to the pathology in other models.

Chronic urticaria is defined as urticaria that lasts for over 6 weeks with near daily symptoms [212]. Inflammation initiated by dermal mast cell degranulation is thought to contribute significantly to this disorder. In autoimmune chronic urticaria, the presence of IgG that reacts with the IgE receptor alpha subunit is detected in 35–40% of patients and IgG anti-IgE in an additional 5–10%, while the etiology in 55% of patients with chronic urticaria is unknown

[212]. In autoimmune chronic urticaria, mast cells are activated by cross-linking of FcεRI by the IgG anti-IgE receptor α chain or IgG anti-IgE. Dermal mast cell activation via complement receptors, primarily the C5aR, may also contribute to mast cell mediator release in this setting [212,213].

The mechanisms of mast cell activation in idiopathic chronic urticaria are not clear. However, skin mast cell-derived IL-1β has been implicated in histamine-independent urticaria in patients with cryopyrin-associated periodic syndrome (CAPS), a disease caused by a mutation of NLRP3 [214]. Transfer of mast cells expressing CAPS disease-associated mutant NLRP3, but not wild-type NLRP3, in mice induced neutrophil recruitment and vascular leakage [214].

Manipulation of mast cell effector function

Many allergic diseases are treated with agents that target mediators which can be derived from mast cells (and other cell types), such as antihistamines and anticysteinyl leukotrienes. However, additional approaches, such as those targeting the IgE-dependent activation of mast cells, are also in use or under investigation. For example, treatment with the anti-IgE antibody omalizumab has shown benefit in some patients with moderate to severe asthma and in patients with intermittent (seasonal) and persistent (perennial) allergic rhinitis [215]. Omalizumab also has been used successfully for the treatment of one patient with a severe case of apparently "idiopathic" cold-induced urticaria, strongly suggesting some role for IgE in that patient's disorder [216].

Administration of anti-IgE reduces free IgE in the serum and tissues, results in reduction in the numbers of FcεRI on mast cells and basophils, and may have other beneficial effects as well [217]. The reduction in numbers of FcεRI expressed by mast cells following anti-IgE therapy (as assessed by immunohistochemistry) is associated with a substantially reduced acute wheal response, as well as, in two out of three individuals, a reduction in the size of the subsequent late-phase reaction) upon intra-dermal challenge with antigen, presumably reflecting reduced IgE-dependent activation of dermal mast cells [218,219]. In addition to stabilizing expression of FcεRI on the mast cell surface, the binding of preparations of monomeric

IgE can also promote the survival *in vitro* of populations of human [53] and mouse [49,50,52,220] mast cells. However, in some experiments no effect of monomeric IgE on human mast cell survival *in vitro* could be identified [51], and we are not aware of reports documenting changes in levels of tissue mast cells in human subjects treated with anti-IgE antibodies [219].

Death receptors (e.g., tumor necrosis factor alpha-related apoptosis-inducing ligand receptor [TRAIL-R]) and inhibitory receptors (FcεRIIB, CD300a, Siglec-8, LAIR-1, SIRP-a, CD200R) expressed by human mast cells recently have been proposed as potential targets for suppressing mast cell function and/or survival [221]. One approach for inhibiting mast cell degranulation/activation is to use IgE Fc-IgG Fc fusion proteins to co-engage mast cell FcεRI with the inhibitory receptor, FcγRIIB [222–224]. Similarly, bifunctional antibodies that cross-link FcεRI and other immunoreceptor tyrosine-based inhibition motif (ITIM)-containing molecules (e.g., CD300a) [225], or agents that directly target intracellular tyrosine phosphatases [226], can also reduce mast cell activation (at least *in vitro*). While the potential utility of these approaches is supported by *in vitro* studies [222,224,226,227] and, in some cases, by tests in experimental animals [222,224,227], they so far have not been evaluated in clinical trials.

Syk is a critical intracellular component downstream of FcεRI receptors in mast cells and basophils, as well as in other signaling pathways in T and B cells [228]. Syk kinase inhibitors have been developed using a high-throughput screen that identifies small molecules that can block IgE signaling in primary cultures of human mast cells [229]. The Syk kinase inhibitor R406 has been shown to prevent mouse mast cell activation *in vitro* and to inhibit airway hyperresponsiveness, airway eosinophilia, and goblet cell metaplasia in a mouse model of asthma [230]. In humans, treatment with the Syk kinase inhibitor R112 has been reported to alleviate acute symptoms of allergic rhinitis [231]. Another Syk kinase inhibitor (R343) is currently in phase I clinical trials for treatment of allergic asthma (http://www.rigel.com).

Corticosteroids are widely used to treat allergic disorders [232,233]. It is well established that one of the effects of corticosteroids on allergic inflammation is suppression of the development of the late phase of allergic reactions [234]. Moreover, corticosteroids have a wide spectrum of cellular targets including epithelial cells, components of the vasculature, lymphocytes, DCs, monocytes/macrophages, granulocytes, and mast cells [232]. Dexamethasone can inhibit cytokine and chemokine production in human umbilical cord blood- or peripheral blood-derived mast cells [51,235,236], but does not suppress degranulation and release of stored mediators by tissue derived-human mast cells activated by an IgE-dependent mechanism [237,238]. Long-term application of corticosteroids leads to reductions in the number of tissue mast cells, probably reflecting diminished mast cell progenitor recruitment and increased apoptosis of tissue mast cells [239].

The search for agents that can be used to manipulate mast cell function (or survival) to achieve therapeutic goals is an active one. However, those developing such agents and testing them clinically must keep in mind that, in vertebrates, mast cells can contribute to health, as well as to diseases. Certainly, there is substantial evidence indicating that mast cells have critical roles in initiating and sustaining allergic inflammation, and may even contribute to the changes in tissue structure and function associated with chronic allergic inflammation. However, an increasing body of evidence derived from studies in mice indicates that mast cells also can have protective functions in innate immunity against certain pathogens and in some settings can provide important anti-inflammatory and immunosuppressive functions. In evaluating the effects of existing and newly introduced therapies on mast cells and the disorders in which they have been implicated, it is important to remember that mast cells also can provide benefits to the host, and that not all of these beneficial roles may yet be understood. Indeed, in addition to efforts to suppress mast cells and their functions when they are harmful, it will be of interest to assess whether certain potentially beneficial mast cell activities can be manipulated to achieve therapeutic ends, such as the enhancement of immune responses that promote health or the suppression of those that result in disease.

Acknowledgment

We thank the members of the Galli lab and our collaborators and colleagues for their contributions to some of the work reviewed herein, apologize to the many other contributors to this field whose work was not cited because of space limitations, and acknowledge the support of United States Public Health Service grants (to SJG) AI23990, AI070813, and CA72074.

References

1 Kitamura Y. Heterogeneity of mast cells and phenotypic change between subpopulations. *Annu Rev Immunol* 1989; **7**: 59–76.

2 Metcalfe DD, Baram D, Mekori YA. Mast cells. *Physiol Rev* 1997; **77**: 1033–79.

3 Kawakami T, Galli SJ. Regulation of mast cell and basophil function and survival by IgE. *Nat Rev Immunol* 2002; **2**: 773–86.

4 Galli SJ, Grimbaldeston MA, Tsai M. Immunomodulatory mast cells: negative, as well as positive, regulators of innate and acquired immunity *Nat Rev Immunol* 2008; **8**: 478–86.

5 Benoist C, Mathis D. Mast cells in autoimmune disease. *Nature* 2002; **420**: 875–8.

6 He SH. Key role of mast cells and their major secretory products in inflammatory bowel disease. *World J Gastroenterol* 2004; **10**: 309–18.

7 Theoharides TC, Conti P. Mast cells: the JEKYLL, and HYDE of tumor growth. *Trends Immunol* 2004; **25**: 235–41.

8 Theoharides TC, Cochrane DE. Critical role of mast cells in inflammatory diseases and the effect of acute stress. *J NeuroImmunol* 2004; **146**: 1–12.

9 Royer B, Varadaradjalou S, Saas P, *et al.* Autocrine regulation of cord blood-derived human mast cell activation by IL-10. *J Allergy Clin Immunol* 2001; **108**: 80–6.

10 Miller HR, Wright SH, Knight PA, Thornton EM. A novel function for transforming growth factor-β1: upregulation of the expression and the IgE-independent extracellular release of a mucosal mast cell granule-specific β-chymase, mouse mast cell protease-1. *Blood* 1999; **93**: 3473–86.

11 Ryan JJ, Kashyap M, Bailey D, *et al.* Mast cell homeostasis: a fundamental aspect of allergic disease. *Crit Rev Immunol* 2007; **27**: 15–32.

12 Kashyap M, Bailey DP, Gomez G, Rivera J, Huff TF, Ryan JJ. TGF-β1 inhibits late-stage mast cell maturation. *Exp Hematol* 2005; **33**: 1281–91.

13 Norozian F, Kashyap M, Ramirez CD, *et al.* TGFβ1 induces mast cell apoptosis. *Exp Hematol* 2006; **34**: 579–87.

14 Zhao W, Gomez G, Yu SH, Ryan JJ, Schwartz LB. TGF-β1 attenuates mediator release and de novo Kit expression by human skin mast cells through a Smad-dependent pathway. *J Immunol* 2008; **181**: 7263–72.

15 Lora JM, Al-Garawi A, Pickard MD, *et al.* FcεRI-dependent gene expression in human mast cells is differentially controlled by T helper type 2 cytokines. *J Allergy Clin Immunol* 2003; **112**: 1119–26.

16 Thienemann F, Henz BM, Babina M. Regulation of mast cell characteristics by cytokines: divergent effects of interleukin-4 on immature mast cell lines versus mature human skin mast cells. *Arch Dermatol Res* 2004; **296**: 134–8.

17 Brightling CE, Bradding P, Symon FA, Holgate ST, Wardlaw AJ, Pavord ID. Mast cell infiltration of airway smooth muscle in asthma. *N Engl J Med* 2002; **346**: 1699–705.

18 Berger P, Girodet PO, Begueret H, *et al.* Tryptase-stimulated human airway smooth muscle cells induce cytokine synthesis and mast cell chemotaxis. *FASEB J* 2003; **17**: 2139–41.

19 Brightling CE, Ammit AJ, Kaur D, *et al.* The CXCL10/CXCR3 axis mediates human lung mast cell migration to asthmatic airway smooth muscle. *Am J Respir Crit Care Med* 2005; **171**: 1103–8.

20 Bradding P, Walls AF, Holgate ST. The role of the mast cell in the pathophysiology of asthma. *J Allergy Clin Immunol* 2006; **117**: 1277–84.

21 Hollins F, Kaur D, Yang W, *et al.* Human airway smooth muscle promotes human lung mast cell survival, proliferation, and constitutive activation: cooperative roles for CADM1: stem cell factor, and IL-6. *J Immunol* 2008; **181**: 2772–80.

22 Allakhverdi Z, Comeau MR, Jessup HK, Delespesse G. Thymic stromal lymphopoietin as a mediator of crosstalk between bronchial smooth muscles and mast cells. *J Allergy Clin Immunol* 2009; **123**: 958–60 e2.

23 Galli SJ, Kalesnikoff J, Grimbaldeston MA, Piliponsky AM, Williams CM, Tsai M. Mast cells as "tunable" effector and immunoregulatory cells: recent advances. *Annu Rev Immunol* 2005; **23**: 749–86.

24 Gilfillan AM, Tkaczyk C. Integrated signalling pathways for mast cell activation. *Nat Rev Immunol* 2006; **6**: 218–30.

25 Rivera J, Gilfillan AM. Molecular regulation of mast cell activation. *J Allergy Clin Immunol* 2006; **117**: 1214–25.

26 Kraft S, Kinet JP. New developments in FcεRI regulation, function and inhibition. *Nat Rev Immunol* 2007; **7**: 365–78.

27 Kalesnikoff J, Galli SJ. New developments in mast cell biology. *Nat Immunol* 2008; **9**: 1215–23.

28 Marshall JS. Mast cell responses to pathogens. *Nat Rev Immunol* 2004; **4**: 787–99.

29 Iikura M, Suto H, Kajiwara N, *et al.* IL-33 can promote survival, adhesion and cytokine production in human mast cells. *Lab Invest* 2007; **87**: 971–8.

30 Allakhverdi Z, Smith DE, Comeau MR, Delespesse G. Cutting edge: The ST2 ligand IL-33 potently activates and drives maturation of human mast cells. *J Immunol* 2007; **179**: 2051–4.

31 Galli SJ, Maurer M, Lantz CS. Mast cells as sentinels of innate immunity. *Curr Opin Immunol* 1999; **11**: 53–9.

32 Moormann C, Artuc M, Pohl E, *et al.* Functional characterization and expression analysis of the proteinase-activated receptor-2 in human cutaneous mast cells. *J Invest Dermatol* 2006; **126**: 746–55.

33 Stopfer P, Mannel DN, Hehlgans T. Lymphotoxin-β receptor activation by activated T cells induces cytokine release from mouse bone marrow-derived mast cells. *J Immunol* 2004; **172**: 7459–65.

34 Fischer M, Harvima IT, Carvalho RF, *et al.* Mast cell CD30 ligand is upregulated in cutaneous inflammation and mediates degranulation-independent chemokine secretion. *J Clin Invest* 2006; **116**: 2748–56.

35 Allakhverdi Z, Comeau MR, Jessup HK, *et al.* Thymic stromal lymphopoietin is released by human epithelial cells in response to microbes, trauma, or inflammation and potently activates mast cells. *J Exp Med* 2007; **204**: 253–8.

36 Kurose M, Saeki K. Histamine release induced by neurotensin from rat peritoneal mast cells. *Eur J Pharmacol* 1981; **76**: 129–36.

37 Metz M, Piliponsky AM, Chen CC, *et al.* Mast cells can enhance resistance to snake and honeybee venoms. *Science* 2006; **313**: 526–30.

38 Varsani M, Pearce FL. Role of phospholipase A2 in mast cell activation. *Inflamm Res* 1997; **46** (Suppl. 1): S9–10.

39 Ziai MR, Russek S, Wang HC, Beer B, Blume AJ. Mast cell degranulating peptide: a multi-functional neurotoxin. *J Pharm Pharmacol* 1990; Jul; **42**: 457–61.

40 Weisel-Eichler A, Libersat F. Venom effects on monoaminergic systems. *J Comp Physiol A Neuroethol Sens Neural Behav Physiol* 2004; **190**: 683–90.

41 Graham C, Richter SC, McClean S, O'Kane E, Flatt PR, Shaw C. Histamine-releasing and antimicrobial peptides from the skin secretions of the dusky gopher frog, *Rana sevosa. Peptides* 2006; **27**: 1313–19.

42 Lind NK. Mechanism of action of fire ant (*Solenopsis*) venoms. I. Lytic release of histamine from mast cells. *Toxicon* 1982; **20**: 831–40.

43 Takei M, Nakagawa H, Endo K. Mast cell activation by pedicellarial toxin of sea urchin, *Toxopneustes pileolus. FEBS Lett* 1993; **328**: 59–62.

44 Cormier SM. Physalia venom mediates histamine release from mast cells. *J Exp Zool* 1981; **218**: 117–20.

45 Soter NA, Wasserman SI. Physical urticaria/angioedema: an experimental model of mast cell activation in humans. *J Allergy Clin Immunol* 1980; **66**: 358–65.

46 Stokes AJ, Shimoda LM, Koblan-Huberson M, Adra CN, Turner H. A TRPV2-PKA signaling module for transduction of physical stimuli in mast cells. *J Exp Med* 2004; **200**: 137–47.

47 Yamaguchi M, Lantz CS, Oettgen HC, *et al.* IgE, enhances mouse mast cell Fc(ε)RI expression *in vitro* and *in vivo*: evidence for a novel amplification mechanism in IgE-dependent reactions. *J Exp Med* 1997; **185**: 663–72.

48 Yamaguchi M, Sayama K, Yano K, *et al.* IgE enhances Fcε receptor I expression and IgE-dependent release of histamine and lipid mediators from human umbilical cord blood-derived mast cells: synergistic effect of IL-4 and IgE on human mast cell Fcε receptor I, expression and mediator release. *J Immunol* 1999; **162**: 5455–65.

49 Kitaura J, Song J, Tsai M, *et al.* Evidence that IgE molecules mediate a spectrum of effects on mast cell survival and activation via aggregation of the FcεRI. *Proc Natl Acad Sci USA* 2003; **100**: 12911–16.

50 Kalesnikoff J, Huber M, Lam V, *et al.* Monomeric IgE stimulates signaling pathways in mast cells that lead to cytokine production and cell survival. *Immunity* 2001; **14**: 801–11.

51 Matsuda K, Piliponsky AM, Iikura M, *et al.* Monomeric IgE enhances human mast cell chemokine production: IL-4 augments and dexamethasone suppresses the response. *J Allergy Clin Immunol* 2005; **116**: 1357–63.

52 Asai K, Kitaura J, Kawakami Y, *et al.* Regulation of mast cell survival by IgE. *Immunity* 2001; **14**: 791–800.

53 Cruse G, Cockerill S, Bradding P. IgE alone promotes human lung mast cell survival through the autocrine production of IL-6. *BMC Immunol* 2008; **9**: 2.

54 Woolhiser MR, Brockow K, Metcalfe DD. Activation of human mast cells by aggregated IgG through FcγRI: additive effects of C3a. *Clin Immunol* 2004; **110**: 172–80.

55 Varadaradjalou S, Feger F, Thieblemont N, *et al.* Toll-like receptor 2 (TLR2) and TLR4 differentially activate human mast cells. *Eur J Immunol* 2003; **33**: 899–906.

56 McCurdy JD, Olynych TJ, Maher LH, Marshall JS. Cutting edge: distinct Toll-like receptor 2 activators selectively induce different classes of mediator production from human mast cells. *J Immunol* 2003; **170**: 1625–9.

57 Okumura S, Yuki K, Kobayashi R, *et al.* Hyperexpression of NOD2 in intestinal mast cells of Crohn's disease patients: preferential expression of inflammatory cell-recruiting molecules via NOD2 in mast cells. *Clin Immunol* 2009; **130**: 175–85.

58 Metz M, Grimbaldeston MA, Nakae S, Piliponsky AM, Tsai M, Galli SJ. Mast cells in the promotion and limitation of chronic inflammation. *Immunol Rev* 2007; **217**: 304–28.

59 Mekori YA, Metcalfe DD. Mast cells in innate immunity. *Immunol Rev* 2000; **173**: 131–40.

60 Grimbaldeston MA, Metz M, Yu M, Tsai M, Galli SJ. Effector and potential immunoregulatory roles of mast cells in IgE-associated acquired immune responses. *Curr Opin Immunol* 2006; **18**: 751–60.

61 Dawicki W, Marshall JS. New and emerging roles for mast cells in host defence. *Curr Opin Immunol* 2007; **19**: 31–8.

62 Blank U, Rivera J. The ins and outs of IgE-dependent mast cell exocytosis. *Trends Immunol* 2004; **25**: 266–73.

63 Sayed BA, Brown MA. Mast cells as modulators of T-cell responses. *Immunol Rev* 2007; **217**: 53–64.

64 Theoharides TC, Kempuraj D, Tagen M, Conti P, Kalogeromitros D. Differential release of mast cell mediators and the pathogenesis of inflammation. *Immunol Rev* 2007; **217**: 65–78.

65 Kandere-Grzybowska K, Letourneau R, Kempuraj D, *et al.* IL-1 induces vesicular secretion of IL-6 without degranulation from human mast cells. *J Immunol* 2003; **171**: 4830–6.

66 Gagari E, Tsai M, Lantz CS, Fox LG, Galli SJ. Differential release of mast cell interleukin-6 via c-kit. *Blood* 1997; **89**: 2654–63.

67 Leal-Berumen I, Conlon P, Marshall JS. IL-6 production by rat peritoneal mast cells is not necessarily preceded by histamine release and can be induced by bacterial lipopolysaccharide. *J Immunol* 1994; **152**: 5468–76.

68 Varadaradjalou S, Feger F, Thieblemont N, *et al.* Toll-like receptor 2 (TLR2) and TLR4 differentially activate human mast cells. *Eur J Immunol* 2003; **33**: 899–906.

69 Kulka M, Alexopoulou L, Flavell RA, Metcalfe DD. Activation of mast cells by double-stranded RNA: evidence for activation through Toll-like receptor 3. *J Allergy Clin Immunol* 2004; **114**: 174–82.

70 Huber M, Helgason CD, Damen JE, Liu L, Humphries RK, Krystal G. The src homology 2-containing inositol phosphatase (SHIP) is the gatekeeper of mast cell degranulation. *Proc Natl Acad Sci USA* 1998; **95**: 11330–5.

71 Kalesnikoff J, Rios EJ, Chen CC, , *et al.* RabGEF1 regulates stem cell factor/c-Kit-mediated signaling events and biological responses in mast cells. *Proc Natl Acad Sci USA* 2006; **103**: 2659–64.

72 Tam SY, Tsai M, Snouwaert JN, *et al.* RabGEF1 is a negative regulator of mast cell activation and skin inflammation. *Nat Immunol* 2004; **5**: 844–52.

73 Kalesnikoff J, Rios EJ, Chen CC, , *et al.* Roles of RabGEF1/Rabex-5 domains in regulating FcεRI surface expression and FcεRI-dependent responses in mast cells. *Blood* 2007; **109**: 5308–17.

74 Kepley CL, Youssef L, Andrews RP, Wilson BS, Oliver JM. Syk deficiency in nonreleaser basophils. *J Allergy Clin Immunol* 1999; **104**: 279–84.

75 Gomez G, Schwartz L, Kepley C. Syk deficiency in human nonreleaser lung mast cells. *Clin Immunol* 2007; **125**: 112–15.

76 Patella V, de Crescenzo G, Ciccarelli A, Marino I, Adt M, Marone G. Human heart mast cells: a definitive case of mast cell heterogeneity. *Int Arch Allergy Immunol* 1995; **106**: 386–93.

77 Stellato C, de Crescenzo G, Patella V, Mastronardi P, Mazzarella B, Marone G. Human basophil/mast cell releasability. XI. Heterogeneity of the effects of contrast media on mediator release. *J Allergy Clin Immunol* 1996; **97**: 838–50.

78 Chong HJ, Andrew Bouton L, Bailey DP, *et al.* IL-4 selectively enhances FcγRIII expression and signaling on mouse mast cells. *Cell Immunol* 2003; **224**: 65–73.

79 Grimbaldeston MA, Nakae S, Kalesnikoff J, Tsai M, Galli SJ. Mast cell-derived interleukin 10 limits skin pathology in contact dermatitis and chronic irradiation with ultraviolet B. *Nat Immunol* 2007; **8**: 1095–104.

80 Tkaczyk C, Okayama Y, Woolhiser MR, Hagaman DD, Gilfillan AM, Metcalfe DD. Activation of human mast cells through the high affinity IgG receptor. *Mol Immunol* 2002; **38**: 1289–93.

81 Hart PH, Grimbaldeston MA, Swift GJ, Jaksic A, Noonan FP, Finlay-Jones JJ. Dermal mast cells determine susceptibility to ultraviolet B-induced systemic suppression of contact hypersensitivity responses in mice. *J Exp Med* 1998; **187**: 2045–53.

82 Hochegger K, Siebenhaar F, Vielhauer V, *et al.* Role of mast cells in experimental anti-glomerular basement membrane glomerulonephritis. *Eur J Immunol* 2005; **35**: 3074–82.

83 Depinay N, Hacini F, Beghdadi W, Peronet R, Mecheri S. Mast cell-dependent downregulation of antigen-specific immune responses by mosquito bites. *J Immunol* 2006; **176**: 4141–6.

84 Lu LF, Lind EF, Gondek DC, *et al.* Mast cells are essential intermediaries in regulatory T-cell tolerance. *Nature* 2006; **442**: 997–1002.

85 Norman MU, Hwang J, Hulliger S, *et al.* Mast cells regulate the magnitude and the cytokine microenvironment of the contact hypersensitivity response. *Am J Pathol* 2008; **172**: 1638–49.

86 Sayed BA, Christy A, Quirion MR, Brown MA. The master switch: the role of mast cells in autoimmunity and tolerance. *Annu Rev Immunol* 2008; **26**: 705–39.

87 Bischoff SC. Role of mast cells in allergic and nonallergic immune responses: comparison of human and murine data. *Nat Rev Immunol* 2007; 7: 93–104.

88 Valent P, Spanblochl E, Sperr WR, *et al.* Induction of differentiation of human mast cells from bone marrow and peripheral blood mononuclear cells by recombinant human stem cell factor/kit-ligand in long-term culture. *Blood* 1992; 80: 2237–45.

89 Saito H, Ebisawa M, Tachimoto H, *et al.* Selective growth of human mast cells induced by Steel factor, IL-6: and prostaglandin E2 from cord blood mononuclear cells. *J Immunol* 1996; 157: 343–50.

90 Saito H. Culture of human mast cells from hemopoietic progenitors. *Methods Mol Biol* 2006; 315: 113–22.

91 Galli SJ, Nakae S, Tsai M. Mast cells in the development of adaptive immune responses. *Nat Immunol* 2005; 6: 135–42.

92 Kirshenbaum AS, Akin C, Wu Y, *et al.* Characterization of novel stem cell factor responsive human mast cell lines LAD 1 and 2 established from a patient with mast cell sarcoma/leukemia; activation following aggregation of FcεRI or FcγRI. *Leuk Res* 2003; 27: 677–82.

93 Butterfield JH, Weiler D, Dewald G, Gleich GJ. Establishment of an immature mast cell line from a patient with mast cell leukemia. *Leuk Res* 1988; 12: 345–55.

94 Bradding P, Okayama Y, Howarth PH, Church MK, Holgate ST. Heterogeneity of human mast cells based on cytokine content. *J Immunol* 1995; 155: 297–307.

95 Barata LT, Ying S, Meng Q, *et al.* IL-4- and IL-5-positive T lymphocytes, eosinophils, and mast cells in allergen-induced late-phase cutaneous reactions in atopic subjects. *J Allergy Clin Immunol* 1998; 101: 222–30.

96 Anderson DF, Zhang S, Bradding P, McGill JI, Holgate ST, Roche WR. The relative contribution of mast cell subsets to conjunctival TH2-like cytokines. *Invest Ophthalmol Vis Sci* 2001; 42: 995–1001.

97 Brightling CE, Symon FA, Holgate ST, Wardlaw AJ, Pavord ID, Bradding P. Interleukin-4 and -13 expression is co-localized to mast cells within the airway smooth muscle in asthma. *Clin Exp Allergy* 2003; 33: 1711–16.

98 Newlands GF, Miller HR, MacKellar A, Galli SJ. Stem cell factor contributes to intestinal mucosal mast cell hyperplasia in rats infected with *Nippostrongylus brasiliensis* or *Trichinella spiralis*, but anti-stem cell factor treatment decreases parasite egg production during *N. brasiliensis* infection. *Blood* 1995; 86: 1968–76.

99 Brandt EB, Strait RT, Hershko D, *et al.* Mast cells are required for experimental oral allergen-induced diarrhea. *J Clin Invest* 2003; 112: 1666–77.

100 Gekara NO, Weiss S. Mast cells initiate early anti-*Listeria* host defences. *Cell Microbiol* 2008; 10: 225–36.

101 Storms W, Kaliner MA. Cromolyn sodium: fitting an old friend into current asthma treatment. *J Asthma* 2005; 42: 79–89.

102 Soucek L, Lawlor ER, Soto D, Shchors K, Swigart LB, Evan GI. Mast cells are required for angiogenesis and macroscopic expansion of Myc-induced pancreatic islet tumors. *Nat Med* 2007; 13: 1211–18.

103 Sun J, Sukhova GK, Yang M, *et al.* Mast cells modulate the pathogenesis of elastase-induced abdominal aortic aneurysms in mice. *J Clin Invest* 2007; 117: 3359–68.

104 Arumugam T, Ramachandran V, Logsdon CD. Effect of cromolyn on S100P interactions with RAGE, and pancreatic cancer growth and invasion in mouse models. *J Natl Cancer Inst* 2006; 98: 1806–18.

105 Norris AA. Pharmacology of sodium cromoglycate. *Clin Exp Allergy* 1996; 26 (Suppl. 4): 5–7.

106 Grimbaldeston MA, Chen CC, Piliponsky AM, Tsai M, Tam SY, Galli SJ. Mast cell-deficient W-sash c-kit mutant Kit$^{W-sh/W-sh}$ mice as a model for investigating mast cell biology *in vivo. Am J Pathol* 2005; 167: 835–48.

107 Zhou JS, Xing W, Friend DS, Austen KF, Katz HR. Mast cell deficiency in Kit^{W-sh} mice does not impair antibody-mediated arthritis. *J Exp Med* 2007; 204: 2797–802.

108 Chervenick PA, Boggs DR. Decreased neutrophils and megakaryocytes in anemic mice of genotype W/W^v. *J Cell Physiol* 1969; 73: 25–30.

109 Nigrovic PA, Gray DH, Jones T, *et al.* Genetic inversion in mast cell-deficient (W^{sh}) mice interrupts corin and manifests as hematopoietic and cardiac aberrancy. *Am J Pathol* 2008; 173: 1693–701.

110 Piliponsky AM, Chen C-C, Grimbaldeston MA, *et al.* Mast cell-derived TNF can exacerbate mortality during severe bacterial infections in C57BL/6-Kit$^{W-sh/W-sh}$ mice. *Am J Pathol* 2010; 176: 926–38.

111 Tchougounova E, Pejler G, Abrink M. The chymase, mouse mast cell protease 4: constitutes the major chymotrypsin-like activity in peritoneum and ear tissue. A role for mouse mast cell protease 4 in thrombin regulation and fibronectin turnover. *J Exp Med* 2003; 198: 423–31.

112 Feyerabend TB, Hausser H, Tietz A, *et al.* Loss of histochemical identity in mast cells lacking carboxypeptidase A. *Mol Cell Biol* 2005; 25: 6199–210.

113 McNeil HP, Adachi R, Stevens RL. Mast cell-restricted tryptases: structure and function in inflammation and pathogen defense. *J Biol Chem* 2007; 282: 20785–9.

114 Scholten J, Hartmann K, Gerbaulet A, *et al.* Mast cell-specific Cre/loxP-mediated recombination *in vivo. Transgenic Res* 2008; 17: 307–15.

115 Boyce JA. The role of mast cells in asthma. *Prostaglandins Leukot Essent Fatty Acids* 2003; **69**: 195–205.

116 Robinson DS. The role of the mast cell in asthma: induction of airway hyperresponsiveness by interaction with smooth muscle? *J Allergy Clin Immunol* 2004; **114**: 58–65.

117 Marone G, Triggiani M, de Paulis A. Mast cells and basophils: friends as well as foes in bronchial asthma? *Trends Immunol* 2005; **26**: 25–31.

118 Galli SJ, Tsai M, Piliponsky AM. The development of allergic inflammation. *Nature* 2008; **454**: 445–54.

119 Caughey GH. Mast cell tryptases and chymases in inflammation and host defense. *Immunol Rev* 2007; **217**: 141–54.

120 Stevens RL, Adachi R. Protease-proteoglycan complexes of mouse and human mast cells and importance of their β-tryptase–heparin complexes in inflammation and innate immunity. *Immunol Rev* 2007; **217**: 155–67.

121 Pejler G, Abrink M, Ringvall M, Wernersson S. Mast cell proteases. *Adv Immunol* 2007; **95**: 167–255.

122 Bradding P, Holgate ST. The mast cell as a source of cytokines in asthma. *Ann N Y Acad Sci* 1996; **796**: 272–81.

123 Saito H, Nakajima T, Matsumoto K. Human mast cell transcriptome project. *Int Arch Allergy Immunol* 2001; **125**: 1–8.

124 Boyce JA. Mast cells and eicosanoid mediators: a system of reciprocal paracrine and autocrine regulation. *Immunol Rev* 2007; **217**: 168–85.

125 Williams CMM, Galli SJ. The diverse potential effector and immunoregulatory roles of mast cells in allergic disease. *J Allergy Clin Immunol* 2000; **105**: 847–59.

126 Kay AB. Allergy and allergic diseases. First of two parts. *N Engl J Med* 2001; **344**: 30–7.

127 Wershil BK, Wang ZS, Gordon JR, Galli SJ. Recruitment of neutrophils during IgE-dependent cutaneous late phase reactions in the mouse is mast cell-dependent. Partial inhibition of the reaction with antiserum against tumor necrosis factor-α. *J Clin Invest* 1991; **87**: 446–53.

128 Marone G, Triggiani M, Genovese A, Paulis AD. Role of human mast cells and basophils in bronchial asthma. *Adv Immunol* 2005; **88**: 97–160.

129 Mukai K, Matsuoka K, Taya C, *et al*. Basophils play a critical role in the development of IgE-mediated chronic allergic inflammation independently of T cells and mast cells. *Immunity* 2005; **23**: 191–202.

130 Larché M, Robinson DS, Kay AB. The role of T lymphocytes in the pathogenesis of asthma. *J Allergy Clin Immunol* 2003; **111**: 450–63.

131 Schleimer RP, Kato A, Kern R, Kuperman D, Avila PC. Epithelium: at the interface of innate and adaptive immune responses. *J Allergy Clin Immunol* 2007; **120**: 1279–84.

132 Holgate ST. Epithelium dysfunction in asthma. *J Allergy Clin Immunol* 2007; **120**: 1233–44.

133 Doherty T, Broide D. Cytokines and growth factors in airway remodeling in asthma. *Curr Opin Immunol* 2007; **19**: 676–80.

134 Mauad T, Bel EH, Sterk PJ. Asthma therapy and airway remodeling. *J Allergy Clin Immunol* 2007; **120**: 997–1009.

135 Holgate ST. Pathogenesis of asthma. *Clin Exp Allergy* 2008; **38**: 872–97.

136 Yu M, Tsai M, Tam SY, Jones C, Zehnder J, Galli SJ. Mast cells can promote the development of multiple features of chronic asthma in mice. *J Clin Invest* 2006; **116**: 1633–41.

137 Brown JM, Wilson TM, Metcalfe DD. The mast cell and allergic diseases: role in pathogenesis and implications for therapy. *Clin Exp Allergy* 2008; **38**: 4–18.

138 Gordon JR, Galli SJ. Release of both preformed and newly synthesized tumor necrosis factor α (TNF-α)/cachectin by mouse mast cells stimulated via the Fc ε RI. A mechanism for the sustained action of mast cell-derived TNF-α during IgE-dependent biological responses. *J Exp Med* 1991; **174**: 103–7.

139 Kendall JC, Li XH, Galli SJ, Gordon JR. Promotion of mouse fibroblast proliferation by IgE-dependent activation of mouse mast cells: role for mast cell tumor necrosis factor-α and transforming growth factor-β 1. *J Allergy Clin Immunol* 1997; **99**: 113–23.

140 Jawdat DM, Albert EJ, Rowden G, Haidl ID, Marshall JS. IgE-mediated mast cell activation induces Langerhans cell migration *in vivo*. *J Immunol* 2004; **173**: 5275–82.

141 Taube C, Stassen M. Mast cells and mast cell-derived factors in the regulation of allergic sensitization. *Chem Immunol Allergy* 2008; **94**: 58–66.

142 Theiner G, Gessner A, Lutz MB. The mast cell mediator PGD2 suppresses IL-12 release by dendritic cells leading to Th2 polarized immune responses *in vivo*. *Immunobiology* 2006; **211**: 463–72.

143 Xue L, Gyles SL, Wettey FR, *et al*. Prostaglandin D2 causes preferential induction of proinflammatory Th2 cytokine production through an action on chemoattractant receptor-like molecule expressed on Th2 cells. *J Immunol* 2005; **175**: 6531–6.

144 Jutel M, Watanabe T, Klunker S, *et al*. Histamine regulates T-cell and antibody responses by differential expression of H1 and H2 receptors. *Nature* 2001; **413**: 420–5.

145 Kashiwakura J, Yokoi H, Saito H, Okayama Y. T-cell proliferation by direct cross-talk between OX40 ligand on human mast cells and OX40 on human T cells:

comparison of gene expression profiles between human tonsillar and lung-cultured mast cells. *J Immunol* 2004; **173**: 5247–57.

146 Nakae S, Suto H, Iikura M, *et al.* Mast cells enhance T-cell activation: importance of mast cell co-stimulatory molecules and secreted TNF. *J Immunol* 2006; **176**: 2238–48.

147 Gri G, Piconese S, Frossi B, *et al.* CD4$^+$CD25$^+$ regulatory T cells suppress mast cell degranulation and allergic responses through OX40–OX40L interaction. *Immunity* 2008; **29**: 771–81.

148 Eisenbarth SC, Piggott DA, Huleatt JW, Visintin I, Herrick CA, Bottomly K. Lipopolysaccharide-enhanced, toll-like receptor 4-dependent T helper cell type 2 responses to inhaled antigen. *J Exp Med* 2002; **196**: 1645–51.

149 Nigo YI, Yamashita M, Hirahara K, *et al.* Regulation of allergic airway inflammation through Toll-like receptor 4-mediated modification of mast cell function. *Proc Natl Acad Sci USA* 2006; **103**: 2286–91.

150 Bryce PJ, Miller ML, Miyajima I, Tsai M, Galli SJ, Oettgen HC. Immune sensitization in the skin is enhanced by antigen-independent effects of IgE. *Immunity* 2004; **20**: 381–92.

151 Gould HJ, Sutton BJ. IgE in allergy and asthma today. *Nat Rev Immunol* 2008; **8**: 205–17.

152 Ghaffar O, Durham SR, Al-Ghamdi K, *et al.* Expression of IgE heavy chain transcripts in the sinus mucosa of atopic and nonatopic patients with chronic sinusitis. *Am J Respir Cell Mol Biol* 1998; **18**: 706–11.

153 KleinJan A, Vinke JG, Severijnen LW, Fokkens WJ. Local production and detection of (specific) IgE in nasal B-cells and plasma cells of allergic rhinitis patients. *Eur Respir J* 2000; **15**: 491–7.

154 Ying S, Humbert M, Meng Q, *et al.* Local expression of ε germline gene transcripts and RNA for the ε heavy chain of IgE in the bronchial mucosa in atopic and nonatopic asthma. *J Allergy Clin Immunol* 2001; **107**: 686–92.

155 Takhar P, Corrigan CJ, Smurthwaite L, *et al.* Class switch recombination to IgE in the bronchial mucosa of atopic and nonatopic patients with asthma. *J Allergy Clin Immunol* 2007; **119**: 213–18.

156 James LK, Durham SR. Rhinitis with negative skin tests and absent serum allergen-specific IgE: more evidence for local IgE? *J Allergy Clin Immunol* 2009; **124**: 1012–13.

157 McLachlan JB, Shelburne CP, Hart JP, *et al.* Mast cell activators: a new class of highly effective vaccine adjuvants. *Nat Med* 2008; **14**: 536–41.

158 Heib V, Becker M, Warger T, *et al.* Mast cells are crucial for early inflammation, migration of Langerhans cells, and CTL responses following topical application of TLR7 ligand in mice. *Blood* 2007; **110**: 946–53.

159 McKee AS, Munks MW, MacLeod MK, *et al.* Alum induces innate immune responses through macrophage and mast cell sensors, but these sensors are not required for alum to act as an adjuvant for specific. *Immunity J Immunol* 2009; **183**: 4403–14.

160 Okayama Y, Saito H, Ra C. Targeting human mast cells expressing G-protein-coupled receptors in allergic diseases. *Allergol Int* 2008; **57**: 197–203.

161 Feoktistov I, Garland EM, Goldstein AE, *et al.* Inhibition of human mast cell activation with the novel selective adenosine A(2B) receptor antagonist 3-isobutyl-8-pyrrolidinoxanthine (IPDX)(2). *Biochem Pharmacol* 2001; **62**: 1163–73.

162 Ryzhov S, Goldstein AE, Matafonov A, Zeng D, Biaggioni I, Feoktistov I. Adenosine-activated mast cells induce IgE synthesis by B lymphocytes: an A2B-mediated process involving Th2 cytokines IL-4 and IL-13 with implications for asthma. *J Immunol* 2004; **172**: 7726–33.

163 Polosa R, Ng WH, Crimi N, *et al.* Release of mast cell-derived mediators after endobronchial adenosine challenge in asthma. *Am J Respir Crit Care Med* 1995; **151**: 624–9.

164 Bochenek G, Nizankowska E, Gielicz A, Szczeklik A. Mast cell activation after adenosine inhalation challenge in patients with bronchial asthma. *Allergy* 2008; **63**: 140–1.

165 Polosa R. Adenosine-receptor subtypes: their relevance to adenosine-mediated responses in asthma and chronic obstructive pulmonary disease. *Eur Respir J* 2002; **20**: 488–96.

166 Zhong H, Shlykov SG, Molina JG, *et al.* Activation of murine lung mast cells by the adenosine A3 receptor. *J Immunol* 2003; **171**: 338–45.

167 Tilley SL, Tsai M, Williams CM, *et al.* Identification of A3 receptor- and mast cell-dependent and -independent components of adenosine-mediated airway responsiveness in mice. *J Immunol* 2003; **171**: 331–7.

168 Hua X, Chason KD, Fredholm BB, Deshpande DA, Penn RB, Tilley SL. Adenosine induces airway hyper-responsiveness through activation of A3 receptors on mast cells. *J Allergy Clin Immunol* 2008; **122**: 107–13, e1–7.

169 Carroll NG, Mutavdzic S, James AL. Increased mast cells and neutrophils in submucosal mucous glands and mucus plugging in patients with asthma. *Thorax* 2002; **57**: 677–82.

170 Carroll NG, Mutavdzic S, James AL. Distribution and degranulation of airway mast cells in normal and asthmatic subjects. *Eur Respir J* 2002; **19**: 879–85.

171 Casolaro V, Galeone D, Giacummo A, Sanduzzi A, Melillo G, Marone G. Human basophil/mast cell releasability. V. Functional comparisons of cells obtained from peripheral blood, lung parenchyma, and bron-

choalveolar lavage in asthmatics. *Am Rev Respir Dis* 1989; **139**: 1375–82.

172 Miyata M, Hatsushika K, Ando T, *et al*. Mast cell regulation of epithelial TSLP expression plays an important role in the development of allergic rhinitis. *Eur J Immunol* 2008; **38**: 1487–92.

173 Cairns JA, Walls AF. Mast cell tryptase is a mitogen for epithelial cells. Stimulation of IL-8 production and intercellular adhesion molecule-1 expression. *J Immunol* 1996; **156**: 275–83.

174 Okumura S, Sagara H, Fukuda T, Saito H, Okayama Y. FcεRI-mediated amphiregulin production by human mast cells increases mucin gene expression in epithelial cells. *J Allergy Clin Immunol* 2005; **115**: 272–9.

175 Gern JE, Busse WW. Relationship of viral infections to wheezing illnesses and asthma. *Nat Rev Immunol* 2002; **2**: 132–8.

176 Bradding P, Roberts JA, Britten KM, *et al*. Interleukin-4: -5: and -6 and tumor necrosis factor-α in normal and asthmatic airways: evidence for the human mast cell as a source of these cytokines. *Am J Respir Cell Mol Biol* 1994; **10**: 471–80.

177 Bradding P. The role of the mast cell in asthma: a reassessment. *Curr Opin Allergy Clin Immunol* 2003; **3**: 45–50.

178 Woodman L, Siddiqui S, Cruse G, *et al*. Mast cells promote airway smooth muscle cell differentiation via autocrine upregulation of TGF-β 1. *J Immunol* 2008; **181**: 5001–7.

179 Berger P, Perng DW, Thabrew H, *et al*. Tryptase and agonists of PAR-2 induce the proliferation of human airway smooth muscle cells. *J Appl Physiol* 2001; **91**: 1372–9.

180 Brown JK, Jones CA, Rooney LA, Caughey GH, Hall IP. Tryptase's potent mitogenic effects in human airway smooth muscle cells are via nonproteolytic actions. *Am J Physiol Lung Cell Mol Physiol* 2002; **282**: L197–206.

181 Wills-Karp M. Immunologic basis of antigen-induced airway hyperresponsiveness. *Annu Rev Immunol* 1999; **17**: 255–81.

182 Tunon-de-Lara JM, Berger P, Marthan R. Chymase-positive mast cells: a double-edged sword in asthma? *Am J Respir Crit Care Med* 2005; **172**: 647–8, author reply 8.

183 Balzar S, Chu HW, Strand M, Wenzel S. Relationship of small airway chymase-positive mast cells and lung function in severe asthma. *Am J Respir Crit Care Med* 2005; **171**: 431–9.

184 Smith DE. IL-33: a tissue derived cytokine pathway involved in allergic inflammation and asthma. *Clin Exp Allergy* 2009; **40**: 200–8.

185 Moulin D, Donze O, Talabot-Ayer D, Mezin F, Palmer G, Gabay C. Interleukin (IL)-33 induces the release of proinflammatory mediators by mast cells. *Cytokine* 2007; **40**: 216–25.

186 Ho LH, Ohno T, Oboki K, *et al*. IL-33 induces IL-13 production by mouse mast cells independently of IgE-FcepsilonRI signals. *J Leukoc Biol* 2007; **82**: 1481–90.

187 Chen CC, Grimbaldeston MA, Tsai M, Weissman IL, Galli SJ. Identification of mast cell progenitors in adult mice. *Proc Natl Acad Sci USA* 2005; **102**: 11408–13.

188 Navi D, Saegusa J, Liu FT. Mast cells and immunological skin diseases. *Clin Rev Allergy Immunol* 2007; **33**: 144–55.

189 Kawakami T, Ando T, Kimura M, Wilson BS, Kawakami Y. Mast cells in atopic dermatitis. *Curr Opin Immunol* 2009; **21**: 666–78.

190 Liu FT, Goodarzi H, Chen WY. IgE, mast cells, and eosinophilic in atopic dermatitis. *Clin Rev Allergy Immunol* 2011 [Epub ahead of print.]

191 Oyoshi MK, He R, Kumar L, Yoon J, Geha RS. Cellular and molecular mechanisms in atopic dermatitis. *Adv Immunol* 2009;**102**: 135–226.

192 Groneberg DA, Bester C, Grutzkau A, *et al*. Mast cells and vasculature in atopic dermatitis—potential stimulus of neoangiogenesis. *Allergy* 2005; **60**: 90–7.

193 Kohda F, Koga T, Uchi H, Urabe K, Furue M. Histamine-induced IL-6 and IL-8 production are differentially modulated by IFN-γ and IL-4 in human keratinocytes. *J Dermatol Sci* 2002; **28**: 34–41.

194 Kanda N, Watanabe S. Histamine enhances the production of nerve growth factor in human keratinocytes. *J Invest Dermatol* 2003; **121**: 570–7.

195 Giustizieri ML, Albanesi C, Fluhr J, Gisondi P, Norgauer J, Girolomoni G. H1 histamine receptor mediates inflammatory responses in human keratinocytes. *J Allergy Clin Immunol* 2004; **114**: 1176–82.

196 Gschwandtner M, Purwar R, Wittmann M, *et al*. Histamine upregulates keratinocyte MMP-9 production via the histamine H1 receptor. *J Invest Dermatol* 2008; **128**: 2783–91.

197 Badertscher K, Bronnimann M, Karlen S, Braathen LR, Yawalkar N. Mast cell chymase is increased in chronic atopic dermatitis but not in psoriasis. *Arch Dermatol Res* 2005; **296**: 503–6.

198 Mao XQ, Shirakawa T, Yoshikawa T, *et al*. Association between genetic variants of mast cell chymase and eczema. *Lancet* 1996; **348**: 581–3.

199 Tanaka K, Sugiura H, Uehara M, Sato H, Hashimoto-Tamaoki T, Furuyama J. Association between mast cell chymase genotype and atopic eczema: comparison between patients with atopic eczema alone and those with atopic eczema and atopic respiratory disease. *Clin Exp Allergy* 1999; **29**: 800–3.

200 Weidinger S, Rummler L, Klopp N, *et al*. Association study of mast cell chymase polymorphisms with atopy. *Allergy* 2005; **60**: 1256–61.

201 Cox HE, Moffatt MF, Faux JA, *et al.* Association of atopic dermatitis to the β subunit of the high affinity immunoglobulin E receptor. *Br J Dermatol* 1998; **138**: 182–7.

202 Jarvikallio A, Harvima IT, Naukkarinen A. Mast cells, nerves and neuropeptides in atopic dermatitis and nummular eczema. *Arch Dermatol Res* 2003; **295**: 2–7.

203 Church MK, Lowman MA, Robinson C, Holgate ST, Benyon RC. Interaction of neuropeptides with human mast cells. *Int Arch Allergy Appl Immunol* 1989; **88**: 70–8.

204 Church MK, el-Lati S, Caulfield JP. Neuropeptide-induced secretion from human skin mast cells. *Int Arch Allergy Appl Immunol* 1991; **94**: 310–18.

205 Huttunen M, Harvima IT, Ackermann L, Harvima RJ, Naukkarinen A, Horsmanheimo M. Neuropeptide- and capsaicin-induced histamine release in skin monitored with the microdialysis technique. *Acta Derm Venereol* 1996; **76**: 205–9.

206 Okayama Y, Ono Y, Nakazawa T, Church MK, Mori M. Human skin mast cells produce TNF-α by substance P. *Int Arch Allergy Immunol* 1998; **117** (Suppl. 1): 48–51.

207 Kulka M, Sheen Ch, Tancowny BP, Grammer LC, Schleimer RP. Neuropeptides activate human mast cell degranulation and chemokine production. *Immunology* 2008; **123**: 398–410.

208 Steinhoff M, Neisius U, Ikoma A, *et al.* Proteinase-activated receptor-2 mediates itch: a novel pathway for pruritus in human skin. *J Neurosci* 2003; **23**: 6176–80.

209 Alenius H, Laouini D, Woodward A, *et al.* Mast cells regulate IFN-γ expression in the skin and circulating IgE levels in allergen-induced skin inflammation. *J Allergy Clin Immunol* 2002; **109**: 106–13.

210 Abboud G, Staumont-Salle D, Kanda A, *et al.* FcεRI, and FcγRIII/CD16 differentially regulate atopic dermatitis in mice. *J Immunol* 2009; **182**: 6517–26.

211 Oiwa M, Satoh T, Watanabe M, *et al.* CRTH2-dependent, STAT6-independent induction of cedar pollen dermatitis. *Clin Exp Allergy* 2008; **38**: 1357–66.

212 Kaplan AP, Greaves M. Pathogenesis of chronic urticaria. *Clin Exp Allergy* 2009; **39**: 777–87.

213 el-Lati SG, Dahinden CA, Church MK. Complement peptides C3a- and C5a-induced mediator release from dissociated human skin mast cells. *J Invest Dermatol* 1994; **102**: 803–6.

214 Nakamura Y, Kambe N, Saito M, *et al.* Mast cells mediate neutrophil recruitment and vascular leakage through the NLRP3 inflammasome in histamine-independent urticaria. *J Exp Med* 2009; **206**: 1037–46.

215 Holgate ST, Djukanovic R, Casale T, Bousquet J. Anti-immunoglobulin E treatment with omalizumab in allergic diseases: an update on anti-inflammatory activity and clinical efficacy. *Clin Exp Allergy* 2005; **35**: 408–16.

216 Boyce JA. Successful treatment of cold-induced urticaria/anaphylaxis with anti-IgE. *J Allergy Clin Immunol* 2006; **117**: 1415–18.

217 Chang TW, Shiung YY. Anti-IgE as a mast cell-stabilizing therapeutic agent. *J Allergy Clin Immunol* 2006; **117**: 1203–12; quiz 13.

218 MacGlashan DW, Jr., Bochner BS, Adelman DC, *et al.* Downregulation of FcεRI, expression on human basophils during *in vivo* treatment of atopic patients with anti-IgE, antibody. *J Immunol* 1997; **158**: 1438–45.

219 Beck LA, Marcotte GV, MacGlashan D, Togias A, Saini S. Omalizumab-induced reductions in mast cell FcεRI expression and function. *J Allergy Clin Immunol* 2004; **114**: 527–30.

220 Kohno M, Yamasaki S, Tybulewicz VL, Saito T. Rapid and large amount of autocrine IL-3 production is responsible for mast cell survival by IgE in the absence of antigen. *Blood* 2005; **105**: 2059–65.

221 Karra L, Berent-Maoz B, Ben-Zimra M, Levi-Schaffer F. Are we ready to downregulate mast cells? *Curr Opin Immunol* 2009; **21**: 708–14.

222 Zhu D, Kepley CL, Zhang K, Terada T, Yamada T, Saxon A. A chimeric human–cat fusion protein blocks cat-induced allergy. *Nat Med* 2005; **11**: 446–9.

223 Kalesnikoff J, Galli SJ. Nipping cat allergy with fusion proteins. *Nat Med* 2005; **11**: 381–2.

224 Mertsching E, Bafetti L, Hess H, *et al.* A mouse Fcγ-Fcε protein that inhibits mast cells through activation of FcγRIIB, SH2 domain-containing inositol phosphatase 1: and SH2 domain-containing protein tyrosine phosphatases. *J Allergy Clin Immunol* 2008; **121**: 441–7 e5.

225 Bachelet I, Munitz A, Levi-Schaffer F. Abrogation of allergic reactions by a bispecific antibody fragment linking IgE to CD300a. *J Allergy Clin Immunol* 2006; **117**: 1314–20.

226 Ong CJ, Ming-Lum A, Nodwell M, *et al.* Small-molecule agonists of SHIP1 inhibit the phosphoinositide 3-kinase pathway in hematopoietic cells. *Blood* 2007; **110**: 1942–9.

227 Zhang K, Kepley CL, Terada T, Zhu D, Perez H, Saxon A. Inhibition of allergen-specific IgE reactivity by a human Ig Fcγ-Fcε bifunctional fusion protein. *J Allergy Clin Immunol* 2004; **114**: 321–7.

228 Gilfillan AM, Rivera J. The tyrosine kinase network regulating mast cell activation. *Immunol Rev* 2009; **228**: 149–69.

229 Rossi AB, Herlaar E, Braselmann S, *et al.* Identification of the Syk kinase inhibitor R112 by a human mast cell screen. *J Allergy Clin Immunol* 2006; **118**: 749–55.

230 Matsubara S, Li G, Takeda K, *et al.* Inhibition of spleen tyrosine kinase prevents mast cell activation and airway hyperresponsiveness. *Am J Respir Crit Care Med* 2006; **173**: 56–63.

231 Masuda ES, Schmitz J. Syk inhibitors as treatment for allergic rhinitis. *Pulm Pharmacol Ther* 2008; **21**: 461–7.

232 Barnes PJ, Adcock IM. How do corticosteroids work in asthma? *Ann Intern Med* 2003; **139**: 359–70.

233 Holgate ST, Polosa R. Treatment strategies for allergy and asthma. *Nat Rev Immunol* 2008; **8**: 218–30.

234 Fokkens WJ, Godthelp T, Holm AF, Blom H, Klein-Jan A. Allergic rhinitis and inflammation: the effect of nasal corticosteroid therapy. *Allergy* 1997; **52** (Suppl. 36): 29–32.

235 Smith SJ, Piliponsky AM, Rosenhead F, Elchalal U, Nagler A, Levi-Schaffer F. Dexamethasone inhibits maturation, cytokine production and FcεRI, expres-sion of human cord blood-derived mast cells. *Clin Exp Allergy* 2002; **32**: 906–13.

236 Kato A, Chustz RT, Ogasawara T, *et al.* Dexamethasone and FK506 inhibit expression of distinct subsets of chemokines in human mast cells. *J Immunol* 2009; **182**: 7233–43.

237 Schleimer RP, Schulman ES, MacGlashan DW, Jr., *et al.* Effects of dexamethasone on mediator release from human lung fragments and purified human lung mast cells. *J Clin Invest* 1983; **71**: 1830–5.

238 Cohan VL, Undem BJ, Fox CC, Adkinson NF, Jr., Lichtenstein LM, Schleimer RP. Dexamethasone does not inhibit the release of mediators from human mast cells residing in airway, intestine, or skin. *Am Rev Respir Dis* 1989; **140**: 951–4.

239 Cole ZA, Clough GF, Church MK. Inhibition by glu-cocorticoids of the mast cell-dependent weal and flare response in human skin *in vivo*. *Br J Pharmacol* 2001; **132**: 286–92.

8 Eosinophils

Nancy A. Lee, Mark V. Dahl, Elizabeth A. Jacobsen, and Sergei I. Ochkur

Mayo Clinic Arizona, Samuel C. Johnson Medical Research Building, Scottsdale, AZ, USA

Introduction

Studies abound linking the presence of eosinophils and/or eosinophil secondary granule proteins with disease or inflammation, including, but not limited to, asthma [1], atopic dermatitis [2,3], cancer [4–6], sinusitis [7], and endometriosis [8]. Eosinophils are traditionally viewed as either end-stage effector cells contributing to disease pathology or simple bystander cells correlating with disease symptoms. However, recent studies have demonstrated that eosinophils are playing a much larger and more robust role in both health and disease. In particular, the development of genetically modified lines of mice deficient of eosinophils has provided invaluable insights that have led this paradigm shift.

For decades, the classical view of eosinophils as destructive effector cells killing cells or tissues indiscriminately by discharging their toxic eosinophil granule proteins has prominently shaped the widespread view as to the perceived roles of these granulocytes. Electron micrographs of the eosinophil secondary granule from wild-type and genetically modified strains are shown in Figure 8.1, in which the genetic deletions of MBP and EPO affect the appearance of the secondary granule (Figure 8.1). However, in this review we will discuss whether eosinophils also have a more constructive role, regulating local immune responses as well as tissue remodeling events. Studies within the last decade have demon-

strated that eosinophils are capable of a multitude of functions, including secretion of immune and remodeling factors (e.g., cytokines, growth factors, proteases, lipases) and interactions with other immune cells (e.g., T cells, mast cells, and dendritic cells). As a result, eosinophils are likely a significant part of a cascade that leads to inflammation and other pathologies. Specifically, in addition to secreting various immune agonist cytokines, eosinophils appear to interact with T cells and possibly dendritic cells as part of a cascade leading to inflammation and other pathologies. They are involved in remodeling, bone synthesis [9] and intimately interact with T cells to modulate the immune response. For example, several of these eosinophil-dependent phenomena have been described in mouse models that are deficient in eosinophils [10]. Indeed, these mouse models as well as human studies have demonstrated that allergies and eosinophils seem to be intertwined in that the presence of allergies coincides with increases in eosinophil numbers. The same could be said for parasites and eosinophils. Despite these specific disease associations, eosinophils are typically such a rare cell type that increases in their numbers generally bear additional scrutiny in all clinical settings.

In this review, we will present studies that document the presence of eosinophils in airway allergic disease and inflammation in the respiratory tract. We will describe the three types of asthma: (i) allergic, nonatopic asthma, (ii) atopic asthma, and (iii)

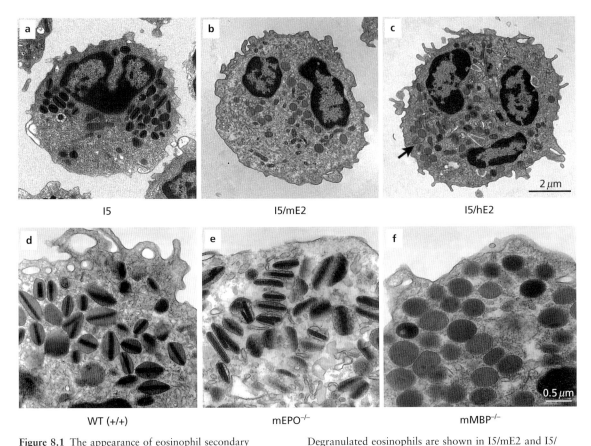

Figure 8.1 The appearance of eosinophil secondary granules in transgenic mice. Electron micrographs showing eosinophil granules from NJ.1638 mice (A, I5), from degranulated eosinophils in I5E2 double transgenic mice (B and C, I5/mE2 and I5/HE2), from wild-type mice (D, WT(+/+)), and from mice with knockouts of the granule proteins eosinophil peroxidase (E, mEPO$^{-/-}$) and major basic protein (panel F, mMBP$^{-/-}$). The eosinophil secondary granules are intact and seen in I5 and WT mice. Degranulated eosinophils are shown in I5/mE2 and I5/hE2. Granules missing the key eosinophil granule proteins are shown in mEPO$^{-/-}$, where the matrix of the secondary granule is decreased leaving the granules thinner and less full, and in mMBP$^{-/-}$, where the granules are lacking the core MBP structural protein. The arrow in C denotes the ghost images of the core of the eosinophil secondary granule showing that the granule and its core proteins have been dispersed.

refractory steroid-resistant asthma. We will discuss mouse models of asthma, airway allergic disease, and respiratory inflammation. Finally, we will also discuss reports of interactions between eosinophils and other cells in the immune system.

Eosinophils and asthma

Asthma is a human disease of the lungs and airways that can encompass pathologies outside the lungs as well. Individuals with asthma have reversible shortness of breath, episodes of wheezing and chest congestion, and feel that they cannot get enough air. In severe cases, asthma can result in death if not treated. Frequently, asthma is found in people with allergies. The Allergy and Asthma Foundation of America reports that approximately 20 million Americans have asthma, with 50% of these individuals reporting allergic asthma symptoms. An allergic reaction in the airways and lungs causes the musculature around the airways to constrict, causing breathlessness and wheezing. There is also increased mucus accumulation, causing congestion and productive coughing, and diminished lung capacity.

Research scientists and physicians who study asthma can mimic many of these asthmatic symptoms in animals. However, in animal models, this syndrome is referred to as allergic airway inflammation or allergic respiratory inflammation. Airway hyperresponsiveness to molecular stimulation (e.g., methacholine) can be demonstrated in animal models of allergic airway inflammation. Studies using mice have provided insights regarding many of the fundamental mechanisms underlying asthma. However, the word "asthma" is reserved to describe human patients with reversible, reproducible, and diminished respiratory capacity, and is not used for animals.

Asthma in humans

Asthma in humans can be divided into three predominant groups: (i) nonatopic allergic asthma, e.g., asthma associated with allergies, (ii) atopic asthma associated with persistently high immunoglobulin E (IgE), levels, hay fever, and atopic dermatitis (AD), and (ii) nonallergic asthma, which is asthma that is not associated with allergies and is refractory to steroids like prednisone. Other subclasses of asthma such as exercise-induced asthma, nocturnal asthma, or emotional asthma are often included within these three overall categories.

Asthma is precipitated by the immune system. Notably, T cells, which can be divided into two major categories, helper (Th) and cytotoxic (Tc), are exceptionally important. In addition to Th and Tc cells, a third subclass of T cells called T regulatory (Treg) cells act to suppress activation of the immune system. Th cells are often subdivided into two functionally distinct subsets, Th1 and Th2 cells, based on the cytokines secreted by the Th cell [11]. Th1 cells are associated with interferon gamma (IFN-γ) production, immune responses to bacterial and viral infections, autoimmune diseases, and are found to be associated with tumors, albeit in a dormant, nonactive state. Th2 cells are active producers of the proinflammatory cytokine interleukin 4 (IL-4), which is also necessary for Th2 differentiation. Th2 cells also produce IL-5 and IL-13, key inflammatory cytokines that are important for eosinophil survival and proliferation. Importantly, the increase in mucus produc-

tion by IL-13 [12,13] blocks the airway and decreases the lung capacity in asthma.

In addition to T cells, eosinophils are key immune modulators and remodeling agents in asthma. Their numbers are increased by IL-5, permitting significant accumulation of a rare cell type in the lungs of asthmatics [14,15]. Eosinophil numbers are increased in the presence of allergic disease, such as asthma, AD, and hay fever. Eosinophil granule proteins are increased in the sputum and are found in the interstitial areas of the airways of asthmatics. In addition, the deposition of eosinophil secondary granule proteins may be responsible for much of the epithelial desquamation that occurs in asthma [16]. This sloughing of epithelial cells together with mucus accumulation contributes to airway obstruction and decreases lung capacity. In addition to these lung remodeling events, eosinophils produce many cytokines that alter the local immune microenvironment. For example, eosinophils in individuals with asthma produce significant levels of IL-4 [17,18] and IL-13 [19].

Eosinophils express several Fc receptors, which may also be involved in signaling cascades that trigger the eosinophil to express certain cytokines and inflammatory mediators [20]. Eosinophils are known to express the low affinity Fcγ receptor, FcγRII (CD32), and can also express FcγRIII (CD16) under certain conditions [20,21]. Eosinophils express the low affinity IgE receptor, FcεRII (CD23) [22], and they may express the high affinity IgE receptor [22,23]. In addition, eosinophils express a lectin-like protein, eBP/Mac2, which has low affinity for IgE, as well [24]. Eosinophils also express the IgA receptor, FcαRI (CD89), and are involved in mucosal IgA responses [25]. Signaling cascades involving the Fc receptors are obviously important to eosinophil functions, survival, and cytokine expression, especially with regards to eosinophil modulation of the immune microenvironment. The possible importance of signaling through the Fc receptors will be discussed below.

Allergic nonatopic asthma

Allergic asthma is frequently observed in atopic patients, but is also seen in nonatopic individuals. Patients can be allergic without being atopic; however, atopic patients are always allergic, as discussed in more detail below. Allergic nonatopic asthma has been referred to in the past as "extrinsic asthma;" however, the use of extrinsic and intrinsic asthma to denote allergic and nonallergic asthma is now outdated. Allergies to airborne or tactile substances are generally the precipitating event in allergic asthma and atopic individuals. Thus, many of the same medications are used for allergic, nonatopic asthma and atopic asthma because the initiation of breathing difficulty can usually be traced to exposure to a specific allergen with both allergic, nonatopic and atopic asthma.

These medications are designed to manipulate the immune system or relax the muscles lining the airways. Prednisone and related anti-inflammatory steroids, which are well known for their many and myriad side-effects, decreases eosinophil and T-cell viability [26]. Inhaled corticosteroids (ICS) largely avoid many of the side-effects associated with oral steroids and reduce the inflammation in the lungs and airways of asthmatics. Medications that stimulate the β_2-adrenergic receptor and relax the smooth muscles surrounding the airways, sometimes referred to as "rescue" inhalants, can provide relief in urgent situations as a last resort before calling the emergency room or physician. Epinephrine works along the same molecular pathway, although they must be injected to be effective.

Leukotriene modifiers are cysteinyl leukotriene receptor (cys-LT1) antagonists (montelukast [Singulair, Merck & Co. Inc. Whitehouse Station, NJ, USA], zafirlukast [Accolate®, AstraZeneca Pharmaceuticals, Wilmington, DE, USA]) or inhibitors of 5-lipoxygenase (zileuton [Zyflo, Abbot Laboratories, Abbott Park, IL, USA]) which are often prescribed for asthma. The cys-LTs (LTC [4], LTD [4], LTE [4]), are released by eosinophils, basophils, and mast cells. Montelukast and zafirlukast bind to the cys-LT1 receptor on mast cells and eosinophils. Zileuton inhibits production of the cys-LTs, as well as leukotriene B by inhibition of the 5-lipoxygenase pathway. Montelukast and other leukotriene antagonists have been effective in treating eosinophilic esophagitis [27] as well as AD [28], a skin disease (discussed below) characterized by dermal deposition of eosinophil granule proteins. Leukotrienes act to attract and recruit eosinophils, constrict smooth muscle, cause swelling of the airways and mucous hypersecretion, and reduce ciliary motility [29]. The exact mechanism of leukotriene inhibitors is not known, although their known effects on leukotrienes and inflammation have been well documented [30].

It is unclear if they have more specific effects on eosinophils, although some studies suggest that inhibition of these pathways reduces eosinophil survival [31,32]. For example, their effects on eosinophilic esophagitis and AD are compelling.

Mepolizumab (Bosatria, anti-IL-5, GlaxoSmith-Kline, Waltham, MA, USA) and other anti-IL-5 therapeutics (SCH55700) are monoclonal antibodies against IL-5, which is required for eosinophil proliferation and survival. Surprisingly, early reports showed that anti-IL-5 treatment of asthmatics did not increase lung function [33–35]. However, two recent reports suggest that mepolizumab treatment of asthmatics will increase lung function and reduce exacerbations [36,37]. The differences in these results is probably a result of the patient selection criteria, where the latter experiments focus on allergic asthmatic patients with defined levels of eosinophils in the sputum. Ultimately, these new results suggest that anti-IL-5 therapy is efficacious in individuals with high levels of eosinophils. Interestingly, separate studies also suggest that imatinib mesylate (Gleevec, Novartis, Basel, Switzerland) is another medication that can result in decreased eosinophils, whether or not individuals have a fusion of the Fip1-like 1 gene (*FIG1L1*) and the gene encoding platelet-derived growth factor receptor alpha (PDGFRA) [38,39]. Imatinib has also been shown to reduce eosinophils in a mouse model of asthma [40]. These findings leave open a role for an unidentified tyrosine kinase in the pathways involving eosinophil survival and IL-5. Additional clinical trials with individuals with asthma using mepolizumab or imatinib mesylate remain to be conducted.

Omalizumab (Xolair®, rhuMAb-E25, IgE 025; Genentech/Novartis, South San Francisco, CA, USA, and Tanox, Inc., Houston, TX, USA) is a humanized monoclonal antibody consisting of 95% human IgG1 and 5% murine IgG, and is believed to work by binding free serum IgE, thus blocking the binding of IgE with its receptor [41]. It binds to the IgE molecule in solution and thus inhibits the binding of the IgE antibody to the high affinity receptor on basophils and mast cells as well as eosinophils [23,42]. Omalizumab treatment of allergic asthmatics has been shown to reduce airway inflammation in asthmatic individuals [43]. It has been shown in atopic patients that omalizumab treatment actually reduces the number of receptors for IgE on basophils [44]. Saini *et al.* [45] have shown that the lack of IgE binding to its surface receptor decreases the cell surface presentation of the high-affinity receptor (CD16) on basophils, but that the level of expression of the low affinity IgE receptor (CD23) did not correlate with serum IgE levels.

Omalizumab treatment has also been shown to prevent anaphylaxis during rush immunotherapy [46,47]. Presumably, omalizumab has not been used in emergency rooms to treat anaphylaxis due to an allergic reaction because it has been reported that one or two individuals out of 1000 will experience anaphylaxis due to the omalizumab itself. Interestingly, studies are under way to determine if omalizumab can be used during immunotherapy for substances that ordinarily lead to anaphylaxis. For example, patients had reduced sensitivity to peanut allergen after omalizumab treatment [48]. Further studies are ongoing, but the potential for patients with anaphylactic reactions to insect stings and peanut antigen is encouraging. The potential for a high-affinity inhibitor of the Fcε receptor is extremely promising.

Atopy and atopic asthma

Ten to twenty percent of infants develop an allergic syndrome soon after birth called "atopy." Pierce *et al.* [49] have estimated that as many as 40% of individuals with asthma have atopy. The word "atopy" is derived from the Greek word *atopos*, meaning "out of place," "special" or "unusual." The word "eczema" is derived from the German, *ekzein*, to erupt, or *Zein* (Boil) and *ex* (out). Atopic patients have very high IgE, levels, and their immune system is characterized by a tendency to develop allergies and is Th2 dominant. AD, also termed atopic eczema, is a chronic relapsing skin condition with an underlying genetic component. Commonly, patients with atopy have the "allergic triad"—eczema or AD, hay fever or allergic rhinitis, and asthma. At present, there is no molecular or diagnostic test for atopy. Diagnosis of atopy is usually made after careful consideration of all the presenting signs, followed by an understanding of the family medical history and the accompanying medical issues. Atopy is essentially a genetic disease of the immune system, although environmental factors are key in its manifestation. Notably, eosinophils or the eosinophil granule proteins can usually be found in association with allergies and AD (reviewed by Martin *et al.* [50] and Gleich and Leiferman [51]).

As mentioned, there is no clinical test or molecular diagnosis for atopy. However, there are several significant and key features that are associated with atopy. The inclusive criteria used in clinical studies of atopic patients varies, but generally include total serum IgE levels, skin tests indicative of atopic allergy, and family histories. Some physicians have also used specific T-cell responses or skin responses as an indication of atopy. For example, a wheal and flare reaction to *Staphylococcus aureus* is indicative of atopy.

Atopy is associated with a Th2-dominant phenotype. Because atopic asthma is a familial syndrome, researchers have tried to map susceptibility genes for atopy in the human genome. Based on these studies, they have identified a number of candidate genes (reviewed in Ober and Moffatt [52]). Not surprisingly, these genes tend toward histocompatibility genes, cytokine genes such as IL-4, or genes that could be involved in the Th2 or IgE response to an allergen (reviewed by Blumenthal [53]). Six major regions have been described which correspond to genes known to be involved with histocompatibility genes (chromosome 6p21), cytokine genes such as IL-13 (chromosome 5q) or IL-4 (chromosome 16p12), CD4, a cell surface molecule important for Th2 CD4$^+$ cells (chromosome 2q), the IgE receptor, FcεRIβ, (chromosome 11q) [54], STAT6 and NOS1, important in Th2 responses (chromosome 12q), and eotaxin, an eosinophil chemoattractant (chromosome 17q). Comprehensive reviews of the literature have been published by Blumenthal [53] and Hoffjan *et al.* [55]

Multiple cells, genes, and environmental factors are involved in atopy, including eosinophils

Multiple factors are important in the development of atopy and AD. First, there must be a genetic defect in the signaling pathway to activate Th2 cells and Th2 immune responses, leading to heightened eosinophil activation, increased eosinophil numbers, and correspondingly lowered Th1 responses (fungal and viral infections). Second, a defective skin barrier in atopic patients leads to increased colonization by *S. aureus* [56]. Concomitantly, there is an allergic response to *S. aureus* colonization on the skin, resulting in the characteristic lesions of atopic eczema and the classical wheal and flare response to *S. aureus* in a skin test [57–60]. Third, there may be an Epstein–Barr virus (EBV) infection of the B cells in atopic patients such that extremely high levels of IgE are produced in the absence of antigen stimulation [61,62]. We believe that these factors, taken together, constitute the atopic pathology and phenotype. The role of eosinophils, which play an integral role in Th2 inflammation and immunity, remains to be determined. However, studies with transgenic mice [63] have indicated that eosinophils are required elements of Th2 immunity in airway inflammation. A transgenic mouse line has recently been created that causes inducible loss of eosinophils (iPHIL; EA Jacobsen, NA Lee, JJ Lee, unpublished data). Studies using iPHIL are under way to explore the role of eosinophils in the induction of Th2 inflammation in asthma and other allergic diseases such as atopy.

Atopic asthma, therefore, is essentially a disease of the immune system. Pharmaceuticals could be developed that target the Th2 dominance of the immune system in atopy. For example, pharmaceuticals that address the altered signaling pathway in atopic patients, such as the major histocompatibility complex (MHC), IL-4, or Fc receptor genes, could be targeted. In addition, pharmaceuticals that address the allergic response to *S. aureus* on the skin, and presumably cause the itching and eczema, in addition to the asthma associated with atopy, could also be developed. The importance of signaling through the Fcε receptor expressed on various cell types, including eosinophils [23], basophils, mast cells [64], and other antigen-presenting cells such as Langerhans cells [65,66], has yet to be fully realized for nonatopic allergic asthma (as mentioned above) and for atopic allergies as well.

Pharmaceuticals, such as omalizumab, that target this Fc receptor signaling pathway may well be promising. Physicians have been reluctant to use omalizumab with atopic patients because they frequently show very high levels of serum IgE and it would be impractical to administer enough omalizumab to bind all the free IgE. However, Sheinkopf *et al.* [67] have found that positive results are obtained even when omalizumab was administered to atopic patients with very high levels of serum IgE—too high to be bound by the administered omalizumab. They have postulated that that the efficacious action of omalizumab may be by a mechanism distinct from its binding of free IgE molecules. Since there are two independent binding sites for omalizumab on each IgE and each omalizumab can bind two independent IgE molecules, there is potential to form interlocking complexes with omalizumab and IgE. It is also important to note that the Fc portion of omalizumab is intact and free to bind to the Fcγ receptors. Zhang *et al.* [68] have reported that coaggregation of the Fcγ receptor with the Fcε receptor inhibits IgE-mediated reactivity. Similarly, Bruhns *et al.* [69] report that FcεRI coengagement with the Fcγ receptor can dampen IgE-induced allergic inflammation. Thus, omalizumab binding to the Fcγ receptor, and possibly FcγRII (CD32) on eosinophils, may be an alternate pathway by which omalizumab regulates the allergic response. Binding to the Fcγ receptor on immune cells may activate a second pathway or downregulate the allergic response pathway that is triggered by binding to the Fcε receptor by IgE. Omalizumab could bind to (and cross-link or coaggregate) the Fcγ receptors and thus provide a signal that would subsequently downregulate the allergic response. This omalizumab–Fcγ binding may initiate an alternate mechanism by which omalizumab might be acting. This would explain why omalizumab can be effective in spite of the high and various serum IgE levels in atopic patients [67]. Such a mechanism would also explain the efficacy of omalizumab in patients with eosinophil esophagitis (EE) as well as other eosinophil-associated gastrointestinal disorders [70]. It is also noteworthy that an alternate pathway utilizing Fcγ receptors explains one of the goals of immunodesensitization therapy—to generate IgG antibodies instead of IgE. Triggering the Fcγ receptor or coaggregating the Fcγ and Fcε receptors may turn out to be invaluable in regulating runaway allergic responses triggered by binding to the Fcε receptor. Such a mechanism could represent a long sought after goal of treating food allergies, bee stings, and seasonal allergies by fundamentally downregulating the allergic response. That is, if triggering or coaggregating the Fcγ receptor blunts IgE-mediated responses, a pharmaceutical designed to bind the Fcγ receptor might be useful in treating patients with potentially fatal allergic reactions to bee stings and food allergies such as peanuts and shrimp. A different anti-IgE antibody, TNX-901, distinct from the better known omalizumab, has been shown to increase the tolerated dose of peanut antigen in one trial [71]. Further investigation into the ramifications and benefits of anti-IgE antibodies as well as drugs designed to bind and cross-link the Fcγ receptors is certainly warranted.

The data from Scheinkopf et al. [67] show that omalizumab can be effective even in atopic patients with very high serum IgE levels. Since the constant itching of atopic eczema could be due primarily to an IgE-mediated allergy to S. aureus (as discussed above), and since omalizumab may blunt the allergic response in atopic children notwithstanding their persistently high serum IgE levels, a clinical trial of omalizumab in children with AD could prove its effectiveness with the lesions and itching of atopic eczema. Omalizumab treatment may act as "rush immunotherapy" when the antigen is ubiquitous like S. aureus. Similarly, if omalizumab works by triggering the Fcγ receptor, and if this will blunt the IgE-mediated allergenic response, pharmaceuticals that bind and aggregate the Fcγ receptor are worth developing. These possibilities, coupled with omalizumab's effectiveness with nonatopic allergic patients illustrates the need for an orally active small-molecule antagonist of the IgE receptor, which remains to be developed. Human IgE-producing B cells would also be a target for potential therapy. Chang and others have described a monoclonal antibody specific for human IgE-producing B cells [72]. This antibody, or a small molecule that binds to the same epitope, should be very useful to counter IgE in atopic and other patients.

Nonallergic asthma

Nonallergic asthma is often not responsive to prednisone treatment. Tedeschi and Asero [73] have proposed that some asthmas, especially nonallergic asthma, could be due to autoimmune pathology related to other disorders, such as chronic autoimmune urticaria. For example, an autoantibody could bind to the high-affinity IgE receptor, thus causing chronic release of histamine and resulting in chronic urticaria and asthma [73]. In addition, Churg–Strauss syndrome is associated with autoimmune antibodies and asthma [74]. Interestingly, a population-based study of individuals with Crohn disease, an autoimmune disorder of the intestine, showed that sufferers had greater likelihood of having asthma [75]. Mansi et al. [76] also found bronchial hyperresponsiveness in children and adolescents with Crohn disease.

Steroid-resistant asthma patients pose a difficult problem for physicians because the pathology of their asthma is markedly different than the allergic, steroid-sensitive patient. Thus, this refractory asthma should be responsive to one of the newer anti-TNF (tumor necrosis factor) medications that have been so successfully used against other autoimmune diseases such as rheumatoid arthritis [77]. In fact, some recent clinical studies show that asthmatics who do not respond to prednisone often breathe better when treated with etanercept (Enbrel, Amgen, Thousand Oaks, CA, USA/Wyeth, now Pfizer, New York, NY, USA) or infliximab (Remicade, Centocor Ortho Biotech Inc., Horsham, PA, USA) [78]. In addition, it should be possible to identify the target of the presumed autoantibodies that result in asthma, and to further refine our understanding of the smooth muscles and airways affected during asthma.

Animal models of asthma

Animal models that display many of the pathologies associated with asthma, as well as airway hyperresponsiveness, often have induced allergic respiratory inflammation, either via immunologic stimulation or genetically through transgenic technology. Using these methods, investigators have focused on the cell types that are required elements in airway hyperresponsiveness and the pathologies associated with asthma. On the basis of this evidence, the significant cell populations that most affect asthma are eosinophils and T cells, discussed below, although other cell types, such as dendritic cells, can still be important.

Eosinophils are required elements in mouse models of asthma

A common feature in human asthma is that eosinophils can be found in the airways and lungs as well as the expectorant phlegm. We created mouse models of asthma that were designed to simulate the increase in eosinophils in the lungs. NJ.1726 [79] was created by using the lung-specific Clara cell promoter CC10 to drive the expression of IL-5 in the lungs. This NJ.1726 mouse reproduced many, but not all, of the pathologies associated with asthma as shown in Table 8.1. Notably, airway hyperresponsiveness was apparent in these mice, but was not as high as the increased order of magnitude as is

Table 8.1 Asthmatic pathologies in humans and mice.

	Induced pulmonary pathologies	Wild type	Acute OVA challenge	Constitutive IL-5 transgenic model	Human asthma patient	IL-5/eotaxin-2 transgenic model (I5E2)	I5E2/PHIL
Pulmonary remodeling events	Goblet cell metaplasia with increased airway epithelial mucin accumulation	–	+	+	++	++	–
	Airway epithelial desquamation and mucus accumulation leading to obstruction	–	–	–	+++	++++	–
	Extracellular matrix deposition around central airways (e.g., collagen)	–	–	+	++	++	–
	Airway epithelial hypertrophy	–	+	+	++	++	–
	Airway smooth muscle thickening (i.e., hyperplasia)	–	–	+/–	++++	++	–
	Increased numbers of tissue myofibroblasts	–	–	+	+++	+++	–
	Pulmonary eosinophilia in both the airway lumen and interstitial lung tissues	–	+++	++	++	+++	–
	Extensive eosinophil degranulation	–	+/–	+/–	+++	+++	–
	Progressive pathology leading to the breakdown of alveolar septa	–	–	–	+++	+++	–
Pulmonary dysfunction	Airway hyperresponsiveness and hyperreactivity	–	+	+	+++	+++	–

This table shows the various major pathologies expected in asthma or allergic airways disease in mice on the vertical axis. Humans as well as different mouse models of asthma are shown on the horizontal axis. Acute ovalbumin (OVA) challenge lists pathologies observed in wild-type mice undergoing OVA sensitization and challenge [79]. Constitutive IL-5 transgenic models refers to NJ.1726 [79]; IL-5/eotaxin-2 transgenic model (I5E2) refers to the CD3delta-IL-5 transgenic crossed to the CC10-eotaxin 2 transgenic [80]. The I5E2/PHIL data refer to the I5E2 mouse crossed to the PHIL mouse [10].

observed in humans. Similarly, there was no evidence of eosinophil degranulation or epithelial desquamation. In human asthma, the degranulation of eosinophils leads to the deposition of the toxic, highly basic granule proteins on the airway epithelium. This may then lead to a sloughing-off of the epithelial layer, or "desquamation." Our most recent mouse model of asthma expresses both IL-5 and eotaxin2 (I5E2) [80]. This mouse expresses IL-5 from the T-cell-specific promoter CD3delta, such that all T cells now express IL-5 [81]. In addition, this double transgenic mouse also carries a gene that expresses I5E2 specifically in the lungs from the lung-specific promoter CC10. I5E2 is a powerful eosinophil chemoattractant. The result is that the T cells induce very high levels of eosinophils in the blood and bone marrow, and the I5E2 draws them into the lung tissues. This I5E2 mouse now duplicates many of the pathologic features of asthma as well as greatly increased airway hyperresponsiveness, eosinophil degranulation, and epithelial desquamation (Table 8.1 and Figure 8.2). The I5E2 mouse has severe lung dysfunction during methacholine challenge, not unlike humans who undergo fatal asthma exacerbations (see below).

In addition to the I5E2 mouse, we have also been able to create a mouse in which there are no eosinophils (PHIL) [82]. This mouse does not develop allergic airway inflammation or airway hyperresponsiveness, even when crossed to the I5E2 mouse (I5E2, PHIL; triple transgenic). Thus, we have definitively shown that eosinophils are required for the allergic airway inflammation indicative of asthma in humans. Future experiments with PHIL are ongoing, including the creation of an inducible PHIL (iPHIL) in which the presence or absence of eosinophils can be manipulated in a temporal manner in the same animal (iPHIL, EA Jacobsen, NA Lee, JJ Lee, unpublished data).

Fatal asthma is often associated with extensive eosinophil degranulation and epithelial desquamation (see Figure 8.2d). We observe a very similar histopathology in our double transgenic I5E2 using T-cell-expressed IL-5 with lung-specific I5E2 expression (Figure 8.2a and b). These double transgenic mice sometimes die when undergoing methacholine treatment to measure lung function [80]. Sergei Ochkur, the author of this study, is continuing this work to examine the double transgenic phenotype on a major basic protein (MBP) knockout and on an eosinophil peroxidase (EPO) knockout background. If these animals are able to survive the methacholine treatment, this may point toward the use of monoclonal antibodies directed toward specific eosinophil granule proteins like MBP or EPO as a treatment for near-fatal asthma or anaphylaxis on a emergency basis or in the emergency room.

Eosinophils in Δdb/GATA mice

GATA is widely acknowledged as a transcription factor that is important in the expression of the eosinophil granule proteins (e.g., see Hirasawa et al. [83]). Mice with a knockout of the GATA upstream region seem to have a deficiency of eosinophils [84]. However, we believe the GATA deletion in the Δdb/GATA mice may be deleting the eosinophil granule, but not the eosinophil itself. All current eosinophil-specific stains depend on the presence of the granule proteins; thus, a granule-deficient eosinophil would not be identified as an eosinophil by commonly used stains. In fact, the original description of the Δdb/GATA mice shows a significantly important piece of data in Figure 8.2 [85].

Yu et al. [85] clearly show the presence of cells marked "EO" in the single transgenic Δdb/GATA in the fluorescence-activated cell sorting (FACS) data. These cells, which include the eosinophils resulting from the presence of the wild-type allele but could also be any eosinophils lacking granule proteins, are absent in the double transgenic (Δdb/GATA, IL-5 transgene), and there are also additional cells marked "MONO (mononuclear cells)" as well as "large unclassified cells" (LUC). The percentages of cells in each population are not stated; thus, no comparison is given between the number of cells marked EO, MONO, or LUC in the Δdb/GATA single transgenic and the wild-type mouse.

Humbles et al. [84] and others who have subsequently used these mice do not present FACS or other data that would highlight these problematic cells. For example, they do not use CCR3 to identify eosinophils when they present their data. The cell population marked EO is absent in the double transgenic Δdb/GATA IL-5 transgene. At first appearance, this would seem to agree with the Yu et al. hypothesis that the eosinophils are deleted in Δdb/GATA mice. However, an alternate possibility is that the Δdb/GATA granuleless eosinophils mature in the presence of the IL-5 transgene and have moved into the

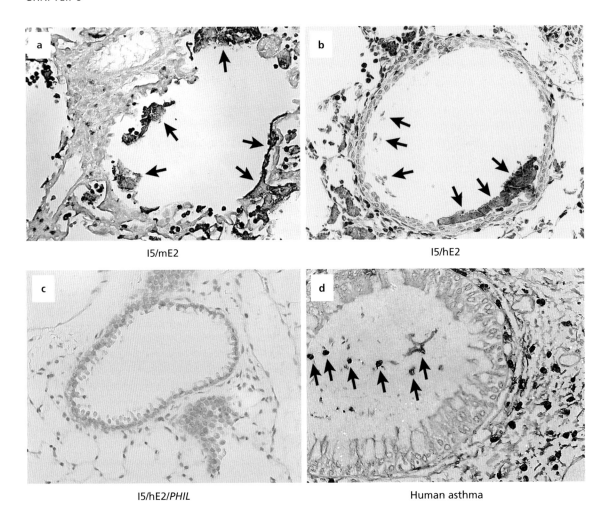

Figure 8.2 Eosinophil degranulation in transgenic mice. Eosinophil degranulation and epithelial desquamation in transgenic mice showing airway pathology and eosinophil degranulation in mouse and human airway disease and asthma). A and B are lung sections from mice transgenic for T-cell-specific IL-5 and lung-specific (A) mouse eotaxin 2 and (B) human eotaxin 2. C is a lung section from a triple transgenic for T-cell-specific IL-5, lung-specific human eotaxin 2, and eosinophil-specific diphtheria toxin. A and B show double transgenic I5/mE2 and I5/hE2 mice, respectively, showing airways with epithelial desquamation and infiltration of eosinophils; C shows an airway from a triple transgenic I5/hE2 with PHIL lacking any eosinophils; panel D shows a tissue section from a patient who died of fatal asthma. The airway disruption and epithelial desquamation is evident in A, B, and D. C shows that the airway in the triple transgenic mouse with the PHIL transgene is devoid of eosinophils and lacking in any airway pathology or epithelial desquamation even in the presence of the I5hE2 transgenes. Dark black and gray indicate eosinophils and presence of degranulation. Arrows show airway epithelial desquamation. Reproduced from Ochkur *et al.* (2007), with permission from the publisher.

windows marked MONO or LUC. Again, the histology stains would not identify eosinophils without granule proteins.

In figure 4 of Yu *et al.*, the authors show reverse transcription polymerase chain reaction (RT-PCR) analysis of gene expression in wild-type and Δdb/GATA mutant male mice. Interestingly, CCR3 is expressed in both wild-type and Δdb/GATA mice, which could be expected even in mice in which eosinophils are deleted because CCR3 expression is not exclusive to eosinophils. However, once again, no quantitative information is provided to determine if CCR3 is proportionately lower in the Δ*db*/GATA mice, which would be expected if the eosinophils are deleted.

Our hypothesis is that the eosinophils in the Δ*db*/GATA mice may not be deleted, even though the granule proteins are absent. The eosinophil could still be there, but not be recognizable by common methods of detection. Eosinophils are important cells that help to regulate the Th2 immune response [63]. Until a more thorough analysis of the reported lack of eosinophils in the Δ*db*/GATA mice is completed, investigators using the Δ*db*/GATA mice are cautioned that it is possible the GATA deletion is removing the eosinophil *granule* and all of the eosinophil granule proteins, but the eosinophil *cell* is left intact although it is not recognizable by commonly used stains (which depend on the presence of the eosinophil granule proteins). Cytokine expression by a granule-deficient eosinophil, rather than unexplained "strain differences," could account for the discrepancies in airway inflammation obtained by Humbles *et al.* [84] and Lee *et al.* [82].

T cells play an integral role in asthmatic inflammation

Numerous investigators have used animal models to study asthma. Many of these models use antigen stimulation followed by a respiratory challenge of the same antigen. Ovalbumin has been used as the stimulating antigen commonly, as well as dust mite antigen, fungal antigens (e.g., *Aspergillus, Alternaria*), cockroach, and ragweed. All of these antigens induce a Th2 response followed by the onset of allergic respiratory inflammation and airway hyperresponsiveness. Guinea-pigs have been used because of the similarity between their and human airways, as well as their neuronal physiology. However, mice have been increasingly used for research, primarily because of the wealth of genotypically modified strains, which are different by only one or a few chosen genes.

Mice deficient in CD4+ T cells do not develop allergic airways disease [86]. RAG mice reconstituted with various cells developed allergic airways disease only when CD4+ T cells were reintroduced [87]. Similarly, STAT6 deficiency, which controls Th2 cytokine expression, abolished airway hyperresponsiveness

[88]. In addition, Mattes *et al.* [89] showed that IL-13 produced by CD4+ T cells was essential in producing airway inflammation and hyperresponsiveness.

Eosinophils and T cells cooperate in asthmatic inflammation

Jacobsen *et al.* [63] used adoptive cell transfers into the PHIL mice to show that restoration of the Th2 inflammation required both the transfer of eosinophils and ovalbumin-specific effector T cells. The PHIL mice treated with ovalbumin did not accumulate CD4+ and CD8+ T cells in the airways, lungs, or regional lymph nodes. We [90,91] and others [92,93] have previously documented the need for CD4+ T cells in the development of allergic airway inflammation. Jacobsen *et al.* showed conclusively that both eosinophils and T cells had to be adoptively transferred into ovalbumin-treated PHIL mice in order to restore allergen-mediated Th2 inflammatory lung responses completely. Additionally, eosinophils may modulate T-cell function through antigen presentation to T cells, thus inducing the production of effector Th2 cells [94,95].

Conclusion

Eosinophils have long been thought to be "mere" end-stage effector cells that are involved in reactions to parasites and allergies. However, we believe that they are much more important regulators of the immune response. Previous work and our own studies have shown that they are intimately involved in T-cell responses. Eosinophils can modulate the immune response by secreting different cytokines, such as IL-4, IL-13, TNF-α, or transforming growth factor beta (TGF-β). Investigators have yet to unravel the mysteries of eosinophilic infiltration of tumors, the thymus, or the uterus and their association with remodeling and bone formation. Eosinophils already have one quality associated with regulatory cells—they are rare. For the moment, they are mysterious as well.

Acknowledgment

The authors would like to thank Linda Mardel and Eric Meek for their help in proofreading and assembling this manuscript, and Marvin Ruona and Nikki Boruff for their work with the graphics and illustrations. NAL would like to thank Dr. Jamie Lee for helpful discussions and proofreading, and Ralph Pero, Cheryl Protheroe, and the entire Lee laboratories for their tireless assistance.

References

1 Rothenberg ME, Hogan SP. The eosinophil. *Annu Rev Immunol* 2006; **24**: 147–74.

2 Leiferman KM. A role for eosinophils in atopic dermatitis. *J Am Acad Dermatol* 2001; **45**: S21–4.

3 Miyasato M, Tsuda S, Nakama T, *et al.* Serum levels of eosinophil cationic protein reflect the state of *in vitro* degranulation of blood hypodense eosinophils in atopic dermatitis. *J Dermatol* 1996; **23**: 382–8 8708149.

4 Tepper RI. The anti-tumour and proinflammatory actions of Il4. *Res Immunol* 1993; **144**: 633–7.

5 Hanamoto H, Nakayama T, Miyazato H, *et al.* Expression of Ccl28 by Reed-Sternberg cells defines a major subtype of classical Hodgkin's disease with frequent infiltration of eosinophils and/or plasma cells. *Am J Pathol* 2004; **164**: 997–1006.

6 Lotfi R, Lee JJ, Lotze MT. Eosinophilic granulocytes and damage-associated molecular pattern molecules (DAMPS): Role in the inflammatory response within tumors. *J Immunother* 2007; **30**: 16–28.

7 Appenroth E, Gunkel AR, Muller H, Volklein C, Schrott-Fischer A. Activated and non-activated eosinophils in patients with chronic rhinosinusitis. *Acta Otolaryngol* 1998; **118**: 240–2.

8 Blumenthal RD, Samoszuk M, Taylor AP, Brown G, Alisauskas R, Goldenberg DM. Degranulating eosinophils in human endometriosis. *Am J Pathol* 2000; **156**: 1581–8.

9 Macias MP, Fitzpatrick LA, Brenneise I, McGarry MP, Lee JJ, Lee NA. Expression of Il-5 alters bone metabolism and induces ossification of the spleen in transgenic mice. *J Clin Invest* 2001; **107**: 949–59.

10 Lee JJ, Dimina D, Macias MP, *et al.* Defining a link with asthma in mice congenitally deficient in eosinophils. *Science* 2004; **305**: 1773–6.

11 Mosmann TR, Coffman RL. Th1 and Th2 cells: Different patterns of lymphokine secretion lead to different functional properties [Review]. *Annu Rev Immunol* 1989; **7**: 145–73.

12 Therien AG, Bernier V, Weicker S, *et al.* Adenovirus Il-13-induced airway disease in mice: a corticosteroid-resistant model of severe asthma. *Am J Respir Cell Mol Biol* 2008; **39**: 26–35.

13 Cohn L. Mucus in chronic airway diseases: sorting out the sticky details. *J Clin Invest* 2006; **116**: 306–8.

14 Heaton T, Rowe J, Turner S, *et al.* An immunoepidemiological approach to asthma: identification of in-vitro T-Cell response patterns associated with different wheezing phenotypes in children. *Lancet* 2005; **365**: 142–9.

15 Umetsu DT. Revising the immunological theories of asthma and allergy. *Lancet* 2005; **365**: 98–100.

16 Gleich GJ, Motojima S, Frigas E, Kephart GM, Fujisawa T, Kravis LP. The eosinophilic leukocyte and the pathology of fatal bronchial asthma: Evidence for pathologic heterogeneity. *J Allergy Clin Immunol* 1987; **80**: 412–15.

17 Moqbel R, Ying S, Barkans J, *et al.* Identification of messenger RNA for IL-4 in human eosinophils with granule localization and release of the translated product. *J Immunol* 1995; **155**: 4939–47.

18 Durham SR, Ying S, Varney VA, *et al.* Cytokine messenger RNA expression for IL-3: IL-4: IL-5: and granulocyte/macrophage-colony-stimulating factor in the nasal mucosa after local allergen provocation: relationship to tissue eosinophilia. *J Immunol* 1992; **148**: 2390–4.

19 Schmid-Grendelmeier P, Altznauer F, Fischer B, *et al.* Eosinophils express functional IL-13 in eosinophilic inflammatory diseases. *J Immunol* 2002; **169**: 1021–7.

20 Kim JT, Schimming AW, Kita H. Ligation of Fc gamma Rii (Cd32) pivotally regulates survival of human eosinophils. *J Immunol* 1999; **162**: 4253–9.

21 Davoine F, Lavigne S, Chakir J, Ferland C, Boulay ME, Laviolette M. Expression of Fcgammariii (Cd16) on human peripheral blood eosinophils increases in allergic conditions. *J Allergy Clin Immunol* 2002; **109**: 463–9.

22 Kita H, Kaneko M, Bartemes KR, *et al.* Does Ige bind to and activate eosinophils from patients with allergy? *J Immunol* 1999; **162**: 6901–11.

23 Gounni AS, Lamkhioued B, Ochiai K, *et al.* High-affinity Ige receptor on eosinophils is involved in defence against parasites. *Nature* 1994; **367**: 183–6.

24 Truong MJ, Gruart V, Liu FT, Prin L, Capron A, Capron M. IgE-binding molecules (Mac-2/Epsilon Bp) expressed by human eosinophils. Implication in Ige-dependent eosinophil cytotoxicity. *Eur J Immunol* 1993; **23**: 3230–5 .

25 Pleass RJ, Andrews PD, Kerr MA, Woof JM. Alternative splicing of the human IgA Fc receptor Cd89 in neutrophils and eosinophils. *Biochem J* 1996; **318**: 771–7.

26 Wallen N, Kita H, Weiler D, Gleich GJ. Glucocorticoids inhibit cytokine-mediated eosinophil survival. *J Immunol* 1991; **147**: 3490–5.

27 Attwood SE, Lewis CJ, Bronder CS, Morris CD, Armstrong GR, Whittam J. Eosinophilic oesophagitis: a novel treatment using montelukast. *Gut* 2003; **52**: 181–5.

28 Rackal JM, Vender RB. The treatment of atopic dermatitis and other dermatoses with leukotriene antagonists. *Skin Therapy Lett* 2004; **9**: 1–5.

29 Bandeira-Melo C, Weller PF. Eosinophils and cysteinyl leukotrienes. *Prostaglandins Leukot Essent Fatty Acids* 2003; **69**: 135–43.

30 Busse W, Kraft M. Cysteinyl leukotrienes in allergic inflammation: Strategic target for therapy. *Chest* 2005; **127**: 1312–26.

31 Lee E, Robertson T, Smith J, Kilfeather S. Leukotriene receptor antagonists and synthesis inhibitors reverse survival in eosinophils of asthmatic individuals. *Am J Respir Crit Care Med* 2000; **161**: 1881–6.

32 Braccioni F, Dorman SC, O'Byrne MP, *et al.* The effect of cysteinyl leukotrienes on growth of eosinophil progenitors from peripheral blood and bone marrow of atopic subjects. *J Allergy Clin Immunol* 2002; **110**: 96–101.

33 Kips JC, O'Connor BJ, Langley SJ, *et al.* Effect of Sch55700: a humanized anti-human interleukin-5 antibody, in severe persistent asthma: A pilot study. *Am J Respir Crit Care Med* 2003; **167**: 1655–9.

34 Flood-Page PT, Menzies-Gow AN, Kay AB, Robinson DS. Eosinophil's role remains uncertain as anti-interleukin-5 only partially depletes numbers in asthmatic airway. *Am J Respir Crit Care Med* 2003; **167**: 199–204.

35 Flood-Page P, Swenson C, Faiferman I, *et al.* A study to evaluate safety and efficacy of mepolizumab in patients with moderate persistent asthma. *Am J Respir Crit Care Med* 2007; **176**: 1062–71.

36 Nair P, Pizzichini MM, Kjarsgaard M, *et al.* Mepolizumab for prednisone-dependent asthma with sputum eosinophilia. *N Engl J Med* 2009; **360**: 985–93.

37 Haldar P, Brightling CE, Hargadon B, *et al.* Mepolizumab and exacerbations of refractory eosinophilic asthma. *N Engl J Med* 2009; **360**: 973–84.

38 Pardanani A, Reeder T, Porrata LF, *et al.* Imatinib therapy for hypereosinophilic syndrome and other eosinophilic disorders. *Blood* 2003; **101**: 3391–7.

39 Cortes J, Ault P, Koller C, *et al.* Efficacy of imatinib mesylate in the treatment of idiopathic hypereosinophilic syndrome. *Blood* 2003; **101**: 4714–16.

40 Berlin AA, Lukacs NW. Treatment of cockroach allergen asthma model with imatinib attenuates airway responses. *Am J Respir Crit Care Med* 2005; **171**: 35–9.

41 Tarantini F, Baiardini I, Passalacqua G, Braido F, Canonica GW. Asthma treatment: "magic bullets which seek their own targets". *Allergy* 2007; **62**: 605–10.

42 Maurer D, Fiebiger E, Reininger B, *et al.* Expression of functional high affinity immunoglobulin E receptors (Fc epsilon Ri) on monocytes of atopic individuals. *J Exp Med* 1994; **179**: 745–50.

43 van Rensen EL, Evertse CE, van Schadewijk WA, *et al.* Eosinophils in bronchial mucosa of asthmatics after allergen challenge: effect of anti-Ige treatment. *Allergy* 2009; **64**: 72–80.

44 MacGlashan DW, Jr., Bochner BS, Adelman DC, *et al.* Downregulation of Fc(epsilon)Ri expression on human basophils during *in vivo* treatment of atopic patients with anti-Ige antibody. *J Immunol* 1997; **158**: 1438–45.

45 Saini SS, Klion AD, Holland SM, Hamilton RG, Bochner BS, Macglashan DW, Jr. The relationship between serum Ige and surface levels of fcepsilonr on human leukocytes in various diseases: Correlation of expression with Fcepsilonri on basophils but not on monocytes or eosinophils. *J Allergy Clin Immunol* 2000; **106**: 514–20.

46 Casale TB, Busse WW, Kline JN, *et al.* Omalizumab pretreatment decreases acute reactions after rush immunotherapy for ragweed-induced seasonal allergic rhinitis. *J Allergy Clin Immunol* 2006; **117**: 134–40.

47 Schulze J, Rose M, Zielen S. Beekeepers anaphylaxis: successful immunotherapy covered by omalizumab. *Allergy* 2007; **62**: 963–4.

48 Berg S. A New weapon against asthma and allergies? *Asthma Mag* 2002; 7: 33–6.

49 Pearce N, Pekkanen J, Beasley R. How much asthma is really attributable to atopy? *Thorax* 1999; **54**: 268–72.

50 Martin LB, Kita H, Leiferman KM, Gleich GJ. Eosinophils in allergy: role in disease, degranulation, and cytokines. *Int Arch Allergy Immunol* 1996; **109**: 207–15.

51 Gleich GJ, Leiferman KM. Role of Eosinophils in Atopic Dermatitis. In: Leung DYM (ed). *Atopic Dermatitis: From Pathogensis to Treatment.* Springer-Verlag, RG Landes Co.: Austin, New York, 1996. p. 226.

52 Ober C, Moffatt MF. Contributing factors to the pathobiology. The genetics of asthma. *Clin Chest Med* 2000; **21**: 245–61.

53 Blumenthal MN. The role of genetics in the development of asthma and atopy. *Curr Opin Allergy Clin Immunol* 2005; **5**: 141–5.

54 Sandford AJ, Moffatt MF, Daniels SE, *et al.* A genetic map of chromosome 11q, including the atopy locus. *Eur J Hum Genet* 1995; **3**: 188–94.

55 Hoffjan S, Nicolae D, Ober C. Association studies for asthma and atopic diseases: A comprehensive review of the literature. *Respir Res* 2003; **4**: 14.

56 Breuer K, Kapp A, Werfel T. Bacterial infections and atopic dermatitis. *Allergy* 2001; **56**: 1034–41.

57 Dahl MV. *Staphylococcus aureus* and atopic dermatitis. *Arch Dermatol* 1983; **119**: 840–6.

58 Abramson JS, Dahl MV, Walsh G, Blumenthal MN, Douglas SD, Quie PG. Antistaphylococcal Ige in patients with atopic dermatitis. *J Am Acad Dermatol* 1982; 7: 105–10.

59 Parish WE, Welbourn E, Champion RH. Hypersensitivity to bacteria in eczema. Ii. titre and immunoglobulin class

of antibodies to staphylococci and micrococci. *Br J Dermatol* 1976; **95**: 285–93.

60 Motala C, Potter PC, Weinberg EG, Malherbe D, Hughes J. Anti-*Staphylococcus aureus*-specific Ige in atopic dermatitis. *J Allergy Clin Immunol* 1986; **78**: 583–9.

61 Rystedt I, Strannegard IL, Strannegard O. Increased serum levels of antibodies to Epstein–Barr virus in adults with history of atopic dermatitis. *Int Arch Allergy Appl Immunol* 75: 1984; 179–83.

62 Calvani M, Alessandri C, Paolone G, Rosengard L, Di Caro A, De Franco D. Correlation between Epstein Barr virus antibodies, serum Ige and atopic disease. *Pediatr Allergy Immunol* 1997; **8**: 91–6.

63 Jacobsen EA, Ochkur SI, Pero RS, *et al.* Allergic pulmonary inflammation in mice is dependent on eosinophil-induced recruitment of effector T cells. *J Exp Med* 2008; **205**: 699–710.

64 Sutton BJ, Gould HJ. The human IgE network. *Nature* 1993; **366**: 421–8.

65 Wang B, Rieger A, Kilgus O, *et al.* Epidermal Langerhans cells from normal human skin bind monomeric Ige Via Fc epsilon Ri. *J Exp Med* 1992; **175**: 1353–65.

66 Bieber T, de la Salle H, Wollenberg A, *et al.* Human epidermal Langerhans cells express the high affinity receptor for immunoglobulin E (Fc epsilon Ri). *J Exp Med* 1992; **175**: 1285–90.

67 Sheinkopf LE, Rafi AW, Do LT, Katz RM, Klaustermeyer WB. Efficacy of omalizumab in the treatment of atopic dermatitis: A pilot study. *Allergy Asthma Proc* 2008; **29**: 530–7.

68 Zhang K, Kepley CL, Terada T, Zhu D, Perez H, Saxon A. Inhibition of allergen-specific IgE reactivity by a human Ig Fcgamma-Fcepsilon bifunctional fusion protein. *J Allergy Clin Immunol* 2004; **114**: 321–7.

69 Bruhns P, Fremont S, Daeron M. Regulation of allergy by Fc receptors. *Curr Opin Immunol* 2005; **17**: 662–9.

70 Foroughi S, Foster B, Kim N, *et al.* Anti-IgE treatment of eosinophil-associated gastrointestinal disorders. *J Allergy Clin Immunol* 2007; **120**: 594–601.

71 Leung DY, Sampson HA, Yunginger JW, *et al.* Effect of anti-IgE therapy in patients with peanut allergy. *N Engl J Med* 2003; **348**: 986–93.

72 Chang TW, Davis FM, Sun N-C, Sun CRY, McGlashan DW, Jr., Hamilton RG. Monoclonal antibodies specific for human IgE-producing B cells: A potential therapeutic for IgE-mediated allergic diseases. *Nat Biotechnol* 1990; **8**: 122–6.

73 Tedeschi A, Cottini M, Asero R. Simultaneous occurrence of chronic autoimmune urticaria and non-allergic asthma: A common mechanism? *Eur Ann Allergy Clin Immunol* 2009; **41**: 56–9.

74 Keogh KA, Specks U. Churg–Strauss syndrome. *Semin Respir Crit Care Med* 2006; **27**: 148–57.

75 Bernstein CN, Wajda A, Blanchard JF. The clustering of other chronic inflammatory diseases in inflammatory bowel disease: A population-based study. *Gastroenterology* 2005; **129**: 827–36.

76 Mansi A, Cucchiara S, Greco L, *et al.* Bronchial hyperresponsiveness in children and adolescents with Crohn's disease. *Am J Respir Crit Care Med* 2000; **161**: 1051–4.

77 Barnes PJ. Cytokine-directed therapies in asthma. *Allergol Int* 2008; **52**: 53–63.

78 Berry MA, Hargadon B, Shelley M, *et al.* Evidence of a role of tumor necrosis factor alpha in refractory asthma. *N Engl J Med* 2006; **354**: 697–708.

79 Lee JJ, McGarry MP, Farmer SC, *et al.* Interleukin-5 expression in the lung epithelium of transgenic mice leads to pulmonary changes pathognomonic of asthma. *J Exp Med* 1997; **185**: 2143–56.

80 Ochkur SI, Jacobsen EA, Protheroe CA, *et al.* Co-expression of Il-5 and eotaxin-2 in mice creates an eosinophil-dependent model of respiratory inflammation with characteristics of severe asthma. *J Immunol* 2007; **178**: 7879–89.

81 Lee NA, McGarry MP, Larson KA, Horton MA, Kristensen AB, Lee JJ. Expression of Il-5 in thymocytes/T cells leads to the development of a massive eosinophilia, extramedullary eosinophilopoiesis, and unique histopathologies. *J Immunol* 1997; **158**: 1332–44.

82 Lee JJ, Dimina D, Macias MP, *et al.* Som: Defining a link with asthma in mice congenitally deficient in eosinophils. *Science* 2004; **305**: 1773–6.

83 Hirasawa R, Shimizu R, Takahashi S, *et al.* Essential and instructive roles of Gata factors in eosinophil development. *J Exp Med* 2002; **195**: 1379–86.

84 Humbles AA, Lloyd CM, McMillan SJ, *et al.* A critical role for eosinophils in allergic airways remodeling. *Science* 2004; **305**: 1776–9.

85 Yu C, Cantor AB, Yang H, *et al.* Targeted deletion of a high-affinity Gata-binding site in the Gata-1 promoter leads to selective loss of the eosinophil lineage *in vivo*. *J Exp Med* 2002; **195**: 1387–95.

86 Hogan SP, Matthaei KI, Young JM, Koskinen A, Young IG, Foster PS. A novel T cell-regulated mechanism modulating allergen-induced airways hyperreactivity in Balb/C mice independently of Il-4 and Il-5. *J Immunol* 1998; **161**: 1501–9.

87 Corry DB, Grunig G, Hadeiba H, *et al.* Requirements for allergen-induced airway hyperreactivity in T, and B cell-deficient mice. *Mol Med* 1998; **4**: 344–55.

88 Miyata S, Matsuyama T, Kodama T, *et al.* Stat6 deficiency in a mouse model of allergen-induced airways inflammation abolishes eosinophilia but induces infiltration of Cd8+ T cells. *Clin Exp Allergy* 1999; **29**: 114–23.

89 Mattes J, Yang M, Siqueira A, *et al.* Il-13 Induces airways hyperreactivity independently of the Il-4r alpha chain in the allergic lung. *J Immunol* 2001; **167**: 1683–92.

90 Crosby JR, Shen HH, Borchers MT, *et al.* Ectopic expression of Il-5 identifies an additional Cd4($^+$) T cell mechanism of airway eosinophil recruitment. *Am J Physiol LCMP* 2002; **282**: L99–L108.

91 Justice JP, Borchers MT, Lee JJ, Rowan WH, Shibata Y, Van Scott MR. Ragweed-induced expression of Gata-3: Il-4: and Il-5 by eosinophils in the lungs of allergic C57bl/6j mice. *Am J Physiol Lung Cell Mol Physiol* 2002; **282**: L302–9.

92 Gavett SH, Chen X, Finkelman F, Wills-Karp M. Depletion of murine Cd4[+] T lymphocytes prevents antigen-induced airway hyperreactivity and pulmonary eosinophilia. *Am J Respir Cell Mol Biol* 1994; **10**: 587–93.

93 Mould AW, Ramsay AJ, Matthaei KI, Young IG, Rothenberg ME, Foster PS. The effect of Il-5 and eotaxin expression in the lung on eosinophil trafficking and degranulation and the induction of bronchial hyperreactivity. *J Immunol* 2000; **164**: 2142–50.

94 Wang H-B, Ghiran I, Matthaei K, Weller PF. Airway eosinophils: allergic inflammation recruited professional antigen-presenting cells. *J Immunol* 2007; **179**: 7585–92.

95 Shi HZ, Humbles A, Gerard C, Jin Z, Weller PF. Lymph node trafficking and antigen presentation by endobronchial eosinophils. *J Clin Invest* 2000; **105**: 945–53.

9 Basophils in inflammation and allergy drug design

Donald MacGlashan, Jr.
Johns Hopkins University Baltimore, Baltimore, MD, USA

Basophils versus mast cells

In humans there are two cells that both express a high affinity for immunoglobulin E (IgE) and express granules that contain histamine. The mast cell is a tissue-resident cell, although its immature forms are produced in the bone marrow and disseminate to the tissues. The basophil matures in the bone marrow and enters the circulation, where it resides for a relatively short period time before migrating to locations that are not yet fully described. A variety of tissue conditions induce the chemotaxis of basophils into tissue sites where they can rapidly accumulate. A rough calculation predicts that the bone marrow generates a nearly equal number of basophils and mast cells but that the life span of the mast cell appears much longer, with estimates at as long as 3 months in some tissues, and therefore the body of resident mast cells is 50- to 100-fold greater than circulating basophils. However, the equal rate of marrow generation means that basophils can rapidly become the dominant histamine-containing cell at specific tissue sites when recruited.

There is no question that mast cells have a role in immediate hypersensitivity reactions, but the precise role of the basophil is still undecided. Numerous studies have demonstrated the accumulation of basophils in the inflammatory responses that follow a mast cell response. Cell morphology, response characteristics, and mediators have clearly demonstrated

their presence. Two antibodies (2D7 and BB1) have been generated that specifically identify basophils [1–3], and tissue sections labeled with either of these antibodies visually demonstrate the accumulation of basophils [4–6]. However, their relative functional contribution to the reaction is not so clear. In a recent clinical study, the new therapeutic agent, omalizumab (Xolair®; Genentech/Novartis, South San Francisco, CA, USA), was used to selectively suppress the basophil response. It was known that during the first weeks of treatment with this drug the expression of FcεRI on basophil was suppressed but the expression on mast cells was not [7]. This result is most likely a consequence of the relative rates of turnover of the two cell compartments. Because IgE does not rapidly dissociate from the cell-surface receptor, the loss of cell-surface IgE on mast cells is slow. Yet, basophils turnover so rapidly that the decrease in cell-surface receptor expression actually reflects not IgE dissociation but cell replacement with basophils that had never experienced upregulation of receptor in the bone marrow [8]. The consequence is that for a window of time lasting several weeks, challenge of mucosal tissue—in this study, the nose—results in mediator release that looks very similar to pretreatment levels. In contrast, it was demonstrated that the IgE-mediated basophil response was markedly suppressed and during this temporal window of differential suppression of basophils versus mast cells, the nasal symptoms that followed antigen challenge were suppressed. While there are several interpretations of this experiment, one possibility is that the basophil normally contributed a significant component of the response and it was this component that was suppressed in the early weeks of treatment with omalizumab.

Studies performed several decades ago also showed a good correlation between the basophil response and the symptoms experienced by atopic patients [6,9–16]. Therefore, it is tentatively concluded that in atopic patients, an immediate hypersensitivity reaction is composed of the response from both basophils and mast cells. The basophils presumably are resident in the tissue because of past chronic exposure to allergens and once there contribute to the reaction.

Mediators of the inflammatory response

There are three described classes of mediators secreted from basophils. The canonical mediator is histamine, which falls into the first class of preformed substances that are stored in the granules of these cells. Release is therefore both coincident with degranulation and rapid. The human basophil contents are not very well studied, although it contains proteoglycans and enzymes that have been partially characterized. For example, chondroitin sulfate is predominant (MacGlashan, Jr., unpublished results and Metcalfe et al. [17]) and there is some tryptase [18,19], although it is a small fraction of the tryptase found in mast cells. Major basic protein is also present [20], although to a lesser extent than that found in eosinophils.

A second class of mediators are also rapidly released but not preformed. The dominant mediator type in this class are the metabolites of arachidonic acid. The profile of AA metabolites from basophils is relatively restricted, at least compared with the mast cell. A broad screen of ^{3}H-AA metabolites profiled by high performance liquid chromatography generated from human basophils and stimulated with anti-IgE antibody resulted in only one identifiable peak, LTC4 [21,22]. There are no cyclooxygenase products and no LTB4 appears to be produced. There is a mixed conclusion regarding platelet-activating factor (PAF), with most studies suggesting that basophils do not produce PAF [23] but do generate the acyl derivative of PAF.

The third class of mediators are neither preformed or rapidly released but represent a rapidly growing and diverse list of molecules. Any secreted protein would fall into this category, and for the basophil this includes interleukin 4 (IL-4), IL-13, IL-3 (see below), IL-8, chemokines such as macrophage inflammatory protein 5 (MIP-5), eotaxin, and MIP-1α, and growth factors such vascular endothelial growth factor (VEGF) [24]. There is an undefined class of proteins represented by granzyme B that do not appear to be present in circulating basophils but do appear after treatment of the cells with IL-3 [25]. The unique aspect of these proteins is their inclusion into already mature granules for rapid release when the cell degranulates. The implication of results like these is that the granule in a mature circulating basophil is not necessarily static in composition. The composition can be modified along with other phenotypic changes that the basophil experiences when exposed to cytokines like IL-3.

Basophils and the innate immune response

The IgE-mediated response in basophils is but one way that these cells can be stimulated to secrete mediators or initiate other functionality. The list of receptors continues to expand but currently consists of chemokine receptors that induce adhesion, migration, and sometimes mediator release (see Table 9.1). There are several other important transmembrane receptors that can be considered to be part of the innate immune response. Another receptor class that has been recently identified is the LIL (leukocyte immunoglobulin-like) receptors. One of these, LILRA-2, has been studied in some detail and has been shown to generate basophil responses that are very similar to IgE-mediated release [26]. Preliminary indications are that it shares many of the same early signaling steps [27]. Its role in modulating the basophil is not yet known. Not all ligands induce histamine release and not all ligands that induce histamine release induce the release of later mediators. A well-studied example is C5a. This secretagogue generates a very strong initial elevation in cytosolic calcium that is very transient. During this window of time, histamine release is fast and marked. But the cytosolic calcium elevation is not sustained long enough to allow secretion of either LTC4 or

Table 9.1 Functionally active ligands (or their receptors) on human basophils.

Function	Ligand (receptor)
Adhesion	Mac-1, P150–95, $\alpha_d\beta_2$, $\alpha_4\beta_7$, VLA-6
Histamine receptors	H2, (H3, H4)
Leukotriene receptors	cys-LT1, cys-LT2
Chemokine receptors	CXCR2, CXCR4 CCR2, CCR4, CCR7, CXCR1
Active chemokines	MCP-2, -3, -4, eotaxin-1, -2, -3 RANTES, TECK, SDF-1α, MCP-1, MIP-3, HCC-4, MIP-3β, SLC, 1-309 GCP-2
Other chemotactic receptors	C5a, C3a, PAF, LTB4, PGD2, FMLP, antigen
LIR	LILRA-2, LILRB-3, LILRB-2
Siglec	Siglec-8 (very weak)
Cytokine receptors	IL-3, IL-5, GM-CSF, IL-33 (ST2), NGF, IL-1, IFN α/β

VLA-6, very late antigen 6; RANTES, regulated on activation, normal T cell-expressed and secreted; MCP, mast cell protease; MIP, macrophage inflammatory protein; FMLP, formyl-met-leu-phe; IL, interleukin; GM-CSF, granulocyte–macrophage colony-stimulating factor; IFN, interferon; cys-LT, cysteinyl leukotrienes.

IL-4. If the cell is primed with a cytokine like IL-3, then C5a becomes a more complete secretagogue [28]. In the case of LTC4 release, the proposed model is that IL-3 preconditions the Erk pathway and establishes a state of cPLA2 phosphorylation that allows this enzyme to respond to the very transient cytosolic calcium response [29,30]. Therefore, the activity of a particular secretagogue is likely to be dependent on the cytokine environment of the basophil. With sufficient exposure to cytokines, the mediator release profile may become complete.

Cytokines are released from basophils late in the reaction. Release of IL-4, while slow compared with histamine release, is one of the fastest cytokines to be released. Substantial release can occur within 1 h and there is evidence for a small amount of IL-4 associated with granules, so that a small portion can be released as quickly as histamine. IL-13 is also secreted by basophils, but much more slowly than IL-4, requiring many hours [31,32]. It has recently been shown that much of the IL-13 secretion is dependent on the release of IL-3 from basophils [33]. IL-3 alone is capable of inducing IL-13 release and IgE-mediated stimulation induces IL-3 secretion. This may be the first clear example of an autocrine response in basophils; blocking the IgE-mediated release of IL-3 with an anti-IL-3 blocking antibody blunts the IgE-mediated secretion of IL-13.

Basophils express a least three Toll-like receptors (TLRs): TLR-2, -4, and -9 [34,35]. Thus far, only TLR-2 has been shown to modify basophil function. Peptidoglycan (PGN) alone has been shown to induce both IL-4 and IL-13 secretion and to augment the secretion of IL-4 and IL-13 during IgE- or IL-3-mediated stimulation. Alone, PGN did not induce histamine or LTC4 release but did augment IgE-mediated release of these mediators. Although basophils express TLR-4, no experiments have shown that activation of TLR-4 modifies measured basophil responses. For example, LPS does not modulate the basophil response, but this behavior is speculated to result from the absence of CD14 expression on basophils. CD14 is thought to bind LPS and facilitate its interaction with TLR-4.

As described above, the basophil possesses many elements of the innate immune response: TLR receptors, complement, and FMLP receptors. In addition, the secretion of IL-4 from basophils is unique. Activation of T cells leads to IL-4 secretion, but the reaction is slow and occurs in only the very small fraction of T cells with the proper antigen specificity. In contrast, essentially all basophils sensitized with the proper antigen-specific IgE or responding to complement products in the presence of IL-3 [28,36] secrete large amounts of IL-4 and IL-13. The secretion can occur any time, within minutes to hours, and with the rapid recruitment of basophils, the basophil becomes a likely source of early IL-4 and IL-13 to modulate other ongoing adaptive immune responses [37,38]. This possibility has now been extensively studied in mice. Within the last few years, the basophil has been identified as a critical component of immune reactions that were once thought the domain of T

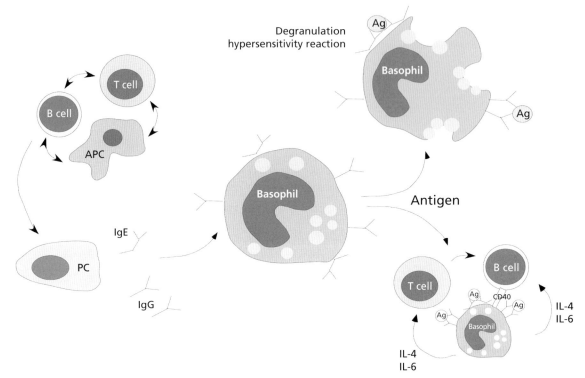

Figure 9.1 Roles of basophils in the immune response. The classic primary immune response (T cells, B cells, and antigen-presenting cells [APCs]) is initiated with the first presentation of antigen to the host. The basophil binds immunoglobulin E (IgE) and IgG antibodies generated by plasma cells (PC): IgG to the inhibitory IgG receptor, FcγRIIb, and IgE to FcεRI. Following a second presentation with antigen, antigen-loaded basophils may begin producing cytokines, interleukin (IL) 4, and IL-6. The presentation of antigen and the production of cytokines by basophils (upper right) enhances the secondary immune response. Alternatively, non-IgE-dependent activation of basophils may induce some IL-4 secretion. This role for basophils has been demonstrated clearly only in mice. The normal effector role of basophils is to respond to antigen with secretion of inflammatory mediators. The circumstances that differentiate this participatory role for basophils and its traditional ability to react like a mast cell with full degranulation, lipid mediator release, and cytokine release to generate an anaphylactic reaction are not yet clear.

cells (Figure 9.1). First, the basophil was identified as an initiator of the primary immune response [39]. Basophils were found in draining lymph nodes and secreted IL-4, which modulated the immune response. Basophils in mice also secrete thymic stromal lymphopoietin (TSLP), a cytokine that has not been identified from human basophils. But in mice the secretion of TSLP also raises the possibility not only that it can modulate dendritic cell responses but that the basophil itself can assume some abilities of the dendritic cell. Indeed, recent studies in mice have suggested that the basophil can present antigen to mediate T-cell activation [40,41]. It is notable in these studies that IL-4 and TSLP secretion are not dependent on IgE-mediated activation. Instead, these studies note that papain can regulate this response. The significance is that proteases are now thought to be an important component of many allergens. If a protease can induce IL-4 secretion then it may also modulate the immune response through the basophil. More recently, a similar line of investigation has shown that basophils also mediate the secondary immune response, augmenting the magnitude of antibody production during a second exposure to antigen [42].

Positive and negative modulation

As noted above and below, IL-3 has a central role in both the development and modulation of human basophils (Figure 9.2; Table 9.1). The receptor for this cytokine (CD123) is expressed at 10–100 times the level of its sister cytokine receptors, IL-5Rα and granulocyte–macrophage colony-stimulating factor (GM-CSF) Rα [43]. This high level of expression allows the receptor to be used to selectively gate basophils from remaining leukocytes in flow cytometric studies. However, it is a property that is also shared with plasmacytoid dendritic cells, which can be removed from analysis by their forward- and side-scatter characteristics or expression of the major histocompatibility complex HLA-DR. There are a plethora of functions modulated by IL-3 in mature basophils, some of which are qualitatively different than the effects of IL-5, GM-CSF, or nerve growth factor (NGF).

Recently, it has been shown that IL-33 has significant effects on basophil function [44,45]. Most notably, IL-33 can alter even the strong effects of IL-3. This IL-1 family member binds to its receptor, ST2, which is upregulated on basophils after their exposure to IL-3. Indeed, ST2 protein is not detectable on basophils before exposure to IL-3 even when IL-33 is shown to markedly alter function [46]. Priming basophils with both IL-3 and IL-33 increases the release of a variety of cytokines, IL-4 and IL-13 for example, 5- to 10-fold. Although IL-33 can replicate many of the effects of IL-3, it appears to use some distinct signaling pathways to accomplish its effects. For example, IL-3 operates through the activation of STAT5 and Erk pathways while IL-33 does not. In this context, the absence of Erk activation means that IL-33 does not lead to cytosolic PLA2 phosphorylation and consequently does not augment the release of LTC4 induced by C5a [46]. In contrast, IL-3 does not induce phosphorylation of the MAP kinase p38

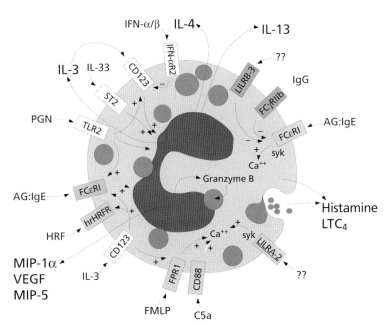

Figure 9.2 Modulation of basophil function. There are many receptors in basophils that induce mediator release, several that induce only cytokine release, and a wide variety of identified receptors that modulate the actions of activating receptors. Interleukin (IL) 3, 4, 13, or 33, FMLP (formyl-met-leu-phe, tripeptide), PGN (peptidoglycan), VEGF (vascular endothelial growth factor), CD123 (IL-3 receptor), TLR2 (Toll-like receptor 2), IFNα/β (interferon α/β), LILRB-3 and LILRA-2 (leukocyte immunoglobulin-like receptor subfamily B-3 and A-2), FPR1 (FMLP high-affinity receptor), CD88 (C5a receptor), HRF (histamine releasing factor), Syk (spleen tyrosine kinase), ST2 (IL-33 receptor), LTC4 (leukotriene C4).

while IL-33 does. IL-33 also induces phosphorylation of IkB.

While a variety of studies have explored the enhancing or priming characteristics of several cytokines, there have been few examples where cytokines or other ligands downregulate basophil responses. Interferons α and β have been shown to blunt the IL-3-dependent secretion of IL-4 and IL-13 [47]. Preliminary studies suggest that the mechanism involves the STAT1-dependent induction of SOCS-1 expression, which is likely to suppress the STAT5 response following IL-3 exposure.

The leukocyte inhibitory receptor family has activating and inhibitory members. As noted previously, LIR-7 (LILRA-2) is an activator of basophils. In contrast, aggregation of LIR-3 (LILRB-3) with antibodies (the ligand being unknown) suppresses IgE-mediated activation of basophils [26]. Basophils also express the inhibitory receptor, FcγRIIb. In other cell models, this receptor can downregulate the IgE-mediated response by recruiting to the reaction complex, SHIP. There are indications that a similar reaction occurs in human basophils, although coaggregation of FcεRI and FcγRIIb does not appear to be necessary [48]. The inhibition of IgE-mediated signaling can be significant and a therapeutic chimera of IgG and IgE or IgG and antigen [49–51] has been developed that is reported to suppress mediator release from basophils (and other cells that express both FcεRI and FcγRIIb).

Receptor expression as a target

Basophils, both murine and human, express high densities of FcεRI. This receptor has the unusual property, although not unique among receptors, of being stabilized on the cell surface by its ligand, monomeric IgE [52–56]. There is no apparent limitation to its expression—densities as high as 1 million per cell have been observed, although this high density is rare. The median level of expression is approximately 100,000 per cell. Since monomeric IgE stabilizes receptor expression, the cell surface density of FcεRI varies as a function of serum IgE [57,58]. Therefore, since atopy is associated with higher levels of IgE expression, it is also associated with higher levels of FcεRI expression.

While IgE prevents the loss of unoccupied FcεRI from the cell surface by endocytotic mechanisms,

it has no effect on synthesis of FcεRI [55]. This process is, however, regulated by extrinsic cytokines. Therefore, cell-surface receptor expression represents a balance of loss by lack of occupancy and synthesis owing to the cytokine environment of the cell. Correlations between serum IgE, titers, and receptor expression suggest that at least 25% of the variance in receptor expression is not due to the protective effects of IgE [58]. Therefore, a large fraction of FcεRI expression might be modulated by exerting control on the synthetic rate of the receptor.

The information on FcεRI synthesis is not detailed but there has been a variety of studies exploring this biology. Beginning with the gene itself, there are some indications that polymorphisms are associated with gene expression. The most extensively studied polymorphisms are those found in the beta subunit of FcεRI, the MS4A2 gene. There are three coding variants, I181L, V183L, and E237G, that have received considerable attention because they have associations with atopy that are defined by several metrics [59–61,62]. However, in vitro studies of variants transfected into model cells have not revealed any functional differences [63], so it remains unclear why these single nucleotide polymorphism (SNP) associations exist. In all, there are 38 polymorphisms associated with this gene: some are in linkage disequilibrium with the coding variants [64], so the noncoding variants may modify the expression of the beta subunit, which in humans is variable in potentially important ways (see below). There are only three identified polymorphisms in the alpha subunit and none is in the coding region. However, in some populations two of these SNPs have been associated with metrics of atopy [65]. In one case, the association relates to increased total IgE levels and in the second case it relates to an increased transcriptional rate of the subunit. Interestingly there are no validated polymorphisms in the gamma subunit gene. For each of these subunits, there is only rudimentary information on the cis- and trans-factors that control their expression. Generally, the known transcriptional factors are rather generic factors that are also known to modulate the generation of mast cells and basophils such as GATA-1 [66–70]. There is evidence that Elf-1, FOG-1, and Oct-1 modulate expression of either FcεRIα or FcRβ.

In humans, expression of the beta subunit, MS4A2, can be dissociated from expression of the alpha and gamma subunits. This property leads to some non-mast cell/basophil types expressing the alpha–gamma form of the receptor without the beta subunit. However, even in basophils, it appears that there is differential expression of the beta subunit [71]. It remains to be demonstrated in wild-type cells that the absence of the beta subunit in an aggregated receptor has a functional consequence, but studies using transfected cells suggest that the generated signal is weaker [72]. The reasons for this will be explored in the next section. Studies in transfected cells also suggest that the presence of the beta subunit, which acts as a chaperone for the alpha subunit, influences the level of receptor expression [73]. There is suggestive evidence that this effect is responsible for the correlation between FcεRβ:FcεRIα ratio and total cell surface FcεRI in peripheral blood basophils [71]. With this as background, one can conclude that regulation of FcRβ expression might be a therapeutic target. The FcRβ gene has an alternate splice site that generates a "spoiler" version of the beta subunit, the so-called β_T. The protein that is generated is highly unstable and, once produced, is rapidly degraded. However, before being lost it acts to scavenge generated alpha subunit, thereby shunting its production to degradative pathways [74]. The consequence is lower FcεRI expression levels. One study has found β_T in peripheral blood basophils while another has not [71]. Since the protein cannot be detected easily, these measurements must rely on the presence of mRNA for the two forms, and handling of the basophils results in a rapid loss of FcRβ mRNA expression. Therefore, it is not yet clear whether β_T is an important element in the control of FcεRI expression. The expression of full-length FcRβ is very sensitive to the condition of the cell, and cell isolation alone results in rapid loss of FcRβ mRNA. IL-3 slows this loss but does not prevent it. Once the mRNA settles down to a level of one or two copies per cell, reintroduction of IL-3 can induce levels of expression that are 3- to 10-fold higher [75]. Therefore, the evidence suggests that IL-3 is one factor that can regulate expression of FcRβ and indirectly influence expression of FcεRI on the cell surface.

IL-3 has also been shown to regulate the pre-Golgi pool of FcεRIα. Recent studies suggest that there is an intermediate steady-state in the sequence of steps that leads to cell-surface expression of FcεRIα. Before expression on the cell surface, FcεRIα is heavily gly-cosylated. The core peptide has a molecular weight of approximately 28 kDa while cell-surface receptor has a very heterogeneous molecular weight with a median of 60 kDa [71]. The glycosylation occurs in the Golgi, but before entering the Golgi apparatus an endoplasmic reticulum (ER)-generated form of FcεRIα is also homogeneously glycosylated to produce a protein with a molecular weight of 46 kDa [76–80]. All of this glycosylation is removed in the first stage of Golgi processing. However, the p46 form of FcεRIα is heavily retained in circulating basophils [71]. The p46 form accumulates to levels that are consistent across preparations of basophils from different donors. Approximately 100,000 molecules per cell are stored this way and isolation of the basophils results in its rapid loss. It is not understood why there is such a significant accumulation at this intermediate step, but it appears that this point in processing represents another steady-state. In this case, there is newly synthesized p46 and two pathways of further processing, movement through the Golgi apparatus. or degradation [81]. IL-3 appears to control the degradation pathway and it is speculated that the presence of FcεRβ, also regulated by IL-3, regulates movement into the Golgi. For reasons not yet understood, the heterogeneity of glycosylation is minimal when receptor expression is low, as if the relative presence of FcεRβ also determines the glycosylation process [82].

The basophil has a very short half-life in circulation. Several studies have provided a rough approximation of a circulation time of 12 h. It is not known what happens to circulating basophils, whether they are lost by apoptosis or sequestered into other tissue compartments such as the spleen, but the majority of receptor upregulation occurs before basophils reach the circulation. Because IgE dissociates from the receptor slowly, at a half-life of approximately 10 days [55], the receptor expression that is observed in peripheral blood basophils results from several factors. The first is that during maturation, receptor accumulation occurs linearly during interphase, G1, and probably G2, but cell division halves the density of receptor. The numerical progression of linear accumulation and division by two results in a plateau of receptors accumulated that is two times the density of receptors accumulated in one cell cycle. This limitation means that in order to accumulate 250,000 receptors before emergence into the circulation, the accumulation rate must be 125,000 per cell cycle, implying a very fast synthetic rate during maturation, much faster than *in vitro* studies have measured [83]. A second feature of this dynamic is that the receptor expression level observed in circulating basophils reflects events happening in the bone marrow, not the circulation. Notably, if the IgE concentration is decreased by an agent like omalizumab, the decrease in cell surface IgE and receptor (that follow initiation of treatment) reflects the accumulation curve in the marrow [8], not the loss of receptor due to IgE dissociation [8,83]. *In vivo* studies demonstrate that this process, with receptor expression decreasing with a half-life of 3 days [84], is three or four times faster than expected based on IgE dissociation rates. In effect, receptor dynamics are a measure of cell replacement dynamics rather than the underlying dynamics of protein accumulation. The dynamics of receptor expression in basophils would apply to any cell that shows similar cell cycle dynamics, for example an intestinal mast cell that turns over rapidly.

IgE-mediated signaling as a target

As an immunoreceptor, FcεRI has no intrinsic enzymatic activity but relies on closely associated tyrosine kinases to initiate the signaling cascade that results in activation of its myriad functions. The requirements for inducing an increase in the activity of these associated kinases are complex. Early studies established that aggregation was one way to start the reaction [85], but in the ensuing years it has become apparent that this view is too simplistic. In ways not yet understood, the process requires a shift in the balance between constitutively active phosphatases and the kinases that initiate the cascade. Antigen aggregation is simply one way that this balance is altered in favor of initiating the reaction. It is most clear that a noncovalent linkage (IgE–antigen–IgE) is not necessary because Cooper *et al.* [86] demonstrated that a univalent ligand mobile in an artificial membrane could induce signaling. This experiment demonstrated that simply raising the density of receptors and possibly slowing down their relative movement might shift the balance between suppression and activation. In fact, recent studies showing that monomeric IgE itself can induce signaling may represent a different form of the same experiment [87,88]. The ability of monomeric IgE to induce signaling is not universal, it is a

property of only some IgE antibodies [89]. It seems likely that these so-called cytokinergic IgE antibodies interact with a membrane structure or each other. For example, one of the most strongly cytokinergic monoclonal IgE antibodies, SPE7, has been shown to only induce signaling if monovalent hapten, DNP1, is not present [87,89]. Furthermore, in the absence of DNP1, this particular Fab binding site can interact with completely unrelated antigens [90]. It is not known whether these properties are generalizable to other IgE antibodies, but slowing of the receptor is demonstrated upon binding [89].

A further complication is that the membrane has a structure that determines whether signaling is initiated. Many studies have demonstrated that there is a dynamic partitioning of the lipid membrane that is dependent on the presence of cholesterol [91]. The receptor-associated kinases in the src family localize to these membrane domains [92,93]. Whether these localized partitions in the membrane composition are dynamic and form in response to aggregation (or localization of the receptor) or whether they are preformed before aggregation remains to be determined. However, proper association of the various components of the early reaction require these membrane "structures" [93]. The src family kinases appear to start this reaction. In the canonical reaction, lyn kinase has a weak association with and phosphorylates the beta subunit [94]. Subsequent binding of the SH2 domain of lyn to the beta subunit allows lyn to phosphorylate the gamma subunit, which permits the recruitment of Syk to the reaction complex that is forming [95]. Syk is obligatory and nonredundant, and many of the reactions that have been documented to follow stimulation are dependent on the recruitment and activity of Syk [96–98]. Therefore, Syk represents a therapeutic target to turn off this reaction. Targeting lyn is more problematic. In some strains of mice, knocking out lyn results in a more reactive mast cell [99]. This is not always true, and the reasons are still being explored, but it may have to do with the relative presence of other src family kinases that also participate in the reaction. In addition, there are data that indicate that lyn initiates some of the self-termination reactions that ultimately serve to quell the activation cascade (more on this below) [100]. The src family kinase fyn also participates in the early reaction and may represent a target for pharmacologic inhibition. However, it is also a practical matter that each of these kinases is a critical participant in many other receptor-mediated events in nonbasophilic leukocytes.

The complexity of the reaction following the activation of Syk is still undefined. The receptor is thought to be a point of reactant accumulation as proteins build a scaffold of enzymes linked to adaptor proteins. The plasma membrane is also both a scaffold and a substrate for enzymes that are recruited to it and the reaction complex. For example, Syk phosphorylates several adaptor proteins like LAT1 or LAT2, which recruit PI3 (phosphatidyl inositol 3′) kinases to the reaction. There are several isozymes of this family of kinases that can participate (α, β, or δ), but evidence suggests that PI3Kδ is the major player in the IgE-mediated reaction [101]. This kinase phosphorylates PIP2 to produce PIP3, which attracts proteins containing PH domains to the plasma membrane. One example is btk (Bruton's tyrosine kinase) [102,103], which is thought to phosphorylate PLCγ1 (phospholipase C) or PLCγ2. These latter enzymes catalyze the generation of IP3 (inositol 3,4,5 trisphosphate) from PIP3 in the plasma membrane, and the released IP3 initiates the elevation of cytoplasmic calcium by interacting with the IP3 receptor and releasing calcium from internal stores [104]. Since an elevation in cytosolic calcium is critical to the release of many mediators (although not necessarily degranulation), this initial sequence of events represents a focal point for therapeutic intervention. In this context, relatively specific inhibitors of PI3Kδ and btk have been developed. These agents are currently in various stages of development for clinical trials.

While it is now clear that complete inhibition of Syk, PI3K, or btk results in complete ablation of mediator secretion, this approach to inhibiting the IgE-mediated reaction has two pitfalls. First, it is relevant only to the IgE-mediated reaction, leaving untouched other receptor-mediated reactions in basophils or mast cells. Second, the enzymes are critical to the function of nearly all cells of the immune system, certainly those relevant to the adaptive immune response. This raises the likelihood of unwanted side-effects if the goal is to simply treat allergic diseases.

It has recently been suggested that there is one way that these agents could be used without necessitating chronic administration. Like all receptor-mediated activation cascades, the IgE-mediated cascade involves self-terminating mechanisms that limit secre-

tion [105]. Some of these termination mechanisms are constitutively active. For example, it is speculated that PTEN serves as a constitutive break on the accumulation of PIP3 (reversing the phosphorylation caused by PI3K) [106]. However, there are also several identified termination mechanisms that are induced by the aggregation of FcεRI. In aggregate, these activation-terminating mechanisms have been termed desensitization. The ultimate result is that the cell stops secreting and is anergic to further activation through the same receptor and in a complicated way also anergic to activation through other noninvolved FcεRI (so-called nonspecific desensitization). Three mechanisms have been identified in human basophils and several additional mechanisms have been identified in nonhuman mast cells [107–110]. The three mechanisms are downregulation of aggregated receptor, downregulation of Syk, and activation of SHIP. There is a fourth process which occurs rapidly and controls the earliest steps in the reaction but does not appear to involve loss of the receptor in human cells. The mechanism involved is unknown. In human cells, but not rodent mast cells [111], loss of the aggregated receptor is very slow, ranging from many hours to days [112]. The loss of Syk is also relatively slow, requiring many hours [113]. The activation of SHIP is rapid but transient [98]. However, recent studies have shown that activation of Syk is not required for any of these events to occur. In other words, inhibition of Syk with third-generation inhibitors results in basophils and mast cells that do not secrete in response to anti-IgE antibody cross-linking but continue to downregulate FcεRI and Syk and continue to activate SHIP [114]. In addition, the functional desensitization that occurs during stimulation, that is, the anergy that can be induced, is also not sensitive to inhibition of Syk. A similar result occurs if there is inhibition of PI3 kinase [114] or btk [115]. In other words, it may be possible to administer a dose of inhibitor followed by antigen after a brief period of time and induce anergy of mast cells and basophils without inducing an allergic reaction (e.g., anaphylaxis). It is not known how long this anergic state would persist, but at a minimum this approach to using drugs that would otherwise be considered risky might have application to preventing iatrogenic reactions. This strategy would likely work for any critical signaling enzyme that is downstream of Syk in the activation cascade.

There is a second area where understanding the regulation of Syk may have future therapeutic application. The IgE-mediated histamine release response of basophils obtained from individuals in the general population has shown a wide variance. For example, there is a phenotype of basophils that has been called the "nonreleaser" phenotype [116]. Basophils with this phenotype express normal levels of FcεRI and secrete normally to non-IgE-dependent stimuli (i.e., they have functional activation cascades leading to standard mediator release for non-IgE-dependent secretagogues). However, activation through FcεRI leads to little or no secretion or function. The deficiency appears to result from a very low level of Syk expression [117,118]. For example, the typical nonreleasing basophil will have less than 2500 molecules of Syk and 100,000 molecules of FcεRI per cell. These studies suggested that Syk expression can be a determinant of IgE-dependent mediator release, and it was found that in the general population Syk expression is a good predictor of histamine release. The variance of Syk expression and variance of histamine release are similar and correlated [119]. A similar variance or correlation was not observed for 18 additional signaling proteins that are part of the early reaction [120]. For basophils, there is another unique feature of Syk expression. Syk expression in all other circulating leukocytes, except T cells, is much greater than in basophils [121]. For example, neutrophils, eosinophils, and B cells express 10 times more Syk than basophils. Monocytes and dendritic cells express 30-fold more Syk. Natural killer (NK) cells are intermediate with only 5-fold more Syk. There is no correlation between Syk expression in basophils and Syk expression in any other type of leukocyte, suggesting that the regulation of Syk is unique in basophils. These levels of Syk expression in basophils are interesting for their relationship to FcεRI expression. On average, a typical basophil contains 25,000 molecules of Syk and 150,000 molecules of FcεRI, i.e., the EC50 for Syk expression is about 25,000 per cell. This ratio of 6–7 molecules of FcεRI per molecule of Syk suggests that Syk expression is tuned to be a rate-limiting step. On average, the ratio will not be this extreme because any given antigen-specific IgE will occupy only 1–5% of the available receptors, but distributed across the entire cell the concentration of Syk may still be rate-limiting.

CD34+ progenitor stem cells express 11-fold more Syk than peripheral blood basophils [121], so in order to mature into a basophil, as opposed to maturing into any other type of leukocyte, they require a significant downregulation of Syk expression. There are in vitro models of basophil maturation from CD34 progenitors that provide some guidance for this process. The established model is to treat CD34 cells with IL-3 for 3 weeks [122,123]. The cell that results has many characteristics of basophils, for example high levels of IL-3R and FMLP-R [121]. However, it has been found that Syk expression is similar to the progenitor, that is, 11-fold greater than peripheral blood basophils. But, if a cell is cultured with IL-3 and an aggregating stimulus throughout the 3 weeks, the resulting cell is phenotypically the same (histamine content, morphology, FcεRI expression) but Syk expression in a subpopulation of cells is suppressed to levels observed in normal peripheral blood basophils [121].

These experiments suggest that Syk expression in vivo might represent a case where the interesting biology of signal element expression is occurring during maturation of the basophil. If there were some endogenous means of aggregating receptor in vivo during maturation, it might lead to the ultimate levels of Syk expression that are observed in subjects. This idea was recently tested by treating patients with omalizumab. This drug markedly reduces free IgE levels and FcεRI expression (owing to the absence of IgE to raise receptor levels) and consequently could relieve a maturing basophil from any endogenous mechanism of chronic aggregation (if it exists) [84]. Patients treated with omalizumab did, on average, produce basophils expressing levels of Syk that were nearly 2-fold greater [82]. Histamine release induced by anti-IgE antibody also increased, while specific antigen-induced release decreased owing to the overall reduction in receptor expression. In other words, there was enough remaining total IgE on the cell surface to take advantage of the higher levels of Syk expression when the stimulus was a panaggregating stimulus like anti-IgE antibody.

However, the increase in Syk expression was not 11-fold (the level found on progenitors). Indeed, there was an excellent inverse correlation between the starting level of Syk and the fold increase in its expression during treatment, but the maximum expression was still well under the expression levels in other leukocytes. In conjunction with other studies that indicate that Syk expression has a weak correlation with levels of Syk mRNA [120], these results suggest that there may be another operative mechanism of regulating Syk in basophils, one that is pretranslational. But regardless of the relative merits of the various interpretations of these results, it is apparent that Syk regulation on basophils is unique to these cells and as such represents an opportunity for selective manipulation by a more sophisticated therapeutic.

References

1 Kepley CL, Craig SS, Schwartz LB. Identification and partial characterization of a unique marker for human basophils. *J Immunol* 1995; **154**: 6548–55.

2 McEuen AR, Buckley MG, Compton SJ, Walls AF. Development and characterization of a monoclonal antibody specific for human basophils and the identification of a unique secretory product of basophil activation. *Lab Invest* 1999; **79**: 27–38.

3 McEuen AR, Calafat J, Compton SJ, *et al*. Mass, charge, and subcellular localization of a unique secretory product identified by the basophil-specific antibody BB1. *J Allergy Clin Immunol* 2001; **107**: 842–8.

4 Macfarlane AJ, Kon OM, Smith SJ, *et al*. Basophils, eosinophils, and mast cells in atopic and nonatopic asthma and in late-phase allergic reactions in the lung and skin. *J Allergy Clin Immunol* 2000; **105**: 99–107.

5 Nouri-Aria KT, Irani AM, Jacobson MR, *et al*. Basophil recruitment and IL-4 production during human allergen-induced late asthma. *J Allergy Clin Immunol* 2001; **108**: 205–11.

6 Irani AM, Huang C, Xia HZ, *et al*. Immunohistochemical detection of human basophils in late-phase skin reactions. *J Allergy Clin Immunol* 1998; **101**: 354–62.

7 Eckman JA, Sterba PM, Kelly D, *et al*. The effect of omalizumab on basophil and mast cell responses using an intranasal cat allergen challenge. *J Allergy Clin Immunol* 2009; **125**: 889–95.

8 MacGlashan D. Loss of receptors and IgE *in vivo* during treatment with anti-IgE antibody. *J Allergy Clin Immunol* 2004; **114**: 1472–4.

9 Norman PS, Lichtenstein LM, Ishizaka K. Diagnostic tests in ragweed hay fever. A comparison of direct skin tests, IgE, antibody measurements, and basophil histamine release. *J Allergy Clin Immunol* 1973; **52**: 210–24.

10 Naclerio RM, Proud D, Togias AG, *et al*. Inflammatory mediators in late antigen-induced rhinitis. *N Engl J Med* 1985; **313**: 65–70.

11 Togias A, Naclerio RM, Proud D, *et al*. Mediator release during nasal provocation. A model to investigate the pathophysiology of rhinitis. *Am J Med* 1985; **79**: 26–33.

12 Bascom R, Wachs M, Naclerio RM, Pipkorn U, Galli SJ, Lichtenstein LM. Basophil influx occurs after nasal antigen challenge: effects of topical corticosteroid pretreatment. *J Allergy Clin Immunol* 1988; **81**: 580–9.

13 Charlesworth EN, Hood AF, Soter NA, Kagey SA, Norman PS, Lichtenstein LM. Cutaneous late-phase response to allergen. Mediator release and inflammatory cell infiltration. *J Clin Invest* 1989;**83**: 1519–26.

14 Irani AA, Huang C, Zweiman B, Schwartz LB. Immunohistochemical detection of basophil infiltration in the skin during the IgE-mediated late phase reaction. *J All Clin Immunol* 1997; **99**: S92.

15 von Allmen C, Zweiman B, Irani AM, Baron M, Schwartz LB. Temporal pattern of basophil accumulation in cutaneous late-phase reactions. *J Allergy Clin Immunol* 2000; **105**: S61.

16 Marone G, Spadaro G, Patella V, Genovese A. The clinical relevance of basophil releasability. *J Allergy Clin Immunol* 1994; **94**: 1293–303.

17 Metcalfe DD, Bland CE, Wasserman SI. Biochemical and functional characterization of proteoglycans isolated from basophils of patients with chronic myelogenous leukemia. *J Immunol* 1984; **132**: 1943–50.

18 Foster B, Schwartz LB, Metccalfe DD, Prussin C. Tryptase is expressed by human basophils independent of disease status. *J Allergy Clin Immunol* 2000; **105**: S89.

19 Xia H-Z, Kepley CL, Sakai K, Chelliah J, Irani A-MA, Schwartz LB. Quantitation of tryptase, chymase, FcεRIα and FcεRIg mRNAs in human mast cells and basophils by competitive reverse transcription-polymerase chain reaction. *J Immunol* 1995; **154**: 5472–80.

20 Leiferman KM, Gleich GJ, Kephart GM, *et al*. Differences between basophils and mast cells: failure to detect Charcot-Leyden crystal protein (lysophospholipase) and eosinophil granule major basic protein in human mast cells. *J Immunol* 1986; **136**: 852–5.

21 Warner JA, Peters SP, Lichtenstein LM, *et al*. Differential release of mediators from human basophils: differences in arachidonic acid metabolism following activation by unrelated stimuli. *J Leukoc Biol* 1989; **45**: 558–71.

22 Warner JA, Freeland HS, MacGlashan DW, Jr., Lichtenstein LM, Peters SP. Purified human basophils do not generate LTB4. *Biochem Pharmacol* 1987; **36**: 3195–9.

133

23 Triggiani M, Schleimer RP, Warner JA, Chilton FH. Differential synthesis of 1-acyl-2-acetyl-sn-glycero-3-phosphocholine and platelet-activating factor by human inflammatory cells. *J Immunol* 1991; **47**: 660–6.

24 de Paulis A, Prevete N, Fiorentino I, *et al.* Expression and functions of the vascular endothelial growth factors and their receptors in human basophils. *J Immunol* 2006; **177**: 7322–31.

25 Tschopp CM, Spiegl N, Didichenko S, *et al.* Granzyme B, a novel mediator of allergic inflammation: its induction and release in blood basophils and human asthma. *Blood* 2006; **108**: 2290–9.

26 Sloane DE, Tedla N, Awoniyi M, *et al.* Leukocyte immunoglobulin-like receptors: novel innate receptors for human basophil activation and inhibition. *Blood* 2004; **104**: 2832–9.

27 MacGlashan DW, Jr., Ishmael S, Macdonald SM, Langdon JM, Arm JP, Sloane DE. Induced loss of Syk in human basophils by non-IgE-dependent stimuli. *J Immunol* 2008; **180**: 4208–17.

28 Ochensberger B, Rihs S, Brunner T, Dahinden CA. IgE-independent interleukin-4 expression and induction of a late phase of leukotriene C4 formation in human blood basophils. *Blood* 1995; **86**: 4039–49.

29 Miura K, Hubbard WC, MacGlashan DW, Jr. Phosphorylation of cytosolic PLA2 (cPLA2) by Interleukin-3 (IL-3) is associated with increased free arachidonic acid and LTC4 release in human basophils. *J Allergy Clin Immunol* 1998; **102**: 512–20.

30 Miura K, MacGlashan DW, Jr. Dual phase priming by interleukin-3 for leukotriene C4 generation in human basophils. *J Immunol* 2000; **164**: 3026–34.

31 Sin AZ, Roche EM, Togias A, Lichtenstein LM, Schroeder JT. Nerve growth factor or IL-3 induces more IL-13 production from basophils of allergic subjects than from basophils of nonallergic subjects. *J Allergy Clin Immunol* 2001; **108**: 387–93.

32 Schroeder JT, MacGlashan DW, Jr., Lichtenstein LM. Mechanisms and pharmacologic control of basophil-derived IL-4 and IL-13. *Int Arch Allergy Immunol* 1999; **118**: 87–9.

33 Schroeder JT, Chichester KL, Bieneman AP. Human basophils secrete IL-3: evidence of autocrine priming for phenotypic and functional responses in allergic disease. *J Immunol* 2009; **182**: 2432–8.

34 Komiya A, Nagase H, Okugawa S, *et al.* Expression and function of toll-like receptors in human basophils. *Int Arch Allergy Immunol* 2006; **140** (Suppl 1): 23–7.

35 Bieneman AP, Chichester KL, Chen YH, Schroeder JT. Toll-like receptor 2 ligands activate human basophils for both IgE-dependent and IgE-independent secretion. *J Allergy Clin Immunol* 2005; **115**: 295–301.

36 Ochensberger B, Daepp GC, Rihs S, Dahinden CA. Human blood basophils produce interleukin-13 in response to IgE-receptor-dependent and -independent activation. *Blood* 1996; **88**: 3028–32.

37 Voehringer D, Shinkai K, Locksley RM. Type 2 immunity reflects orchestrated recruitment of cells committed to IL-4 production. *Immunity* 2004; **20**: 267–77.

38 Min B, Prout M, Hu-Li J, *et al.* Basophils produce IL-4 and accumulate in tissues after infection with a Th2-inducing parasite. *J Exp Med* 2004; **200**: 507–17.

39 Sokol CL, Barton GM, Farr AG, Medzhitov R. A mechanism for the initiation of allergen-induced T helper type 2 responses. *Nat Immunol* 2008; **9**: 310–18.

40 Sokol CL, Chu NQ, Yu S, Nish SA, Laufer TM, Medzhitov R. Basophils function as antigen-presenting cells for an allergen-induced T helper type 2 response. *Nat Immunol* 2009; **10**: 713–20.

41 Perrigoue JG, Saenz SA, Siracusa MC, *et al.* MHC class II-dependent basophil-CD4+ T cell interactions promote T(H)2 cytokine-dependent immunity. *Nat Immunol* 2009; **10**: 697–705.

42 Denzel A, Maus UA, Gomez MR, *et al.* Basophils enhance immunological memory responses. *Nat Immunol* 2008; **9**: 733–42.

43 Yamaguchi M, Koketsu R, Suzukawa M, Kawakami A, Iikura M. Human basophils and cytokines/chemokines. *Allergol Int* 2009; **58**: 1–10.

44 Smithgall MD, Comeau MR, Yoon BR, Kaufman D, Armitage R, Smith DE. IL-33 amplifies both Th1- and Th2-type responses through its activity on human basophils, allergen-reactive Th2 cells, iNKT, and NK cells. *Int Immunol* 2008; **20**: 1019–30.

45 Suzukawa M, Iikura M, Koketsu R, *et al.* An IL-1 cytokine member, IL-33: induces human basophil activation via its ST2 receptor. *J Immunol* 2008; **181**: 5981–9.

46 Pecaric-Petkovic T, Didichenko SA, Kaempfer S, Spiegl N, Dahinden CA. Human basophils and eosinophils are the direct target leukocytes of the novel IL-1 family member IL-33. *Blood* 2009; **113**: 1526–34.

47 Chen YH, Bieneman AP, Creticos PS, Chichester KL, Schroeder JT. IFN-alpha inhibits IL-3 priming of human basophil cytokine secretion but not leukotriene C4 and histamine release. *J Allergy Clin Immunol* 2003; **112**: 944–50.

48 Kepley CL, Cambier JC, Morel PA, *et al.* Negative regulation of FcepsilonRI signaling by FcgammaRII costimulation in human blood basophils. *J Allergy Clin Immunol* 2000; **106**: 337–48.

49 Zhu D, Kepley CL, Zhang M, Zhang K, Saxon A. A novel human immunoglobulin Fc gamma Fc epsilon bifunctional fusion protein inhibits Fc epsilon RI-mediated degranulation. *Nat Med* 2002; **8**: 518–21.

50 Zhu D, Kepley CL, Zhang K, Terada T, Yamada T, Saxon A. A chimeric human–cat fusion protein blocks cat-induced allergy. *Nat Med* 2005; **11**: 446–9.

51 Allen LC, Kepley CL, Saxon A, Zhang K. Modifications to an Fcgamma–Fcvarepsilon fusion protein alter its effectiveness in the inhibition of FcvarepsilonRI-mediated functions. *J Allergy Clin Immunol* 2007; **120**: 462–8.

52 Stallman PJ, Aalberse RC, Bruhl PC, van Elven EH. Experiments on the passive sensitization of human basophils, using quantitative immunofluorescence microscopy. *Int Arch Allergy Appl Immunol* 1977; **54**: 364–73.

53 Furuichi K, Rivera J, Isersky C. The receptor for immunoglobulin E on rat basophilic leukemia cells: effect of ligand binding on receptor expression. *Proc Natl Acad Sci USA* 1985; **82**: 1522–5.

54 Hsu C, MacGlashan DW, Jr. IgE Antibody upregulates high affinity IgE binding on murine bone marrow derived mast cells. *Immunol Lett* 1996; **52**: 129–34.

55 MacGlashan DW, Jr., Xia HZ, Schwartz LB, Gong JP. IgE-regulated expression of FceRI in human basophils: Control by regulated loss rather than regulated synthesis. *J Leuk Biol* 2001; **70**: 207–18.

56 Borkowski TA, Jouvin MH, Lin SY, Kinet JP. Minimal requirements for IgE-mediated regulation of surface Fc epsilon RI. *J Immunol* 2001; **167**: 1290–6.

57 Malveaux FJ, Conroy MC, Adkinson NFJ, Lichtenstein LM. IgE receptors on human basophils. Relationship to serum IgE concentration. *J Clin Invest* 1978; **62**: 176–81.

58 Saini SS, Klion AD, Holland SM, Hamilton RG, Bochner BS, MacGlashan DW, Jr. The relationship between serum IgE, and surface levels of FcepsilonR on human leukocytes in various diseases: Correlation of expression with FcepsilonRI on basophils but not on monocytes or eosinophils. *J Allergy Clin Immunol* 2000; **106**: 514–20.

59 Cookson WO, Sharp PA, Faux JA, Hopkin JM. Linkage between immunoglobulin E responses underlying asthma and rhinitis and chromosome 11q. *Lancet* 1989; **1**: 1292–5.

60 Shirakawa T, Li A, Dubowitz M, et al. Association between atopy and variants of the beta subunit of the high-affinity immunoglobulin E receptor. *Nature Genet* 1994; **7**: 125–9.

61 Shirakawa T, Mao XQ, Sasaki S, et al. Association between atopic asthma and a coding variant of Fc epsilon RI beta in a Japanese population. *Hum Mol Genet* 1996; **5**: 2068.

62 Palmer LJ, Pare PD, Faux JA, et al. Fc epsilon R1-beta polymorphism and total serum IgE, levels in endemically parasitized Australian aborigines. *Am J Hum Genet* 1997; **61**: 182–8.

63 Donnadieu E, Cookson WO, Jouvin MH, Kinet JP. Allergy-associated polymorphisms of the FcepsilonRIbeta subunit do not impact its two amplification functions [In Process Citation]. *J Immunol* 2000; **165**: 3917–22.

64 Nishiyama C, Akizawa Y, Nishiyama M, et al. Polymorphisms in the Fc epsilon RI beta promoter region affecting transcription activity: a possible promoter-dependent mechanism for association between Fc epsilon RI beta and atopy. *J Immunol* 2004; **173**: 6458–64.

65 Hasegawa M, Nishiyama C, Nishiyama M, et al. A novel −66T/C polymorphism in Fc epsilon RI, alpha-chain promoter affecting the transcription activity: possible relationship to allergic diseases. *J Immunol* 2003; **171**: 1927–33.

66 Nishiyama C, Yokota T, Okumura K, Ra C. The transcription factors elf-1 and GATA-1 bind to cell-specific enhancer elements of human high-affinity IgE receptor alpha-chain gene. *J Immunol* 1999; **163**: 623–30.

67 Maeda K, Nishiyama C, Tokura T, et al. FOG-1 represses GATA-1-dependent FcepsilonRI beta-chain transcription: transcriptional mechanism of mast cell-specific gene expression in mice. *Blood* 2006; **108**: 262–9.

68 Akizawa Y, Nishiyama C, Hasegawa M, et al. Regulation of human FcepsilonRI beta chain gene expression by Oct-1. *Int Immunol* 2003; **15**: 549–56.

69 Wang QH, Nishiyama C, Nakano N, et al. Suppressive effect of Elf-1 on FcepsilonRI, alpha-chain expression in primary mast cells. *Immunogenetics* 2008; **60**: 557–63.

70 Maeda K, Nishiyama C, Tokura T, et al. Regulation of cell type-specific mouse Fc epsilon RI beta-chain gene expression by GATA-1 via four GATA motifs in the promoter. *J Immunol* 2003; **170**: 334–40.

71 Saini S, Richardson J, Wofsy J, Lavens-Phillips C, Bochner B, MacGlashan DW, Jr. Expression and modulation of FceRIa and FceRIb in human blood basophils. *J. All. Clin. Immunol* 2001; **107**: 832–41.

72 Lin S, Cicaia C, Scharenberg AM, Kinet JP. The FceRIb subunit functions as an amplifier of FceRIg-mediated cell activation signals. *Cell* 1996; **85**: 985–95.

73 Donnadieu E, Jouvin MH, Kinet JP. A second amplifier function for the allergy-associated Fc(epsilon)RI-beta subunit. *Immunity* 2000; **12**: 515–23.

74 Donnadieu E, Jouvin MH, Rana S, et al. Competing functions encoded in the allergy-associated F(c)epsilon-RIbeta gene. *Immunity* 2003; **18**: 665–74.

75 Miura K, Saini SS, Gauvreau G, MacGlashan DW, Jr. Differences in functional consequences and signal transduction induced by IL-3: IL-5 and NGF in human basophils. *J Immunol* 2001; **167**: 2282–91.

76 Albrecht B, Woisetschlager M, Robertson MW. Export of the high affinity IgE receptor from the endoplasmic reticulum depends on a glycosylation-mediated quality control mechanism. *J Immunol* 2000; **165**: 5686–94.

77 Cauvi DM, Tian X, von Loehneysen K, Robertson MW. Transport of the IgE receptor alpha-chain is controlled by a multicomponent intracellular retention signal. *J Biol Chem* 2006; **281**: 10448–60.

78 Fiebiger E, Tortorella D, Jouvin MH, Kinet JP, Ploegh HL. Cotranslational endoplasmic reticulum assembly of FcepsilonRI controls the formation of functional IgE-binding receptors. *J Exp Med* 2005; **201**: 267–77.

79 Letourneur O, Sechi S, Willette-Brown J, Robertson MW, Kinet JP. Glycosylation of human truncated Fc epsilon RI alpha chain is necessary for efficient folding in the endoplasmic reticulum. *J Biol Chem* 1995; **270**: 8249–56.

80 Letourneur F, Hennecke S, Demolliere C, Cosson P. Steric masking of a dilysine endoplasmic reticulum retention motif during assembly of the human high affinity receptor for immunoglobulin E. *J Cell Biol* 1995; **129**: 971–8.

81 Zaidi A, MacGlashan DW, Jr. IgE-dependent and IgE-independent stimulation of human basophils increased the presence of immature FcεRIα by reversing degradative pathways. *Int Arch Allergy Appl Immunol* 2010; **154**: 15–24.

82 Zaidi AK, Saini SS, MacGlashan DW, Jr. Regulation of Syk kinase and FcRbeta expression in human basophils during treatment with omalizumab. *J Allergy Clin Immunol* 2010; **125**: 902–8.

83 Zaidi AK, MacGlashan DW, Jr. Regulation of FceRI expression during murine basophil maturation: The interplay between IgE cell division and FceRI synthetic rate. *J Immunol* 2010; **184**: 1463–74.

84 MacGlashan DW, Jr., Bochner BS, Adelman DC, *et al.* Downregulation of FceRI expression on human basophils during *in vivo* treatment of atopic patients with anti-IgE antibody. *J Immunol* 1997; **158**: 1438–45.

85 Segal DM, Taurog JD, Metzger H. Dimeric immunoglobulin E serves as a unit signal for mast cell degranulation. *Proc Natl Acad Sci USA* 1977; **74**: 2993–7.

86 Cooper AD, Balakrishnan K, McConnell HM. Mobile haptens in liposomes stimulate serotonin release by rat basophil leukemia cells in the presence of specific immunoglobulin E. *J Biol Chem* 1981; **256**: 9379–81.

87 Kalesnikoff J, Huber M, Lam V, *et al.* Monomeric IgE stimulates signaling pathways in mast cells that lead to cytokine production and cell survival. *Immunity* 2001; **14**: 801–11.

88 Asai K, Kitaura J, Kawakami Y, *et al.* Regulation of mast cell survival by IgE. *Immunity* 2001; **14**: 791–800.

89 Kitaura J, Song J, Tsai M, *et al.* Evidence that IgE molecules mediate a spectrum of effects on mast cell survival and activation via aggregation of the FcepsilonRI. *Proc Natl Acad Sci USA* 2003; **100**: 12911–16.

90 James LC, Roversi P, Tawfik DS. Antibody multispecificity mediated by conformational diversity. *Science* 2003; **299**: 1362–7.

91 Chang EY, Zheng Y, Holowka D, Baird B. Alteration of lipid composition modulates Fc epsilon RI signaling in RBL-2H3 cells. *Biochemistry* 1995; **34**: 4376–84.

92 Field KA, Holowka D, Baird B. Fc epsilon RI-mediated recruitment of p53/56lyn to detergent-resistant membrane domains accompanies cellular signaling. *Proc Natl Acad Sci USA* 1995; **92**: 9201–5.

93 Ortega E, Lara M, Lee I, *et al.* Lyn dissociation from phosphorylated Fc epsilon RI subunits: a new regulatory step in the Fc epsilon RI signaling cascade revealed by studies of Fc epsilon RI dimer signaling activity. *J Immunol* 1999; **162**: 176–85.

94 Vonakis BM, Chen H, Haleem-Smith H, Metzger H. The unique domain as the site on Lyn kinase for its constitutive association with the high affinity receptor for IgE. *J Biol Chem* 1997; **272**: 24072–80.

95 Kihara H, Siraganian RP. Src homology 2 domains of Syk and Lyn bind to tyrosine-phosphorylated subunits of the high affinity IgE receptor. *J Biol Chem* 1994; **269**: 22427–32.

96 Zhang J, Berenstein EH, Evans RL, Siraganian RP. Transfection of Syk protein tyrosine kinase reconstitutes high affinity IgE receptor-mediated degranulation in a Syk-negative variant of rat basophilic leukemia RBL-2H3 cells. *J Exp Med* 1996; **184**: 71–9.

97 Vilarino N, MacGlashan DW, Jr. Transient transfection of human peripheral blood basophils. *J Immunol Methods* 2005; **296**: 11–18.

98 MacGlashan DW, Jr., Vilarino N. Nonspecific desensitization, functional memory and the characteristics of SHIP phosphorylation following IgE-mediated stimulation of human basophils. *J Immunol* 2006; **177**: 1040–51.

99 Odom S, Gomez G, Kovarova M, *et al.* Negative regulation of immunoglobulin E-dependent allergic responses by Lyn kinase. *J Exp Med* 2004; **199**: 1491–502.

100 Lavens-Phillips SE, Miura K, MacGlashan DW, Jr. Pharmacology of IgE-mediated desensitization of human basophils: Effects of protein kinase C, and Src-family kinase inhibitors. *Biochem Pharmacol* 2000; **60**: 1717–227.

101 Smith AJ, Surviladze Z, Gaudet EA, Backer JM, Mitchell CA, Wilson BS. p110beta and p110delta phosphatidylinositol 3-kinases upregulate Fc(epsilon) RI-activated Ca2+ influx by enhancing inositol 1,4,5-trisphosphate production. *J Biol Chem* 2001; **276**: 17213–20.

102 Iwaki S, Tkaczyk C, Satterthwaite AB, *et al.* Btk plays a crucial role in the amplification of Fc epsilonRI-mediated mast cell activation by kit. *J Biol Chem* 2005; **280**: 40261–70.

103 Hata D, Kawakami Y, Inagaki N, *et al*. Involvement of Bruton's tyrosine kinase in FcepsilonRI-dependent mast cell degranulation and cytokine production. *J Exp Med* 1998; **187**: 1235–47.

104 Tkaczyk C, Beaven MA, Brachman SM, Metcalfe DD, Gilfillan AM. The phospholipase C gamma 1-dependent pathway of Fc epsilon RI-mediated mast cell activation is regulated independently of phosphatidylinositol 3-kinase. *J Biol Chem* 2003; **278**: 48474–84.

105 MacGlashan DW, Jr. Self-termination/anergic mechanisms in human basophils and mast cells. *Int Arch Allergy Immunol* 2009; **150**: 109–21.

106 Vazquez F, Devreotes P. Regulation of PTEN function as a PIP3 gatekeeper through membrane interaction. *Cell Cycle* 2006; **5**: 1523–7.

107 Mao SY, Pfeiffer JR, Oliver JM, Metzger H. Effects of subunit mutation on the localization to coated pits and internalization of cross-linked IgE-receptor complexes. *J Immunol* 1993; **151**: 2760–74.

108 Oliver JM, Seagrave J, Stump RF. Two Distinct States of Cross-linked IgE Receptors that may Trigger and Terminate Secretion from RBL-2H3 Mast Cells. In: Perelson AL, (ed). *Studies in the Science of Complexity*. Addison-Wesley: Redwood City, CA, 1987. p. 61–82.

109 Itoh K, Sakakibara M, Yamasaki S, *et al*. Cutting edge: negative regulation of immune synapse formation by anchoring lipid raft to cytoskeleton through Cbp-EBP50-ERM assembly. *J Immunol* 2002; **168**: 541–4.

110 Ozawa T, Nakata K, Mizuno K, Yakura H. Negative autoregulation of Src homology region 2-domain-containing phosphatase-1 in rat basophilic leukemia-2H3 cells. *Int Immunol* 2007; **19**: 1049–61.

111 Isersky C, Rivera J, Segal DM, Triche T. The fate of IgE bound to rat basophilic leukemia cells. II. Endocytosis of IgE oligomers and effect on receptor turnover. *J Immunol* 1983; **131**: 388–96.

112 MacGlashan DW, Jr. Endocytosis, re-cycling and degradation of unoccupied FcεRI in human basophils. *J Leukoc Biol* 2007; **82**: 1003–10.

113 MacGlashan D,W, Jr., Miura K. Loss of Syk kinase during IgE-mediated stimulation of human basophils. *J Allergy Clin Immunol* 2004; **114**: 1317–24.

114 MacGlashan DW, Jr., Undem BJ. Inducing an anergic state in mast cells and basophils without secretion. *J Allergy Clin Immunol* 2008; **121**: 1500–6.

115 MacGlashan DW, Jr., Honigberg LA, Smith A, Buggy J, Schroeder JT. Inhibition of IgE-mediated secretion from human basophils with a highly selective Bruton's tyrosine kinase, Btk, inhibitor. *Int Immunopharmacol* 2011; **11**: 475–9.

116 Nguyen KL, Gillis S, MacGlashan DW, Jr. A comparative study of releasing and nonreleasing human basophils: nonreleasing basophils lack an early component of the signal transduction pathway that follows IgE cross-linking. *J Allergy Clin Immunol* 1990; **85**: 1020–9.

117 Kepley CL, Youssef L, Andrews RP, Wilson BS, Oliver JM. Syk deficiency in nonreleaser basophils. *J Allergy Clin Immunol* 1999; **104**: 279–84.

118 Lavens-Phillips SE, MacGlashan DW, Jr. The tyrosine kinases, p53/56lyn and p72syk are differentially expressed at the protein level but not at the mRNA, level in nonreleasing human basophils. *Am J Resp Cell Mol Biol* 2000; **23**: 566–71.

119 MacGlashan DW, Jr. Relationship between Syk and SHIP expression and secretion from human basophils in the general population. *J Allergy Clin Immunol* 2007; **119**: 626–33.

120 Ishmael S, MacGlashan DW, Jr. Early signal protein expression profiles in basophils: a population study. *J Leukoc Biol* 2009; **86**: 313–25.

121 Ishmael S, MacGlashan DW, Jr. Syk expression in peripheral blood leukocytes, CD34+ progenitors and CD34-derived basophils. *J Leuk Biol* 2010; **87**: 291–300.

122 Kepley CL, Pfeiffer JR, Schwartz LB, Wilson BS, Oliver JM. The identification and characterization of umbilical cord blood-derived human basophils. *J Leukoc Biol* 1998; **64**: 474–83.

123 Langdon JM, Schroeder JT, Vonakis BM, Bieneman AP, Chichester K, Macdonald SM. Histamine-releasing factor/translationally controlled tumor protein (HRF/TCTP)-induced histamine release is enhanced with SHIP-1 knockdown in cultured human mast cell and basophil models. *J Leukoc Biol* 2008; **84**: 1151–8.

10 Epithelial cells

Tillie-Louise Hackett,[1,2] *Stephanie Warner,*[1] *Dorota Stefanowicz,*[1] *and Darryl Knight*[1,2]

[1]UBC James Hogg Research Centre, Providence Heart and Lung Institute, St Paul's Hospital, Vancouver, BC, Canada

[2]Department of Anesthesiology, Pharmacology, and Therapeutics, University of British Columbia, Vancouver, BC, Canada

Introduction

Asthma has been traditionally considered as a disease of immune origin. However, a more recent and compelling hypothesis suggests that alterations in the structural cells of the airways, particularly the epithelium, act in concert with abnormal immune responses leading to the development of the disease. This chapter describes our current understanding of the airway epithelium in terms of phenotype and repair, immune and inflammatory pathways, and genetic and epigenetic regulation. We highlight how these processes are dysfunctional in asthma and what key molecules or pathways may provide future novel therapeutic targets.

The epithelial barrier

The epithelium constitutes the interface between the external environment and the internal milieu of the lung, and as such is the point of first contact with respirable particles, respiratory viruses, and airborne allergens. Under normal circumstances, the airway epithelium forms a highly regulated, semipermeable barrier comprising multiple cell types. This barrier function is maintained by cell-to-cell contacts termed the apical junction complex (AJC), consisting of tight junctions (TJs), gap junctions (GJs), adherens junctions (AJs), and desmosomes (Des), as shown in

Figure 10.1 [1,2]. Epithelial damage and denudation in individuals with asthma has been observed for many years [3]. Indeed it is now accepted that the asthmatic epithelium is fragile and displays a loss of columnar ciliated cells in both adults [4] and children [5]. This coincides with reduced and altered expression of AJC proteins such as E-cadherin [6]. Epithelial damage is not confined to the lower airways; disrupted desmosome formation has also been shown in nasal polyps from children with asthma [7]. Allergens with proteolytic activity, such as Der p 1 from the house dust mite and proteases from pollen, can disrupt mucosal integrity through direct extracellular cleavage of intracellular TJs [8,9]. Oxidant pollutants such as ozone, nitrogen dioxide, and to a lesser extent sulfur dioxide and formaldehyde have been shown to significantly increase the permeability of epithelial monolayers [10,11]. In addition, interleukin 4 (IL-4), interferon gamma (IFN-γ) and tumor necrosis factor alpha (TNF-α) produced by inflammatory cells in response to injury may decrease the expression of zonula occludin (ZO)-1 and γ-catenin in human airway cells [12–15]. The effects of increased epithelial permeability are unknown but may provide allergens with a mechanism for enhanced antigen presentation to dendritic cells, thereby promoting allergic sensitization.

The composition of the asthmatic airway epithelium itself is different from nondiseased airways (Figure 10.2). For example, airway epithelial cells

Inflammation and Allergy Drug Design, First Edition. Edited by Kenji Izuhara, Stephen T. Holgate, Marsha Wills-Karp.

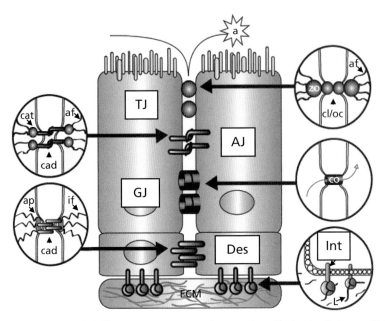

Figure 10.1 Epithelial adhesion. Inhaled allergens (a) are unable to travel between the epithelium because of adhesion complexes. Tight junctions (TJ) are composed of claudins/occludins (cl/oc) that interact with zonula occludins (zo), which are then tethered to actin filaments (af). Gap junctions (GJ) are portholes from cell to cell and are composed of connexins (co). Adherens junctions (AJ) contain cadherins (cad) that are linked to actin filaments (af) via catenins (cat). Desmosomes (Des) also contain cadherins (cad), which are held together through an adhesion plaque (ap) that interacts with intermediate filaments (if). Cells are tethered to the extracellular matrix (ECM) via integrins (Int) bound to their ligands (l).

obtained by bronchial brushings from children with asthma display decreased expression of the differentiation marker cytokeratin 19 with concurrent increased expression of the basal epithelial marker cytokeratin-5 compared with atopic and nonatopic children [16–18]. Goblet cell hyperplasia and excessive mucus production are common features of asthma and contribute significantly to related morbidity and mortality. Recent studies have shown that IL-13- and epidermal growth factor receptor (EGFR)-dependent expression of Forkhead transcription factors Fox-A2 and Fox-A3 is a central step in epithelial cell mucin production in asthma [19]. Another potential mediator of this process is the SAM pointed domain containing ETS transcription factor (SPDEF), which in mice induces the differentiation of Clara cells into goblet cells in response to house dust mite allergen or IL-13 [20,21].

These morphologic changes are also mirrored at the molecular level in cultured asthmatic epithelial cells, which are more susceptible to oxidant-induced "stress" and display abnormal expression of proinflammatory transcription factors (nuclear factor κB [NFκB], AP-1, STAT1, and STAT6) as well as heat shock proteins [22–24]. The overall proliferative rate also appears to be increased in the epithelium of asthmatics and particularly in those with more severe disease [18,25,26]. However, somewhat surprisingly, asthmatic epithelial cells display attenuated and dysregulated wound repair *in vitro*, concurrent with elevations in PAI-1 expression [27] and decreased fibronectin expression [28]. In the asthmatic epithelium, expression of EGFR is markedly increased, especially in areas where columnar cells have been shed. This is seen in both adults [29] and children with moderate/severe asthma [30], although its ligands were not found to be upregulated under nonstimulated conditions [31]. Furthermore, increased expression of EGFR in asthmatics occurs even in areas of intact epithelium and does not correlate with the pro-

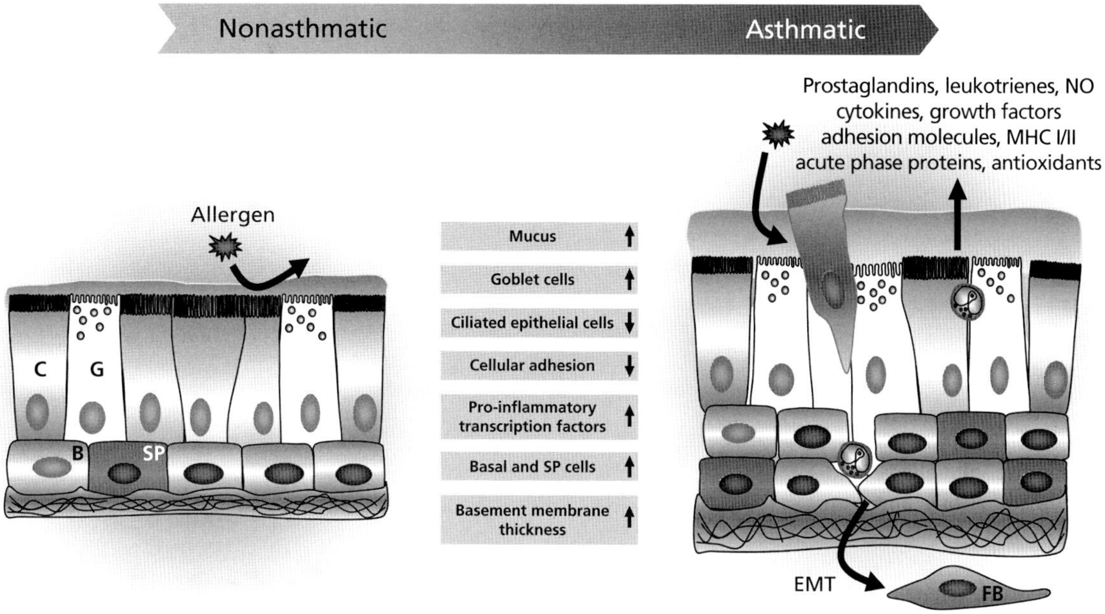

Figure 10.2 The airway epithelium is intrinsically altered in asthma. Loss of ciliated cells and expansion of the basal cell population may indicate an abnormal repair or proliferative response of repairing cells [32]. However, differentiation process such as EMT. FB, fibroblast; EMT, epithelial-mesenchymal transition; C, ciliated cells; G, goblet cells; B, basal cells; SP, side population cells.

proliferative response of repairing cells [32]. However, increased expression of the cyclin-dependent kinase inhibitor p21$^{WAF1/CIP1}$ in the asthmatic epithelium [33] may provide some explanation for the discrepancy between EGFR levels and the proliferative response.

Epithelial cells obtained from children with mild asthma also express greater levels of PGE$_2$ and IL-6 than those obtained from nonasthmatic individuals [18]. Thus, the available evidence suggests that the asthmatic epithelium is fragile, has an altered phenotype, and has dysregulated repair, which could arise from repeated and excessive damage or a compromised ability to differentiate.

The epithelial immune barrier

As a result of persistent exposure to the external environment, the airway epithelium must not only function as a barrier to and react to inhaled agents, but must also be able to communicate and signal to other cells. This capacity permits the epithelium to act as a functional interface between innate and adaptive immune regulation (Figure 10.3).

The innate immune system is the first line of host defense providing protection against a broad spectrum of microbial threats. Thus, in addition to the well-known functions of mucociliary clearance and the provision and maintenance of a physical barrier, epithelial cells can kill or neutralize microbes through the production of several families of molecules including defensins, lysozymes, cathepsins, etc. (reviewed in Bals and Hiemstra [34]). The innate immune response also relies on pattern-recognition receptors (PRRs), which recognize highly conserved microbial structures called pathogen-associated molecular patterns (PAMPs) and enables the host to recognize a broad range of pathogens quickly, bypassing T- and B-cell activation. Epithelial cells express several PRRs including nucleotide-binding oligomerization domains (NODS) and Toll-like receptors (TLRs) [35]. Activation of both Nod1 and Nod2 in epithelial cells induces NF-κB, activation, although Nod1 can also activate the JNK pathway, resulting in an inflammatory response [36–38]. TLRs are PRRs that identify PAMPs such as single-stranded and double-stranded RNA from viruses, lipoproteins from bacteria and yeasts, and lipopolysaccharide, flagellar proteins, and

141

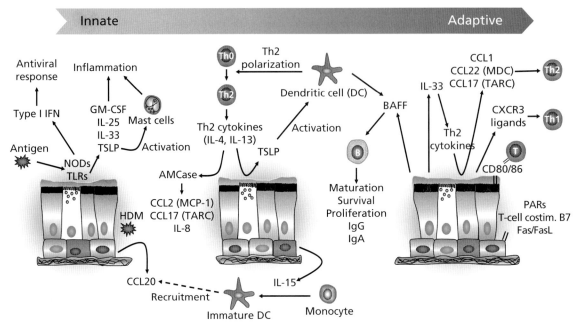

Figure 10.3 The epithelium acts as a functional interface between innate and adaptive immune regulation through expression of a multitude of cytokines, chemokines, receptors, ligands and enzymes, both endogenously and in response to external stimuli. NOD, nucleotide oligomerization domain; TSLP, thymic stromal lymphopoietin; IL, interleukin; IFN, interferon, Th, T helper cell; TLR, Toll-like receptor; Ig, immunoglobulin; GM-CSF, granulocyte–macrophage colony-stimulating factor; AMCase, acidic mammalian chitinase; BAFF, B-cell activating factor; DC, dendritic cell; CCL, chemokine (C-C motif) ligand; TARC, thymus and activation-regulated chemokine; CXCR, chemokine (CXC motif) receptor; PAR, protease-activated receptor.

unmethylated CpG DNA from bacteria [39]. Under normal conditions, the predominant TLR expressed on the surface of airway epithelial cells *in vivo* is TLR2, whereas TLR3, TLR4, and TLR5 reside primarily intracellularly. However, these TLRs can be rapidly mobilized to the cell surface following stimulation [40–42]. Depending on the TLRs activated, the result can be proinflammatory cytokine and chemokine release via NF-κB or JNK induction, or antiviral type I-interferon release via IRF-3/5/7 activation [43–45]. For example, activation of TLR4 by house dust mite allergen induces an innate cytokine immune response through production of granulocyte–macrophage colony-stimulating factor (GM-CSF), IL-25, IL-33, and thymic stromal lymphopoietin (TSLP) by airway epithelial cells. TLSP expression is also upregulated in epithelial cells in response to dsRNA

viruses, such as rhinovirus, through TLR3-mediated activation of other TLRs, including TLR2, TLR8, and TLR9, NF-κB, and Th2 cytokines such as IL-4 and IL-13 [46–48]. The release of TSLP by the epithelium in inflammatory conditions can activate mast cells, resulting in the release of proinflammatory cytokines, chemokines, and lipid mediators [47] and effectively bypassing the traditional T cell-mediated allergic reaction. Thus, TSLP coupled with antigenic stimulation is capable of initiating both innate and adaptive immune responses resulting in allergic airway inflammation [49].

The epithelium is also ideally situated to orchestrate and influence adaptive immune responses. For example, the epithelium can act as an antigen-presenting cell itself, expressing low levels of major histocompatibility complex (MHC) class I and II under resting conditions but is rapidly upregulated by allergens and other inflammatory stimuli [50,51]. The epithelium also produces a number of cytokines that act in a paracrine fashion to regulate the recruitment, maturation, and activity of dendritic cells, the major antigen-presenting cells in the airway mucosa [52–57].

Airway epithelial cells produce a multitude of chemokines and cytokines that influence recruitment, activation, and polarization of T lymphocytes; they are the main producers of the IFN-γ-induced Th-1 cell-attracting CXCR3 ligands CXCL9 (Mig), CXCL10 (IP-10), and CXCL11 (I-TAC) [58], and more recently the T-cell chemoattractant CXCL16 [59]. Epithelial cells are also potent directors of Th2 cells, mainly through production of CCL1, CCL17, (TARC) and CCL22 (MDC). These chemokines are induced by Th2 cytokines such as IL-4 and IL-13, and expression is increased in the airways of atopic asthmatics [60]. Airway epithelial cells also produce the ST-2 ligand IL-33, which induces an allergic inflammation in the lung and gut [61]. Direct interaction with T lymphocytes is facilitated by expression of CD40, Fas and Fas ligand, as well as the T-cell co-stimulatory B7 family of molecules on epithelial cells [58]. Furthermore, viral exposure increases the expression of the co-stimulatory molecules CD80 and CD86, further promoting direct interaction between the epithelium and T cells [62]. Airway epithelial cells also express intercellular adhesion molecule 1 (ICAM-1/CD54), the expression of which is enhanced following exposure to proinflammatory cytokines as well as in response to respiratory viral infections [63]. Expression of epithelial cell adhesion molecule (Ep-CAM) is seen as a general marker of epithelial lineage but its role in leukocyte–epithelial interactions is unknown [64].

The airway epithelium can also produce the enzyme acidic mammalian chitinase (AMCase), which degrades the protective chitin coating of certain organisms [65]. Chitin is a ubiquitous biopolymer that is found in fungi, helminths, crustaceans, and insects [65,66], and is thus encountered by the body on a recurring basis. Although chitin induces AMCase expression in sinonasal epithelial cells [67], investigations into activity and expression in the lung have been limited to an inflammatory model in which IL-13-induced Th2 inflammation effectively increased AMCase expression [68]. AMCase is also capable of acting in an autocrine and/or paracrine manner, resulting in production of the chemokines CCL2, CCL17, and CXCL8 [69], making it an important part of both the innate and adaptive immune responses to the inhaled environment. Interestingly, blocking AMCase abolishes Th2 inflammation and airway hyperresponsiveness [68], suggesting that it may be a novel target for asthma therapy.

Epithelial repair and stem cells

Under normal conditions, the turnover of the epithelium is slow compared with other mucosal surfaces such as the skin and gut [70]. However, when injured, it has the capacity to rapidly repair. In these situations, secretory and ciliated cells surrounding the wound site lose cilia and migrate rapidly to cover the wound area, while progenitor cells proliferate and differentiate. This is associated with delayed recruitment and proliferation of mesenchymal cells in the subepithelial tissues [71]. These processes are spatially and temporally controlled by local signals generated by a plethora of mediators released initially by the epithelium and subsequently by the underlying mesenchymal cells. In this regard epithelial repair resembles reactivation of lung development programs [72].

Despite the observations of epithelial repair both *in vivo* and *in vitro*, the cues, signals, and mechanisms of how the epithelium replenishes itself after damage remain unknown. Many reports have suggested that circulating stem cells localize to various tissues and differentiate into tissue-specific cells [73,74]. More recently, a population of circulating epithelial progenitor cells that aided airway epithelial reconstitution was identified in mice [75]. The findings of several murine experimental models developed to mimic epithelial injury and repair following environmental challenges have demonstrated that different regions within the respiratory system (conducting airways, distal bronchioles, and alveoli) contain different stem cell populations and different repair mechanisms [76]. To date, the cells reported to be enriched for stem/progenitor cell activity include cytokeratin 5/14-expressing basal cells, Clara cells, cells residing in submucosal glands, and neuroepithelial bodies (NEBs) [77–79]. More recently, GATA-6/Wnt has been shown to temporally control the appearance of bronchoalveolar stem cells (BASC) [80], although other studies have suggested that another molecule downstream of Wnt signaling, β-catenin, may not be necessary for maintenance or repair of the bronchiolar epithelium [81]. These cells may or may not reside within stem/progenitor niches such as the bronchoalveolar duct junction (BADJ) [82,83]. More recently, single randomly distributed progenitor cells were shown to maintain epithelial homeostasis in healthy and modestly injured airways [84]. In contrast, repair following severe injury resulted from large clonal cell patches associated with stem cell niches residing within NEBs and BADJs. Importantly, repair mediated through the activation of local stem cells led to a loss of progenitor cell diversity. Thus, following extensive or repeated injury or damage to the epithelium, such as in asthma, repair through stem cell niches may have important implications for the resultant phenotype of epithelial cells.

Little is known about resident epithelial stem/progenitor cells in human airways. Transit amplifying cells expressing CD151 and tissue factor have been shown to have the capacity to generate a differentiated epithelium *in vitro* and in xenograft models *in vivo* [85–87]. A so-called resident side population (SP), characterized by the ability to actively efflux the DNA-binding dye Hoechst 33342, has also been identified in the basal cell compartment of human airways [16]. These cells are rare, making up less than 0.1% of the total epithelial cell number, do not express CD45, and exhibit several key features of stem/progenitor cell function, including sustained colony-forming capacity, stable telomere length, and, importantly, the ability to form a multilayered differentiated epithelium. Of interest, the asthmatic airway epithelium harbors 40 times more SP cells than do normal airways. The capacity of epithelial SP cells to differentiate into other nonepithelial tissues has not been formally examined. However, it appears that once these cells take up residence in a specific tissue, they become committed to lineage decisions appropriate for that tissue [88].

Genetic and epigenetic factors influencing the airway epithelium

Recent studies using genetic techniques such as positional cloning and genome-wide association have identified numerous genes that are associated with asthma and preferentially expressed in the epithelium.

These include genes that encode dipeptidyl peptidase (DPP10) [89,90], TSLP [91–93], AMCase [94], and protocadherin (PCDH-1) [95].

The DPP10 gene encodes an enzyme that cleaves the terminal two peptides from specific proinflammatory chemokines, but the functional significance of this activity is still unknown—the result could be activation or deactivation of the individual chemokines [89,96]. If they are activated, as has been suggested for a subset of chemokines [89], then DPP10 has the potential to be a new target for asthma therapy.

In an experimental murine asthma model, TSLP was shown to be upregulated in the asthmatic airway [97], which was confirmed in bronchial biopsies from human asthmatic airways [91,98]. Interestingly, a study investigating gene variants in asthmatic populations identified a single nucleotide polymorphism near the TSLP gene which is associated with both asthma and airway hyperresponsiveness [93].

AMCase is strongly upregulated in the epithelium of asthmatics [68], and haplotype analysis of genetic variants in the AMCase gene has revealed an association of certain haplotypes with asthma [94]. Investigations into the functional effects of polymorphisms in the AMCase gene in American ethnic populations found that a variant isoform of the gene has a protective effect against asthma [99].

PCDH1 has only recently been identified as an asthma susceptibility gene. In multiple populations, genetic variations in the PCDH1 gene have been associated with both bronchial hyperresponsiveness and asthma [95]. Given that PCDH1 is a structural protein involved in cell adhesion and barrier function, the discovery of an association to asthma highlights the importance of the structural barrier that the epithelium provides [96]. Novel adhesion molecules genes such as catenin α-like 1, which is linked to asthma susceptibility, also appear to play a role in epithelial wound repair and proliferation [100].

In addition to the genetic abnormalities listed above, epigenetic regulation of gene expression has generated much recent attention. For example, the asthmatic epithelium has been shown to have diminished expression of certain histone deacetylases (HDACs) such as HDAC1 and HDAC2 [101], which can modify proteins and chromatin structure, effecting protein function and gene transcription. In this context, histone acetyl transferases (HATs) and HDACs may play a significant role in steroid resistance as in order for the glucocorticoid receptor (GR) to associate with and suppress the NF-κB complex, it must be deacetylated. Therefore, in an environment where HDAC2 is limited, GRs cannot function to their full capacity [102].

Summary

From the evidence presented, the epithelium is far more than a physical barrier. It expresses a large and expanding repertoire of receptors, cytokines, chemokines, growth factors, and lipid mediators that impact on airway function. Importantly, it is becoming increasingly recognized as a central component of both the innate and adaptive immune responses. As such, the airway epithelium almost certainly contributes to both inflammation and remodeling and should be considered as a target for novel asthma medications.

Acknowledgment

TLH is the recipient of CIHR/CLA/GSK, CIHR/ IMPACT strategic training and Michael Smith Foundation postdoctoral fellowships; DS is the recipient of an NSERC Graduate Student Scholarship; SW is the recipient of an NSERC Alexander Graham Bell Canada Graduate Scholarship; DAK is the Canada Research Chair in Airway Disease, a Michael Smith Foundation for Health Research Career Investigator and a William Thurlbeck Distinguished Researcher. This work is funded by CIHR and an unrestricted educational grant from the Corporate Office of Science & Technology at Johnson & Johnson.

References

1 Schneeberger EE, Lynch RD. Structure, function, and regulation of cellular tight junctions. *Am J Physiol Lung Cell Mol Physiol* 1992; **262**: L647–61.

2 Evans MJ, Cox RA, Shami SG, et al. Junctional adhesion mechanisms in airway basal cells. *Am J Respir Cell Mol Biol* 1990; **3**: 341–7.

3 Dunnill MS. The pathology of asthma, with special reference to changes in the bronchial mucosa. *J Clin Pathol* 1960; **13**: 27–33.

4 Trautmann A, Kruger K, Akdis M, et al. Apoptosis and loss of adhesion of bronchial epithelial cells

5 Barbato A, Turato G, Baraldo S, et al. Epithelial damage and angiogenesis in the airways of children with asthma. *Am J Respir Crit Care Med* 2006; **174**: 975–81.

6 de Boer WI, Sharma HS, Baelemans SM, et al. Altered expression of epithelial junctional proteins in atopic asthma: possible role in inflammation. *Can J Physiol Pharmacol* 2008; **86**: 105–12.

7 Shahana S, Jaunmuktane Z, Asplund MS, et al. Ultrastructural investigation of epithelial damage in asthmatic and nonasthmatic nasal polyps. *Respir Med* 2006; **100**: 2018–28.

8 Hassim Z, Maronese SE, Kumar RK. Injury to murine airway epithelial cells by pollen enzymes. *Thorax* 1998; **53**: 368–71.

9 Winton HL, Wan H, Cannell MB, et al. Class specific inhibition of house dust mite proteinases which cleave cell adhesion, induce cell death and which increase the permeability of lung epithelium. *Br J Pharmacol* 1998; **124**: 1048–59.

10 Bayram H, Rusznak C, Khair OA, et al. Effect of ozone and nitrogen dioxide on the permeability of bronchial epithelial cell cultures of nonasthmatic and asthmatic subjects. *Clin Exp Allergy* 2002; **32**: 1285–92.

11 Chitano P, Hosselet JJ, Mapp CE, et al. Effect of oxidant air pollutants on the respiratory system: insights from experimental animal research. *Eur Respir J* 1995; **8**: 1357–71.

12 Kampf C, Roomans GM. Effects of hypochlorite on cultured respiratory epithelial cells. *Free Radic Res* 2001; **34**: 499–511.

13 Shahana S, Kampf C, Roomans GM. Effects of the cationic protein poly L-arginine on airway epithelial cells *in vitro*. *Mediators Inflamm* 2002; **11**: 141–8.

14 Relova AJ, Kampf C, Roomans GM. Effects of Th-2 type cytokines on human airway epithelial cells: interleukins-4, -5, and -13. *Cell Biol Int* 2001; **25**: 563–6.

15 Jang AS, Choi IS, Koh YI, et al. The relationship between alveolar epithelial proliferation and airway obstruction after ozone exposure. *Allergy* 2002; **57**: 737–40.

16 Hackett TL, Shaheen F, Johnson A, et al. Characterization of side population cells from human airway epithelium. *Stem Cells* 2008; **26**: 2576–85.

17 Hackett TL, Warner SM, Stefanowicz D, et al. Induction of epithelial-mesenchymal transition in primary airway epithelial cells from patients with asthma by transforming growth factor-beta1. *Am J Respir Crit Care Med* 2009; **180**: 122–33.

18 Kicic A, Sutanto EN, Stevens PT, et al. Intrinsic biochemical and functional differences in bronchial

epithelial cells of children with asthma. *Am J Respir Crit Care Med* 2006; **174**: 1110–18.

19 Zhen G, Park SW, Nguyenvu LT, *et al.* IL-13 and epidermal growth factor receptor have critical but distinct roles in epithelial cell mucin production. *Am J Respir Cell Mol Biol* 2007; **36**: 244–53.

20 Park KS, Korfhagen TR, Bruno MD, *et al.* SPDEF regulates goblet cell hyperplasia in the airway epithelium. *J Clin Invest* 2007; **117**: 978–88.

21 Chen G, Korfhagen TR, Xu Y, *et al.* SPDEF is required for mouse pulmonary goblet-cell differentiation and regulates a network of genes associated with mucus production. *J Clin Invest* 2009; **119**: 2914–24.

22 Mullings RE, Wilson SJ, Puddicombe SM, *et al.* Signal transducer and activator of transcription 6 (STAT6) expression and function in asthmatic bronchial epithelium. *J Allergy Clin Immunol* 2001;**108**: 832–8.

23 Sampath D, Castro M, Look DC, *et al.* Constitutive activation of an epithelial signal transducer and activator of transcription (STAT) pathway in asthma. *J Clin Invest* 1999; **103**: 1353–61.

24 Holgate ST, Lackie P, Wilson S, *et al.* Bronchial epithelium as a key regulator of airway allergen sensitization and remodeling in asthma. *Am J Respir Crit Care Med* 2000; **162**: S113–17.

25 Cohen L, E X, Tarsi J, *et al.* Epithelial cell proliferation contributes to airway remodeling in severe asthma. *Am J Respir Crit Care Med* 2007; **176**: 138–45.

26 Ricciardolo FL, Di Stefano A, van Krieken JH, *et al.* Proliferation and inflammation in bronchial epithelium after allergen in atopic asthmatics. *Clin Exp Allergy* 2003; **33**: 905–11.

27 Stevens PT, Kicic A, Sutanto EN, *et al.* Dysregulated repair in asthmatic paediatric airway epithelial cells: the role of plasminogen activator inhibitor-1. *Clin Exp Allergy* 2008; **38**: 1901–10.

28 Kicic A, Hallstrand TS, Sutanto EN, *et al.* Decreased fibronectin production significantly contributes to dysregulated repair of asthmatic epithelium. *Am J Respir Crit Care Med* 2010; **181**: 889–98.

29 Amishima M, Munakata M, Nasuhara Y, *et al.* Expression of epidermal growth factor and epidermal growth factor receptor immunoreactivity in the asthmatic human airway. *Am J Respir Crit Care Med* 1998; **157**: 1907–12.

30 Fedorov IA, Wilson SJ, Davies DE, *et al.* Epithelial stress and structural remodelling in childhood asthma. *Thorax* 2005; **60**: 389–94.

31 Polosa R, Puddicombe SM, Krishna MT, *et al.* Expression of c-erbB receptors and ligands in the bronchial epithelium of asthmatic subjects. *J Allergy Clin Immunol* 2002; **109**: 75–81.

32 Puddicombe SM, Polosa R, Richter A, *et al.* Involvement of the epidermal growth factor receptor

in epithelial repair in asthma. *Faseb J* 2000; **14**: 1362–74.

33 Puddicombe SM, Torres-Lozano C, Richter A, *et al.* Increased expression of p21(waf) cyclin-dependent kinase inhibitor in asthmatic bronchial epithelium. *Am J Respir Cell Mol Biol* 2003; **28**: 61–8.

34 Bals R, Hiemstra PS. Innate immunity in the lung: how epithelial cells fight against respiratory pathogens. *Eur Resp J* 2004; **23**: 327–33.

35 Palm NW, Medzhitov R. Pattern recognition receptors and control of adaptive immunity. *Immunol Rev* 2009; **227**: 221–33.

36 Inohara N, Koseki T, del Peso L, *et al.* Nod1: an Apaf-1-like activator of caspase-9 and nuclear factor-kappaB. *J Biol Chem* 1999; **274**: 14560–7.

37 Girardin SE, Tournebize R, Mavris M, *et al.* CARD4/Nod1 mediates NF-kappaB, and JNK, activation by invasive *Shigella flexneri*. *EMBO Rep* 2001; **2**: 736–42.

38 Opitz B, Puschel A, Schmeck B, *et al.* Nucleotide-binding oligomerization domain proteins are innate immune receptors for internalized *Streptococcus pneumoniae*. *J Biol Chem* 2004;**279**: 36426–32.

39 Takeda K, Kaisho T, Akira S. Toll-like receptors. *Annu Rev Immunol* 2003; **21**: 335–76.

40 Ciencewicki JM, Brighton LE, Jaspers I. Localization of type I interferon receptor limits interferon-induced TLR3 in epithelial cells. *J Interferon Cytokine Res* 2009; **29**: 289–97.

41 Adamo R, Sokol S, Soong G, *et al.* Pseudomonas aeruginosa flagella activate airway epithelial cells through asialoGM1 and toll-like receptor 2 as well as toll-like receptor 5. *Am J Respir Cell Mol Biol* 2004; **30**: 627–34.

42 Monick MM, Yarovinsky TO, Powers LS, *et al.* Respiratory syncytial virus upregulates TLR4 and sensitizes airway epithelial cells to endotoxin. *J Biol Chem* 2003; **278**: 53035–44.

43 Takeuchi O, Kawai T, Sanjo H, *et al.* TLR6: A novel member of an expanding toll-like receptor family. *Gene* 1999; **231**: 59–65.

44 Cario E, Rosenberg IM, Brandwein SL, *et al.* Lipopolysaccharide activates distinct signaling pathways in intestinal epithelial cell lines expressing Toll-like receptors. *J Immunol* 2000; **164**: 966–72.

45 Takeuchi O, Akira S. Toll-like receptors; their physiological role and signal transduction system. *Int Immunopharmacol* 2001; **1**: 625–35.

46 Kato A, Favoreto S, Jr., Avila PC, *et al.* TLR3- and Th2 cytokine-dependent production of thymic stromal lymphopoietin in human airway epithelial cells. *J Immunol* 2007; **179**: 1080–7.

47 Allakhverdi Z, Comeau MR, Jessup HK, *et al.* Thymic stromal lymphopoietin is released by human epithelial cells in response to microbes, trauma, or inflammation

and potently activates mast cells. *J Exp Med* 2007; **204**: 253–8.

48 Lee HC, Ziegler SF. Inducible expression of the proallergic cytokine thymic stromal lymphopoietin in airway epithelial cells is controlled by NFkappaB. *Proc Natl Acad Sci USA* 2007; **104**: 914–19.

49 Headley MB, Zhou B, Shih WX, *et al.* TSLP conditions the lung immune environment for the generation of pathogenic innate and antigen-specific adaptive immune responses. *J Immunol* 2009; **182**: 1641–7.

50 Cunningham AC, Zhang JG, Moy JV, *et al.* A comparison of the antigen-presenting capabilities of class II MHC-expressing human lung epithelial and endothelial cells. *Immunology* 1997; **91**: 458–63.

51 Kalb Th, Chuang MT, Marom Z, *et al.* Evidence for accessory cell function by class II MHC antigen-expressing airway epithelial cells. *Am J Respir Cell Mol Biol* 1991; **4**: 320–9.

52 Stick SM, Holt PG. The airway epithelium as immune modulator: the LARC ascending. *Am J Respir Cell Mol Biol* 2003; **28**: 641–4.

53 van Rijt LS, Jung S, Kleinjan A, *et al.* In vivo depletion of lung CD11c⁺ dendritic cells during allergen challenge abrogates the characteristic features of asthma. *J Exp Med* 2005; **201**: 981–91.

54 Lambrecht BN, Hammad H. Taking our breath away: dendritic cells in the pathogenesis of asthma. *Nat Rev Immunol* 2003; **3**: 994–1003.

55 Holt PG, Stumbles PA. Characterization of dendritic cell populations in the respiratory tract. *J Aerosol Med* 2000; **13**: 361–7.

56 Upham JW, Stick SM. Interactions between airway epithelial cells and dendritic cells: implications for the regulation of airway inflammation. *Curr Drug Targets* 2006; **7**: 541–5.

57 Regamey N, Obregon C, Ferrari-Lacraz S, *et al.* Airway epithelial IL-15 transforms monocytes into dendritic cells. *Am J Respir Cell Mol Biol* 2007; **37**: 75–84.

58 Kato A, Schleimer RP. Beyond inflammation: airway epithelial cells are at the interface of innate and adaptive immunity. *Curr Opin Immunol* 2007; **19**: 711–20.

59 Day C, Patel R, Guillen C, *et al.* The chemokine CXCL16 is highly and constitutively expressed by human bronchial epithelial cells. *Exp Lung Res* 2009; **35**: 272–83.

60 Montes-Vizuet R, Vega-Miranda A, Valencia-Maqueda E, *et al.* CC chemokine ligand 1 is released into the airways of atopic asthmatics. *Eur Respir J* 2006; **28**: 59–67.

61 Schmitz J, Owyang A, Oldham E, *et al.* IL-33: an interleukin-1-like cytokine that signals via the IL-1 receptor-related protein ST2 and induces T helper type 2-associated cytokines. *Immunity* 2005; **23**: 479–90.

62 Stanciu LA, Bellettato CM, Laza-Stanca V, *et al.* Expression of programmed death-1 ligand (PD-L) 1, PD-L2, B7-H3, and inducible costimulator ligand on human respiratory tract epithelial cells and regulation by respiratory syncytial virus and type 1 and 2 cytokines. *J Infect Dis* 2006; **193**: 404–12.

63 Vignola AM, Campbell AM, Chanez P, *et al.* HLA-DR and ICAM-1 expression on bronchial epithelial cells in asthma and chronic bronchitis. *Am Rev Respir Dis* 1993; **148**: 689–94.

64 Winter MJ, Nagtegaal ID, van Krieken JHJM, *et al.* The epithelial cell adhesion molecule (Ep-CAM) as a morphoregulatory molecule is a tool in surgical pathology. *Am J Pathol* 2003; **163**: 2139–48.

65 Shuhui L, Mok YK, Wong WS. Role of mammalian chitinases in asthma. *Int Arch Allergy Immunol* 2009; **149**: 369–77.

66 Boot RG, Blommaart EF, Swart E, *et al.* Identification of a novel acidic mammalian chitinase distinct from chitotriosidase. *J Biol Chem* 2001; **276**: 6770–8.

67 Lalaker A, Nkrumah L, Lee WK, *et al.* Chitin stimulates expression of acidic mammalian chitinase and eotaxin-3 by human sinonasal epithelial cells in vitro. *Am J Rhinol Allergy* 2009; **23**: 8–14.

68 Zhu Z, Zheng T, Homer RJ, *et al.* Acidic mammalian chitinase in asthmatic Th2 inflammation and IL-13 pathway activation. *Science* 2004; **304**: 1678–82.

69 Hartl D, He Ch, Koller B, *et al.* Acidic mammalian chitinase is secreted via an ADAM17/epidermal growth factor receptor-dependent pathway and stimulates chemokine production by pulmonary epithelial cells. *J Biol Chem* 2008; **283**: 33472–82.

70 Rawlins EL, Hogan BL. Ciliated epithelial cell lifespan in the mouse trachea and lung. *Am J Physiol Lung Cell Mol Physiol* 2008; **295**: L231–4.

71 Erjefalt JS, Erjefalt I, Sundler F, *et al.* In vivo restitution of airway epithelium. *Cell Tissue Res* 1995; **281**: 305–16.

72 Demayo F, Minoo P, Plopper CG, *et al.* Mesenchymal–epithelial interactions in lung development and repair: are modeling and remodeling the same process? *Am J Physiol Lung Cell Mol Physiol* 2002; **283**: L510–17.

73 Leblond AL, Naud P, Forest V, *et al.* Developing cell therapy techniques for respiratory disease: intratracheal delivery of genetically engineered stem cells in a murine model of airway injury. *Hum Gene Ther* 2009; **20**: 1329–43.

74 Liebler JM, Lutzko C, Banfalvi A, *et al.* Retention of human bone marrow-derived cells in murine lungs following bleomycin-induced lung injury. *Am J Physiol Lung Cell Mol Physiol* 2008; **295**: L285–92.

75 Wong AP, Keating A, Lu W-Y, *et al.* Identification of a bone marrow derived epithelial-like population capable

of repopulating injured mouse airway epithelium. *J Clin Invest* 2009; **119**: 336–48.

76 McQualter JL, Yuen K, Williams B, *et al.* Evidence of an epithelial stem/progenitor cell hierarchy in the adult mouse lung. *Proc Natl Acad Sci USA* 2010; **107**: 1414–19.

77 Hong KU, Reynolds SD, Watkins S, *et al.* Basal cells are a multipotent progenitor capable of renewing the bronchial epithelium. *Am J Pathol* 2004; **164**: 577–88.

78 Reynolds SD, Giangreco A, Power JH, *et al.* Neuroepithelial bodies of pulmonary airways serve as a reservoir of progenitor cells capable of epithelial regeneration. *Am J Pathol* 2000; **156**: 269–78.

79 Rock JR, Onaitis MW, Rawlins EL, *et al.* Basal cells as stem cells of the mouse trachea and human airway epithelium. *Proc Natl Acad Sci USA* 2009; **106**: 12771–5.

80 Zhang Y, Goss AM, Cohen ED, *et al.* A Gata6-Wnt pathway required for epithelial stem cell development and airway regeneration. *Nat Genet* 2008; **40**: 862–70.

81 Zemke AC, Teisanu RM, Giangreco A, *et al.* {beta}-Catenin is not necessary for maintenance or repair of the bronchiolar epithelium. *Am J Respir Cell Mol Biol* 2009; **41**: 535–43.

82 Giangreco A, Reynolds SD, Stripp BR. Terminal bronchioles harbor a unique airway stem cell population that localizes to the bronchoalveolar duct junction. *Am J Pathol* 2002; **161**: 173–82.

83 Tiozzo C, De Langhe S, Yu M, *et al.* Deletion of Pten expands lung epithelial progenitor pools and confers resistance to airway injury. *Am J Respir Crit Care Med* 2009; **180**: 701–12.

84 Giangreco A, Arwert EN, Rosewell IR, *et al.* Stem cells are dispensable for lung homeostasis but restore airways after injury. *Proc Natl Acad Sci USA* 2009; **106**: 9286–91.

85 Hajj R, Baranek T, Le Naour R, *et al.* Basal cells of the human adult airway surface epithelium retain transit-amplifying cell properties. *Stem Cells* 2007; **25**: 139–48.

86 Ford JR, Terzaghi-Howe M. Basal cells are the progenitors of primary tracheal epithelial cell cultures. *Exp Cell Res* 1992; **198**: 69–77.

87 Engelhardt JF, Schlossberg H, Yankaskas JR, *et al.* Progenitor cells of the adult human airway involved in submucosal gland development. *Development* 1995; **121**: 2031–46.

88 Redvers RP, Li A, Kaur P. Side population in adult murine epidermis exhibits phenotypic and functional characteristics of keratinocyte stem cells. *Proc Natl Acad Sci USA* 2006; **103**: 13168–73.

89 Allen M, Heinzmann A, Noguchi E, *et al.* Positional cloning of a novel gene influencing asthma from chromosome 2q14. *Nat Genet* 2003; **35**: 258–63.

90 Rogers AJ, Raby BA, Lasky-Su JA, *et al.* Assessing the reproducibility of asthma candidate gene associations, using genome-wide data. *Am J Respir Crit Care Med* 2009; **179**: 1084–90.

91 Ying S, O'Connor B, Ratoff J, *et al.* Thymic stromal lymphopoietin expression is increased in asthmatic airways and correlates with expression of Th2-attracting chemokines and disease severity. *J Immunol* 2005; **174**: 8183–90.

92 Hunninghake GM, Lasky-Su J, Soto-Quiros ME, *et al.* Sex-stratified linkage analysis identifies a female-specific locus for IgE to cockroach in Costa Ricans. *Am J Respir Crit Care Med* 2008; **177**: 830–6.

93 He JQ, Hallstrand TS, Knight D, *et al.* A, thymic stromal lymphopoietin gene variant is associated with asthma and airway hyperresponsiveness. *J Allergy Clin Immunol* 2009; **124**: 222–9.

94 Bierbaum S, Nickel R, Koch A, *et al.* Polymorphisms and haplotypes of acid mammalian chitinase are associated with bronchial asthma. *Am J Respir Crit Care Med* 2005; **172**: 1505–9.

95 Koppelman GH, Meyers DA, Howard TD, *et al.* Identification of PCDH1 as a novel susceptibility gene for bronchial hyperresponsiveness. *Am J Respir Crit Care Med* 2009; **180**: 929–35.

96 Cookson W. The immunogenetics of asthma and eczema: a new focus on the epithelium. *Nat Rev Immunol* 2004; **4**: 978–88.

97 Zhou B, Comeau MR, De Smedt T, *et al.* Thymic stromal lymphopoietin as a key initiator of allergic airway inflammation in mice. *Nat Immunol* 2005; **6**: 1047–53.

98 Ying S, O'Connor B, Ratoff J, *et al.* Expression and cellular provenance of thymic stromal lymphopoietin and chemokines in patients with severe asthma and chronic obstructive pulmonary disease. *J Immunol* 2008; **181**: 2790–8.

99 Seibold MA, Reese TA, Choudhry S, *et al.* Differential enzymatic activity of common haplotypic versions of the human acidic mammalian chitinase protein. *J Biol Chem* 2009; **284**: 19650–8.

100 Xiang Y, Tan Y-R, Zhang J-S, *et al.* Wound repair and proliferation of bronchial epithelial cells regulated by CTNNAL1. *J Cell Biochem* 2008; **103**: 920–30.

101 Ito K, Caramori G, Lim S, *et al.* Expression and activity of histone deacetylases in human asthmatic airways. *Am J Respir Crit Care Med* 2002; **166**: 392–6.

102 Ito K, Yamamura S, Essilfie-Quaye S, *et al.* Histone deacetylase 2-mediated deacetylation of the glucocorticoid receptor enables NF-kappaB suppression. *J Exp Med* 2006; **203**: 7–13.

11 Fibroblasts

Alastair G. Stewart,[1] Lilian Soon,[2] and Michael Schuliga[1]
[1]Department of Pharmacology, University of Melbourne, Parkville, VIC, Australia
[2]Australian Centre for Microscopy and Microanalysis, University of Sydney, Sydney, NSW, Australia

Airway remodeling

The structural changes that characterize chronic asthma include an increase in the number of goblet cells, loss of contiguous epithelial cell lining of the airways, subepithelial thickening of the lamina reticularis, infiltration of the subepithelial region with inflammatory cells, and an increase in the number and activation of fibroblasts. There is also an increase in the numerical density of blood vessels. The smooth muscle lies closer to the epithelium, and there are more, larger airway smooth muscle (ASM) cells. More recently, remodeling of the adventitial aspect of the asthmatic airway has been described. The remodeling literature has recently been reviewed (see for example Fixman *et al.* [1], Boxall *et al.* [2], and James and Wenzel [3]). Our focus in this chapter will be on the structural and functional roles of the fibroblast and on the potential to target the remodeling capacity of this cell type with new drugs.

The overall impact of the above-described changes at a functional level includes an amplified increase in airway resistance for a given degree of smooth muscle shortening that contributes to airway hyperresponsiveness. This amplification of airway narrowing is attributable to the thickening of the airway wall. Thickening is mainly due to hyperplasia of the smooth muscle, but an increase in vascular density and inflammatory mediator-induced vasodilator responses also contribute. The airway may be further compromised by hypersecretion of mucus. In addition to these structural influences of the remodeling, it is widely believed that the phenotype of many of the structural cells changes in the asthmatic airway wall. Fibroblasts, epithelial cells, and smooth muscle cells express the capacity to produce and secrete small molecule and cytokine mediators of inflammation to an extent rivaling that of the infiltrating or resident inflammatory cells [4].

Consideration of the notion that there should be a focus on fibroblasts as targets of intervention in airway remodeling requires some discussion of the relative roles of smooth muscle and fibroblasts in remodeling. Holgate and colleagues [5] have advanced the idea that remodeling is initiated and perpetuated by a defect in the response to injury of the epithelial mesenchymal trophic unit (EMTU) in which physical and paracrine communication between epithelium and fibroblasts is thought to maintain the integrity of the repair process. In longstanding asthma, airway biopsies have failed to reveal proliferating smooth muscle cells [6–9]. The frequency of smooth muscle proliferation may be too low to be evident in the random sampling used in these biopsy studies. Proliferation may be confined to short periods following the inflammation associated with asthma exacerbations. However, smooth muscle proliferation can be detected readily in experimental mouse [10], rat [11], and horse [12] models. The proliferation may have already occurred in the early history of the asthma. In biopsy studies of the small number of available cases in children, certain features of remodeling are evident before the development of asthma, a phenomenon referred to as "premodeling" [13,14]. Alternatively, the idea of a key contribution from fibroblasts to ASM hyperplasia needs to be considered.

Allergen challenge increases the number and activity of subepithelial myofibroblasts within 24 h, a period of time too brief for any significant proliferation, which has led the authors to suggest that pre-existing fibroblasts had been activated to a myofibroblast phenotype [15]. This activation can be mimicked *in vitro* by exposure to transforming growth factor beta (TGF-β), which initiates a broad pattern of gene expression changes including the upregulation of contractile protein expression that is normally associated with the smooth muscle phenotype [16]. Conversely, when smooth muscle cells are cultured in growth factor-containing media, levels of expression of contractile proteins are greatly reduced [17]. The continuum of phenotype between smooth muscle and fibroblast has been discussed previously [18]. The full extent of the phenotypic plasticity of these mesenchymal cells remains to be established, but it is conceivable that myofibroblasts could reach the end of the spectrum to become functionally and immunohistochemically indistinguishable from smooth muscle cells. Thus, this alternate mechanism for ASM hyperplasia could comprise an agglomeration of extensively differentiated myofibroblasts or their migration to the boundary of the original smooth muscle bundles. An implicit component of this alternate mechanism for hyperplasia is the requirement for a migratory response from the subepithelial region to the smooth muscle bundle. While such a migration has yet to be established *in vivo*, there is abundant evidence of the migratory behavior of the (myo) fibroblasts in cell culture studies [19].

Are there major impediments to target validation in airway remodelling?

There are a number of uncertainties regarding the remodeling process, which creates a risk for unequivocal declaration of drug targets. Animal models suggest that functionally important airway remodeling can be induced within several weeks [20]. However, the period over which remodeling develops in asthmatics remains unclear. The recent findings of early life remodeling [13,14] raise the possibility that the most dynamic period, during which one expects the greatest benefit from effective drug treatment, may not be currently accessible because it occurs before asthma is diagnosed. Indeed, some data suggest that remodeling may precede the disease itself. Furthermore, post-mortem studies indicate that the remodeling is related to severity but unrelated to duration of disease or age at onset, providing direct support for the early development of remodeling [21]. The fibrosis and remodeling in asthma seems to reach a natural limit in terms of overall thickening of the airway and the extent of subepithelial fibrosis, even in severe asthma. This self-limiting aspect of the asthmatic airway remodeling contrasts with inexorably progressive forms of fibrosis and remodeling such as idiopathic pulmonary fibrosis (IPF) and bronchiolitis obliterans. Understanding the distinct pathophysiology of fibrosis in asthma and IPF may give clues to distinct therapeutic approaches.

If a dynamic equilibrium is reached in the remodeled asthmatic airway, then the flux of cell division/death/ apoptosis/migration will determine how quickly an effective drug intervention would result in structural change and functional improvement. A slow turnover would require very long clinical trial periods to detect significant change. This challenge has beset attempts to find an effective treatment for IPF in which many interventions shown to be effective in animal models of remodeling have failed in clinical trials. The discordance in response to different treatment strategies between animal models of remodeling and human IPF may reflect the timing of treatment in relation to disease progression, a lack of understanding of key molecular drivers of the progression, species differences, and/or the fact that animal models are too synchronous, linear, and rapid in comparison with the temporal and spatial complexities of IPF in humans. In asthma, the remodeling is but one of a number of components of the pathophysiology underlying the loss of airway/lung function. The evaluation of antiremodeling strategies in asthma is rendered more uncertain by the lack of well-established surrogates of remodeling. Technology for direct measurement of airway size is somewhat limited in resolution [22]. Biopsies of central airways are informative, but distinct patterns of remodeling in the more distal resistance-determining airways have been observed [23,24]. Surrogate measures, such as the presence of fixed airway obstruction or airway hyperresponsiveness, may correlate with structural change, but their use for this purpose remains speculative.

Are there beneficial effects of remodelling?

There are a number of findings that suggest that aspects of remodeling may represent an adaptive response to limit dynamic airway obstruction. Treatment of rabbit ASM preparation with collagenase accelerates smooth muscle shortening in response to contractile agonists, consistent with the provision of internal resistance by collagen and other elements of the extracellular matrix (ECM) [25]. Airway fibrosis may limit airway narrowing (owing to the folding of the subepithelial region internal to the smooth layer that is required to accommodate shortening and airway narrowing) and the need to deform the elastic tissue external to the shortening smooth muscle layer [26]. Of course, the converse argument that fibrosis limits lung volume-dependent broncho-dilation is also true, and may well be important in determining airway responsiveness [27]. Despite numerous studies on the volume and composition of the ECM, the impact of inflammation and remodeling on the dynamic biophysical and biochemical influences of changes in ECM on smooth muscle and fibroblasts is largely unknown.

Remodelling activities of airway fibroblasts

The increased abundance of fibroblasts and myofibroblasts in the airway wall in asthma has been attributed to proliferation and differentiation of pre-existing subepithelial fibroblasts. Additional mechanisms include the recruitment of fibrocytes from the circulation, whereupon they differentiate in the inflamed airway wall to mature fibroblasts [28,29]. This mechanism is well documented in animal models of pulmonary fibrosis and in biopsy tissue from patients with IPF, although its importance relative to epithelial mesenchymal transition (EMT) remains controversial. EMT should also be considered as a potential source of fibroblasts in the asthmatic airway wall. Epithelium cultured from asthmatics readily expresses a mixed phenotype (colocalized expression of fibroblasts and epithelial cell markers) upon exposure to TGF-β, whereas cells from nonasthmatic

donors show a much-reduced EMT response [30]. The EMT response appears to be resistant to glucocorticoid (GC) treatment in *in vitro* studies of epithelial cells [31]. Nevertheless, there is no clear evidence for EMT in asthmatic biopsy.

Fibroblasts from asthmatic and nonasthmatic donors

Many studies designed to address fibroblast function in asthma have used cells grown from lung parenchyma. These data may be useful, but the particular tissue origin of the fibroblast population is a determinant of their phenotype, and the differences between lung and airway fibroblasts are known [32]. Not only are there differences in fibroblast phenotype in different organs, but the fibroblast populations within organs also show heterogeneity related to whether they are derived from wounded or normal tissue [33]. In IPF, the corollary of this heterogeneity is reflected by reports of both hyper- and hypoproliferative behaviors of fibroblasts, possibly as a consequence of heterogeneous patterns of fibrosis in the source tissue [34]. Similar determinants may be important in the behavior of cultured fibroblasts from asthmatic airways.

The mechanisms that subserve remodeling in the transition from normal cells to asthma cells need to be understood in order to judge whether the normal cell phenotype, or those cells that have adopted an asthmatic phenotype, should be used to define the pharmacology of cellular responses to mediators and drugs intended to treat remodeling. Asthmatic-derived airway fibroblasts are reported to show greater differentiation in response to TGF-β1 or TGF-β2, as measured by accumulation of α-smooth muscle actin [35]. Moreover, mixed cell cultures of BEAS2B, epithelial cells, fibroblasts, and T cells show increased TGF-β1 production in parallel with diminished T-cell apoptosis [36]. In severe asthma, fibroblasts express greater levels of platelet-derived growth factor (PDGF)$_{BB}$, its receptor PDGFR-β, and procollagen I [37]. Fibroblasts from asthmatics are hyperproliferative to PDGF but have a shorter time to become senescent than nonasthmatic fibroblasts [38]. Our findings also indicated that asthmatic fibroblasts are hypoproliferative in response to thrombin but that normal responses were obtained with serum

[6]. This mitogen-dependent variation in proliferation merits further investigation because contrasts in the responses to different stimuli may reveal new insights into asthma-related changes in specific signal transduction systems. In ASM derived from asthmatics, the C/EBPα transcription factor, which functions as a negative regulator of proliferation, is deficient. Conversely, C/EBPβ, which serves to increase transcription of a number of cytokines, is overexpressed [39]. Whether these C/EBP defects are also present in asthma-derived fibroblasts is unknown.

The mediator production profile of airway fibroblasts also indicates an effect of asthma status, with asthma-derived fibroblasts generating higher levels of several cytokines including stem cell factor, interleukin 6 (IL-6), IL-8, and granulocyte–macrophage colony-stimulating factor (GM-CSF) [6,40,41]. Unlike human ASM from asthmatics, cytokine production by airway fibroblasts shows normal sensitivity to the regulatory actions of GCs [6,40].

Models used to assess fibroblast function

Many of the studies on potential targets in remodeling activity of fibroblasts have been carried out with cells in two-dimensional (2D) culture. However, some three-dimensional (3D) models, including those with multiple cell types, have been described. For example, the mast cell, HMC-1, has been co-cultured with lung fibroblasts in a collagen extracellular matrix [42]. These studies have established a role for matrix metalloproteinases (MMPs) in the activation of latent TGF-β to elicit remodeling (contraction) of the collagen gel. A co-culture model involving a monolayer of epithelial cells overlaying fibroblasts imbedded in a 3D matrix has been used to establish that polycation-mediated epithelial injury releases remodeling cytokines, including insulin-like growth factor (IGF), basic fibroblast growth factor (bFGF), and TGF-β [43].

Drug targets: processes mediators and receptors

As the process of myofibroblast activation is established in the asthmatic airway and its consequences can be readily rationalized as being detrimental to airway remodeling and inflammation, it is reasonable to consider that suppression of myofibroblast activation is a desirable target activity for a novel anti-asthma agent. Is the process targetable, or is it more logical to target specific inducers of myofibroblast activation? We will first consider individual activators and then signaling processes that may provide a common downstream target with the required breadth of activity to provide a potentially useful site of intervention.

Transforming growth factor beta

The best-characterized fibroblast activator is TGF-β [44]. This cytokine is made by a number of cell types within the airway wall, released in a latent form, and subsequently activated by a variety of exposures including certain integrin subtypes, MMPs, plasmin, and an acidic environment. All three isoforms of TGF-β (1,2,3) have been identified in the airway wall, but TGF-β2 appears to be selectively upregulated following allergen challenge [45]. Once activated, TGF-β binds to the type II receptor (TGFBRII) in a complex with the type I receptor that acquires kinase activities as a result of phosphorylation by TGFBRII. There are several isoforms of the type I receptor that belong to the activin receptor-like kinases (ALK) family: the particular type I receptor to which TGF-β binds is known as ALK5.

TGF-β mimics many aspects of remodeling in the airways through fibroblast activation [46]. TGF-β increases the expression of genes associated with the myocyte phenotype such as α-smooth muscle actin, myosin, and desmin [47]. The postreceptor signaling involves competition between serum response factor (SRF) and myocardin that regulate the SRF element in the gene promoters of these "contractile" proteins [48]. The migration of airway fibroblasts may also be increased by TGF-β. The growth effects of TGF-β on most cell types show some biphasic features. Low concentrations of TGF-β usually stimulate a small degree of proliferation. In several cell types TGF-β has shown antiproliferative effects when a strong proliferative stimulus such as fetal calf serum is used [49]. In addition, a prominent effect of TGF-β in many cell types is to increase cell size, as some groups have reported for ASM [50,51]. The hypertrophy and differentiation with increased expression of contractile proteins is consistent with the antiproliferative activity of TGF-β. However, few of these mechanisms have been investigated specifically in airway fibroblasts.

Several studies in mice address the extent to which TGF-β may contribute to fibroblast activation in chronic allergic inflammation. The loss of the anti-inflammatory actions of TGF-β1 leads to increased interferon gamma (IFN-γ), higher immunoglobulin (Ig) E levels, increased eosinophilia, and mucus hypersecretion, but airway hyperresponsiveness is not changed, which unmasks a possible beneficial antiremodeling consequence of the gene deletion [52]. Allergen-induced inflammation, remodeling, smooth muscle thickening, and associated airway hyperresponsiveness in the Brown Norway rat is reduced by the ALK5 inhibitor, SD-208 [53]. These inhibitory effects of the ALK5 inhibitor suggest a substantial role of TGF-β and support its targeting to inhibit remodeling. However, there are reasons to be cautious in providing a blanket inhibition of TGF-β activity. Mice with limited TGF-β expression in T cells show an autoimmune colitis [54]. Moreover, TGF-β may mediate some functions of T regulatory cells (Tregs) that are likely to limit the degree of allergic sensitization [55]. Identification of downstream signals that block some of the fibrogenic activity of TGF-β, but spare these beneficial actions, may prove to be the only viable way to exploit TGF-β as a target in chronic inflammatory disease.

TGF-β signaling has considerable complexity with a number of branching independent signal transduction pathways in addition to the so-called canonical Smad pathway. Selective targeting of specific branches could possibly avoid loss of immunoregulatory actions that would engender adverse consequences. Mitogen-activated protein kinases (MAPKs) are activated by the TGF-β receptor ALK5. The p38[MAPK] pathway has been implicated in many pathways of inflammatory cytokine production. One of its downstream kinase targets, MK2, is specifically implicated in myofibroblast formation. Unexpectedly, in transgenic MK2[−/−] mice, bleomycin-induced pulmonary fibrosis was exacerbated, which is consistent with myofibroblast formation being part of the repair process [56]. However, fibroblast-independent MK2 functions could influence the extent of fibrosis. These findings in MK2[−/−] mice lessen interest in the p38[MAPK] pathway as a strategy for inhibition of fibrosis. Although targeting p38[MAPK] reduces remodeling and airway inflammation in asthma models [57], toxicity of this class of kinase inhibitors remains to be an issue.

Endothelin

The vaso/bronchoactive peptide endothelin (ET), produced in hypoxic blood vessels, has been investigated for its potential contribution to obstructive airway diseases and more specifically to fibroblast activation. ET-1 induces the myofibroblast phenotype and contractility of lung fibroblasts [58] as well as airway fibroblasts [59]. There is also evidence for a synergistic interaction between TGF-β and PDGF in ET-1-mediated activation of proliferation and collagen synthesis by airway fibroblasts derived from either asthmatic or nonasthmatic individuals [60] and for a TGF-β-independent promotion of survival [61]. If current trials evaluating the ET receptor A/B antagonist, bosentan (Tracleer®, Actelion Pharmaceuticals, Allschwil, Switzerland), in IPF [62] are successful, then interest in its use in asthma would be increased.

Urokinase plasminogen activator

The plasminogen activation system has a wide range of potential contributions to fibroblast function (Figure 11.1), but few have been explored specifically in airway fibroblasts. In lung fibroblasts, apoptosis is promoted by the plasmin-mediated proteolysis of pericellular fibronectin through an MMP-independent mechanism that is delayed, but not blocked, by TGF-β [63]. Plasmin directly elicits important cellular remodeling and inflammatory responses including proliferation, migration, and cytokine release in ASM [64,65] and in airway fibroblasts (Schuliga, Che, Harris, and Stewart, University of Melbourne, Australia, unpublished observations). These responses involve the p38[MAPK], ERK1/2, and PI3K/AKT pathways that are regulated by plasmin via binding to the annexin A2 tetramer [66,67]. Urokinase plasminogen activator (uPA)/uPA receptor (uPAR)-dependent signaling has a role in the migration of airway and vascular smooth muscle cells [68,69]. Cleavage of uPAR is implicated in the TGF-β differentiation of corneal

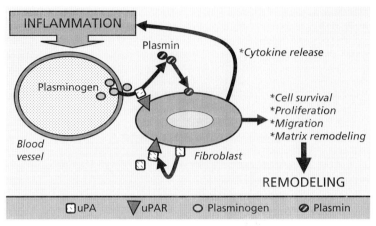

Figure 11.1 Plasminogen released into the airway wall via vascular inflammatory leak is converted by urokinase plasminogen activator (uPA) into plasmin. Each uPA and plasmin is able to independently activate a number of remodeling and inflammatory signals. uPAR, uPA regulator.

fibroblasts to myofibroblasts through the activity of cell-bound cathepsin [70]. The uPAR is truncated to a form that has migration-promoting activity through activation of the FPR2 receptor by its nascent cleaved uPAR N-terminal sequence [71]. The uPA and uPAR genes have multiple single nucleotide polymorphisms (SNPs) of high frequency that link these genes to asthma [72]. Small molecule inhibitors of uPA reduce tumor growth and metastasis. These agents have not yet been evaluated in models of airway inflammation and remodeling.

Integrins

The fibrillar form of type I collagen attenuates the proliferative response of ASM [73] and lung fibroblasts [74] through binding to the α2β1 integrin receptor. These observations argue for an increased emphasis on investigations of fibroblast function in 2D and 3D environments containing ECM components (Figure 11.2). There is a similar effect of fibrillar collagen on airway fibroblast proliferation (Schuliga, Che, Harris, and Stewart, unpublished observations). Thus, the formation of collagen fibrils has an important regulatory role in wound-healing processes by limiting the extent of fibrosis through negative feedback on fibrogenesis. Furthermore, aberrations in the signaling processes between the matrix and cell may contribute to a dys-

regulated repair. IPF-derived lung fibroblasts cultured in fibrillar collagen exhibit pathologic β1-integrin signaling involving the phosphoinositide 3 kinase/Akt cell survival pathway [75]. These IPF fibroblasts, unlike those from normal lung, are resistant to the antiproliferative effect of fibrillar collagen. Asthmatic airway fibroblasts exhibit increased expression of the β1 integrin collagen receptor [37], increased collagen production [37], and a reduced capacity to degrade collagen by phagocytosis [76].

Relaxin

Relaxin is a hormone that acts to soften the pubic symphysis during pregnancy. The remodeling actions of relaxin on bone extend to impact on fibrotic processes in a multitude of target tissues including the heart and lung [77,78]. In murine models of allergic inflammation, relaxin administration ameliorates remodeling and reduces airway hyperresponsiveness [79,80]. The fibroblast is a proximal target for some of these actions because relaxin is known to act on fibroblasts to diminish collagen production. The impact of relaxin on airway fibroblast responses is not yet described. Importantly, relaxin treatment is one of the few interventions shown to reverse, rather than merely prevent, allergen-induced airway wall remodeling in murine models [81].

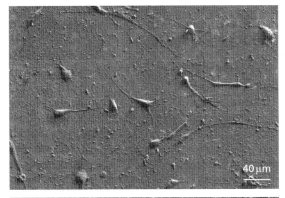

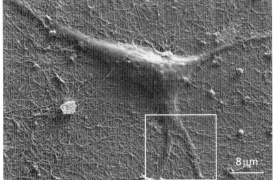

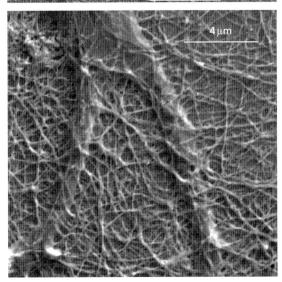

Figure 11.2 Human airway fibroblasts grown on a three-dimensional matrix. The fibroblasts display a spindle-shaped morphology and the presence of elongated protrusions. The latter are imbedded in the matrix and appear to anchor the cell to the substrate and lead the process of cell invasion (inset).

Follistatin

The superfamily of TGF-β cytokines has many members, with bone morphogenic protein (BMP) and activins being prominent subclasses that share some of the biologic activities of TGF-β. Activin has a similar wound-repair/inflammation-resolution profile to TGF-β [82]. In addition, there are endogenous inhibitors of the TGF-β superfamily, including follistatin and inhibin. Follistatin has documented antifibrotic effects in a number of models. Follistatin binds to activin and prevents activation of activin RIIa receptors [83]. Therapeutic exploitation of this peptide carries the usual challenges with peptide/protein therapeutics, and it is likely that the same cautions that apply to small molecule modulators of the TGF-β signaling pathway regarding loss of anti-inflammatory effects will be relevant to loss of activin activity.

Chemokines

Chemokine receptor antagonists are at an advanced stage of clinical development, and a number of the receptor subclasses already have approved clinical indications. Allergic disease has been a major focus of preclinical investigations in order to identify the potential of these compounds. There is now substantial literature that supports additional roles for chemokines in regulating the migration and activity of cellular targets other than lymphocytes/leukocytes, such as mesenchymal cells. The circulating fibrocyte expresses the CXCR4 receptor that contributes to the trafficking of this fibroblast precursor to the fibrotic lung [84].

Cyclooxygenase

The antifibrotic actions of the cyclooxygenase (COX) product, prostaglandin E_2 (PGE$_2$), may be significant as it is a highly abundant airway prostaglandin (PG). However, in the bleomycin model of lung fibrosis, PGF$_2\alpha$ acting via FP receptors promotes fibrosis independently of TGF-β [85]. The FP PGF$_{2\alpha}$ receptors mediate contraction of hepatic fibroblasts [86]. Selective antagonists of FP receptors have been developed recently [87] and have been used together with FP gene deletion to establish a role for PGF$_{2\alpha}$

in fibrosis [86]. Despite clear evidence of a role for PGE_2, individual gene deletion of the EP receptors or their antagonism by a small molecule blocker had no effect in the bleomycin model. The lack of impact of knockout of the individual receptors for PGE_2 may reflect complex mutual antagonism in the effects of the different receptors, or simply that PGE_2 production is diminished in the fibrotic lesions. Conventional nonsteroidal anti-inflammatory drugs (NSAIDs) precipitate asthma symptoms in the 10% of individuals with aspirin-induced asthma, an effect not shared by COX-2-selective inhibitors (Coxibs). Nevertheless, with safety concerns over the Coxibs, exploitation of the recent findings with $PGF_{2\alpha}$ will require an FP-selective antagonist.

The epidermal growth factor receptor

Epithelial injury disrupts physical and functional communication between the cell types that comprise the epithelial mesenchymal trophic unit. Restitution of epithelium following injury is impaired by a deficient response to epidermal growth factor (EGF) [88,89]. Acute asthma, triggered by allergen inhalation, is associated with increased levels of the EGF receptor (EGFR), ligands, EGF, and, for a much shorter period, amphiregulin. Acute exposure of epithelial cells in culture to either of these growth factors results in proliferation, but more protracted exposure causes mucus cell metaplasia [90]. Both amphiregulin and EGF are also mitogenic for ASM. It is possible that these short-term increases in EGFR activation contribute to epithelial restitution, whereas ongoing activation may promote remodeling. In chronic obstructive pulmonary disease (COPD), the rationale for targeting EGFR is driven by the established role of EGF in inducing mucus cell metaplasia. However, recent clinical evaluation of a small molecule EGFR kinase inhibitor showed minimal impact on epithelial remodeling [91]. The concurrent exacerbation of airway function observed in this trial makes the evaluation of EGF kinase inhibitors in asthma unlikely.

Fibroblast proliferation

There is a vast array of mediators and growth factors with proliferative effects on fibroblasts from various tissue sources. The examination of this array of potential mediators of fibroproliferation in asthma has been limited by the difficulty of obtaining and propagating airway fibroblast cultures. Nevertheless, our own studies have established activity of thrombin and bFGF. The cysteinyl leukotrienes (cys-LTs) synergize with tyrosine kinase growth factor receptor stimulants to activate proliferation through a mechanism that is resistant to blockade of both of the known high-affinity cys-LT receptors [92], which is similar to observations made on ASM.

Administration of bFGF diminishes airway wall remodeling in a mouse model [93] despite extensive evidence that it promotes proliferation of both ASM [94] and fibroblasts in cell culture [6]. The more important influence of bFGF may be in antagonizing the effects of TGF-β. Our studies suggest that these cytokines behave as mutual antagonists in ASM and lung fibroblasts.

Fibroblast apoptosis

The regulation of (myo)fibroblast numbers is multifaceted (Figure 11.3). Apoptosis in healing wounds reduces the burden of myofibroblasts [95]. In cell culture studies, dermal fibroblasts show rapid induction of apoptosis after the release of isometric tension in contracted (remodeled) collagen gels [96]. Concurrent with tension release, fibroblast growth (survival) factor production declines sharply. Phosphatase and tensin homolog on chromosome 10 (PTEN) is activated during collagen gel remodeling [97]. PTEN dephosphorylates the membrane phospholipid phosphatidylinositol 3,4,5-phosphate (PIP3) that is a substrate of phosphatidylinositol 3-kinase (PI3K), thereby reducing activation of the survival pathway, PI3K/Akt.

Leukocyte and lymphocyte apoptosis is reduced in asthmatic airways [98], but there are no studies that specifically explore airway fibroblast or smooth muscle apoptosis. However, proliferation and apoptosis markers have been localized to smooth muscle α-actin-expressing cells in airways from horses with an asthma-like airway disease called heaves [12]. The *in vitro* studies of fibroblast apoptosis to date have focused on tension applied by gel-imbedded fibroblasts. Other studies using ASM have examined strain applied externally to cells grown on flexible silastic

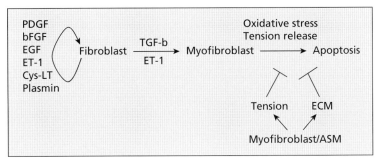

Figure 11.3 The airway fibroblast is subjected to a variety of cytokine stimuli that cause cell proliferation. A more restricted set of influences have been identified as mediating myofibroblast differentiation. The survival of this phenotype is under the control of tension, oxidative environment, and the extracellular matrix (ECM) as described in the text. PDGF, platelet-derived growth factor; bFGF, basic fibroblast growth factor; EGF, epidermal growth factor; ET, endothelin; cys-LT, cysteinyl leukotriene; TGF, transforming growth factor; ASM, airway smooth muscle.

coated with ECM proteins [99,100]. *In situ* fibroblasts may be too sparse to play a major role in determining the local tension. Nevertheless, those fibroblasts adjacent to bundles of smooth muscle could be influenced by ASM contractile state. ASM tension may act as a survival signal to (myo)fibroblasts. Conversely, during periods of inflammation, increased remodeling of the ECM by leukocyte-derived proteases could generate a tension release for subepithelial fibroblasts by disengaging them from the tension applied by ASM and transmitted through the ECM. This disengagement could protect against worsening fibrosis by promoting fibroblast apoptosis.

Functional antagonists of fibroblast function

There is an overwhelming case for multivalent treatments in asthma. The antecedents are the endogenous adrenal products cortisol and epinephrine. The mediator-independent functional nature of the antagonism of these natural anti-asthma agents confers their efficacy. β_2-Agonists and GCs are able to functionally antagonize the proliferative and some of the cytokine responses of airway fibroblasts. PGE$_2$ limits collagen gel remodeling [101] and migration of fetal lung fibroblasts, actions that are linked to upregulation of PTEN activity [102]. PGE$_2$ promotes lung fibroblast apoptosis via activation of PTEN and downregulation of survival signaling via the PI3K/Akt pathway by way of the EP2/EP4 receptors that are

linked to cAMP generation [103]. PGE$_2$ is less active in promoting apoptosis in IPF-derived fibroblasts than in normal lung fibroblasts [104]. Moreover, PGE$_2$ production by mesenchymal cells, and specifically fibroblasts, is decreased in asthma [6,105]. Further definition of the roles of EP receptor subtypes may identify more selective strategies for utilizing beneficial actions of PGE$_2$.

There is some controversy in the literature as to the impact of GCs on airway fibroblast proliferation. Our work shows that the inhibitory effects of GCs are of similar magnitude in both normal and asthma-derived cells, but other studies show augmentation of proliferation by GCs [106,107]. Studies of pulmonary fibroblasts are less controversial, with agreement that GCs have either no effect or promote proliferative responses [108]. Whether this heterogeneity in GC response is related to variable production of PGE$_2$ is not known. GCs and β_2-adrenoceptor agonists, in combination or alone, have suppressive effects on lung fibroblast extracellular matrix synthesis [109,110], myofibroblast differentiation [111], and other proremodeling actions such as gel contraction [112], and a similar finding has been reported in airway fibroblasts [113].

Conclusions

There is sufficient evidence to validate the fibroblast as a suitable target through which to control airway remodeling responses. There is sufficient uncertainty with asthma-related studies *in vitro* human cell cultures and those using various mouse strains to caution that validation is incomplete until a proof of concept in human asthma is achieved. Some targets, such as TGF-β, are too pleiotropic in their actions to be likely to show a desirable safety:efficacy ratio. Others, such as endothelin-1, may have too narrow a contribution to yield clinically meaningful results.

Acknowledgment

The authors' work has been supported by the National Health and Medical Research Council grant number 500901 in addition to grants from the Asthma Foundation of Victoria and the CASS foundation.

References

1 Fixman ED, Stewart A, Martin JG. Basic mechanisms of development of airway structural changes in asthma. *Eur Respir J* 2007; **29**: 379–89.

2 Boxall C, Holgate ST, Davies DE. The contribution of transforming growth factor-beta and epidermal growth factor signalling to airway remodelling in chronic asthma. *Eur Respir J* 2006; **27**: 208–29.

3 James AL, Wenzel S. Clinical relevance of airway remodelling in airway diseases. *Eur Respir J* 2007; **30**: 134–55.

4 Damera G, Tliba O, Panettieri RA, Jr. Airway smooth muscle as an immunomodulatory cell. *Pulm Pharmacol Ther* 2009; **22**: 353–9.

5 Holgate ST, Arshad HS, Roberts GC, Howasth PH, Thurner P, Davis DE. A new look at the pathogenesis of asthma. *Clin Sci (Lond)* 118: 439–50.

6 Ward JE, Harris T, Bamford T, *et al.* Proliferation is not increased in airway myofibroblasts isolated from asthmatics. *Eur Respir J* 2008; **32**: 362–71.

7 Benayoun L, Druilhe A, Dombret MC, Aubier M, Pretolani M. Airway structural alterations selectively associated with severe asthma. *Am J Respir Crit Care Med* 2003; **167**: 1360–8.

8 Benayoun L, Leture S, Druilhe A, *et al.* Regulation of peroxisome proliferator-activated receptor gamma expression in human asthmatic airways: relationship with proliferation, apoptosis, and airway remodeling. *Am J Respir Crit Care Med* 2001; **164**: 1487–94.

9 Druilhe A, Wallaert B, Tsicopoulos A, *et al.* Apoptosis, proliferation, and expression of Bcl-2: Fas and Fas ligand in bronchial biopsies from asthmatics. *Am J Respir Cell Mol Biol* 1998; **19**: 747–57.

10 Tormanen KR, Uller L, Persson CG, Erjefalt JS. Allergen exposure of mouse airways evokes remodeling of both bronchi and large pulmonary vessels. *Am J Respir Crit Care Med* 2005; **171**: 19–25.

11 Labonte I, Hassan M, Risse PA, *et al.* The effects of repeated allergen challenge on airway smooth muscle structural and molecular remodeling in a rat model of allergic asthma. *Am J Physiol Lung Cell Mol Physiol* 2009; **297**: L698–705.

12 Herszberg B, Ramos-Barbon D, Tamaoka M, Mastin JG, Lavoie JP. Heaves, an asthma-like equine disease, involves airway smooth muscle remodeling. *J Allergy Clin Immunol* 2006; **118**: 382–8.

13 Fedorov IA, Wilson SJ, Davies DE, Holgate ST. Epithelial stress and structural remodelling in childhood asthma. *Thorax* 2005; **60**: 389–94.

14 Saglani S, Payne DN, Zhu J, *et al.* Early detection of airway wall remodeling and eosinophilic inflammation in preschool wheezers. *Am J Respir Crit Care Med* 2007; **176**: 858–64.

15 Gizycki MJ, Adelroth E, Rogers AV, O'Byrne PM, Jeffery PK. Myofibroblast involvement in the allergen-induced late response in mild atopic asthma. *Am J Respir Cell Mol Biol* 1997; **16**: 664–73.

16 Wicks J, Haitchi HM, Holgate ST, Davies DE, Powell RM. Enhanced upregulation of smooth muscle related transcripts by TGF beta2 in asthmatic (myo) fibroblasts. *Thorax* 2006; **61**: 313–19.

17 Halayko AJ, Tran T, Gosens R. Phenotype and functional plasticity of airway smooth muscle: role of caveolae and caveolins. *Proc Am Thorac Soc* 2008; **5**: 80–8.

18 Stewart AG. Airway smooth muscle as a target for novel anti-asthma drugs acting airway wall remodelling. In: Howasth P, Wilson JW, Bousquet J, Rak S, Pauwels S (eds). *Airway Remodelling. Lung Biology in Health and Disease*, volume 55. Marcel Dekker Inc: New York, 2000. pp. 245–60.

19 Malmstrom J, Tufvesson E, Lofdahl CG, Hansson L, Masko-Varga G, Westergren-Thorsson G. Activation of platelet-derived growth factor pathway in human asthmatic pulmonary-derived mesenchymal cells. *Electrophoresis* 2003; **24**: 276–85.

20 Southam DS, Ellis R, Wattie J, Inman MD. Components of airway hyperresponsiveness and their associations with inflammation and remodeling in mice. *J Allergy Clin Immunol* 2007; **119**: 848–54.

21 James AL, Bai TR, Mauad T, *et al.* Airway smooth muscle thickness in asthma is related to severity but not duration of asthma. *Eur Respir J* 2009; **34**: 1040–5.

22 Williamson JP, James AL, Phillips MJ, Sampson DD, Hillman DR, Eastwood PR. Quantifying tracheobronchial tree dimensions: methods, limitations and emerging techniques. *Eur Respir J* 2009; **34**: 42–55.

23 Ebina M, Yaegashi H, Chiba T, Motomiya M. Distribution of smooth muscles along the bronchial tree. A morphometric study of ordinary autopsy lungs. *Am Rev Respir Dis* 1990; **141**: 1322–6.

24 Ebina M, Takahashi T, Chiba T, Motomiya M. Cellular hypertrophy and hyperplasia of airway smooth muscles underlying bronchial asthma: a 3-D morphometric study. *Am Rev Respir Dis* 1993; **148**: 720–6.

25 Bramley AM, Roberts CR, Schellenberg RR. Collagenase increases shortening of human bronchial smooth muscle in vitro. *Am J Respir Crit Care Med* 1995; **152**: 1513–17.

26 McParland BE, Macklem PT, Pare PD. Airway wall remodeling: friend or foe? *J Appl Physiol* 2003; **95**: 426–34.

27 King GG, Moore BJ, Seow CY, Pare PD. Airway narrowing associated with inhibition of deep inspiration during methacholine inhalation in asthmatics. *Am J Respir Crit Care Med* 2001; **164**: 216–18.

28 Schmidt M, Sun G, Stacey MA, Mori L, Mattoli S. Identification of circulating fibrocytes as precursors of bronchial myofibroblasts in asthma. *J Immunol* 2003; **171**: 380–9.

29 Wang CH, Huang CD, Lin HC. Increased circulating fibrocytes in asthma with chronic airflow obstruction. *Am J Respir Crit Care Med* 2008; **178**: 583–91.

30 Hackett TL, Warner SM, Stefanowicz D, *et al.* Induction of epithelial-mesenchymal transition in primary airway epithelial cells from patients with asthma by transforming growth factor-beta1. *Am J Respir Crit Care Med* 2009; **180**: 122–33.

31 Doerner AM, Zuraw BL. TGF-beta1 induced epithelial to mesenchymal transition (EMT) in human bronchial epithelial cells is enhanced by IL1beta but not abrogated by corticosteroids. *Respir Res* 2009; **10**: 100.

32 Kotaru C, Schoonover KJ, Trudeau JB. Regional fibroblast heterogeneity in the lung: implications for remodeling. *Am J Respir Crit Care Med* 2006; **173**: 1208–15.

33 Larochelle S, Langlois C, Thibault I, Lopez-Valle CA, Roy M, Moulin V. Sensitivity of myofibroblasts to H2O2-mediated apoptosis and their antioxidant cell network. *J Cell Physiol* 2004; **200**: 263–71.

34 Moodley YP, Scaffidi AK, Misso NL, *et al.* Fibroblasts isolated from normal lungs and those with idiopathic pulmonary fibrosis differ in interleukin-6/gp130-mediated cell signaling and proliferation. *Am J Pathol* 2003; **163**: 345–54.

35 Michalik M, Pierzchalska M, Legutko A, *et al.* Asthmatic bronchial fibroblasts demonstrate enhanced potential to differentiate into myofibroblasts in culture. *Med Sci Monit* 2009; **15**: BR194–201.

36 Darveau ME, Jacques E, Rouabhia M, Wamid Q, Chakir J. Increased T-cell survival by structural bronchial cells derived from asthmatic subjects cultured in an engineered human mucosa. *J Allergy Clin Immunol* 2008; **121**: 692–9.

37 Lewis CC, Chu HW, Westcott JY, *et al.* Airway fibroblasts exhibit a synthetic phenotype in severe asthma. *J Allergy Clin Immunol* 2005; **115**: 534–40.

38 Dube J, Chakir J, Laviolette M, *et al.* In vitro procollagen synthesis and proliferative phenotype of bronchial fibroblasts from normal and asthmatic subjects. *Lab Invest* 1998; **78**: 297–307.

39 Roth M, Black JL. An imbalance in C/EBPs and increased mitochondrial activity in asthmatic airway smooth muscle cells: novel targets in asthma therapy? *Br J Pharmacol* 2009; **157**: 334–41.

40 Zhang S, Howarth PH, Roche WR. Cytokine production by cell cultures from bronchial subepithelial myofibroblasts. *J Pathol* 1996; **180**: 95–101.

41 Zhang S, Mohammed Q, Burbidge A, Morland CM, Roche WR. Cell cultures from bronchial subepithelial myofibroblasts enhance eosinophil survival in vitro. *Eur Respir J* 1996; **9**: 1839–46.

42 Margulis A, Nocka KH, Wood NL, Wolf SF, Goldman SJ, Kasaian MT. MMP dependence of fibroblast contraction and collagen production induced by human mast cell activation in a three-dimensional collagen lattice. *Am J Physiol Lung Cell Mol Physiol* 2009; **296**: L236–47.

43 Zhang S, Smartt H, Holgate ST, Roche WR. Growth factors secreted by bronchial epithelial cells control myofibroblast proliferation: an in vitro co-culture model of airway remodeling in asthma. *Lab Invest* 1999; **79**: 395–405.

44 Margadant C, Sonnenberg A. Integrin–TGF-beta crosstalk in fibrosis, cancer and wound healing. *EMBO Rep* 2010; **11**: 97–105.

45 Balzar S, Chu HW, Silkoff P, *et al.* Increased TGF-beta2 in severe asthma with eosinophilia. *J Allergy Clin Immunol* 2005; **115**: 110–17.

46 Camoretti-Mercado B, Solway J. Transforming growth factor-beta1 and disorders of the lung. *Cell Biochem Biophys* 2005; **43**: 131–48.

47 Chambers RC, Leoni P, Kaminski N, Laurent GJ, Heller RA. Global expression profiling of fibroblast responses to transforming growth factor-beta1 reveals the induction of inhibitor of differentiation-1 and provides evidence of smooth muscle cell phenotypic switching. *Am J Pathol* 2003; **162**: 533–46.

48 Camoretti-Mercado B, Dulin NO, Solway J. Serum response factor function and dysfunction in smooth muscle. *Respir Physiol Neurobiol* 2003; **137**: 223–35.

49 Cohen MD, Ciocca V, Panettieri RA, Jr. TGF-beta 1 modulates human airway smooth-muscle cell proliferation induced by mitogens. *Am J Respir Cell Mol Biol* 1997; **16**: 85–90.

50 Goldsmith AM, Bentley JK, Zhou L, *et al.* Transforming growth factor-beta induces airway smooth muscle hypertrophy. *Am J Respir Cell Mol Biol* 2006; **34**: 247–54.

51 Zhou D, Zheng X, Wang L, *et al.* Expression and effects of cardiotrophin-1 (CT-1) in human airway smooth muscle cells. *Br J Pharmacol* 2003; **140**: 1237–44.

52 Scherf W, Burdach S, Hansen G. Reduced expression of transforming growth factor beta 1 exacerbates pathology in an experimental asthma model. *Eur J Immunol* 2005; **35**: 198–206.

53 Leung SY, Niimi A, Noble A. *et al.* Effect of transforming growth factor-beta receptor I kinase inhibitor 2,4-disubstituted pteridine (SD-208) in chronic allergic airway inflammation and remodeling. *J Pharmacol Exp Ther* 2006; **319**: 586–94.

54 Gorelik L, Flavell RA. Abrogation of TGFbeta signaling in T cells leads to spontaneous T-cell differentiation and autoimmune disease. *Immunity* 2000; **12**: 171–81.

55 Larche M. Regulatory T cells in allergy and asthma. *Chest* 2007; **132**: 1007–14.

56 Liu T, Warburton RR, Guevara OE, *et al.* Lack of MK2 inhibits myofibroblast formation and exacerbates pulmonary fibrosis. *Am J Respir Cell Mol Biol* 2007; **37**: 507–17.

57 Koppelman B, Webb HK, Medicherla S, *et al.* Pharmacological properties of SD-282—an alpha-isoform selective inhibitor for p38 MAP kinase. *Pharmacology* 2008; **81**: 204–20.

58 Sun G, Stacey MA, Bellini A, Manni M, Mattoli S. Endothelin-1 induces bronchial myofibroblast differentiation. *Peptides* 1997; **18**: 1449–51.

59 Shi-Wen X, Chen Y, Denton CP, *et al.* Endothelin-1 promotes myofibroblast induction through the ETA receptor via a rac/phosphoinositide 3-kinase/Akt-dependent pathway and is essential for the enhanced contractile phenotype of fibrotic fibroblasts. *Mol Biol Cell* 2004; **15**: 2707–19.

60 Dube J, Chakir J, Dube C, Grimard Y, Laviolette M, Boulet LP. Synergistic action of endothelin (ET)-1 on the activation of bronchial fibroblast isolated from normal and asthmatic subjects. *Int J Exp Pathol* 2000; **81**: 429–37.

61 Kulasekaran P, Scavone CA, Rogers DS, Arenberg DA, Thannickal VJ, Horowitz JC. Endothelin-1 and transforming growth factor-beta1 independently induce fibroblast resistance to apoptosis via AKT activation. *Am J Respir Cell Mol Biol* 2009; **41**: 484–93.

62 du Bois RM. Strategies for treating idiopathic pulmonary fibrosis. *Nat Rev Drug Discov* 2010; **9**: 129–40.

63 Horowitz JC, Rogers DS, Simon RH, Sisson TH, Thannickal VJ. Plasminogen activation induced pericellular fibronectin proteolysis promotes fibroblast apoptosis. *Am J Respir Cell Mol Biol* 2008; **38**: 78–87.

64 Nicholl SM, Roztocil E, Galaria II, Davies MG. Plasmin induces smooth muscle cell proliferation. *J Surg Res* 2005; **127**: 39–45.

65 Li Q, Laumonnier Y, Syrovets T, Simmet T. Plasmin triggers cytokine induction in human monocyte-derived macrophages. *Arterioscler Thromb Vasc Biol* 2007; **27**: 1383–9.

66 Laumonnier Y, Syrovets T, Burysek L, Simmet T. Identification of the annexin A2 heterotetramer as a receptor for the plasmin-induced signaling in human peripheral monocytes. *Blood* 2006; **107**: 3342–9.

67 Zhang Y, Zhou ZH, Bugge TH, Wahl LM. Urokinase-type plasminogen activator stimulation of monocyte matrix metalloproteinase-1 production is mediated by plasmin-dependent signaling through annexin A2 and inhibited by inactive plasmin. *J Immunol* 2007; **179**: 3297–304.

68 Carlin SM, Resink TJ, Tamm M, Roth M. Urokinase signal transduction and its role in cell migration. *FASEB J* 2005; **19**: 195–202.

69 Kusch A, Tkachuk S, Haller H, *et al.* Urokinase stimulates human vascular smooth muscle cell migration via a phosphatidylinositol 3 kinase–Tyk2 interaction. *J Biol Chem* 2000; **275**: 39466–73.

70 Bernstein AM, Twining SS, Warejcka DJ, Tall E, Masur SK. Urokinase receptor cleavage: a crucial step in fibroblast-to-myofibroblast differentiation. *Mol Biol Cell* 2007; **18**: 2716–27.

71 Mazzieri R, D'Alessio S, Kenmoe RK, Ossowski L, Blasi F. An uncleavable uPAR mutant allows dissection of signaling pathways in uPA-dependent cell migration. *Mol Biol Cell* 2006; **17**: 367–78.

72 Barton SJ, Koppelman GH, Vonk JM, *et al.* PLAUR polymorphisms are associated with asthma, PLAUR levels, and lung function decline. *J Allergy Clin Immunol* 2009; **123**: 1391–400 e17.

73 Schuliga M, Ong SC, Soon L, Zal F, Harris T, Stewart AG. Airway smooth muscle remodels pericellular collagen fibrils: implications for proliferation. *Am J Physiol Lung Cell Mol Physiol* 2010; **298**: L584–92.

74 Schuliga MJ, See I, Ong SC, *et al.* Fibrillar collagen clamps lung mesenchymal cells in a nonproliferative and noncontractile phenotype. *Am J Respir Cell Mol Biol* 2009; **41**: 731–41.

75 Xia H, Diebold D, Nho R, *et al.* Pathological integrin signaling enhances proliferation of primary lung fibroblasts from patients with idiopathic pulmonary fibrosis. *J Exp Med* 2008; **205**: 1659–72.

76 Laliberte R, Rouabhia M, Bosse M, Chakir J. Decreased capacity of asthmatic bronchial fibroblasts to degrade collagen. *Matrix Biol* 2001; **19**: 743–53.

77 Tang ML, Samuel CS, Royce SG. Role of relaxin in regulation of fibrosis in the lung. *Ann N Y Acad Sci* 2009; **1160**: 342–7.

78 Lekgabe ED, Royce SG, Hewitson TD, *et al.* The effects of relaxin and estrogen deficiency on collagen deposition and hypertrophy of nonreproductive organs. *Endocrinology* 2006; **147**: 5575–83.

79 Samuel CS, Royce SG, Burton MD, Zhao C, Tregear GW, Samuel CS, Tang ML. Relaxin plays an important role in the regulation of airway structure and function. *Endocrinology* 2007; **148**: 4259–66.

80 Mookerjee I, Solly NR, Royce SG, Tregear GW, Tang ML. Endogenous relaxin regulates collagen deposition in an animal model of allergic airway disease. *Endocrinology* 2006; **147**: 754–61.

81 Royce SG, Miao YR, Lee M, Samuel CS, Tregear GW, Tang ML. Relaxin reverses airway remodeling and airway dysfunction in allergic airways disease. *Endocrinology* 2009; **150**: 2692–9.

82 Kariyawasam HH, Pegorier S, Barkans J, *et al.* Activin and transforming growth factor-beta signaling pathways are activated after allergen challenge in mild asthma. *J Allergy Clin Immunol* 2009; **124**: 454–62.

83 Hardy CL, O'Connor AE, Yao J, *et al.* Follistatin is a candidate endogenous negative regulator of activin A in experimental allergic asthma. *Clin Exp Allergy* 2006; **36**: 941–50.

84 Strieter RM, Keeley EC, Hughes MA, Burdick MD, Mehrad B. The role of circulating mesenchymal progenitor cells (fibrocytes) in the pathogenesis of pulmonary fibrosis. *J Leukoc Biol* 2009; **86**: 1111–18.

85 Oga T, Matsuoka T, Yao C, *et al.* Prostaglandin F(2alpha) receptor signaling facilitates bleomycin-induced pulmonary fibrosis independently of transforming growth factor-beta. *Nat Med* 2009; **15**: 1426–30.

86 Ayabe S, Murata T, Maruyama T, Hori M, Ozaki H. Prostaglandin E2 induces contraction of liver myofibroblasts by activating EP3 and FP prostanoid receptors. *Br J Pharmacol* 2009; **156**: 835–45.

87 Jones RL, Giembycz MA, Woodward DF. Prostanoid receptor antagonists: development strategies and therapeutic applications. *Br J Pharmacol* 2009; **158**: 104–45.

88 Puddicombe SM, Polosa R, Richter A, *et al.* Involvement of the epidermal growth factor receptor in epithelial repair in asthma. *Faseb J* 2000; **14**: 1362–74.

89 Holgate ST, Lackie PM, Howarth PH, *et al.* Invited lecture: activation of the epithelial mesenchymal trophic unit in the pathogenesis of asthma. *Int Arch Allergy Immunol* 2001; **124**: 253–8.

90 Enomoto Y, Orihara K, Takamasu T, *et al.* Tissue remodeling induced by hypersecreted epidermal growth factor and amphiregulin in the airway after an acute asthma attack. *J Allergy Clin Immunol* 2009; **124**: 913–20 e1–7.

91 Woodruff PG, Wolff M, Hohlfeld JM, *et al.* Safety and efficacy of an inhaled epidermal growth factor receptor inhibitor (BIBW 2948; BS) in chronic obstructive pulmonary disease. *Am J Respir Crit Care Med* 2010; **181**: 438–45.

92 Yoshisue H, Kirkham-Brown J, Healy E, Holgate ST, Sampson SP, Davies DE. Cysteinyl leukotrienes synergize with growth factors to induce proliferation of human bronchial fibroblasts. *J Allergy Clin Immunol* 2007; **119**: 132–40.

93 Jeon SG, Lee CG, Oh MH, *et al.* Recombinant basic fibroblast growth factor inhibits the airway hyperresponsiveness, mucus production, and lung inflammation induced by an allergen challenge. *J Allergy Clin Immunol* 2007; **119**: 831–7.

94 Bonacci J, Schuliga M, Harris T, Stewart A. Collagen impairs glucocorticoid actions in airway smooth muscle through integrin signalling. *Br J Pharmacol* 2006; **149**: 365–73.

95 Desmouliere A, Redard M, Darby I, Gabbiani G. Apoptosis mediates the decrease in cellularity during the transition between granulation tissue and scar. *Am J Pathol* 1995; **146**: 56–66.

96 Grinnell F, Zhu M, Carlson MA, Abrams JM. Release of mechanical tension triggers apoptosis of human fibroblasts in a model of regressing granulation tissue. *Exp Cell Res* 1999; **248**: 608–19.

97 Nho RS, Xia H, Diebold D, *et al.* PTEN regulates fibroblast elimination during collagen matrix contraction. *J Biol Chem* 2006; **281**(44): 33291–301.

98 Lamb JP, James A, Carroll N, Siena L, Elliot J, Vignola AM. Reduced apoptosis of memory T-cells in the inner airway wall of mild and severe asthma. *Eur Respir J* 2005; **26**: 265–70.

99 Hasaneen NA, Zucker S, Lin RZ, Vaday GG, Panattieri RA, Foda HD. Angiogenesis is induced by airway smooth muscle strain. *Am J Physiol Lung Cell Mol Physiol* 2007; **293**: L1059–68.

100 Chaudhuri S, Smith PG. Cyclic strain-induced HSP27 phosphorylation modulates actin filaments in airway smooth muscle cells. *Am J Respir Cell Mol Biol* 2008; **39**: 270–8.

101 Skold CM, Liu XD, Zhu YK, *et al.* Glucocorticoids augment fibroblast-mediated contraction of collagen gels by inhibition of endogenous PGE production. *Proc Assoc Am Physicians* 1999; **111**: 249–58.

102 White ES, Atrasz RG, Dickie EG, *et al.* Prostaglandin E(2) inhibits fibroblast migration by E-prostanoid 2 receptor-mediated increase in PTEN activity. *Am J Respir Cell Mol Biol* 2005; **32**: 135–41.

103 Huang SK, White ES, Wettlaufer SH, *et al.* Prostaglandin E(2) induces fibroblast apoptosis by modulating multiple survival pathways. *FASEB J* 2009; **23**: 4317–26.

104 Maher TM, Evans IC, Bottoms SE, *et al.* Diminished prostaglandin E2 contributes to the apoptosis paradox in idiopathic pulmonary fibrosis. *Am J Respir Crit Care Med* 2010; **182**: 73–82.

105 Pierzchalska M, Szabo Z, Sanak M, Suja J, Szczeklik A. Deficient prostaglandin E2 production by bronchial fibroblasts of asthmatic patients, with special reference to aspirin-induced asthma. *J Allergy Clin Immunol* 2003; **111**: 1041–8.

106 Fouty B, Moss T, Solodushko V, Kraft M. Dexamethasone can stimulate G1-S phase transition in human airway fibroblasts in asthma. *Eur Respir J* 2006; **27**: 1160–7.

107 Lewis CC, Sutherland ER, Moss TA, Metze TL, Rex MD, Kraft M. Interleukin-4 and interleukin-13 augment the proliferative effect of dexamethasone on distal lung fibroblasts. *Chest* 2003; **123** (Suppl3): 356S.

108 Langenbach SY, Wheaton BJ, Fernandes DJ, *et al.* Resistance of fibrogenic responses to glucocorticoid and 2-methoxyestradiol in bleomycin-induced lung fibrosis in mice. *Can J Physiol Pharmacol* 2007; **85**: 727–38.

109 Todorova L, Gurcan E, Westergren-Thorsson G, Miller-Larsson A. Budesonide/formoterol effects on metallo-proteolytic balance in TGFbeta-activated human lung fibroblasts. *Respir Med* 2009; **103**: 1755–63.

110 Todorova L, Gurcan E, Miller-Larsson A, Westergren-Thorsson G. Lung fibroblast proteoglycan production induced by serum is inhibited by budesonide and formoterol. *Am J Respir Cell Mol Biol* 2006; **34**: 92–100.

111 Cazes E, Giron-Michel J, Baouz S, *et al.* Novel anti-inflammatory effects of the inhaled corticosteroid fluticasone propionate during lung myofibroblastic differentiation. *J Immunol* 2001; **167**: 5329–37.

112 Baouz S, Giron-Michel J, Azzarone B, *et al.* Lung myofibroblasts as targets of salmeterol and fluticasone propionate: inhibition of alpha-SMA, and NF-kappaB. *Int Immunol* 2005; **17**: 1473–81.

113 Descalzi D, Folli C, Nicolini G, *et al.* Antiproliferative and anti-remodelling effect of beclomethasone dipropionate, formoterol and salbutamol alone or in combination in primary human bronchial fibroblasts. *Allergy* 2008; **63**: 432–7.

12 Airway smooth muscle cells

Andrew J. Halayko[1-6] and Pawan Sharma[1,5,6]
Departments of [1]Physiology, [2]Internal Medicine, and [3]Pediatrics and Child Health,
[4]Section of Respiratory Disease, and [5]CIHR National Training Program in Allergy
and Asthma, University of Manitoba, Winnipeg, MB, Canada
[6]Biology of Breathing Group, Manitoba Institute of Child Health, Winnipeg, MB,
Canada

Introduction

Airway smooth muscle (ASM) is a primary determinant of lung physiology because its ability to contract affords it dynamic control over airway diameter. Research for improved ways to treat asthma has long focused on factors that determine ASM contractility, including mechanical properties and responsiveness to spasmogens and relaxing factors. However, the scope of research on ASM biology and function has broadened greatly in the past decade and a half, embracing the now-recognized dynamic, multifunctional behavior that equips myocytes to be directly involved with the inflammation and fibroproliferative wound healing that underpins the development of airway remodeling. These cells can control airway diameter both acutely, via reversible contraction, and chronically, by driving fixed changes in structure and function properties of the airway wall. We review the spectrum of ASM phenotype and function in the context of pathobiology in obstructive airways disease and describe the impact of some emerging therapies on the properties of these cells.

Phenotype plasticity and functional diversity of smooth muscle

Work over the past 40 years on arterial smooth muscle *in vitro* and *in vivo* led to the concept that a dynamic phenotypic spectrum of differentiated smooth muscle

cells exists, ranging between so-called "contractile" and "synthetic/proliferative" states [1,2] (Figure 12.1). Contractile myocytes exist in smooth muscle tissues throughout the body and are chiefly designed to stiffen, shorten, or relax in response to chemical and mechanical signals. Synthetic/proliferative cells exhibit what has also been called an immature phenotype that is characterized by a tendency to proliferate and synthesize extracellular matrix (ECM) and other biologically active proteins.

Only after 1980 were primary cultured canine tracheal smooth muscle cells first described [3,4]. Nine years later [5,6] primary human ASM cell cultures were reported, leading to studies on the expression and function of physiologically relevant receptors, ion channels, and factors that regulate cell proliferation [7]. Though investigators recognized that airway myocytes likely modulated from a contractile phenotype when placed in culture, it was not until the late 1990s that systematic descriptions of phenotype and functional switching were published [8,9]. This provided impetus to examine the breadth of ASM function. Studies on biologic and molecular mechanisms that regulate phenotype and function have moved to the forefront, recognizing that ASM cells contribute broadly to the pathobiology of obstructive airways disease.

Phenotype plasticity

Phenotype plasticity is a feature of differentiated smooth muscle cells and is manifest as the reversible

---

Inflammation and Allergy Drug Design, First Edition. Edited by Kenji Izuhara, Stephen T. Holgate, Marsha Wills-Karp.
© 2011 Blackwell Publishing Ltd. Published 2011 by Blackwell Publishing Ltd.

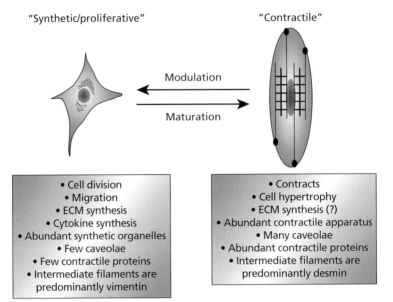

"Synthetic/proliferative"

"Contractile"

Modulation

Maturation

- Cell division
- Migration
- ECM synthesis
- Cytokine synthesis
- Abundant synthetic organelles
- Few caveolae
- Few contractile proteins
- Intermediate filaments are predominantly vimentin

- Contracts
- Cell hypertrophy
- ECM synthesis (?)
- Abundant contractile apparatus
- Many caveolae
- Abundant contractile proteins
- Intermediate filaments are predominantly desmin

Figure 12.1 Reversible phenotypic plasticity of airway smooth muscle. *Modulation* of myocytes to a "synthetic/proliferative" state occurs in primary culture and with exposure to mitogens and extracellular matrix (ECM) proteins such as fibronectin and collagen-1. *Maturation* to a "contractile" state occurs in cell culture at a high cell density in response to mitogen withdrawal, exposure to insulin, and adherence to laminin-rich ECM. "Contractile" myocytes predominate in adult tissues and exhibit variable degrees of maturation based on expression of molecular markers. Key functional, ultrastructural, and biochemical features of the extreme phenotypic states are shown.

modulation and maturation of myocytes both *in vitro* and *in vivo* [10]. Cell culture studies have provided insight on the control of phenotype expression and its regulation by stimuli including growth factors, G protein-coupled receptor ligands, and ECM proteins. Depending on the stimulus, myocytes can be induced to modulate to a synthetic/proliferative phenotype or to undergo maturation to a functionally contractile state.

In primary culture, contractile ASM cells undergo phenotype *modulation* [8], which promotes acquisition of a functional synthetic form marked by abundant organelles for protein and lipid synthesis and numerous mitochondria (Figure 12.1). The cells exhibit a high proliferative index but lose contractile apparatus proteins and responsiveness to contractile agonists [2,11]. The induction of primary cultured airway myocytes to a contractile phenotype is called *maturation* (Figure 12.1). Maturation is marked by the reaccumulation of contractile apparatus proteins, reacquisition of responsiveness to physiologic contractile agonists, and reduced numbers of synthetic organelles [9,12]. An additional ultrastructural

feature of contractile myocytes is the presence of abundant caveolae and their unique structural proteins, caveolin-1 and -2, which modulate signal transduction [13,14]. Molecular markers for the contractile phenotype include smooth muscle (SM) α-actin, SM-myosin heavy chain, calponin, *h*-caldesmon, SM22, desmin, caveolin-1, β-dystroglycan, and integrin α7 [8,9,15–19]. Regulation of the expression of these proteins requires coordinated control of gene transcription and translation [10,20]. Intracellular signaling cascades, including Rho/Rho kinase and phosphatidylinositol 3 kinase (PI3K)-dependent pathways play a central role in smooth muscle specific gene expression and protein synthesis [21–25].

In culture, growth factors, such as TGF-β1 and insulin, and ECM proteins, such as laminins, support the expression of a contractile ASM phenotype, whereas mitogens such as platelet-derived growth factor (PDGF) or fetal serum and extracellular fibronectin matrices support proliferative function [16,26–28]. Maturation requires endogenously expressed laminin-2 and is reliant on cells expressing a unique repertoire of laminin-binding α-integrin subunits [15,16]. Notably, in primary culture only a subset of airway myocytes appear able to reacquire a functionally contractile phenotype, suggesting—and supported by *in situ* evidence [29]—the existence of intrinsic heterogeneity between myocytes and that divergent mesenchymal sublineages may seed the ASM bed during development [9,11]. Notably, the maturation of contractile myocytes parallels the process of cellular hypertrophy, involving an increase in cell size and reliance on PI3K-associated signaling pathways [21,25,30]. Increased smooth muscle mass is a feature of airways remodeling and thus evaluation of myocyte maturation in culture contributes to the understanding of the pathogenesis of obstructive airway disease.

Functional diversity

Although there are molecular and ultrastructural markers for contractile phenotype myocytes, there also exists a broad diversity in the sensitivity and reactivity of smooth muscle to factors that trigger contraction and relaxation. Diversity in functional responses to proliferative and prosynthetic mediators is also seen in cells expressing an immature phenotype [31,32]. Thus, although myocytes may be classified as "contractile" or "immature," there are mechanisms that fine-tune cell function. Moreover, airway myocytes in a contractile phenotype retain a variable capacity to synthesize and express cytokines, chemokines, and ECM proteins [15,16,33]. This indicates that strict designation of airway myocytes as being contractile or synthetic/proliferative is not appropriate, as cells of any phenotype retain diversity in functional responses (Figure 12.2).

One element of functional diversity that is dynamic over relatively short durations is termed mechanical plasticity, which stems from the remodeling of actomyosin filaments in response to changes in muscle length during stretch or contraction [34,35]. A functional capacity of this nature meets the physiologic burden of constantly variable forces, for example in breathing. Mechanical adaptation confers the capacity to retain maximum force generation but can alter shortening velocity, which may contribute to airway hyperresponsiveness [36,37].

An additional mechanism for the functional diversity of mature myocytes is a variation in the expression of proteins that mediate responses to extra-cellular cues. For example, arterial resistance vessels contract after mechanical stretch owing to the activation of inward cation channels, whereas healthy bronchial smooth muscle exhibits little or no myogenic response [38,39]. Indeed, the repertoire of proteins expressed as receptors, receptor regulators, signaling effectors, and ion channels contributes significantly to the functional fine-tuning of smooth muscle cells across the range of phenotypic states [12,13, 40–42].

Functional plasticity airway smooth muscle: role in asthma pathogenesis

Phenotypic plasticity of airway myocytes confers a multifunctional capacity—contraction, proliferation, hypertrophy, migration, and synthesis of inflammation and fibrosis-modulating biomolecules (Figure 12.3) [20]. Thus, myocytes contribute both to bronchial spasm and to structural changes associated with fixed airway obstruction.

That ASM cells can synthesize inflammatory biomolecules and are a rich source of cytokines, chemokines, and growth factors is well documented [43,44]. Cultured myocytes express a number of cytokines (Th1 type: interleukin 2 [IL-2], interferon γ [IFN-γ], IL-12; Th2 type: IL-5, IL-6, granulocyte–macrophage colony-stimulating factor [GM-CSF]) and high levels of RANTES (regulated on activation, normal T cell-expressed, and secreted), eotaxin, IL-8, and IL-11 [45]. This indicates that ASM cells can determine local inflammation and establish a self-regulating mechanism for phenotype plasticity as a determinant of asthma pathogenesis and symptoms.

Cultured ASM cells from asthmatics produce an altered composition of ECM [46,47]. The ECM affects all aspects of the functional repertoire of smooth muscle cells. For instance, seeding ASM onto fibronectin or collagen type I promotes a proliferative phenotype, whereas laminin-rich matrices are needed for maturation of a contractile phenotype [16,26,48]. Laminin-2 and its selective receptor, α7β1 integrin, are required for airway myocyte maturation and hypertrophy [15]. Moreover, laminin-2 is increased in the asthmatic airway [16]. Focus on the role of ECM receptor expression by ASM is warranted as it could yield viable therapeutic targets to combat, and even reverse, airway remodeling.

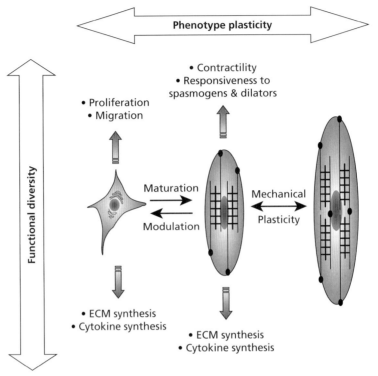

Figure 12.2 Schematic representation of phenotype plasticity and functional diversity of smooth muscle. *Phenotype plasticity* results from reversible modulation and maturation of myocytes. *Mechanical plasticity*, a form of functional diversity, occurs in contractile phenotype myocytes as the result of subcellular reorganization of the contractile filaments in response to changes in muscle length during stretch or contraction. *Functional diversity* exists cells of any phenotype owing to differences in expression of (i) receptor subtypes for growth factors, hormones, neurotransmitters, and extracellular matrix (ECM), (ii) regulators of receptors and receptor-induced signaling proteins (e.g., caveolins and GRKs), (iii) receptor-induced signaling proteins, and (iv) ion channels that determine membrane electrophysiology.

Increased ASM mass in human asthmatics results from cellular hyperplasia and hypertrophy [49,50]. ASM cells cultured from endobronchial biopsies from asthmatics proliferate at a faster rate than those from healthy individuals, and this difference appears to be directly linked to changes in the profile of ECM proteins synthesized by "asthmatic" myocytes [31,47,51]. This suggests the existence of an intrinsic, stable abnormality in the phenotype of myocytes in asthmatics that is associated with altered functional responses to asthma-associated mitogens. Prohypertrophic factors that are increased in asthmatic airways include TGF-β1 and endothelin 1, which induce ASM cell hypertrophy in culture [30,52]. Increased ASM mass, even in mild-to-moderate asthma, is accompanied by increased proteins associated with contraction, such as myosin light chain kinase, which underpins the increased contractility of ASM tissue in asthma and in asthma models [50,53,54].

Additional mechanisms that could account for increased ASM mass in asthma also stem from the multifunctional capacity of these cells. Migration of fibroblasts from the submucosa to the muscle layer with subsequent maturation to a contractile phenotype could promote the accumulation of ASM tissue. A mechanism in which circulating mesenchymal stem cells home and migrate into damaged airways and then undergo differentiation to smooth muscle has also been postulated [55]. Moreover, to account for increases in airway myofibroblasts, ASM cells could undergo phenotype modulation and migrate toward the epithelium [56].

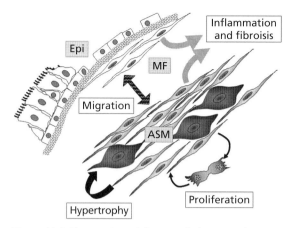

Figure 12.3 Phenotypic and functional plasticity of mesenchymal cells in airway remodeling. Airway smooth muscle (ASM) cells (gray) and myofibroblasts (MF) (white) regulate the local tissue microenvironment by releasing inflammatory mediators and increasing expression of cell adhesion molecules and extracellular matrix (ECM) components. Increased ASM mass results from myocyte proliferation and hypertrophy. Myofibroblasts migrating toward the ASM layer may also contribute to muscle thickening—upon reaching the ASM compartment, mesenchymal cells undergo maturation. The process is likely modulated by local cytokines, chemokines, and ECM. Migration of phenotypically modulated ASM to the submucosal compartment leads to an increased number of myofibroblasts.

Emerging therapies and their impact on airway smooth muscle

Phosphodiesterase inhibitors

Cyclic nucleotide phosphodiesterases (PDE) degrade the phosphodiester bond in cAMP and cGMP, imparting important signal transduction control [57]. Theophylline, a nonspecific PDE inhibitor, has been used to treat airway diseases for over 50 years and has bronchodilating, anti-inflammatory, and antifibrotic effects [58,59]. Subtype-specific PDE inhibitors that minimize unwanted side-effects now exist. PDE-4 is the predominant PDE subtype expressed in the airways [60]. First- and second-generation PDE-4 inhibitors like rolipram (Calbiochem, Alexandria, NSW, Australia), piclamilast, also called RP73401 (Aventis Pharma, Guildford, Surrey), ciclamilast (Aventis), cilomilast (Ariflo®; GlaxoSmithKline),

and roflumilast (Daxas®; Nycomed) show promise for reducing features of airway remodeling [61,62]; largely by raising cAMP in inflammatory, immune, and ASM cells.

PDE-4 inhibitors appear to have effects on the breadth of ASM cell function. Roflumilast directly inhibits TGF-β1-induced ECM protein synthesis by asthmatic and nonasthmatic cultured ASM cells and in tracheal rings *in vitro* [63]. It also reduces subepithelial fibrosis and tracheal epithelial activation in mice that are chronically challenged with allergen [64]. Cilomilast reduces both basal- and PDGF-stimulated migration of human ASM cells *in vitro* [65]. Both rolipram and NIS-62949 reduce airway hyperresponsiveness (AHR) and bronchoconstriction in animal models of allergic asthma AHR [66,67]. Thus, there are compelling data emerging to suggest that PDE-4 inhibitors prevent AHR, airway remodeling, and inflammation via pathways involving ASM.

Rho kinase inhibitors

Rho kinases are effectors of RhoA, a monomeric GTP-binding protein, that cause Ca^{2+} sensitization of ASM by inactivating myosin light chain phosphatase, the enzyme chiefly responsible for tempering contraction and causing relaxation. Two isoforms of Rho kinase exist (ROCK-1 and ROCK-2 [68]), there are no isoform selective inhibitors, and both isoforms are expressed in lung and inflammatory cells. The major roles of Rho kinase in cell physiology include contraction, cell attachment, migration, proliferation, and cell survival. A widely studied Rho kinase inhibitor, Y-27632, is a potent cell-permeable competitive inhibitor with bronchodilatory effects when delivered to the airways in allergen exposed animals [69,70]. In animal models of asthma, Rho kinase inhibitors suppress acute AHR and airway remodeling arising from allergic inflammation [70,71]. Analogs of Y-27632 also promote smooth muscle relaxation [72,73]. Rho kinase is also involved with "activation" of airway fibroblasts to myofibroblasts that contribute to collagen deposition [74]. Based on the links between Rho A and Rho kinase activity with bronchoconstriction, inflammatory cell recruitment, AHR, smooth muscle growth, and myofibroblast activation, Rho kinase inhibitors may be useful for treatment, and abundant research in this area is expected.

Statins

Statins inhibit mevalonate synthesis, the proximal step in cholesterol biosynthesis. They reduce serum cholesterol but emerging evidence indicates that they have an even greater health benefit, thus spawning a growing number of clinical trials of their impact on lung health. The positive effects of statins in asthma control are equivocal [75–77]; however, studies to date are limited because they only included mild asthmatics, statin use was of relatively short duration, and in some cases steroid use was stopped. Reports indicate a direct impact for statins on ASM cell growth, fibrotic function, and cell survival [78–80]. Statins impact cell responses via the indirect inhibition of small GTPase proteins (e.g., Ras, Rac, Rho), mitogen-activated protein (MAP) kinases, and nuclear factor κB; this suppresses airway inflammation in allergen-challenged mice and improves lung physiology [81,82]. Although the investigation into the use of statins to treat asthma is in its infancy, studies to date suggest that these compounds could open doors for new therapeutic approaches as mechanisms for their pleiotropic effects are unraveled.

Bronchial thermoplasty

Bronchial thermoplasty uses radiofrequency energy to reduce ASM mass and attenuate bronchoconstriction [83]. Initial studies in canines show that the application of radiofrequency to the airways, at temperatures of 65°C and 75°C, reduced airway responsiveness to methacholine by ~50% [84]. These effects were maintained for up to 3 years, and histologic analysis revealed complete ablation of ASM with emergence of a thin layer of collagen [84]. The procedure is in clinical trial; to date, patients report decreased numbers of mild and severe exacerbations and increased symptom-free days [85]. The changes to the airway wall and the effectiveness of treatment on long-term asthma control are currently under investigation, and more insight is expected in the foreseeable future.

Concluding remarks

The broad functional behavior of ASM may be at the root of the biologic mechanisms that lead to changes in airway function and structure in obstructive airways disease. Increased bronchial spasm with altered airway structure, which manifests as AHR, are likely linked to the plastic multifunctional behavior of airway myocytes. For instance, increased myocyte contraction due to elevated myosin light chain kinase leads to greater airway narrowing. Similarly, changes in pharmacologic responsiveness of myocytes occur in the face of asthma-associated mediators and thus underpin increased sensitivity to inhaled allergic and nonallergic contractile agonists. Notably, airway myocytes are also rich sources of inflammatory mediators, making them determinants of the local inflammatory environment, and the accumulation of airway ECM is largely the result of altered function of ASM and (myo)fibroblasts. Thus, the role of mesenchymal cells in the pathogenesis of obstructive airways disease is at the forefront of current research in airway biology. Advances expected in the next decade will likely yield significant insight that may dictate the direction for the development of new and more effective pharmacologic interventions.

Acknowledgment

PS holds a Frederick Banting and Charles Best Canadian Graduate Scholarship from Canadian Institute of Health Research (CIHR) and National Training Program in Allergy and Asthma. AJH is supported by the Canada Research Chair program, Canada Foundation for Innovation, and the Manitoba Institute of Child Health.

References

1 Wissler RW. The arterial medial cell, smooth muscle, or multifunctional mesenchyme? *Circulation* 1967; **36**: 1–4.

2 Chamley-Campbell J, Campbell GR, Ross R. The smooth muscle cell in culture. *Physiol Rev* 1979; **59**: 1–61.

3 Avner BP, Delongo J, Wilson S, Ladman AJ. A method for culturing canine tracheal smooth muscle cells *in vitro*: morphologic and pharmacologic observations. *Anat Rec* 1981; **200**: 357–70.

4 Tom-Moy M, Madison JM, Jones CA, de Lanerolle P, Brown JK. Morphologic characterization of cultured smooth muscle cells isolated from the tracheas of adult dogs. *Anat Rec* 1987; **218**: 313–28.

5 Twort Ch, van Breemen C. Human airway smooth muscle in cell culture: control of the intracellular calcium store. *Pulm Pharmacol* 1989; **2**: 45–53.

6 Panettieri RA, Murray RK, DePalo LR, Yadvish PA, Kotlikoff MI. A human airway smooth muscle cell line that retains physiological responsiveness. *Am J Physiol* 1989; **256**: C329–35.

7 Hall IP, Kotlikoff M. Use of cultured airway myocytes for study of airway smooth muscle. *Am J Physiol* 1995; **268**: L1–11.

8 Halayko AJ, Salari H, Ma X, Stephens NL. Markers of airway smooth muscle cell phenotype. *Am J Physiol* 1996; **270**: L1040–51.

9 Halayko AJ, Camoretti-Mercado B, Forsythe SM, *et al.* Divergent differentiation paths in airway smooth muscle culture: induction of functionally contractile myocytes. *Am J Physiol Lung Cell Mol Physiol* 1999; **276**: L197–206.

10 Halayko AJ, Solway J. Molecular mechanisms of phenotypic plasticity in smooth muscle cells. *J Appl Physiol* 2001; **90**: 358–68.

11 Mitchell RW, Halayko AJ, Kahraman S, Solway J, Wylam ME. Selective restoration of calcium coupling to muscarinic M(3) receptors in contractile cultured airway myocytes. *Am J Physiol Lung Cell Mol Physiol* 2000; **278**: L1091–100.

12 Mitchell RW, Halayko AJ, Kahraman S, Solway J, Wylam ME. Selective restoration of calcium coupling to muscarinic M(3) receptors in contractile cultured airway myocytes. *Am J Physiol Lung Cell Mol Physiol* 2000; **278**: L1091–100.

13 Gosens R, Stelmack GL, Dueck G, *et al.* Caveolae facilitate muscarinic receptor-mediated intracellular Ca^{2+} mobilization and contraction in airway smooth muscle. *Am J Physiol Lung Cell Mol Physiol* 2007; **293**: L1406–18.

14 Halayko AJ, Tran T, Gosens R. Phenotype and functional plasticity of airway smooth muscle: role of caveolae and caveolins. *Proc Am Thorac Soc* 2008; **5**: 80–8.

15 Tran T, Ens-Blackie K, Rector ES, *et al.* Laminin-binding Integrin {alpha}7 is required for contractile phenotype expression by human airway myocyte. *Am J Respir Cell Mol Biol* 2007; **37**: 668–80.

16 Tran T, McNeill KD, Gerthoffer WT, Unruh H, Halayko AJ. Endogenous laminin is required for human airway smooth muscle cell maturation. *Respir Res* 2006; **7**: 117.

17 Solway J, Seltzer J, Samaha FF, *et al.*, Structure and expression of a smooth muscle cell-specific gene, SM22 alpha. *J Biol Chem* 1995; **270**: 13460–9.

18 Gosens R, Stelmack GL, Dueck G, *et al.* Role of caveolin-1 in p42/p44 MAP kinase activation and proliferation of human airway smooth muscle. *Am J Physiol Lung Cell Mol Physiol* 2006; **291**: L523–34.

19 Sharma P, Tran T, Stelmack GL, *et al.*, Expression of the dystrophin–glycoprotein complex is a marker for human airway smooth muscle phenotype maturation. *Am J Physiol Lung Cell Mol Physiol* 2008; **294**: L57–68.

20 Halayko AJ, Tran T, Ji SY, Yamasaki A, Gosens R. Airway smooth muscle phenotype and function: interactions with current asthma therapies. *Curr Drug Targets* 2006; **7**: 525–40.

21 Halayko AJ, Kartha S, Stelmack GL, *et al.* Phophatidylinositol-3 kinase/mammalian target of rapamycin/p70S6K regulates contractile protein accumulation in airway myocyte differentiation. *Am J Respir Cell Mol Biol* 2004; **31**: 266–75.

22 Camoretti-Mercado B, Fernandes DJ, *et al.*, Inhibition of transforming growth factor beta-enhanced serum response factor-dependent transcription by SMAD7. *J Biol Chem* 2006; **281**: 20383–92.

23 Camoretti-Mercado B, Liu HW, Halayko AJ, *et al.* Physiological control of smooth muscle-specific gene expression through regulated nuclear translocation of serum response factor. *J Biol Chem* 2000; **275**: 30387–93.

24 Liu HW, Halayko AJ, Fernandes DJ, *et al.*, The RhoA/Rho kinase pathway regulates nuclear localization of serum response factor. *Am J Respir Cell Mol Biol* 2003; **29**: 39–47.

25 Zhou L, Goldsmith AM, Bentley JK, *et al.* 4E-binding protein phosphorylation and eukaryotic initiation factor-4E release are required for airway smooth muscle hypertrophy. *Am J Respir Cell Mol Biol* 2005; **33**: 195–202.

26 Hirst SJ, Twort Ch, Lee Th. Differential effects of extracellular matrix proteins on human airway smooth muscle cell proliferation and phenotype. *Am J Respir Cell Mol Biol* 2000; **23**: 335–44.

27 Schaafsma D, McNeill KD, Stelmack GL, *et al.* Insulin increases the expression of contractile phenotypic markers in airway smooth muscle. *Am J Physiol Cell Physiol* 2007; **293**: C429–39.

28 Dekkers BG, Schaafsma D, Nelemans SA, Zaagsma J, Meurs H. Extracellular matrix proteins differentially regulate airway smooth muscle phenotype and function. *Am J Physiol Lung Cell Mol Physiol* 2007; **292**: L1405–13.

29 Halayko AJ, Stelmack GL, Yamasaki A, McNeill K, Unruh H, Rector E. Distribution of phenotypically disparate myocyte subpopulations in airway smooth muscle. *Can J Physiol Pharmacol* 2005; **83**: 104–16.

30 Goldsmith AM, Bentley JK, Zhou L, *et al.* Transforming growth factor-beta induces airway smooth muscle hypertrophy. *Am J Respir Cell Mol Biol* 2006; **34**: 247–54.

31 Johnson PR, Roth M, Tamm M, *et al.* Airway smooth muscle cell proliferation is increased in asthma. *Am J Respir Crit Care Med* 2001; **164**: 474–7.

32 Burgess JK, Ge Q, Boustany S, Black JL, Johnson PR. Increased sensitivity of asthmatic airway smooth

169

muscle cells to prostaglandin E2 might be mediated by increased numbers of E-prostanoid receptors. *J Allergy Clin Immunol* 2004; **113**: 876–81.

33 Redhu NS, Saleh A, Shan L, *et al.* Proinflammatory and Th2 cytokines regulate the high affinity IgE receptor (FcepsilonRI) and IgE-dependent activation of human airway smooth muscle cells. *PLoS One* 2009; **4**: e6153.

34 Gunst SJ, Tang DD, Opazo Saez A. Cytoskeletal remodeling of the airway smooth muscle cell: a mechanism for adaptation to mechanical forces in the lung. *Respir Physiol Neurobiol* 2003; **137**: 151–68.

35 Ford LE, Seow CY, Pratusevich VR. Plasticity in smooth muscle, a hypothesis. *Can J Physiol Pharmacol* 1994; **72**: 1320–4.

36 Wang L, Pare PD, Seow CY. Changes in force-velocity properties of trachealis due to oscillatory strains. *J Appl Physiol* 2002; **92**: 1865–72.

37 King GG, Pare PD, Seow CY. The mechanics of exaggerated airway narrowing in asthma: the role of smooth muscle. *Respir Physiol* 1999; **118**: 1–13.

38 McGregor E, Gosling M, Beattie DK, Ribbons DM, Davies AH, Powell JT. Circumferential stretching of saphenous vein smooth muscle enhances vasoconstrictor responses by Rho kinase-dependent pathways. *Cardiovasc Res* 2002; **53**: 219–26.

39 Wu X, Davis MJ. Characterization of stretch-activated cation current in coronary smooth muscle cells. *Am J Physiol Heart Circ Physiol* 2001; **280**: H1751–61.

40 Janssen LJ. Ionic mechanisms and Ca(2⁺) regulation in airway smooth muscle contraction: do the data contradict dogma? *Am J Physiol Lung Cell Mol Physiol* 2002; **282**: L1161–78.

41 Borchers MT, Biechele T, Justice JP, *et al.* Methacholine-induced airway hyperresponsiveness is dependent on Galphaq signaling. *Am J Physiol Lung Cell Mol Physiol* 2003; **285**: L114–20.

42 Walker JK, Gainetdinov RR, Feldman DS, *et al.* G protein-coupled receptor kinase 5 regulates airway responses induced by muscarinic receptor activation. *Am J Physiol Lung Cell Mol Physiol* 2004; **286**: L312–19.

43 Howarth PH, Knox AJ, Amrani Y, Tliba O, Panettieri RA, Jr., Johnson M. Synthetic responses in airway smooth muscle. *J Allergy Clin Immunol* 2004; **114**: S32–50.

44 Halayko AJ, Solway J. Molecular mechanisms of phenotypic plasticity in smooth muscle cells. *J Appl Physiol* 2001; **90**: 358–68.

45 Halayko AJ, Amrani Y. Mechanisms of inflammation-mediated airway smooth muscle plasticity and airways remodeling in asthma. *Respir Physiol Neurobiol* 2003; **137**: 209–22.

46 Johnson PR, Black JL, Carlin S, Ge Q, Underwood PA. The production of extracellular matrix proteins by human passively sensitized airway smooth-muscle cells

in culture: the effect of beclomethasone. *Am J Respir Crit Care Med* 2000; **162**: 2145–51.

47 Johnson PR. Role of human airway smooth muscle in altered extracellular matrix production in asthma. *Clin Exp Pharmacol Physiol* 2001; **28**: 233–6.

48 Tran T, Gosens R, Halayko AJ. Effects of extracellular matrix and integrin interactions in airway smooth muscle phenotype and function: it takes two to tango! *Curr Respir Med Rev* 2007; **3**: 193–205.

49 Ebina M, Takahashi T, Chiba T, Motomiya M. Cellular hypertrophy and hyperplasia of airway smooth muscles underlying bronchial asthma. A 3-D morphometric study. *Am Rev Respir Dis* 1993; **148**: 720–6.

50 Benayoun L, Druilhe A, Dombret MC, Aubier M, Pretolani M. Airway structural alterations selectively associated with severe asthma. *Am J Respir Crit Care Med* 2003; **167**: 1360–8.

51 Johnson PR, Burgess JK, Underwood PA, *et al.* Extracellular matrix proteins modulate asthmatic airway smooth muscle cell proliferation via an autocrine mechanism. *J Allergy Clin Immunol* 2004; **113**: 690–6.

52 McWhinnie R, Pechkovsky DV, Zhou D, *et al.* Endothelin-1 induces hypertrophy and inhibits apoptosis in human airway smooth muscle cells. *Am J Physiol Lung Cell Mol Physiol* 2007; **292**: L278–86.

53 Jiang H, Rao K, Halayko AJ, Liu X, Stephens NL. Ragweed sensitization-induced increase of myosin light chain kinase content in canine airway smooth muscle. *Am J Respir Cell Mol Biol* 1992; **7**: 567–73.

54 Ammit AJ, Armour CL, Black JL. Smooth-muscle myosin light-chain kinase content is increased in human sensitized airways. *Am J Respir Crit Care Med* 2000; **161**: 257–63.

55 Stewart AG. Emigration and immigration of mesenchymal cells: a multicultural airway wall. *Eur Respir J* 2004; **24**: 515–17.

56 Kelly MM, O'Connor TM, Leigh R, *et al.* Effects of budesonide and formoterol on allergen-induced airway responses, inflammation, and airway remodeling in asthma. *J Allergy Clin Immunol* 2010; **125**: 349–56, e13.

57 Weiss B, Hait WN. Selective cyclic nucleotide phosphodiesterase inhibitors as potential therapeutic agents. *Annu Rev Pharmacol Toxicol* 1977; **17**: 441–77.

58 Finney MJ, Karlsson JA, Persson CG. Effects of bronchoconstrictors and bronchodilators on a novel human small airway preparation. *Br J Pharmacol* 1985; **85**: 29–36.

59 Yano Y, Yoshida M, Hoshino S, *et al.* Anti-fibrotic effects of theophylline on lung fibroblasts. *Biochem Biophys Res Commun* 2006; **341**: 684–90.

60 Kroegel C, Foerster M. Phosphodiesterase-4 inhibitors as a novel approach for the treatment of respiratory disease: cilomilast. *Expert Opin Investig Drugs* 2007; **16**: 109–24.

61 Bundschuh DS, Eltze M, Barsig J, Wollin L, Hatzelmann A, Beume R. *In vivo* efficacy in airway disease models of roflumilast, a novel orally active PDE4 inhibitor. *J Pharmacol Exp Ther* 2001; **297**: 280–90.

62 Mata M, Sarria B, Buenestado A, Cortijo J, Cerda M, Morcillo EJ. Phosphodiesterase 4 inhibition decreases MUC5AC, expression induced by epidermal growth factor in human airway epithelial cells. *Thorax* 2005; **60**: 144–52.

63 Burgess JK, Oliver BG, Poniris MH, *et al*. A phosphodiesterase 4 inhibitor inhibits matrix protein deposition in airways *in vitro*. *J Allergy Clin Immunol* 2006; **118**: 649–57.

64 Kumar RK, Herbert C, Thomas PS, *et al*. Inhibition of inflammation and remodeling by roflumilast and dexamethasone in murine chronic asthma. *J Pharmacol Exp Ther* 2003; **307**: 349–55.

65 Goncharova EA, Billington CK, Irani C, *et al*. Cyclic AMP-mobilizing agents and glucocorticoids modulate human smooth muscle cell migration. *Am J Respir Cell Mol Biol* 2003; **29**: 19–27.

66 Singh SP, Mishra NC, Rir-Sima-Ah J, *et al*. Maternal exposure to secondhand cigarette smoke primes the lung for induction of phosphodiesterase-4D5 isozyme and exacerbated Th2 responses: rolipram attenuates the airway hyperreactivity and muscarinic receptor expression but not lung inflammation and atopy. *J Immunol* 2009; **183**: 2115–21.

67 Dastidar SG, Ray A, Shirumalla R, *et al*., Pharmacology of a novel, orally active PDE4 inhibitor. *Pharmacology* 2009; **83**: 275–86.

68 Noma K, Oyama N, Liao JK. Physiological role of ROCKs in the cardiovascular system. *Am J Physiol Cell Physiol* 2006; **290**: C661–8.

69 Iizuka K, Shimizu Y, Tsukagoshi H, *et al*. Evaluation of Y-27632: a rho-kinase inhibitor, as a bronchodilator in guinea pigs. *Eur J Pharmacol* 2000; **406**: 273–9.

70 Henry PJ, Mann TS, Goldie RG. A rho kinase inhibitor, Y-27632; inhibits pulmonary eosinophilia, bronchoconstriction and airways hyperresponsiveness in allergic mice. *Pulm Pharmacol Ther* 2005; **18**: 67–74.

71 Schaafsma D, Bos IS, Zuidhof AB, Zaagsma J, Meurs H. Inhalation of the Rho-kinase inhibitor Y-27632; reverses allergen-induced airway hyperresponsiveness after the early and late asthmatic reaction. *Respir Res* 2006; **7**: 121.

72 Uehata M, Ishizaki T, Satoh H, *et al*. Calcium sensitization of smooth muscle mediated by a Rho-associated protein kinase in hypertension. *Nature* 1997; **389**: 990–4.

73 Ishizaki T, Uehata M, Tamechika I, *et al*., Pharmacological properties of Y-27632: a specific inhibitor of rho-associated kinases. *Mol Pharmacol* 2000; **57**: 976–83.

74 Urata Y, Nishimura Y, Hirase T, Yokoyama M. Sphingosine 1-phosphate induces alpha-smooth muscle actin expression in lung fibroblasts via Rho-kinase. *Kobe J Med Sci* 2005; **51**: 17–27.

75 Menzies D, Nair A, Meldrum KT, Fleming D, Barnes M, Lipworth BJ. Simvastatin does not exhibit therapeutic anti-inflammatory effects in asthma. *J Allergy Clin Immunol* 2007; **119**: 328–35.

76 Hothersall EJ, Chaudhuri R, McSharry C, *et al*. Effects of atorvastatin added to inhaled corticosteroids on lung function and sputum cell counts in atopic asthma. *Thorax* 2008; **63**: 1070–5.

77 Ostroukhova M, Kouides RW, Friedman E. The effect of statin therapy on allergic patients with asthma. *Ann Allergy Asthma Immunol* 2009; **103**: 463–8.

78 Ghavami S, Mutawe MM, Hauff K, *et al*. Statin-triggered cell death in primary human lung mesenchymal cells involves p53-PUMA and release of Smac and Omi but not cytochrome c. *Biochim Biophys Acta* 2010; **1803**: 452–67.

79 Schaafsma D, Dueck G, Ghavami S, *et al*. The mevalonate cascade as a target to suppress extracellular matrix synthesis by human airway smooth muscle. *Am J Respir Cell Mol Biol* 2010; **44**: 394–403.

80 Takeda N, Kondo M, Ito S, Ito Y, Shimokata K, Kume H. Role of RhoA inactivation in reduced cell proliferation of human airway smooth muscle by simvastatin. *Am J Respir Cell Mol Biol* 2006; **35**: 722–9.

81 Zeki AA, Franzi L, Last J, Kenyon NJ. Simvastatin inhibits airway hyperreactivity: implications for the mevalonate pathway and beyond. *Am J Respir Crit Care Med* 2009; **180**: 731–40.

82 Kim DY, Joo JK, Ryu SY, Park YK, Kim YJ, Kim SK. Clinicopathological characteristics and prognosis of carcinoma of the gastric cardia. *Dig Surg* 2006; **23**: 313–18.

83 Cox G, Miller JD, McWilliams A, Fitzgerald JM, Lam S. Bronchial thermoplasty for asthma. *Am J Respir Crit Care Med* 2006; **173**: 965–9.

84 Danek CJ, Lombard CM, Dungworth DL, *et al*. Reduction in airway hyperresponsiveness to methacholine by the application of RF energy in dogs. *J Appl Physiol* 2004; **97**: 1946–53.

85 Cox G, Thomson NC, Rubin AS, *et al*. Asthma control during the year after bronchial thermoplasty. *N Engl J Med* 2007; **356**: 1327–37.

Part II
Cytokines contributing to the pathogenesis of allergic diseases in the respiratory tract

13 Interleukin 4, interleukin 13, and interleukin 9

Kenji Izuhara,[1] *Shoichiro Ohta,*[2] *Hiroshi Shiraishi,*[3] *and Shoichi Suzuki*[3]

[1]Division of Medical Biochemistry, Department of Biomolecular Sciences, Saga Medical School, Saga, Japan

[2]Department of Laboratory Medicine, Saga Medical School, Saga, Japan

[3]Division of Medical Biochemistry, Department of Biomolecular Sciences, Saga Medical School, Saga, Japan

IL-4 and IL-13

In the 1990s, it was established that T helper (Th2) cytokines played a key role in bronchial asthma in mice. Later, interest centered on which Th2 cytokine played the most important part in bronchial asthma. During the investigations, it was thought that both interleukin 4 (IL-4) and IL-13 were important in the pathogenesis of bronchial asthma but that the effects of these two interleukins were redundant because they shared receptors and signal pathways. However, it has since been discovered that IL-13 acts as a central mediator in the pathogenesis of asthma in mice, as supported by the results of expression profiling in asthmatic individuals and the genetic association with asthma. Based on these findings, antagonists against IL-4 and in particular IL-13 are currently being developed as therapeutic agents against bronchial asthma.

Signal transduction of IL-4/IL-13

Both IL-4 and IL-13 bind to their specific receptors on their target cells. Two types of IL-4 receptors (IL-4R) exist: type I IL-4R and type II IL-4R [1,2] (Figure 13.1). Type I IL-4R is composed of the IL-4Rα chain and the common γ chain (γc) that is shared by IL-2, IL-7, IL-9, IL-15, and IL-21, whereas type II IL-4R comprises IL-4Rα and the IL-13Rα1 chain. Because IL-13 also binds to type II IL-4R, this receptor acts as the functional IL-13R. Hematopoietic/

immune cells mainly express type I IL-4R, through which IL-4 induces Th2 differentiation and class switching into immunoglobulin E (IgE) and IgG4 (and, in the case of mouse, IgG1). On the other hand, nonhematopoietic cells ubiquitously express type II IL-4R/IL-13R, whose signals play an important role in the setting of bronchial asthma. Another IL-13-binding component that exists in addition to IL-13Rα1 is the IL-13R α2 chain (IL-13Rα2), which cannot transduce signals that act as a decoy receptor, although there is a report that IL-13Rα2 activates jun and Fra-2, inducing expression of tumor growth factor beta (TGF-β) [3].

The Jak/STAT pathways are the main signal pathways for IL-4/IL-13 and other cytokines. In addition to these pathways, MAP kinase and phosphatidylinositol-3 kinase pathways are also involved [1,2]. IL-4Rα, γc, and IL-13Rα1 bind to Jak1, Jak3, and Tyk2, respectively, which activate STAT6, along with STAT1 and STAT3 in some cases, and play a critical role in the IL-4/IL-13 signals.

It is now known that IL-13 is dominant in the pathogenesis of bronchial asthma compared with IL-4. It took a long time to clarify the underlying mechanism that determines whether the effects of IL-13 are dominant *in vivo*, although both IL-4 and IL-13 transduce their signals via the shared pathways; however, biochemical and structural analyses have recently addressed this subject [4–7] (Figure 13.2). In type II IL-4R/IL-13R, IL-4 first binds to IL-4Rα with

Inflammation and Allergy Drug Design, First Edition. Edited by Kenji Izuhara, Stephen T. Holgate, Marsha Wills-Karp.
© 2011 Blackwell Publishing Ltd. Published 2011 by Blackwell Publishing Ltd.

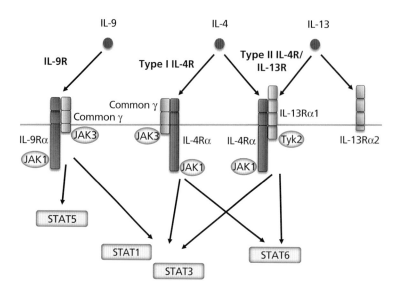

Figure 13.1 The receivers and Jak/STAT pathways of interleukin 4 (IL-4), IL-13, and IL-9. The receptor components of IL-4, IL-13, and IL-9 and the Jak/STAT molecules associated with their signals are depicted.

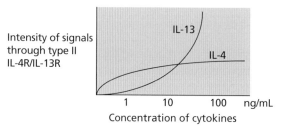

Figure 13.2 The correlation between the concentration of cytokines (interleukin 4 [IL-4] or IL-13) and the intensity of the signals through type II IL-4 receptor (IL-4R)/IL-13R. The intensity of IL-13 signals through type II IL-4R/IL-13R in nonimmune cells is dose dependent, whereas that of IL-4 signals reaches a plateau at low concentration. Modified from Junttila *et al.* (2008).

high affinity (Kd: 100–200 pM) and then to IL-13Rα1 with little contribution to the affinity, generating the functional receptor, whereas IL-13 first binds to IL-13Rα1 with low affinity (Kd: 2–10 nM) and then to IL-4Rα, generating the high-affinity receptor (Kd: 30–400 pM). IL-13Rα1 is expressed more abundantly on nonhematopoietic cells than IL-4Rα. With such characteristics and distribution of the receptor components, IL-13 signals are dose dependent, whereas IL-4 reaches a plateau at low concentrations. In fact, the local concentration of IL-13 in inflamed lesions is high compared with IL-4 [8–10]; therefore, IL-13 dominantly transduces the signals *in vivo*.

The roles of IL-4 and IL-13 in the pathogenesis of bronchial asthma in mice

Many studies using mice that are defective in various IL-4/IL-13 signal-transducing molecules have been performed for the mouse model of allergen-challenged asthma [1,2]. Application of IL-4- or IL-13-deficient mice or administration of neutralizing anti-IL-4 Abs initially showed alleviation, but not complete diminishment, of asthmatic phenotypes such as eosinophilia or enhanced airway hyperreactivity (AHR) [11–15]. In contrast, in mice that are defective in either IL-4Rα or STAT6, signal-transducing components common in IL-4 and IL-13, asthmatic phenotypes were more severely or even completely diminished [16–20]. These results suggested that both IL-4 and IL-13 are important in bronchial asthma and that these two cytokines are redundant. However, it has since been shown that a specific blockage or defect of IL-13 in allergen-challenged mice diminishes asthmatic phenotypes more significantly than that of IL-4, demonstrating that IL-13 is central in the pathogenesis of asthma in mice [16,21–23].

Since then, many studies have been performed to analyze target cells of IL-13 *in vivo* using various gene-manipulated mice [1,2]. Both RAG1-deficient mice and wild type mice showed asthmatic phenotypes after intratracheal administration of IL-13, suggesting that IL-13 causes asthmatic phenotypes, independent of lymphocytes, that act on nonimmune cells [16]. Moreover, mice that specifically expressed IL-13 in the bronchial epithelial cells and STAT6-deficient mice in which STAT6 reconstituted specifically in the bronchial epithelial cells enhanced AHR, indicating that the effect of IL-13 on epithelial cells is important in enhancing AHR [24,25].

The roles of IL-4 and IL-13 in the pathogenesis of bronchial asthma in humans

Expression of IL-4 and IL-13 was higher in individuals with asthma than in those without at the baseline and was greatly upregulated by allergen challenge in bronchial tissues, bronchoalveolar lavage fluids, and sputum, with IL-13 predominantly expressed [8–10]. These results indicate the involvement of IL-4/IL-13 in the pathogenesis of bronchial asthma in humans as well as in mice. The high expression of IL-13 in the inflamed lesions explains why IL-13 plays a dominant role in the pathogenesis of bronchial asthma compared with IL-4.

In addition to the expression profile of IL-4 and IL-13, genetic analyses of the genes coding IL-4 and IL-13 signal-transducing molecules were performed and showed an association between several single nucleotide polymorphisms (SNPs) on IL-4, IL-13, and IL-4RA genes and bronchial asthma with high reproducibility [26,27]. An SNP on the IL-4 gene,

−589(590)C/T, may enhance transcription of IL-4 by modulating the binding of NFAT-1 [28]. The gene products of Arg110(130)Gln on the IL-13 gene are well characterized by biochemical and structural analyses. The Gln110 type showing high incidence in individuals with asthma augments the signals through type II IL-4R/IL-13R, decreases the binding to IL-13Rα2, and enhances its stability, probably by affecting its conformation [29–32]. Among the variants of the IL-4RA gene, Ile50Val and Glu551Arg are reported to affect the affinity with IL-4Rα followed by STAT6 activation or binding to SHP-1, a phosphotyrosine phosphatase associated with IL-4Rα, and allergic airway inflammation *in vivo*, respectively [33–35]. Such an association of genes coding IL-4 and IL-13 signal-transducing molecules in bronchial asthma supports the significance of these signals in the pathogenesis of asthma.

The underlying mechanism of how IL-4 and IL-13 cause asthmatic phenotypes

As described before, IL-4 is an essential factor for Th2-type inflammation because it induces Th2 differentiation and class switching into IgE in B cells. IL-13 also has the potency to induce class switching into IgE (Figure 13.3). These actions of IL-4 and IL-13 on hematopoietic/immune cells are indispensable

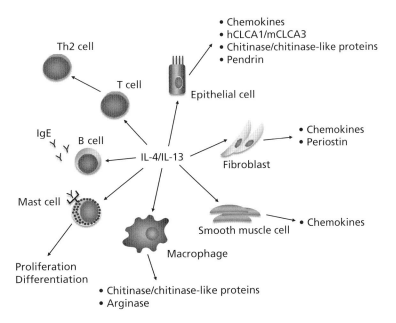

Figure 13.3 Actions of interleukin 4 (IL-4) and IL-13. The actions of IL-4 and IL-13 on immune and nonimmune cells correlated with the pathogenesis of bronchial asthma are depicted.

for type I (immediate) hypersensitivity in bronchial asthma. Additionally, IL-13, and to a lesser extent IL-4, acts on bronchial epithelial cells, endothelial cells, and smooth muscle cells. This induces various chemokines including MCP-1, -2, -5, CCL11 (eotaxin), CCL24 (eotaxin-2), MIP1α, and TARC, followed by the recruitment of inflammatory cells such as eosinophils and Th2 cells [2,36]. Moreover, in order to understand the underlying mechanism of how IL-4 and IL-13 induce asthmatic phenotypes, several trials using DNA microarray have been performed to identify IL-13-inducible genes in bronchial epithelial cells, smooth muscle cells, and lung tissues of mice, monkeys, or humans [37–40]. We describe five molecules, among IL-13-inducible gene products, which are well characterized.

Human calcium-activated chloride channel 1 (hCLCA1)/mouse CLCA3 (mCLCA3, Gob-5)

mCLCA3 was identified as a gene product induced in ovalbumin-challenged mice with asthma, and expression of mCLCA3 was correlated with mucus production and enhanced AHR [41]. The human ortholog of mCLCA3, hCLCA1, was highly expressed in the bronchial tissues of humans with asthma [42]. Both mCLCA3 and hCLCA1 are downstream of IL-9 or IL-13 [39,42,43]. However, the results of the analyses using mCLCA3-deficient mice were inconsistent; one report showed no change in asthmatic phenotypes, whereas the other showed decreased goblet cell hyperplasia (GCH) [44,45]. Moreover, it was realized that mCLCA3 and hCLCA1 are secreted proteins, not membrane-imbedded channels, and their function remain unclear [46].

Chitinase/chitinase-like protein

Several chitinase or chitinase-like proteins, including acidic mammalian chitinase (AMCase), Ym1/2, and YKL-40/BRP-39, are induced by IL-13 in bronchial epithelial cells and macrophages, and play an important role in the pathogenesis of bronchial asthma [47–49]. The chitinase/chitinase-like protein family is assumed to have evolved as a defense mechanism against exogenous microbes such as parasites possessing chitin as components of their bodies. Chitinases such as AMCase sustain chitinase activities, whereas chitinase-like proteins such as Ym1/2 and YKL-40/BRP-39 lose them. Several SNPs on AMCase and CHI3L1 (coding YKL-40) genes associate with bron-

chial asthma, and serum levels of YKL-40 were upregulated in asthmatic individuals [50–52]. The underlying mechanism of how chitinase/chitinase-like proteins cause asthmatic phenotypes remains unclear; however, it is demonstrated that AMCase induced chemokine production in epithelial cells and that YKL-40/BRP-39 augmented antigen presentation, IgE synthesis, and activation of dendritic cells and macrophages, whereas it inhibited apoptosis of inflammatory cells [47,49].

Pendrin

Pendrin is a multispanning anion channel that transports chloride, iodide, and bicarbonate ions and was originally identified as a defective product in Pendred syndrome, which is characterized by deafness and goiter. We found that pendrin was expressed at the apical side of bronchial epithelial cells in mice and humans with asthma downstream of IL-13 signals, and that enforced expression of pendrin in mice caused mucus production and enhanced AHR [53]. Pendrin-defective mice showed alleviation of allergic inflammation [54], demonstrating that pendrin is involved in forming asthmatic phenotypes, particularly mucus production.

Arginase

It is known that IL-13 causes fibrosis, a typical feature of bronchial asthma, via the TGF-β-dependent pathway [2]. In addition to this pathway, IL-13 contributes to the formation of fibrosis by inducing arginase-1/2 in macrophages [40]. Arginase forms ornithine using arginine as a substrate, and ornithine is converted by ornithine aminotransferase into proline, an essential component of collagen production. Moreover, ornithine is converted by ornithine decarboxylase into polyamine, involved in hypertrophy of smooth muscle cells. Both the expression and activities of arginase were high in asthmatic individuals, and several SNPs on ARG1/2 genes were associated with asthma [40,55,56].

Periostin

We found that periostin, an IL-13-inducible gene product, is a component of fibrosis in asthma [38,57,58]. Periostin was deposited in thickened basement membranes in humans or in subepithelial regions in mice. It had a potency to bind to other matrix proteins such as fibronectin, tenascin-C, and

Antagonists	Manufacturer	IL-4 inhibition	IL-13 inhibition	Status of the trial
IL-4 mutein (AEROVANT™)	Bayer/Aerovance	+	+	Phase IIa finished
αIL-13Ab (CAT-354)	MedImmune	–	+	Phase IIa ongoing
αIL-13Ab (lebrikizumab)	Genentech	–	+	Phase IIa ongoing

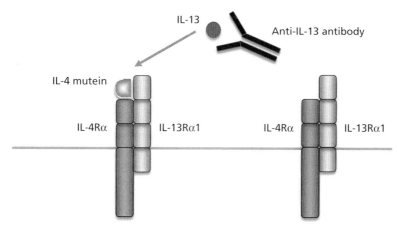

Figure 13.4 Therapeutic reagents against bronchial asthma targeting interleukin 4 (IL-4) and IL-13 currently in development and their actions. The therapeutic reagents against bronchial asthma targeting IL-4 and IL-13 currently being developed are listed. IL-4 mutein inhibits both IL-4 and IL-13 signals by occupying type II IL-13 receptor, and anti-IL-13 antibodies inhibit IL-13 signals by binding to IL-13.

type V collagen, contributing to stable or insoluble fibrinogenesis. Periostin-deficient mice showed improved eosinophilic inflammation because periostin enhanced the binding of fibronectin to eosinophils [59]. Moreover, it has been reported that expression of periostin is associated with responsiveness to steroid therapy [60].

Application of IL-4/IL-13 antagonists to development as therapeutic agents for bronchial asthma

Based on the importance of IL-4 and IL-13, particularly the latter, in the pathogenesis of bronchial asthma, several IL-4 and/or IL-13 antagonists have been applied to development as therapeutic agents for bronchial asthma. To our knowledge, three agents, an IL-4R antagonist called IL-4 mutein and two types of neutralizing anti-IL-13 Abs, are at this moment under development (Figure 13.4).

An IL-4R antagonist, IL-4 mutein (AEROVANT™, Aerovance, Berkeley, CA, USA), is an IL-4 variant in which Arg at the 121st amino acid and Tyr at the 124th amino acid are both replaced with Asp. It sustains a binding activity with IL-4R but not the potency to transduce its signals. IL-4 mutein inhibits not only IL-4 signals but also IL-13 signals by occupying type II IL-4R/IL-13R [61]. Aerovance has finished a phase IIa trial, which showed that AEROVANT improved lung function by either subcutaneous administration or inhalation without significant side effects [62]. MedImmune (Gaithersburg, MD, USA) and Genentech (San Francisco, CA, USA) are now performing phase II trials of anti-IL-13 Ab for individuals with asthma (CAT-354 and Lebrikizumab, respectively, URLs: http://www.medimmune.com and http://www.gene.com/gene/index.jsp).

IL-9

IL-9 was originally identified as a T-cell growth factor [63] and thereafter turned out to be a pleiotropic cytokine acting on B cells, mast cells, other types of hematopoietic cells, and nonhematopoietic cells including bronchial epithelial cells and smooth muscle cells. IL-9 was initially thought to be a member of the Th2 cytokines; many studies have shown involvement of IL-9 in the pathogenesis of bronchial asthma, based on a mouse model, IL-9 expression in humans with asthma, and a genetic association between IL-9 and asthma. However, recently it has been found that naturally occurring regulatory T cells [64] and Th17 cells [65,66] produce IL-9, although the roles of these IL-9-producing cells in asthma have not been examined.

Signal transduction of IL-9

The functional IL-9R is a heterodimeric complex composed of the IL-9Rα chain (IL-9Rα; also known as IL-9R) and the γc (Figure 13.1). The former is the component specific for IL-9 and the latter is shared with IL-2, IL-4, IL-7, IL-15, and IL-21 [67]. Upon engagement of IL-9R with IL-9, Jak1 and Jak3, which associate with IL-9Rα and the common γc, respectively, are activated, followed by activation of STAT1, STAT3, and STAT5, which are essential for proliferative responses by IL-9 [68,69].

The role of IL-9 in the pathogenesis of bronchial asthma in mice

To examine the role of IL-9 in the pathogenesis of bronchial asthma, mice were intratracheally administered with IL-9, and either IL-9-transgenic (IL-9-TG) mice, IL-9-deficient mice, or administration of neutralizing anti-IL-9 Ab was subjected into the analyses of mice with asthma.

Intratracheal administration of IL-9 caused asthma-like phenotypes such as mucus production,

GCH, enhanced AHR, eosinophilia, elevated IgE levels in serum, and upregulation of IL-13 [70,71]. Accordingly, IL-9-TG mice showed similar changes (lung eosinophilia, mucus production, GCH, mastocytosis, elevated IgE levels, enhanced AHR, and fibrosis) either spontaneously or by allergen challenge [72–76]. Particularly, specific expression of IL-9 in the lungs of TG mice caused lung eosinophilia, mucus production, GCH, enhanced AHR, and elevated mast cell numbers in the basal line, demonstrating the importance of IL-9 in the pathogenesis of bronchial asthma [77]. In IL-9-TG mice, expression of other Th2 cytokines such as IL-5 and IL-13 were upregulated in the lungs [78]. To address whether the actions of IL-9 *in vivo* are due to those of other Th2 cytokines induced by IL-9, neutralizing Abs or soluble receptors against these cytokines were administered into IL-9-TG mice and IL-9-TG mice were crossed with IL-13- or IL-4Rα-deficient mice. All administration of soluble IL-13Rα2 into IL-9-TG mice [78], IL-9-TG and IL-13-deficient mice [79], and IL-9-TG and IL-4Rα-deficient mice [80] alleviated mucus production and GCH, and in some cases lung inflammation, whereas the effects of anti-IL-4 and anti-IL-5 Abs were weak [78]. This demonstrated that at least some IL-9 actions, particularly mucus production and GCH, are dependent on IL-13.

The results with the loss-of-function mice mostly were opposite to those of the gain-of-function mice; however, there was some discrepancy between them. IL-9-deficient mice did not show a decrease of GCH or eosinophilia, or enhanced AHR, or elevated IgE levels in allergen-challenged mice with asthma [81]. On the other hand, administration of neutralizing anti-IL-9 Abs into allergen-challenged mice downregulated pulmonary eosinophilia, GCH, enhanced AHR, and expression of IL-4, IL-5, and IL-13 [82,83]. Moreover, anti-IL-9 Abs, but not anti-IL-5 Abs or anti-IL-13 Abs, inhibited mucin production in allergen-challenged dogs [84]. These results support the importance of IL-9; other Th2 cytokines may compensate for the actions of IL-9 in IL-9-deficient mice.

Involvement of IL-9 in the pathogenesis of asthmatic individuals

It has been reported that bronchial tissues from asthmatic individuals show upregulation of IL-9, most of which is lymphocytes [42,85,86]. IL-9Rα, the specific component of functional IL-9R, was also upregulated in bronchial tissues from people with asthma, particularly epithelial cells, and was correlated with PAS+ rates [42,87]. Genetic studies support the involvement of IL-9 in the pathogenesis of asthmatics. The IL-9 gene locus is reported to be associated with IgE levels [88], and several haplotypes of SNPs on the IL-9R and IL-4RA genes show association with childhood wheezing [89]. Genetic association was also observed in mice; the IL-9 gene was identified as a quantitative trait for bronchial responsiveness between DBA/2J and C57BL/6 and bronchial hyper- and hyporesponsive strains, respectively [90]. These results strongly indicate that IL-9 plays a role in the pathogenesis of asthma.

In vitro functions of IL-9

IL-9 was originally identified as a T-cell growth factor [63] and was later found to be a IgE/IgG1-inducing factor in B cells synergizing with IL-4, a growth factor for mast cells [91], hematopoietic progenitors [92], and eosinophils synergizing with IL-5 [93], and an IL-8-producing factor in neutrophils (Figure 13.5) [94]. In addition to these actions on hematopoietic/immune cells, it has been shown that IL-9 acts on nonhematopoietic/nonimmune cells in bronchial

tissues *in vitro*; IL-9 acts on bronchial epithelial cells, inducing production of MCP-1, MCP-3, IL-16, and RANTES [74,95], and on airway smooth muscle cells, inducing production of IL-8 and eotaxin together with TNF-α and IL-13, respectively [96,97]. However, in contrast to the mouse model, it was demonstrated that IL-9 does not directly induce expression of mucin genes in human tracheobronchial epithelial cells [98]. These IL-9 actions found by *in vitro* experiments can provide an underlying mechanism of how IL-9 is involved in bronchial asthma.

Application of IL-9 to development as a therapeutic agent for bronchial asthma

Based on the importance of IL-9 in the pathogenesis of bronchial asthma, anti-IL-9 Abs (MEDI-528, MedImmune) are now currently under development as a therapeutic agent for bronchial asthma. The phase I study for healthy adults has just been finished with an acceptable safety profile [99].

Acknowledgment

The authors have no financial conflict of interest. We thank Dr. Dovie R. Wylie for critical review of this manuscript.

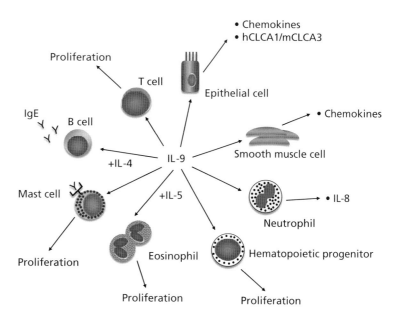

Figure 13.5 Actions of interleukin 9 (IL-9). The actions of IL-9 on immune and nonimmune cells correlated with pathogenesis of bronchial asthma are depicted.

References

1 Izuhara K, Arima K, Yasunaga S. IL-4 and IL-13: their pathological roles in allergic diseases and their potential in developing new therapies. *Curr Drug Targets Inflamm Allergy* 2002; **1**: 263–9.

2 Izuhara K, Arima K, Kanaji S, *et al*. IL-13: a promising therapeutic target for bronchial asthma. *Curr Med Chem* 2006; **13**: 2291–8.

3 Fichtner-Feigl S, Strober W, Kawakami K, *et al*IL-13 signaling through the IL-13α2 receptor is involved in induction of TGF-β1 production and fibrosis. *Nat Med.* 2006; **12**: 99–106.

4 Junttila IS, Mizukami K, Dickensheets H, *et al*. Tuning sensitivity to IL-4 and IL-13: differential expression of IL-4Rα, IL-13Rα1: and γc regulates relative cytokine sensitivity. *J Exp Med* 2008; **205**: 2595–608.

5 Arima K, Sato K, Tanaka G, *et al*. Characterization of the interaction between interleukin-13 and interleukin-13 receptors. *J Biol Chem* 2005; **280**: 24915–22.

6 LaPorte SL, Juo ZS, Vaclavikova J, *et al*. Molecular and structural basis of cytokine receptor pleiotropy in the interleukin-4/13 system. *Cell* 2008; **132**: 259–72.

7 Ito T, Suzuki S, Kanaji S, *et al*. Distinct structural requirements for interleukin-4 (IL-4) and IL-13 binding to the shared IL-13 receptor facilitate cellular tuning of cytokine responsiveness. *J Biol Chem* 2009; **284**: 24289–96.

8 Kotsimbos TC, Ernst P, Hamid QA. Interleukin-13 and interleukin-4 are coexpressed in atopic asthma. *Proc Assoc Am Phys* 1996; **108**: 368–73.

9 Bodey KJ, Semper AE, Redington AE, *et al*. Cytokine profiles of BAL T cells and T-cell clones obtained from human asthmatic airways after local allergen challenge. *Allergy* 1999; **54**: 1083–93.

10 Truyen E, Coteur L, Dilissen E, *et al*. Evaluation of airway inflammation by quantitative Th1/Th2 cytokine mRNA measurement in sputum of asthma patients. *Thorax* 2006; **61**: 202–8.

11 Brusselle G, Kips J, Joos G, *et al*. Allergen-induced airway inflammation and bronchial responsiveness in wild type and interleukin-4-deficient mice. *Am J Respir Cell Mol Biol* 1995; **12**: 254–9.

12 Hogan SP, Mould A, Kikutani H, *et al*. Aeroallergen-induced eosinophilic inflammation, lung damage, and airways hyperreactivity in mice can occur independently of IL-4 and allergen-specific immunoglobulins. *J Clin Invest* 1997; **99**: 1329–39.

13 Hogan SP, Matthaei KI, Young JM, *et al*. A novel T cell-regulated mechanism modulating allergen-induced airways hyperreactivity in BALB/c mice independently of IL-4 and IL-5. *J Immunol* 1998; **161**: 1501–9.

14 Corry DB, Folkesson HG, Warnock ML, *et al*. Interleukin 4: but not interleukin 5 or eosinophils, is required in a murine model of acute airway hyperreactivity. *J Exp Med* 1996; **183**: 109–17.

15 Webb DC, McKenzie AN, Koskinen AM, *et al*. Integrated signals between IL-13: IL-4: and IL-5 regulate airways hyperreactivity. *J Immunol* 2000; **165**: 108–13.

16 Grünig G, Warnock M, Wakil AE, *et al*. Requirement for IL-13 independently of IL-4 in experimental asthma. *Science* 1998; **282**: 2261–3.

17 Akimoto T, Numata F, Tamura M, *et al*. Abrogation of bronchial eosinophilic inflammation and airway hyperreactivity in signal transducers and activators of transcription (STAT)6-deficient mice. *J Exp Med* 1998; **187**: 1537–42.

18 Tomkinson A, Kanehiro A, Rabinovitch N, *et al*. The failure of STAT6-deficient mice to develop airway eosinophilia and airway hyperresponsiveness is overcome by interleukin-5. *Am J Respir Crit Care Med* 1999; **160**: 1283–91.

19 Blease K, Schuh JM, Jakubzick C, *et al*. Stat6-deficient mice develop airway hyperresponsiveness and peribronchial fibrosis during chronic fungal asthma. *Am J Pathol* 2002; **160**: 481–90.

20 Venkayya R, Lam M, Willkom M, *et al*. The Th2 lymphocyte products IL-4 and IL-13 rapidly induce airway hyperresponsiveness through direct effects on resident airway cells. *Am J Respir Cell Mol Biol* 2002; **26**: 202–8.

21 Wills-Karp M, Luyimbazi J, Xu X, *et al*. Interleukin-13: central mediator of allergic asthma. *Science* 1998; **282**: 2258–61.

22 Blease K, Jakubzick C, Westwick J, *et al*. Therapeutic effect of IL-13 immunoneutralization during chronic experimental fungal asthma. *J Immunol* 2001; **166**: 5219–24.

23 Walter DM, McIntire JJ, Berry G, *et al*. Critical role for IL-13 in the development of allergen-induced airway hyperreactivity. *J Immunol* 2001; **167**: 4668–75.

24 Zhu Z, Homer RJ, Wang Z, *et al*. Pulmonary expression of interleukin-13 causes inflammation, mucus hypersecretion, subepithelial fibrosis, physiologic abnormalities, and eotaxin production. *J Clin Invest* 1999; **103**: 779–88.

25 Kuperman DA, Huang X, Koth LL, *et al*. Direct effects of interleukin-13 on epithelial cells cause airway hyperreactivity and mucus overproduction in asthma. *Nat Med* 2002; **8**: 885–9.

26 Hoffjan S, Nicolae D, Ober C. Association studies for asthma and atopic diseases: a comprehensive review of the literature. *Respir Res* 2003; **4**: 14.

27 Vercelli D. Discovering susceptibility genes for asthma and allergy. *Nat Rev Immunol* 2008; **8**: 169–82.

28 Rosenwasser LJ, Borish L. Genetics of atopy and asthma: the rationale behind promoter-based candidate gene studies (IL-4 and IL-10). *Am J Respir Crit Care Med* 1997; **156**: S152–5.

29 Arima K, Umeshita-Suyama R, Sakata Y, *et al.* Upregulation of IL-13 concentration *in vivo* by the IL-13 variant associated with bronchial asthma. *J Allergy Clin Immunol* 2002; **109**: 980–7.

30 Chen W, Ericksen MB, Levin LS, *et al.* Functional effect of the R110Q IL-13 genetic variant alone and in combination with IL-4RA genetic variants. *J Allergy Clin Immunol* 2004; **114**: 553–60.

31 Vladich FD, Brazille SM, Stern D, *et al.* IL-13 R130Q, a common variant associated with allergy and asthma, enhances effector mechanisms essential for human allergic inflammation. *J Clin Invest* 2005; **115**: 747–54.

32 Yoshida Y, Ohkuri T, Takeda C, *et al.* Analysis of internal motions of interleukin-13 variant associated with severe bronchial asthma using (15)N NMR relaxation measurements. *Biochem Biophys Res Commun* 2007; **358**: 292–7.

33 Mitsuyasu H, Izuhara K, Mao XQ, *et al.* Ile50Val variant of IL-4Rα upregulates IgE synthesis and associates with atopic asthma. *Nat Genet* 1998; **19**: 119–20.

34 Hershey GK, Friedrich MF, Esswein LA, *et al.* The association of atopy with a gain-of-function mutation in the α subunit of the interleukin-4 receptor. *N Engl J Med* 1997; **337**: 1720–5.

35 Tachdjian R, Mathias C, Al Khatib S, *et al.* Pathogenicity of a disease-associated human IL-4 receptor allele in experimental asthma. *J Exp Med* 2009; **206**: 2191–204.

36 Wills-Karp M. Interleukin-13 in asthma pathogenesis. *Immunol Rev* 2004; **202**: 175–90.

37 Lee JH, Kaminski N, Dolganov G, *et al.* Interleukin-13 induces dramatically different transcriptional programs in three human airway cell types. *Am J Respir Cell Mol Biol* 2001; **25**: 474–85.

38 Yuyama N, Davies DE, Akaiwa M, *et al.* Analysis of novel disease-related genes in bronchial asthma. *Cytokine* 2002; **19**: 287–96.

39 Zou J, Young S, Zhu F, *et al.* Microarray profile of differentially expressed genes in a monkey model of allergic asthma. *Genome Biol* 2002; **3**: research0020.

40 Zimmermann N, King NE, Laporte J, *et al.* Dissection of experimental asthma with DNA microarray analysis identifies arginase in asthma pathogenesis. *J Clin Invest* 2003; **111**: 1863–74.

41 Nakanishi A, Morita S, Iwashita H, *et al.* Role of gob-5 in mucus overproduction and airway hyperresponsiveness in asthma. *Proc Natl Acad Sci USA* 2001; **98**: 5175–80.

42 Toda M, Tulic MK, Levitt RC, *et al.* A calcium-activated chloride channel (HCLCA1) is strongly related to IL-9 expression and mucus production in bronchial epithelium of patients with asthma. *J Allergy Clin Immunol* 2002; **109**: 246–50.

43 Kuperman DA, Lewis CC, Woodruff PG, *et al.* Dissecting asthma using focused transgenic modeling and functional genomics. *J Allergy Clin Immunol* 2005; **116**: 305–11.

44 Robichaud A, Tuck SA, Kargman S, *et al.* Gob-5 is not essential for mucus overproduction in preclinical murine models of allergic asthma. *Am J Respir Cell Mol Biol* 2005; **33**: 303–14.

45 Long AJ, Sypek JP, Askew R, *et al.* Gob-5 contributes to goblet cell hyperplasia and modulates pulmonary tissue inflammation. *Am J Respir Cell Mol Biol* 2006; **35**: 357–65.

46 Gibson A, Lewis AP, Affleck K, *et al.* hCLCA1 and mCLCA3 are secreted nonintegral membrane proteins and therefore are not ion channels. *J Biol Chem* 2005; **280**: 27205–12.

47 Zhu Z, Zheng T, Homer RJ, *et al.* Acidic mammalian chitinase in asthmatic Th2 inflammation and IL-13 pathway activation. *Science* 2004; **304**: 1678–82.

48 Cai Y, Kumar RK, Zhou J, *et al.* Ym1/2 promotes Th2 cytokine expression by inhibiting 12/15(S)-lipoxygenase: identification of a novel pathway for regulating allergic inflammation. *J Immunol* 2009; **182**: 5393–9.

49 Lee CG, Hartl D, Lee GR, *et al.* Role of breast regression protein 39 (BRP-39)/chitinase 3-like-1 in Th2 and IL-13-induced tissue responses and apoptosis. *J Exp Med* 2009; **206**: 1149–66.

50 Bierbaum S, Nickel R, Koch A, *et al.* Polymorphisms and haplotypes of acid mammalian chitinase are associated with bronchial asthma. *Am J Respir Crit Care Med* 2005; **172**: 1505–9.

51 Ober C, Tan Z, Sun Y, *et al.* Effect of variation in CHI3L1 on serum YKL-40 level, risk of asthma, and lung function. *N Engl J Med* 2008; **358**: 1682–91.

52 Chupp GL, Lee CG, Jarjour N, *et al.* A chitinase-like protein in the lung and circulation of patients with severe asthma. *N Engl J Med* 2007; **357**: 2016–27.

53 Nakao I, Kanaji S, Ohta S, *et al.* Identification of pendrin as a common mediator for mucus production in bronchial asthma and chronic obstructive pulmonary disease. *J Immunol* 2008; **180**: 6262–9.

54 Nakagami Y, Favoreto S, Jr., Zhen G, *et al.* The epithelial anion transporter pendrin is induced by allergy and rhinovirus infection, regulates airway surface liquid, and increases airway reactivity and inflammation in an asthma model. *J Immunol* 2008; **181**: 2203–10.

55 Salam MT, Islam T, Gauderman WJ, *et al.* Roles of arginase variants, atopy, and ozone in childhood asthma. *J Allergy Clin Immunol* 2009; **123**: 596–602: e591–8.

56 Morris CR, Poljakovic M, Lavrisha L, *et al.* Decreased arginine bioavailability and increased serum arginase activity in asthma. *Am J Respir Crit Care Med* 2004; **170**: 148–53.

57 Takayama G, Arima K, Kanaji T, *et al*. Periostin: a novel component of subepithelial fibrosis of bronchial asthma downstream of IL-4 and IL-13 signals. *J Allergy Clin Immunol* 2006; **118**: 98–104.

58 Hayashi N, Yoshimoto T, Izuhara K, *et al*. T helper 1 cells stimulated with ovalbumin and IL-18 induce airway hyperresponsiveness and lung fibrosis by IFN-γ and IL-13 production. *Proc Natl Acad Sci USA* 2007; **104**: 14765–70.

59 Blanchard C, Mingler MK, McBride M, *et al*. Periostin facilitates eosinophil tissue infiltration in allergic lung and esophageal responses. *Mucosal Immunol* 2008; **1**: 289–96.

60 Woodruff PG, Boushey HA, Dolganov GM, *et al*. Genome-wide profiling identifies epithelial cell genes associated with asthma and with treatment response to corticosteroids. *Proc Natl Acad Sci USA* 2007; **104**: 15858–63.

61 Tony HP, Shen BJ, Reusch P, *et al*. Design of human interleukin-4 antagonists inhibiting interleukin-4-dependent and interleukin-13-dependent responses in T-cells and B-cells with high efficiency. *Eur J Biochem* 1994; **225**: 659–65.

62 Wenzel S, Wilbraham D, Fuller R, *et al*. Effect of an interleukin-4 variant on late phase asthmatic response to allergen challenge in asthmatic patients: results of two phase 2a studies. *Lancet* 2007; **370**: 1422–31.

63 Uyttenhove C, Simpson RJ, Van Snick J. Functional and structural characterization of P40: a mouse glycoprotein with T-cell growth factor activity. *Proc Natl Acad Sci USA* 1988; **85**: 6934–8.

64 Lu LF, Lind EF, Gondek DC, *et al*. Mast cells are essential intermediaries in regulatory T-cell tolerance. *Nature* 2006; **442**: 997–1002.

65 Elyaman W, Bradshaw EM, Uyttenhove C, *et al*. IL-9 induces differentiation of TH17 cells and enhances function of FoxP3⁺ natural regulatory T cells. *Proc Natl Acad Sci USA* 2009; **106**: 12885–90.

66 Nowak EC, Weaver CT, Turner H, *et al*. IL-9 as a mediator of Th17-driven inflammatory disease. *J Exp Med* 2009; **206**: 1653–60.

67 Asao H, Okuyama C, Kumaki S, *et al*. The common γ-chain is an indispensable subunit of the IL-21 receptor complex. *J Immunol* 2001; **167**: 1–5.

68 Demoulin JB, Uyttenhove C, Van Roost E, *et al*. A single tyrosine of the interleukin-9 (IL-9) receptor is required for STAT, activation, antiapoptotic activity, and growth regulation by IL-9. *Mol Cell Biol* 1996; **16**: 4710–16.

69 Demoulin JB, Uyttenhove C, Lejeune D, *et al*. STAT5 activation is required for interleukin-9-dependent growth and transformation of lymphoid cells. *Cancer Res* 2000; **60**: 3971–7.

70 Levitt RC, McLane MP, MacDonald D, *et al*. IL-9 pathway in asthma: new therapeutic targets for allergic

71 Reader JR, Hyde DM, Schelegle ES, *et al*. Interleukin-9 induces mucous cell metaplasia independent of inflammation. *Am J Respir Cell Mol Biol* 2003; **28**: 664–72.

72 Godfraind C, Louahed J, Faulkner H, *et al*. Intraepithelial infiltration by mast cells with both connective tissue-type and mucosal-type characteristics in gut, trachea, and kidneys of IL-9 transgenic mice. *J Immunol* 1998; **160**: 3989–96.

73 McLane MP, Haczku A, van de Rijn M, *et al*. Interleukin-9 promotes allergen-induced eosinophilic inflammation and airway hyperresponsiveness in transgenic mice. *Am J Respir Cell Mol Biol* 1998; **19**: 713–20.

74 Dong Q, Louahed J, Vink A, *et al*. IL-9 induces chemokine expression in lung epithelial cells and baseline airway eosinophilia in transgenic mice. *Eur J Immunol* 1999; **29**: 2130–9.

75 Louahed J, Toda M, Jen J, *et al*. Interleukin-9 upregulates mucus expression in the airways. *Am J Respir Cell Mol Biol* 2000; **22**: 649–56.

76 van den Brule S, Heymans J, Havaux X, *et al*. Profibrotic effect of IL-9 overexpression in a model of airway remodeling. *Am J Respir Cell Mol Biol* 2007; **37**: 202–9.

77 Temann UA, Geba GP, Rankin JA, *et al*. Expression of interleukin 9 in the lungs of transgenic mice causes airway inflammation, mast cell hyperplasia, and bronchial hyperresponsiveness. *J Exp Med* 1998; **188**: 1307–120.

78 Temann UA, Ray P, Flavell RA. Pulmonary overexpression of IL-9 induces Th2 cytokine expression, leading to immune pathology. *J Clin Invest* 2002; **109**: 29–39.

79 Steenwinckel V, Louahed J, Orabona C, *et al*. IL-13 mediates *in vivo* IL-9 activities on lung epithelial cells but not on hematopoietic cells. *J Immunol* 2007; **178**: 3244–51.

80 Whittaker L, Niu N, Temann UA, *et al*. Interleukin-13 mediates a fundamental pathway for airway epithelial mucus induced by CD4 T cells and interleukin-9. *Am J Respir Cell Mol Biol* 2002; **27**: 593–602.

81 McMillan SJ, Bishop B, Townsend MJ, *et al*. The absence of interleukin 9 does not affect the development of allergen-induced pulmonary inflammation nor airway hyperreactivity. *J Exp Med* 2002; **195**: 51–7.

82 Kung TT, Luo B, Crawley Y, *et al*. Effect of anti-mIL-9 antibody on the development of pulmonary inflammation and airway hyperresponsiveness in allergic mice. *Am J Respir Cell Mol Biol* 2001; **25**: 600–5.

83 Cheng G, Arima M, Honda K, *et al*. Anti-interleukin-9 antibody treatment inhibits airway inflammation and hyperreactivity in mouse asthma model. *Am J Respir Crit Care Med* 2002; **166**: 409–16.

inflammatory disorders. *J Allergy Clin Immunol* 1999; **103**: S485–91.

84 Longphre M, Li D, Gallup M, *et al*. Allergen-induced IL-9 directly stimulates mucin transcription in respiratory epithelial cells. *J Clin Invest* 1999; **104**: 1375–82.

85 Shimbara A, Christodoulopoulos P, Soussi-Gounni A, *et al*. IL-9 and its receptor in allergic and nonallergic lung disease: increased expression in asthma. *J Allergy Clin Immunol* 2000; **105**: 108–15.

86 Erpenbeck VJ, Hohlfeld JM, Volkmann B, *et al*. Segmental allergen challenge in patients with atopic asthma leads to increased IL-9 expression in bronchoalveolar lavage fluid lymphocytes. *J Allergy Clin Immunol* 2003; **111**: 1319–27.

87 Bhathena PR, Comhair SA, Holroyd KJ, *et al*. Interleukin-9 receptor expression in asthmatic airways *in vivo*. *Lung* 2000; **178**: 149–60.

88 Doull IJ, Lawrence S, Watson M, *et al*. Allelic association of gene markers on chromosomes 5q and 11q with atopy and bronchial hyperresponsiveness. *Am J Respir Crit Care Med* 1996; **153**: 1280–4.

89 Melen E, Umerkajeff S, Nyberg F, *et al*. Interaction between variants in the interleukin-4 receptor α and interleukin-9 receptor genes in childhood wheezing: evidence from a birth cohort study. *Clin Exp Allergy* 2006; **36**: 1391–8.

90 Nicolaides NC, Holroyd KJ, Ewart SL, *et al*. Interleukin 9: a candidate gene for asthma. *Proc Natl Acad Sci USA* 1997; **94**: 13175–80.

91 Renauld JC, Goethals A, Houssiau F, *et al*. Cloning and expression of a cDNA for the human homolog of mouse T cell and mast cell growth factor P40. *Cytokine* 1990; **2**: 9–12.

92 Bourette RP, Royet J, Mouchiroud G, *et al*. Murine interleukin 9 stimulates the proliferation of mouse erythroid progenitor cells and favors the erythroid differentiation of multipotent FDCP-mix cells. *Exp Hematol* 1992; **20**: 868–73.

93 Louahed J, Zhou Y, Maloy WL, *et al*. Interleukin 9 promotes influx and local maturation of eosinophils. *Blood* 2001; **97**: 1035–42.

94 Abdelilah S, Latifa K, Esra N, *et al*. Functional expression of IL-9 receptor by human neutrophils from asthmatic donors: role in IL-8 release. *J Immunol* 2001; **166**: 2768–74.

95 Little FF, Cruikshank WW, Center DM. IL-9 stimulates release of chemotactic factors from human bronchial epithelial cells. *Am J Respir Cell Mol Biol* 2001; **25**: 347–52.

96 Baraldo S, Faffe DS, Moore PE, *et al*. Interleukin-9 influences chemokine release in airway smooth muscle: role of ERK. *Am J Physiol Lung Cell Mol Physiol* 2003; **284**: L1093–102.

97 Gounni AS, Hamid Q, Rahman SM, *et al*. IL-9-mediated induction of eotaxin1/CCL11 in human airway smooth muscle cells. *J Immunol* 2004; **173**: 2771–9.

98 Chen Y, Thai P, Zhao YH, *et al*. Stimulation of airway mucin gene expression by interleukin (IL)–17 through IL-6 paracrine/autocrine loop. *J Biol Chem* 2003; **278**: 17036–43.

99 White B, Leon F, White W, *et al*. Two first-in-human, open-label, phase I dose-escalation safety trials of MEDI-528: a monoclonal antibody against interleukin-9: in healthy adult volunteers. *Clin Ther* 2009; **31**: 728–40.

14 Interleukin 3, interleukin 5, and granulocyte–macrophage colony-stimulating factor

Alba Llop-Guevara, Josip Marcinko, Ramzi Fattouh, and Manel Jordana
Department of Pathology and Molecular Medicine, Centre for Gene Therapeutics, Division of Respiratory Diseases and Allergy, McMaster University, Hamilton, ON, Canada

Introduction

Survival of an organism depends on its ability to mount an immune-inflammatory response that is specific and sufficiently measured to avoid immunopathology. Such a response is highly complex as it involves many exquisitely coordinated steps, from the generation of the set of innate signals that will instruct an effective adaptive response to the mobilization of particular subsets of leukocytes from the bone marrow into the blood and, ultimately, into the tissue, where they are activated to fulfill their effector functions. Interleukin 3 (IL-3), IL-5, and granulocyte–macrophage colony-stimulating factor (GM-CSF) are three cytokines produced by myeloid and structural cells that participate in many steps of this complex process. They exhibit pleiotropic effects, including proliferation, differentiation, survival, and activation of several hematopoietic cell lineages and their precursors, and mediate a number of overlapping and distinct actions in the early and late stages of allergic inflammatory responses. This chapter will first outline some of the structural and functional features of IL-3, IL-5, and GM-CSF. Then, it will examine the expression of these cytokines in clinical settings and follow with a discussion of the immunobiologic functions of each of these cytokines both *in vitro* and *in vivo*. This chapter will conclude with an appraisal of the potential of the therapeutic strategies aimed at inhibiting the activity of IL-3, IL-5, and GM-CSF in allergic diseases.

Structure of IL-3, IL-5, and GM-CSF, and their receptors

IL-3, IL-5, and GM-CSF are 133–166 amino acid-long glycoproteins. IL-3 and GM-CSF are biologically active as monomers, while IL-5 requires homodimer formation given its inactivity as a monomer. They belong to a family of hematopoietic cytokines, with a likely common ancestral relationship given their genetic proximity on chromosome 5 in humans and chromosome 11 in mice. Their gene expression is in part regulated by conserved DNA elements, including cytokine-1 and conserved lymphokine elements, as well as the transcription factors NFAT, AP-1, and NF-GMa, among others. Each of these cytokines, however, can also be differentially regulated by distinct transcription factors and enhancers.

The receptors for IL-3, IL-5, and GM-CSF are glycoproteins belonging to the type I cytokine receptor family. They are composed of a heterodimeric complex of two single span transmembrane polypeptides: a unique α subunit (IL-3 receptor α [IL-3Rα] or CD123, IL-5Rα or CD125, and GM-CSFRα or CD116) and a common β chain (βc or CD131) [1,2]. The α and βc chain genes are encoded on different

Inflammation and Allergy Drug Design, First Edition. Edited by Kenji Izuhara, Stephen T. Holgate, Marsha Wills-Karp.
© 2011 Blackwell Publishing Ltd. Published 2011 by Blackwell Publishing Ltd.

chromosomes and, unlike humans, mice have two different receptors for IL-3 owing to the presence of two β chain genes: a $β_{IL-3}$, which dimerizes only with the mIL-3Rα, and a βc, which functions similarly to the human βc [2,3]. The α chains are cytokine-specific and can bind their cognate ligand with low affinity, forming binary complexes (ligand:Rα). They have conserved motifs in the cytoplasmic domain that seem necessary for signal initiation but do not transduce any biologic activity [4]. It is the recruitment of free β chains that increases the cytokine affinity of intermediate complexes (ligand:Rα:β), which dimerize to form mature hexamer complexes (2ligand:2Rα:2β), and induce signal transduction [4].

A number of *in vitro* studies have suggested hierarchical receptor binding, or cross-competition, of these cytokines in human cells. For example, in eosinophils, GM-CSF is the strongest recruiter of βc followed by IL-3 and then IL-5; in basophils, IL-3 outcompetes GM-CSF and IL-5 for βc binding [5,6]. In addition, different cell types show low- and/or high-affinity receptors based on the α subunit to βc expression ratio. For instance, eosinophils express receptor α chains of GM-CSF, IL-3, and IL-5 in similar numbers to βc, displaying only high-affinity binding; monocytes, which do not bind IL-5, express both low- and high-affinity receptors for GM-CSF and IL-3 since their respective α chains are present in excess over βc [7]. IL-5Rα and GM-CSFRα also exist as secreted soluble isoforms. They may compete with their respective transmembrane Rα for cytokine binding, potentially contributing to downregulation of IL-5 and GM-CSF responses [7,8].

Pleiotropy, redundancy, and specificity of IL-3, IL-5, and GM-CSF

IL-3, IL-5, and GM-CSF are pleiotropic cytokines because they can each elicit multiple functions [9]. Originally classified as hematopoietic cytokines based on a number of *in vitro* and *in vivo* studies demonstrating effects on the differentiation, growth, survival, and activation of progenitor cells, they have been shown also to modulate a variety of activities in mature leukocyte populations. From a molecular perspective, pleiotropy can be explicated by the presence of IL-3R, IL-5R, and GM-CSFR on multiple cell lineages and the ability of these cytokines to activate

multiple signaling pathways, namely Jak/STAT, PI3K/PKB, and several MAP kinase (Ras-Raf-ERK, JNK/SAPK, and p38) pathways [10].

The fact that IL-3, IL-5, and GM-CSF share the βc as well as several signal-transduction pathways leads to a degree of functional redundancy. Teleologically, pleiotropy and redundancy might be viewed as protective fail-safe immune mechanisms to ensure survival in the event of failure of a single pathway. While this is a seemingly undesired sequela in the case of allergic disease, we must be mindful that the underlying mechanisms that operate in response to allergens are likely developed, ontogenically, to fight against pathogens, notably parasites [11]. Despite a degree of redundancy, it is clear that IL-3, IL-5, and GM-CSF retain functional specificity. This functional specificity can be accounted for by several mechanisms, such as the existence of several βc cytoplasmic domains and the distribution of nonshared receptor α subunits in different cell types or at different stages of differentiation. Interestingly, specificity in GM-CSF signaling is plausibly regulated by a phosphotyrosine/phosphoserine binary switch phenomenon [12]. Depending on cytokine concentrations, either one of two mutually exclusive positions in the cytoplasmic tail of the GM-CSFRβ, Ser585 or Tyr577, are phosphorylated to independently promote cell survival alone or cell survival and proliferation, respectively [12].

IL-3, IL-5, and GM-CSF in steady-state and emergency responses

Despite a plethora of findings *in vitro*, IL-3, IL-5, and GM-CSF do not play a major role in steady-state hematopoiesis *in vivo*. Typically, this is illustrated by studies in βc-deficient mice (which allows for IL-3 function via the $β_{IL-3}$ subunit) and βc/IL-3 double-knockout mice [13–16]. Mice lacking the entire IL-3/IL-5/GM-CSF signaling pathway develop normally and have entirely normal hematopoiesis with the exception of decreased basal eosinophil numbers. In addition, these mice show normal hematopoietic recovery after treatment with the cytotoxic drug 5-fluorouracil [13].

In contrast to steady-state hematopoiesis, these cytokines play important roles in pulmonary homeostasis. βc/IL-3 double-knockout mice exhibit evidence of pulmonary peribronchovascular lymphoid infil- trates and pulmonary alveolar proteinosis (PAP)-like disease, which consists of enlarged foamy alveolar macrophages and an overabundance of surfactant proteins and phospholipids [14–16]. Studies in GM-CSF-deficient mice or involving expression of GM-CSF in lung epithelial cells demonstrated that the absence of GM-CSF was the principal cause of this phenotype [17,18]. In accordance with the experi- mental data, patients with point mutations or exon deletions in the gene encoding βc or GM-CSFRα, or with circulating neutralizing autoantibodies to GM- CSF, have no apparent hematopoietic abnormalities but do exhibit PAP [19,20]. Lastly, Uchida et al. [21] provided evidence in humans with PAP and in GM-CSF-deficient mice of neutrophil dysfunction, including reduced bactericidal capability, which could contribute to their increased susceptibility to a wide variety of infections.

Of particular relevance to T helper type 2 (Th2) immunity, βc-deficient mice exhibit a reduced number of eosinophils not only at baseline but also in response to infection with the nematode *Nippostrongylus bra- siliensis* [14]. In addition, βc/β$_{IL-3}$ double-knockout mice exposed to ovalbumin (OVA) fail to mount an eosinophilic response in the lung and have reduced myeloid dendritic cell (DC) numbers, Th2 cell prolif- eration, cytokine- and OVA-specific immunoglobulin E (IgE) production as well as decreased airway hyper- responsiveness (AHR) and mucus hypersecretion [22]. Collectively, the evidence reveals the nonessen- tial role of IL-3/IL-5/GM-CSF signaling in steady- state hematopoiesis but emphasizes its importance in lung homeostasis and response to some pathogens and allergens.

IL-3, IL-5, and GM-CSF in allergic airway disease

At the genetic level, a single nucleotide polymorphism in the IL-3 gene has been significantly associated with the risk of nonatopic asthma and atopy in nonasth- matics. Also, polymorphisms in the GM-CSF gene have been associated with atopy and atopic asthma [23]. Likewise, there have also been reports of pol- ymorphisms in IL-5 and IL-5Rα linked to allergy. Numerous studies have demonstrated the presence of IL-3, IL-5, and GM-CSF in cells, secretions, and

tissues of patients with respiratory allergic diseases. Furthermore, fluctuations in their level of expression in relation to disease severity, natural exacerbations, and experimental allergen challenge have been amply documented. However, these studies establish merely correlative relationships. Investigation of the role of these cytokines in experimental systems of disease, which will be addressed below, aids to advance cau- sality arguments and uncover the specific mechanisms underlying their effects.

Immunobiologic functions of IL-3, IL-5, and GM-CSF

Interleukin 3

IL-3 was originally defined as multilineage colony- stimulating factor (multi-CSF) with potent growth factor activity for both human and murine progeni- tor cells. Subsequently, IL-3 was shown to be a dif- ferentiating and activating factor for a number of cell types, particularly basophils, mast cells, and eosinophils. Several hematopoietic cells, including T cells, NK cells, mast cells, and basophils are capable of secreting IL-3. In particular, both Th1 and Th2 CD4$^+$ T cells can produce substantial amounts of this cytokine upon activation via TCR/CD3. With respect to mast cells and basophils, IL-3 production is linked to IgE/FcεRI-dependent activation or stimula- tion with calcium ionophores.

Short-term treatment of mice with IL-3 specifically induces an expansion of basophils [24]. Similarly, IL-3 administration to healthy nonhuman pri- mates leads to marked increases in blood leukocyte counts, particularly basophils and eosinophils [25]. Additionally, the long-term culture of murine bone marrow cells with IL-3 leads to the emergence of eosinophils and mast cells [26,27]. In regards to *human* mast cells, the role of IL-3 on differentiation is controversial and sometimes discrepant with murine data; indeed, divergent effects have been reported depending on the tissue. Lastly, recent studies have shown that IL-3 is able to promote the development of peripheral blood monocytes to macrophages and myeloid DCs [26,28].

In addition to its effects on cell differentiation and expansion, IL-3 can regulate a number of biologic activities. For example, IL-3 induces accumulation of histamine in basophils [25]; while it does not significantly stimulate its release in basophils from healthy individuals, it does so in basophils from allergic subjects. IL-3 is also capable of enhancing cytokine secretion, including IL-4 and IL-13, from human basophils [29,30]. Interestingly, a recent study has reported a role for IL-3 in the recruitment of basophils into the lymph nodes, but also a dispensable effect in the development of Th2 immunity following helminth infection [31]. Furthermore, studies *in vitro* have demonstrated an effect of IL-3 on eosinophil, plasmacytoid DC, and macrophage survival.

While hematopoiesis is unimpaired in IL-3-deficient mice, some forms of delayed-type hypersensitivity as well as parasite immunity, including worm expulsion, are compromised owing to decreased numbers and activation status of immune-effector cells [32–34]. In an experimental model of allergic asthma, administration of recombinant IL-3 to sensitized rats led to a doubling in the number of mast cells in the airways and increased eosinophilia after OVA challenge, yet lung resistance after challenge was not altered [35]. In mice, IL-3 neutralization after allergen challenge increased leukocyte clearance by apoptosis and reduced eosinophil activation, the number of infiltrating eosinophils to the airways, and AHR [36]. In sharp contrast, Hsiue *et al.* [37] have shown that IL-3 neutralization in guinea pigs sensitized and challenged with a crude mite extract exhibit a similar degree of eosinophilic airway inflammation as similarly treated controls.

Interleukin 5

IL-5 is associated with an array of activities including the promotion of differentiation, proliferation, migration, survival, and activation of several hematopoietic cells, namely B cells, basophils, and eosinophils. While Th2 cells are the main source of this cytokine, several other cell types can also produce IL-5. These include bronchial and nasal epithelial cells in response to NO_2, O_3, and *Staphylococcal* enterotoxin B; mast cells in response to lipopolysaccharide (LPS) and IgE cross-linking; and airway smooth muscle (ASM) cells, basophils, eosinophils, and CD34+ progenitor cells in response to various intrinsic stimuli, such as cytokines and chemokines.

It is well established that IL-5 may drive the differentiation of activated B cells into antibody-secreting plasma cells (ASCs). Correspondingly, complementary DNA microarray analyses showed that IL-5 regulates many Ig-related genes as well as genes involved in B-cell maturation [38]. Additional studies demonstrated that IL-5 also contributes to isotype class switching [38,39]; however, this effect may be limited to the IgG isotype as other isotypes do not appear to be inducible by IL-5 [39,40]. Moreover, many *in vitro*-based studies have demonstrated that IL-5 significantly enhances B-cell antibody secretion, although this effect may too be restricted, in this case to B-1 and not B-2 cells. In agreement, IL-5 overexpressing transgenic mice exhibit markedly elevated levels of serum Igs [41], and loss-of-function studies have demonstrated that, in the absence of IL-5, homeostatic proliferation and survival of mature B-1 cells are significantly reduced [42].

That IL-5 can also induce the differentiation of eosinophil/basophil progenitors and some cell lines into basophils, at least *in vitro*, suggests that IL-5 also acts as a basopoietin [43], although the findings of Saito *et al.* [44] indicate that this effect may not be critical *in vivo*. Arguably, the most significant contribution of IL-5 to allergic airway disease stems from its effects on eosinophils. Initially, IL-5 was shown to induce eosinophil differentiation from human bone marrow, and, accordingly, was named eosinophil differentiation factor. In concordance, IL-5 transgenic mice display a massive increase in the number of circulating eosinophils [41]. In addition, IL-5 is known to be a chemotactic factor for eosinophils and may augment eosinophilic migration toward other chemotactic factors. IL-5 may further contribute to eosinophil migration into the lung by enhancing adhesion to, and diapedesis through, the endothelium. Also, many *in vitro* studies have demonstrated that IL-5 activates eosinophils and induces the production of various compounds including cytokines, growth factors, vasoactive mediators, and toxic products, implying that eosinophils may drive various aspects of the allergic response, including inflammation, remodeling, and bronchoconstriction. Of significance, IL-5 may further influence airways responsiveness in an eosinophil-independent manner by directly affecting ASM cells. Indeed, ASM cells express IL-5Rα substantially [45], and their incubation with IL-5 and acetylcholine results in enhanced contraction compared with acetylcholine alone [45]. IL-5 also acts to promote eosinophil survival by inhibiting the induction of apoptosis [46]. Interestingly, eosinophils were found to downregulate cell-surface expression of the IL-5Rα subunit following stimulation with IL-5, suggesting that, at some point, eosinophils may become insensitive to the effects of IL-5 [47].

Thus, IL-5 is thought to play an important role in allergic airway disease via its effects on eosinophils. The question of whether eosinophils play a role in asthma is perhaps one of the most debated issues in the field. Certainly, a considerable number of experimental studies have examined the role of eosinophils in all facets of the asthmatic response using animal models. Collectively, the evidence suggests that eosinophils are not fundamentally required for the development of allergic sensitization [48,49]. Regarding inflammation, the findings indicate that eosinophils may augment leukocyte recruitment and mediator release, although the exact extent of their contribution appears to vary depending on the experimental system and ranges from little, if any, to considerable. Nearly two-dozen studies in experimental animal models have investigated the involvement of eosinophils in AHR. The results of these studies are split, with half showing that eosinophils do play a role in this process and half do not [49]. Similarly, the impact of eosinophils on the development of airway remodeling remains somewhat unclear [49]. Several explanations have been proposed in an attempt to resolve these discrepancies, although, ultimately, none of these explanations have proven entirely adequate [48,49]. Noteworthy, the use of IL-5-based interference strategies as a means of clarifying the role of eosinophils in allergic airway disease is complicated by the fact that IL-5 is known to be involved in other processes that may impact disease in an eosinophil-independent manner.

Granulocyte–macrophage colony-stimulating factor

In 1977, Burgess *et al.* [50] were the first to purify GM-CSF, also known as CSF2, from mouse lung-conditioned medium. Originally defined by its capability to generate both granulocyte and macrophage colonies from precursor cells in mouse bone marrow, it had become evident that GM-CSF can mediate many biologic effects, including the promotion of differentiation, proliferation, migration, survival, and activation on several hematopoietic cells such as monocytes, macrophages, granulocytes, and DCs.

With respect to cellular sources of GM-CSF, several studies in patients with asthma have detected, in agreement with *in vitro* findings, significant upregulation of GM-CSF, either mRNA or protein, in bronchial epithelial cells, lymphocytes, and alveolar macrophages. There is extensive evidence demonstrating that the production of GM-CSF can be directly as well as indirectly induced by a wide array of stimuli. For example, regarding microbes, several studies have shown that GM-CSF production can be induced by a number of bacteria, fungi, and viruses, including *Mycobacterium tuberculosis*, LPS, *Pneumocystis carinii*, *Aspergillus fumigatus*, rhinovirus, and respiratory syncytial virus. The relevance of the role of GM-CSF in host defense is demonstrated by evidence of impaired macrophage clearance of group B *Streptococcus* or *Pneumocystis carinii* following infection in GM-CSF-deficient mice and recovery after administration of recombinant GM-CSF. Nonbiologic, harmful entities such as urban air pollutants (e.g., ozone, nitrogen dioxide, suspended particulate matter, and its main component, diesel exhaust particles) have been shown to induce expression and production of GM-CSF by airway epithelial cells and alveolar macrophages both *in vitro* and *in vivo* [51]. Common biologic environmental allergens such as the house dust mite (HDM) allergens Der p 1, 3, and 9 can induce GM-CSF production by human bronchial epithelial cell cultures [52]. In addition to microbes, pollutants, and common environmental allergens, a number of *in vitro* studies have shown that GM-CSF production by human hematopoietic progenitor cells, basophils, neutrophils, bronchial epithelial cells, ASM cells, endothelial cells, and fibroblasts can be induced after stimulation with several inflammatory mediators such as TNF-α, IL-1, and IL-33. That GM-CSF can be potentially induced by such a variety of intruders as well as by secondary signals elicited in the tissue intimates that GM-CSF plays a central role in both innate and adaptive immunity.

In animal models of OVA-induced allergic asthma, neutralization of GM-CSF, or the use of GM-CSF knockout mice significantly attenuates key hallmarks, such as inflammation, eosinophilia, mucus production, and AHR [53,54]. On the other hand, GM-CSF overexpression via the delivery of an adenoviral vector expressing the GM-CSF transgene at the time of challenge resulted in a more sustained accumulation of eosinophils, macrophages, neutrophils, and proliferating lymphocytes in both bronchoalveolar lavage and airway tissue [55]. Also, GM-CSF expression in the lungs can subvert the development of inhalation tolerance to OVA and instead facilitate the development of an asthmatic phenotype [56]. More recent studies using common environmental allergens such as HDM and ragweed extracts, which can mimic many features of allergic asthma when delivered to the respiratory mucosa in the absence of exogenous adjuvants, have strengthened the role of GM-CSF in allergic responses [57,58]. Thus, many studies strongly support the notion that GM-CSF plays a central role in facilitating allergic sensitization, plausibly through its effect on antigen-presenting cells (APCs). In addition, GM-CSF contributes to the enhancement and/or maintenance of airway inflammation through its effects on the proliferation, migration, function, and/or survival of immune-inflammatory cells such as eosinophils and lymphocytes and, hence, on allergic responses.

Intervention studies in humans

Inhibition of IL-3 bioactivity using monoclonal anti-IL-3 or anti-IL-3Rα antibodies, IL-3 antisense oligodeoxynucleotides, or a recombinant IL-3 fusion immunotoxin has been investigated in individuals with leukemia with some promising findings. However, to our knowledge, no clinical trials have been reported studying the impact of IL-3 neutralization in allergic diseases. Similarly, no studies have investigated GM-CSF neutralization in allergic diseases, most likely because such an approach could severely hamper host responses to harmful intruders and compromise pulmonary homeostasis.

In contrast, several clinical trials have evaluated the therapeutic potential of IL-5 inhibition [59–64]. As expected, treatment of asthmatic individuals with the anti-IL-5 antibodies exhibited long-term decreases in blood and sputum eosinophils, thus demonstrating a role of IL-5 in human eosinophilopoiesis [60,62,63]. However, this did not translate into clinical or functional improvement since parameters of asthma expression, such as FEV_1, airway responsiveness to histamine, symptom scores, and allergen-induced late asthmatic response, were not affected by the treatment [60,62,63]. This disconnection between decreases in the number of eosinophils and unaltered

clinical and physiologic responses instigated a questioning of the relative importance of eosinophils in asthma pathogenesis [65]. However, alternate explanations have been proposed to clarify that divergence. For example, airway biopsy samples revealed that the decrease in eosinophils in the lung tissue itself was actually modest following anti-IL-5 treatment [60,61]. Additionally, the treatment did not affect levels of eosinophil major basic protein, intimating a further disconnection between eosinophil numbers and degranulation.

While issues of sample size arose with the earlier clinical trials, a recent study involving 300 asthmatic individuals with a spectrum of mild to severe disease generally agreed that anti-IL-5 therapy was unsuccessful [59]. However, this study raised the issue of whether a potential effect of the intervention was diluted by the heterogeneity of the sample population. In this regard, the latest anti-IL-5 antibody trials were performed on a small subset of individuals with asthma who had persistent sputum eosinophilia despite steroid treatment. Patients exhibited a significant reduction in exacerbations, prednisone sparing, and asthma quality of life questionnaire scores [61,64]. Blood and sputum eosinophil levels were, expectedly, significantly decreased, although conventional parameters of disease progression similar to those used in earlier studies again remained unchanged following treatment [61,64]. Ultimately, whether the reduction in exacerbations in this select set of asthmatic individuals is directly the result of eosinophil depletion or of the effects of IL-5 on other cells such as B cells, basophils, and ASM cells remains unsolved.

Given the interplay of IL-3, IL-5, and GM-CSF in contributing to the allergic phenotype, Sun et al. [66] generated a monoclonal antibody, BION-1, against a major cytokine-binding domain of βc. The antagonism of all three cytokines in vitro was shown to greatly reduce human eosinophil production, survival, and activation but its efficacy in vivo is still unknown. In this regard, Gauvreau et al. [67] showed that inhaled TPI ASM8 (Topigen Pharmaceuticals Inc., now part of Pharmaxis Ltd., French Forest, NSW, Australia), a mix of antisense oligonucleotides that downregulate βc and CCR3 mRNA, can attenuate allergen-induced eosinophilia and physiologic responses in individuals with mild allergic asthma.

Concluding remarks

It is clear that, in addition to their roles in emergency hematopoiesis, IL-3, IL-5, and GM-CSF regulate a vast array of activities on APCs, lymphocytes, mast cells, and granulocytes. The evidence indicates that these cytokines play a variety of roles in conditions as diverse as infections, cancer, autoimmunity, neurologic disorders, and allergic inflammation. In regards to the later, IL-3, IL-5, and GM-CSF are undoubtedly involved in the pathogenesis of allergic asthma, contributing to both disease development and progression and having, directly or indirectly, a major impact on the extent of inflammation, airway remodeling, dysfunction, and, ultimately, disease severity. However, the potential of these molecules to become significant therapeutic targets in allergic asthma is, in our view, limited for several reasons.

First, these molecules ontogenically evolved to become elements of the host defense program. Therefore, the potential benefits of neutralizing these molecules or inhibiting their effects must be assessed against the risk of compromising not only host defense but also other homeostatic activities, both in the short and long term. Second, as we have discussed earlier, there is a notable degree of redundancy and, consequently, the blockade of one single cytokine is likely to have modest effects on particular biologic activities. Moreover, there are additional layers of redundancy outside this triad of cytokines. For example, osteopontin and thymic stromal lymphopoietin may have some activities on APCs that are redundant with GM-CSF. Third, asthma is a complex and inherently heterogeneous disease. This implies that the relationships between a specific molecule and a particular biologic activity and, most importantly, a given functional, structural, or clinical outcome are nonlinear. The failure of anti-IL-5 trials in asthma "at large" and, particularly, the disconnection between decreases in eosinophils and unaltered functional parameters in a selected and rare group of steroid-resistant patients illustrates this point.

The development of future therapies for asthma faces an apparent dilemma: specific versus generic strategies. Specific strategies are confronted with the issues outlined above; generic strategies, of which corticosteroids are an archetype, are of limited benefit in patients with moderate or severe disease and must deal with the potential of detrimental adverse effects.

However, the real challenge is to deconstruct the idea of asthma as a single or homogeneous disease. Indeed, the identification of distinct asthma phenotypes underlined by specific cellular and molecular pathways that extend or challenge current dogmas may be the only venue to discover new treatments for asthma.

Acknowledgment

We apologize to the many investigators whose work could not be cited owing to strict space limitations. We are thankful to Derek K. Chu for his critical reading of the manuscript. A.L-G is supported by a doctoral scholarship from Fundación Caja Madrid (Spain) and J.M by a Canadian Institutes of Health Research (CIHR) Frederick Banting and Charles Best Canada Graduate Scholarship. M.J holds a Senior Canada Research Chair in Immunobiology of Respiratory Diseases and Allergy.

References

1 Bagley CJ, Woodcock JM, Stomski FC, et al. The structural and functional basis of cytokine receptor activation: lessons from the common beta subunit of the granulocyte–macrophage colony-stimulating factor, interleukin-3 (IL-3), and IL-5 receptors. *Blood* 2007; **89**: 1471–82.

2 Miyajima A. Molecular structure of the IL-3: GM-CSF, and IL-5 receptors. *Int J Cell Cloning* 1992; **10**: 126–34.

3 Hara T, Miyajima A. Two distinct functional high affinity receptors for mouse interleukin-3 (IL-3). *EMBO J* 1992; **11**: 1875–84.

4 Bazan JF. Structural design and molecular evolution of a cytokine receptor superfamily. *Proc Natl Acad Sci USA* 1990; **87**: 6934–8.

5 Lopez AF, Eglinton JM, Gillis D, et al. Reciprocal inhibition of binding between interleukin 3 and granulocyte–macrophage colony-stimulating factor to human eosinophils. *Proc Natl Acad Sci USA* 1989; **86**: 7022–6.

6 Lopez AF, Vadas MA, Woodcock JM, et al. Interleukin-5: interleukin-3: and granulocyte–macrophage colony-stimulating factor cross-compete for binding to cell-surface receptors on human eosinophils. *J Biol Chem* 1991; **266**: 24741–7.

7 Lopez AF, Elliott MJ, Woodcock J, *et al.* GM-CSF, IL-3 and IL-5: cross-competition on human haemopoietic cells. *Immunol Today* 1992; **13**: 495–500.

8 Martinez-Moczygemba M, Huston DP. Biology of common beta receptor-signaling cytokines: IL-3: IL-5: and GM-CSF. *J Allergy Clin Immunol* 2003; **112**: 653–65; quiz 66.

9 Ozaki K, Leonard WJ. Cytokine and cytokine receptor pleiotropy and redundancy. *J Chem* 1998; **277**: 29355–8.

10 de Groot RP, Coffer PJ, Koenderman L. Regulation of proliferation, differentiation and survival by the IL-3/IL-5/GM-CSF receptor family. *Cell Signal* 1998; **10**: 619–28.

11 Fitzsimmons CM, Dunne DW. Survival of the fittest: allergology or parasitology? *Trends Parasitol* 2009; **25**: 447–51.

12 Guthridge MA, Powell JA, Barry EF, *et al.* Growth factor pleiotropy is controlled by a receptor Tyr/Ser motif that acts as a binary switch. *EMBO J* 2006; **25**: 479–89.

13 Nishinakamura R, Miyajima A, Mee PJ, *et al.* Hematopoiesis in mice lacking the entire granulocyte–macrophage colony-stimulating factor/interleukin-3/interleukin-5 functions. *Blood* 1996; **88**: 2458–64.

14 Nishinakamura R, Nakayama N, Hirabayashi Y, *et al.* Mice deficient for the IL-3/GM-CSF/IL-5 beta c receptor exhibit lung pathology and impaired immune response, while beta IL-3 receptor-deficient mice are normal. *Immunity* 1995; **2**: 211–22.

15 Nishinakamura R, Wiler R, Dirksen U, *et al.* The pulmonary alveolar proteinosis in granulocyte–macrophage colony-stimulating factor/interleukins 3/5 beta c receptor-deficient mice is reversed by bone marrow transplantation. *J Exp Med* 1996; **183**: 2657–62.

16 Robb L, Drinkwater CC, Metcalf D, *et al.* Hematopoietic and lung abnormalities in mice with a null mutation of the common beta subunit of the receptors for granulocyte–macrophage colony-stimulating factor and interleukins 3 and 5. *Proc Natl Acad Sci USA* 1995; **92**: 9565–9.

17 Huffman JA, Hull WM, Dranoff G, *et al.* Pulmonary epithelial cell expression of GM-CSF corrects the alveolar proteinosis in GM-CSF-deficient mice. *J Clin Invest* 1996; **97**: 649–55.

18 Stanley E, Lieschke GJ, Grail D, *et al.* Granulocyte/macrophage colony-stimulating factor-deficient mice show no major perturbation of hematopoiesis but develop a characteristic pulmonary pathology. *Proc Natl Acad Sci USA* 1994; **91**: 5592–6.

19 Kitamura T, Tanaka N, Watanabe J, *et al.* Idiopathic pulmonary alveolar proteinosis as an autoimmune disease with neutralizing antibody against granulocyte/macrophage colony-stimulating factor. *J Exp Med* 1999; **190**: 875–80.

20 Martinez-Moczygemba M, Doan ML, Elidemir O, *et al.* Pulmonary alveolar proteinosis caused by deletion of the GM-CSFRalpha gene in the X chromosome pseudoautosomal region 1. *J Exp Med* 2008; **205**: 2711–16.

21 Uchida K, Beck DC, Yamamoto T, *et al.* GM-CSF, autoantibodies and neutrophil dysfunction in pulmonary alveolar proteinosis. *New Engl J Med* 2007; **356**: 567–79.

22 Asquith KL, Ramshaw HS, Hansbro PM, *et al.* The IL-3/IL-5/GM-CSF common receptor plays a pivotal role in the regulation of Th2 immunity and allergic airway inflammation. *J Immunol* 2008; **180**: 1199–206.

23 Kabesch M, Depner M, Dahmen I, *et al.* Polymorphisms in eosinophil pathway genes, asthma and atopy. *Allergy* 2007; **62**: 423–8.

24 Ohmori K, Luo Y, Jia Y, *et al.* IL-3 induces basophil expansion *in vivo* by directing granulocyte-monocyte progenitors to differentiate into basophil lineage-restricted progenitors in the bone marrow and by increasing the number of basophil/mast cell progenitors in the spleen. *J Immunol* 2009;**182**: 2835–41.

25 Mayer P, Valent P, Schmidt G, *et al.* The in vivo effects of recombinant human interleukin-3: demonstration of basophil differentiation factor, histamine-producing activity, and priming of GM-CSF-responsive progenitors in nonhuman primates. *Blood* 1989; **74**: 613–21.

26 Baumeister T, Rossner S, Pech G, *et al.* Interleukin-3Ralpha⁺ myeloid dendritic cells and mast cells develop simultaneously from different bone marrow precursors in cultures with interleukin-3. *J Invest Dermatol* 2003; **121**: 280–8.

27 Valent P, Schmidt G, Besemer J, *et al.* Interleukin-3 is a differentiation factor for human basophils. *Blood* 1989; **73**: 1763–9.

28 Ebner S, Hofer S, Nguyen VA, *et al.* A novel role for IL-3: human monocytes cultured in the presence of IL-3 and IL-4 differentiate into dendritic cells that produce less IL-12 and shift Th cell responses toward a Th2 cytokine pattern. *J Immunol* 2002; **168**: 6199–207.

29 Brunner T, Heusser Ch, Dahinden CA. Human peripheral blood basophils primed by interleukin 3 (IL-3) produce IL-4 in response to immunoglobulin E receptor stimulation. *J Exp Med* 1993; **177**: 605–11.

30 Ochensberger B, Daepp GC, Rihs S, *et al.* Human blood basophils produce interleukin-13 in response to IgE-receptor-dependent and -independent activation. *Blood* 1996; **88**: 3028–37.

31 Kim S, Prout M, Ramshaw H, *et al.* Cutting edge: basophils are transiently recruited into the draining lymph nodes during helminth infection via IL-3: but infection-induced Th2 immunity can develop without basophil lymph node recruitment or IL-3. *J Immunol* 2010; **184**: 1143–7.

32 Kimura K, Song Ch, Rastogi A, *et al.* Interleukin-3 and c-Kit/stem cell factor are required for normal eosinophil responses in mice infected with *Strongyloides venezue-*

lensis. Lab Investig; J Tech Methods Pathol 2006; **86**: 987–96.

33 Lantz CS, Boesiger J, Song Ch, *et al.* Role for interleukin-3 in mast cell and basophil development and in immunity to parasites. *Nature* 1998; **392**: 90–3.

34 Mach N, Lantz CS, Galli SJ, *et al.* Involvement of interleukin-3 in delayed-type hypersensitivity. *Blood* 1998; **91**: 778–83.

35 Du T, Martin JG, Xu LJ, *et al.* IL-3 does not affect the allergic airway responses and leukotriene production after allergen challenge in rats. *Eur Resp J* 1999; **13**: 970–5.

36 Lloyd CM, Gonzalo JA, Nguyen T, *et al.* Resolution of bronchial hyperresponsiveness and pulmonary inflammation is associated with IL-3 and tissue leukocyte apoptosis. *J Immunol* 2001; **166**: 2033–40.

37 Hsiue TR, Lei HY, Hsieh AL, *et al.* Time course of pharmacological modulation of peak eosinophilic airway inflammation after mite challenge in guinea pigs: a therapeutic approach. *Int Arch Allergy Immunol* 1999; **11**: 297–303.

38 Horikawa K, Takatsu K. Interleukin-5 regulates genes involved in B-cell terminal maturation. *Immunology* 2006; **118**: 497–508.

39 Purkerson JM, Isakson PC. Interleukin 5 (IL-5) provides a signal that is required in addition to IL-4 for isotype switching to immunoglobulin (Ig) G1 and IgE. *J Exp Med* 1992; **175**: 973–82.

40 Schoenbeck S, McKenzie DT, Kagnoff MF. Interleukin 5 is a differentiation factor for IgA B cells. *Eur J Immunol* 1989; **19**: 965–9.

41 Tominaga A, Takaki S, Koyama N, *et al.* Transgenic mice expressing a B cell growth and differentiation factor gene (interleukin 5) develop eosinophilia and autoantibody production. *J Exp Med* 1991; **173**: 429–37.

42 Moon BG, Takaki S, Miyake K, *et al.* The role of IL-5 for mature B-1 cells in homeostatic proliferation, cell survival, and Ig production. *J Immunol* 2004; **172**: 6020–9.

43 Denburg JA. Cytokine-induced human basophil/mast cell growth and differentiation *in vitro*. *Springer Semin Immunopathol* 1990; **12**: 401–14.

44 Saito H, Hatake K, Dvorak AM, *et al.* Selective differentiation and proliferation of hematopoietic cells induced by recombinant human interleukins. *Proc Natl Acad Sci USA* 1988; **85**: 2288–92.

45 Rizzo CA, Yang R, Greenfeder S, *et al.* The IL-5 receptor on human bronchus selectively primes for hyperresponsiveness. *J Allergy Clin Immunol* 2002; **109**: 404–9.

46 Simon HU, Yousefi S, Schranz C, *et al.* Direct demonstration of delayed eosinophil apoptosis as a mechanism causing tissue eosinophilia. *J Immunol* 1997; **158**: 3902–8.

47 Liu LY, Sedgwick JB, Bates ME, *et al.* Decreased expression of membrane IL-5 receptor alpha on human eosi-

nophils: II. IL-5 down-modulates its receptor via a proteinase-mediated process. *J Immunol* 2002; **169**: 6459–66.

48 Walsh ER, Sahu N, Kearley J, *et al.* Strain-specific requirement for eosinophils in the recruitment of T cells to the lung during the development of allergic asthma. *J Exp Med* 2008; **205**: 1285–92.

49 Fattouh R, Jordana M. TGF-beta, eosinophils and IL-13 in allergic airway remodeling: a critical appraisal with therapeutic considerations. *Inflamm Allergy—Drug Targets* 2008; **7**: 224–36.

50 Burgess AW, Metcalf D. The nature and action of granulocyte–macrophage colony stimulating factors. *Blood* 1980; **56**: 947–58.

51 Saxon A, Diaz-Sanchez D. Air pollution and allergy: you are what you breathe. *Nat Immunol* 2005; **6**: 223–6.

52 Cates EC, Fattouh R, Johnson JR, *et al.* Modeling responses to respiratory house dust mite exposure. *Contributions Microbiol* 2007; **14**: 42–67.

53 Su YC, Rolph MS, Hansbro NG, *et al.* Granulocyte–macrophage colony-stimulating factor is required for bronchial eosinophilia in a murine model of allergic airway inflammation. *J Immunol* 2008; **180**: 2600–7.

54 Yamashita N, Tashimo H, Ishida H, *et al.* Attenuation of airway hyperresponsiveness in a murine asthma model by neutralization of granulocyte–macrophage colony-stimulating factor (GM-CSF). *Cell Immunol* 2002; **219**: 92–7.

55 Lei XF, Ohkawara Y, Stampfli MR, *et al.* Compartmentalized transgene expression of granulocyte–macrophage colony-stimulating factor (GM-CSF) in mouse lung enhances allergic airways inflammation. *Clin Exp Immunol* 1998; **113**: 157–65.

56 Stampfli MR, Wiley RE, Neigh GS, *et al.* GM-CSF transgene expression in the airway allows aerosolized ovalbumin to induce allergic sensitization in mice. *J Clin Invest* 1998; **102**: 1704–14.

57 Cates EC, Gajewska BU, Goncharova S, *et al.* Effect of GM-CSF on immune, inflammatory, and clinical responses to ragweed in a novel mouse model of mucosal sensitization. *J Allergy Clin Immunol* 2003; **111**: 1076–86.

58 Cates EC, Fattouh R, Wattie J, *et al.* Intranasal exposure of mice to house dust mite elicits allergic airway inflammation via a GM-CSF-mediated mechanism. *J Immunol* 2004; **173**: 6384–92.

59 Flood-Page P, Swenson C, Faiferman I, *et al.* A study to evaluate safety and efficacy of mepolizumab in patients with moderate persistent asthma. *Am J Respir Crit Care Med* 2007; **176**: 1062–71.

60 Flood-Page PT, Menzies-Gow AN, Kay AB, *et al.* Eosinophil's role remains uncertain as anti-interleukin-5 only partially depletes numbers in asthmatic airway. *Am J Respir Crit Care Med* 2003; **167**: 199–204.

61 Haldar P, Brightling CE, Hargadon B, *et al*. Mepolizumab and exacerbations of refractory eosinophilic asthma. *New Engl J Med* 2009; **360**: 973–84.

62 Kips JC, O'Connor BJ, Langley SJ, *et al*. Effect of SCH55700: a humanized anti-human interleukin-5 antibody, in severe persistent asthma: a pilot study. *Am J Respir Crit Care Med* 2003; **167**: 1655–9.

63 Leckie MJ, ten Brinke A, Khan J, *et al*. Effects of an interleukin-5 blocking monoclonal antibody on eosinophils, airway hyperresponsiveness, and the late asthmatic response. *Lancet* 2000; **356**: 2144–8.

64 Nair P, Pizzichini MM, Kjarsgaard M, *et al*. Mepolizumab for prednisone-dependent asthma with sputum eosinophilia. *New Engl J Med* 2009; **360**: 985–93.

65 Boushey HA, Fahy JV. Targeting cytokines in asthma therapy: round one. *Lancet* 2000; **356**: 2114–16.

66 Sun Q, Jones K, McClure B, *et al*. Simultaneous antagonism of interleukin-5: granulocyte–macrophage colony-stimulating factor, and interleukin-3 stimulation of human eosinophils by targetting the common cytokine binding site of their receptors. *Blood* 1999; **94**:1943–51.

67 Gauvreau GM, Boulet LP, Cockcroft DW, *et al*. Antisense therapy against CCR3 and the common beta chain attenuates allergen-induced eosinophilic responses. *Am J Respir Crit Care Med* 2008; **177**: 952–8.

15 Interleukin 15, interleukin 17, and interleukin 25

Hiroshi Nakajima[1,2] and Itsuo Iwamoto[3]

[1]Department of Molecular Genetics, Graduate School of Medicine, Chiba University, Chiba, Japan
[2]Department of Allergy and Clinical Immunology, Chiba University Hospital, Chiba, Japan
[3]Research Center for Allergy and Clinical Immunology, Asahi General Hospital, Chiba, Japan

Introduction

It is well established that a strong correlation exists between the presence of eosinophils and the presence of T helper 2 (Th2) cells in the asthmatic airways and that classical Th2 cell-derived cytokines, namely interleukin 4 (IL-4), IL-5, and IL-13, play critical roles in orchestrating and amplifying allergic inflammation in asthma. However, accumulating evidence suggests that the regulation of allergic inflammation is more complex. In this chapter, our current understanding of the roles of nonclassical cytokines including IL-15, IL-17, IL-21, IL-23, and IL-25 in the pathogenesis of allergic airway inflammation will be summarized.

IL-23–Th17 cell axis

The basis of IL-23–Th17 cell axis

The original member of IL-17 family cytokines, IL-17A, was identified in 1995, subsequently followed by five other cytokines, IL-17B, IL-17C, IL-17D, IL-17E (also known as IL-25), and IL-17F [1] (Table 15.1). IL-17 family cytokines are disulfide-linked homodimeric proteins that possess a characteristic cysteine knot structure [2]. IL-17A and IL-17F, the most closely related protein to IL-17A, are mainly expressed in a recently identified subpopulation of CD4[+] T cells, namely Th17 cells, which are believed to be involved in the pathogenesis of autoimmune diseases [3,4]. IL-17A and IL-17F homodimers and IL-17F/IL-17A heterodimers transduce their signals through the receptor composed of IL-17RA and IL-17RC (Table 15.1) [5,6].

IL-23 has been identified as a novel IL-12 family cytokine that is composed of a p19 subunit specific for IL-23 and a p40 subunit shared with IL-12 [7]. Despite a structural similarity between IL-12 and IL-23, it is apparent that IL-23, rather than IL-12, plays a pathogenic role in chronic inflammation in a number of disease models, including experimental autoimmune encephalomyelitis, psoriasis, collagen-induced arthritis, and inflammatory bowel diseases [3,4]. In addition, studies using IL-23 p19-deficient mice have revealed that IL-23 is crucial for the maintenance of Th17 cells [8,9]. Moreover, McGeachy *et al.* [10] have shown that IL-23 is required for full acquisition of an effector function of Th17 cells. These findings indicate that the IL-23–Th17 cell axis plays a crucial role in the development of inflammatory diseases.

The role of IL-23–Th17 cell axis in neutrophilic airway inflammation

While it is believed that pathognomonic features of asthma, including intense eosinophilic infiltration,

Inflammation and Allergy Drug Design, First Edition. Edited by Kenji Izuhara, Stephen T. Holgate, Marsha Wills-Karp.
© 2011 Blackwell Publishing Ltd. Published 2011 by Blackwell Publishing Ltd.

Table 15.1 Interleukin 17 (IL-17) family cytokines and their receptors.

Family member	Alternate names	% Homology with IL-17A	Cellular source	Receptor
IL-17A	IL-17	100	Th17, CD8 T, NK, γδT, neutrophil	IL-17RA, IL-17RC
IL-17B	CX1	21	?	IL-17RB
IL-17C	CX2	24	?	?
IL-17D	–	16	?	?
IL-17E	IL-25	16	Th2, mast cells, eosinophil, basophil, epithelium	IL-17RB, IL-17RA
IL-17F	ML-1	45	Th17, CD8 T, NK, γδT, neutrophil	IL-17RC, IL-17RA
IL–17A/F heterodimer	–	–	?	IL-17RC, IL-17RA

airway remodeling, and airway hyperresponsiveness (AHR), are mediated by antigen-specific Th2 cells and their cytokines, such as IL-4, IL-5, and IL-13 [11–13], several lines of evidence suggest that IL-17A and IL-17F are involved in airway inflammation [14,15]. It has been shown that IL-17A is expressed in the airways of asthmatic individuals [15] and its expression is correlated with the severity of asthma [16]. IL-17A has also been shown to stimulate bronchial fibroblasts, epithelial cells, and smooth muscle cells to induce the expression of a variety of cytokines and chemokines, which are important for granulopoiesis and neutrophil recruitment [17]. The ability of IL-17A to evoke migration of neutrophils makes it likely that IL-17A is involved in severe asthma, of which neutrophil infiltration is one of the hallmarks (Figure 15.1) [18,19]. Moreover, it has been shown that Th17 cell-mediated airway inflammation is steroid-resistant [20] and it has also been demonstrated that IL-23 p19 mRNA is induced upon antigen inhalation in the lung of antigen-sensitized mice [21,22]. Together with recent observations suggesting the critical role of IL-23 in the maintenance of Th17 cells [3,4,10], it is speculated that IL-23–Th17 cell axis plays some roles in causing airway inflammation, especially neutrophilic inflammation, in severe asthma. Consistent with this notion, the enforced expression of IL-23 in the lung or the transfer of antigen-specific Th17 cells enhances antigen-induced neutrophil recruitment into

the airways [22]. Further studies identifying the cellular and molecular targets of IL-23 and Th17 cell-derived cytokines in the regulation of neutrophilic airway inflammation could help to develop a novel therapeutic approach against severe asthma and/or steroid-resistant asthma.

The role of IL-23–Th17 cell axis in eosinophilic airway inflammation

Recently, we have shown that the administration of anti-p19 antibody, which neutralizes the activity of IL-23 but not of IL-12, attenuates not only antigen-induced neutrophil recruitment but also antigen-induced eosinophil recruitment into the airways [22]. The administration of anti-p19 antibody also decreases antigen-induced Th2 cytokine production in the airways [22]. In addition, it has been shown that resolvin E1, an endogenous lipid mediator, inhibits the development of allergic airway inflammation by suppressing the expression of IL-23 in the lung [23]. Moreover, enforced expression of IL-23 in the lung enhances not only antigen-induced IL-17A production and neutrophil recruitment in the airways but also antigen-induced Th2 cytokine production and eosinophil recruitment into the airways [22]. Together, these findings reveal a substantial role of IL-23 in causing eosinophilic airway inflammation (Figure 15.1).

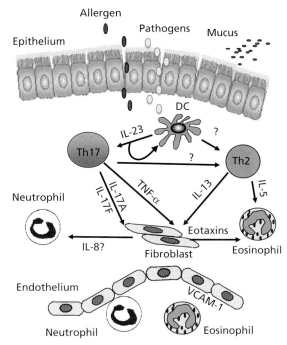

Figure 15.1 Schema of the roles of interleukin 23 (IL-23)–T helper (Th) 17 cell axis in causing airway inflammation. Upon stimulation with antigens and some pathogens, dendritic cells (DCs) produce IL-23, which enhances the development and maintenance of Th17 cells. IL-23 may also enhance the ability of DCs to induce antigen-specific Th2 cells in an autocrine manner. The effector cytokines of Th17 cells such as tumor necrosis factor α (TNF-α) may collaborate with IL-13 to recruit more eosinophils into the airways through the production of eotaxins. Th17 cells may also directly activate Th2 cells by producing some cytokines. On the other hand, Th17 cell-derived cytokines such as IL-17A and IL-17F enhance the recruitment of neutrophils into the airways.

The mechanism of IL-23-mediated enhancement of eosinophilic airway inflammation is still unclear. Although the production of IL-17A is enhanced by the enforced expression of IL-23 in the lung, the enhancement of eosinophilic inflammation by the expression of IL-23 is still observed in the absence of IL-17A [22], which is consistent with the previous findings that antigen-induced airway inflammation is induced normally in IL-17A-deficient mice [24,25]. In addition, it has been demonstrated that IL-17F-deficient mice exhibit rather exacerbated antigen-induced eosinophilic airway inflammation [26]. These

findings suggest that IL-23 enhances antigen-induced eosinophilic airway inflammation by the mechanism independent of IL-17A and IL-17F.

IL-21, a type I cytokine with significant homology to IL-2, IL-15, and IL-4 [27,28], has been reported to be a product of Th17 cells and functions as an autocrine/paracrine growth factor for Th17 cells [29–32]. IL-21 has pleiotropic effects on the proliferation, differentiation, and effector functions of T cells, B cells, natural killer (NK) cells, and dendritic cells (DCs) [27,28]. However, we have previously shown that the administration of recombinant IL-21 rather decreases antigen-induced immunoglobulin E (IgE) production and eosinophil recruitment into the airways in antigen-sensitized mice [33], suggesting that IL-21 may not be responsible for the IL-23-mediated enhancement of eosinophilic airway inflammation. IL-22, an IL-10-related cytokine, is also expressed in CD4+ T cells in Th17-polarizing conditions and mediates IL-23-induced dermal inflammation and hyperplasia of the epidermis in psoriasis [34]. The role of IL-22 in eosinophilic airway inflammation needs to be determined in future.

The role of Th17 cells themselves in the induction of eosinophilic airway inflammation has been addressed by adoptive transfer experiments [22]. Although the transfer of antigen-specific Th17 cells to nonsensitized mice does not effect antigen-induced eosinophil recruitment into the airways, co-transfer of antigen-specific Th17 cells with antigen-specific Th2 cells significantly enhances antigen-induced, Th2 cell-mediated eosinophil recruitment into the airways [22]. When antigen-specific Th17 cells are transferred to antigen-sensitized mice in which endogenous antigen-specific Th2 cells are present, Th17 cells significantly enhance antigen-induced eosinophil recruitment into the airways [22]. Therefore, it is indicated that Th17 cells themselves do not induce eosinophilic airway inflammation but cooperate to enhance Th2 cell-mediated eosinophilic airway inflammation. Interestingly, co-transfer of Th17 cells with Th2 cells enhances the expression of eotaxin-1/eotaxin-2 and neutralization of eotaxins before the inhaled antigen challenge decreases the eosinophil recruitment into the airways of the mice transferred with a combination of Th2 cells and Th17 cells [22]. These findings suggest that Th17 cells may enhance eosinophilic airway inflammation through the upregulation of eotaxins. In this regard, it has been demonstrated

199

that STAT6 and nuclear factor κB (NF-κB) synergistically induce eotaxin expression in fibroblasts and epithelial cells [35]. Because Th17 cells produce tumor necrosis factor α (TNF-α) [8], which activates NF-κB pathways, it is possible that the induction of eotaxins by the coactivation of Th2 cells and Th17 cells is mediated by IL-4/IL-13 and TNF-α. These findings are consistent with the recent report showing the effectiveness of TNF-α neutralization on severe asthma [36].

The pathophysiologic situations in which IL-23–Th17 cell axis plays a crucial role in asthmatic individuals remain unclear. Importantly, it has been demonstrated that antigen-presenting cells including DCs produce IL-23 upon a variety of stimuli such as TNF-α, CD40L, lipopolysaccharide, and CpG-ODN. IL-23 is also induced in the lung upon viral or bacterial infection. Thus, IL-23–Th17 cell axis may be involved in the exacerbation of asthma upon viral or bacterial infection. In addition, it has been reported that the engagement of dectin-1 by fungal component β-glucan activates DCs to produce IL-23 [37,38]. Therefore, it is speculated that IL-23–Th17 cell axis is involved in the immune responses in allergic bronchopulmonary aspergillosis (ABPA), in which chronic colonization of fungus such as *Aspergillus fumigatus* is found in the bronchial mucus of asthmatics. These findings suggest that IL-23 and/or Th17 cells could be a novel therapeutic target of asthma exacerbation or severe asthma including ABPA.

IL-25

The basis of IL-25

Among IL-17 family cytokines, IL-25 is less homologic to other members (Table 15.1) [1]. In addition, the receptor for IL-25 (IL-25R, also known as IL-17RB) is different from that for IL-17A and IL-17F (Table 15.1) [1]. Consequently, *in vivo* and *in vitro* biologic activities of IL-25 are markedly different from those described for IL-17A and other IL-17 family cytokines [1]. For example, the systemic administration of IL-25 causes eosinophilia through the production of IL-5 [39–41], whereas other IL-17 family cytokines induce neutrophilia [14,15]. Moreover, IL-25 induces elevated gene expression of IL-4 and IL-13 in multiple tissues and subsequent Th2-type immune responses including increased serum IgE levels and pathologic

changes in multiple tissues [39–41]. Interestingly, previous studies have demonstrated that IL-25-induced Th2 cytokine production is observed even in Rag-2-defcient mice, suggesting that non-T-cell/non-B-cell populations could produce Th2 cytokines in response to IL-25 [39,41].

Regarding IL-25-producing cells, an original report has demonstrated that IL-25 mRNA is expressed in polarized Th2 cells [39]. However, quantitative reverse-transcriptase polymerase chain reaction (RT-PCR) analyses have revealed that IL-25 mRNA is detected in multiple tissues, including colon, uterus, stomach, small intestine, kidney, and lung [39,40,42]. In this regard, we have shown that bone marrow-derived mast cells express IL-25 mRNA upon IgE cross-linking at levels comparable to activated Th2 cells [43]. Subsequently, several cell types including allergen-stimulated epithelial cells [44], IgE-activated basophils [45], and IL-5-activated eosinophils [45] have been shown to produce IL-25. Future studies are required for identifying the cell types that produce IL-25 in each allergic disease.

Role of IL-25 in allergic airway inflammation

Although the cell types that produce IL-25 in the site of allergic airway inflammation remains unclear, we have recently shown that IL-25 mRNA is expressed in the lung upon antigen inhalation [46]. We have also shown that the neutralization of endogenously produced IL-25 by soluble IL-25 receptor decreases antigen-induced eosinophil recruitment into the airways [46]. Recently, Ballantyne *et al.* [47] have shown that the administration of anti-IL-25 antibody inhibits antigen-induced airway inflammation. These findings suggest that IL-25 is involved in the induction and/or enhancement of allergic airway inflammation (Figure 15.2).

In addition, we have shown that the enforced expression of IL-25 in the lung significantly enhances antigen-induced Th2 cytokine production and eosinophil recruitment in the airways [46]. Importantly, IL-25-induced enhancement of antigen-induced eosinophil recruitment into the airways is inhibited by the addition of anti-CD4 antibody [46], suggesting that cells expressing CD4 such as CD4+ T cells and natural killer T (NKT) cells are involved in IL-25-mediated enhancement of antigen-induced eosinophil recruitment into the airways. Furthermore, the enhanced

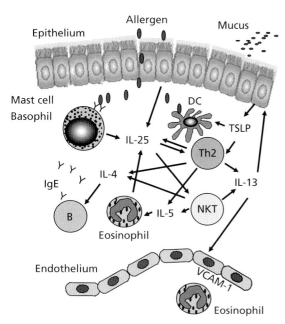

Figure 15.2 Schema of the roles of interleukin 25 (IL-25) in causing airway inflammation. T helper (Th) 2 cells, mast cells, basophils, eosinophils, and epithelial cells produce IL-25 upon activation. IL-25 activates thymic stromal lymphopoietin (TSLP)-stimulated memory Th2 cells or a subset of natural killer T (NKT) cells that expresses IL-25 receptor and CD4 and then induces Th2-type immune responses through the production of Th2 cytokines from these cells. IgE, immunoglobulin E.

expression of IL-25 in the airways of humans with asthma has recently been reported [48]. Together, these findings raise the possibility that IL-25 is involved in the enhancement and/or prolongation of allergic inflammation in asthma and suggest that IL-25 could be a therapeutic target of allergic diseases.

IL-25-responding cells in allergic inflammation

Recently, much progress has been made in identifying IL-25-responding cells during allergic inflammation. Wang et al. [45] have shown that when memory Th2 cells are stimulated with thymic stromal lymphopoietin (TSLP)-activated DCs or by the combination of IL-7 and IL-15, Th2 cells express IL-25R and produce more Th2 cytokines in respond to IL-25. More recently, Taniguchi and colleagues [49] have identified a novel subset of NKT cells that express IL-25R and CD4 and produce predominantly IL-13

upon stimulation with IL-25 *in vitro. In vivo,* IL-25R$^+$ CD4$^+$ NKT cells are mainly detected in the lung and are responsible for IL-25-mediated AHR [49]. These findings suggest that memory Th2 cells and/or IL-25R$^+$ CD4$^+$ NKT cells are involved in IL-25-mediated enhancement of allergic airway inflammation. On the other hand, previous studies have demonstrated that the intranasal administration of large amounts of recombinant IL-25 or the systemic expression of IL-25 could induce Th2 cytokine production and eosinophil infiltration in Rag-2-deficient mice that lack CD4$^+$ T cells and NKT cells [39–41]. Recently, with regard to IL-25-responding non-T/non-B cells in lung, Claudio et al. [50] have shown that CD11c$^+$ macrophage-like cells in the lung express IL-25R and produce IL-5 and IL-13 in response to IL-25. Together, these findings suggest that IL-25 evokes allergic airway inflammation by at least two distinct mechanisms. In a situation where IL-25 is abundant, it causes allergic inflammation through the induction of Th2 cytokines from non-T/non-B cells. In contrast, in other situation where the amounts of IL-25 are limited, collaboration with memory Th2 cells or IL-25R$^+$ CD4$^+$ NKT cells is required for the induction of allergic inflammation by IL-25. Because the amounts of the endogenously produced IL-25 in the lung are limited, it is suggested that, in a physiologic setting, IL-25 needs memory Th2 cells and/or IL-25R$^+$ CD4$^+$ NKT cells to exert its function on allergic inflammation.

IL-15

The basis of IL-15

Two groups have independently discovered IL-15 to be a cytokine with IL-2-like action on T cells [51,52]. In contrast with IL-2, which is mainly produced by activated T cells, IL-15 is produced by monocytes, macrophages, DCs, and epithelial cells in the thymus, kidney, skin, and intestines [53], and the production is regulated by transcriptional as well as posttranscriptional mechanisms [54].

IL-15 binds to a receptor complex that consists of the IL-15Rα, IL-2Rβ, and the common cytokine receptor γ chain (γc), and activates Jak1/Jak3 and STAT5 [55]. IL-15R is expressed on CD8$^+$ T cells, NK cells, NKT cells, γδT cells, monocytes, macrophages, DCs, and neutrophils [53]. Consistent with

201

the pattern of the receptor expression, IL-15 plays important roles in the innate and adaptive immune system [53] and is essential for the development, proliferation, function, and survival of CD8+ T cells, NK cells, and NKT cells. On the other hand, IL-15 does not affect CD4+ T cells [56]. Indeed, IL-15-deficient mice [57] as well as IL-15Rα-deficient mice [58] show a marked reduction in the number of CD8+ T cells (especially CD44[high] memory CD8+ T cells), NK cells, NKT cells, and γδT cells, but show normal numbers of CD4+ T cells and B cells.

The role of IL-15 in allergic airway inflammation

The role of IL-15 in allergic diseases including asthma remains controversial. It has been shown that enforced expression of IL-15 by transgene attenuates antigen-induced Th2 cytokine production and eosinophil recruitment in the airways through the induction of IFN-γ-producing CD8+ T cells [59]. However, while antigen-induced Th2 cytokine production and antigen-specific IgE production are normally induced in IL-15-deficient mice after sensitization with antigen, eosinophil infiltration into the nasal mucosa and antigen-induced Th2 cytokine production by regional lymph node cells are aggravated in antigen-sensitized IL-15-deficient mice after intranasal challenge with antigen [60]. Transfer experiments of antigen-specific CD8+ T cells then suggest that IL-15 attenuates Th2 responses at the effector phase of experimental allergic rhinitis by activation of antigen-specific CD8+ T cells [60]. On the contrary, a recent study has shown that the blocking of endogenous IL-15 during the sensitization phase by a soluble IL-15Rα attenuates the induction of antigen-specific Th2 cell differentiation and subsequent antigen-induced, Th2 cell-mediated airway inflammation [61]. These discrepancies could be accounted for by the broad distribution of IL-15Rα. IFN-γ-producing CD8+ T cells, which are major IL-15-responding cells, are potent suppressor for Th2 cell-mediated allergic inflammation, whereas DCs, the function of which depends on IL-15, are required for the mounting of antigen-specific Th2 cells.

In human asthmatics, Komai-Koma *et al.* [62] have reported that IL-15 levels are increased in sputum fluid from steroid-treated asthmatics and that the expression of IL-15 is localized specifically to macrophages. By contrast, the other group has shown that

the number of IL-15-producing cells is normal in the airways of steroid-treated asthmatics [63]. The association between the single nucleotide polymorphism of IL-15 gene and asthma is reported by one group [64] but other groups deny the association [65,66]. Further studies are required in order to understand the role of IL-15 in asthma.

Acknowledgment

This work was supported in part by Grants-in-Aids for Scientific Research from the Ministry of Education, Culture, Sports, Science and Technology, the Japanese Government, and by the Global COE Program (Global Center for Education and Research in Immune System Regulation and Treatment), MEXT, Japan.

References

1 Moseley TA, Haudenschild DR, Rose L, *et al.* Interleukin-17 family and IL-17 receptors. *Cytokine Growth Factor Rev* 2003; **14**: 155–74.

2 Hymowitz SG, Filvaroff EH, Yin JP, *et al.* IL-17s adopt a cysteine knot fold: structure and activity of a novel cytokine, IL-17F, and implications for receptor binding. *EMBO J* 2001; **20**: 5332–41.

3 McGeachy MJ, Cua DJ. Th17 cell differentiation: the long and winding road. *Immunity* 2008; **28**: 445–53.

4 Korn T, Bettelli E, Oukka M, *et al.* IL-17 and Th17 cells. *Annu Rev Immunol* 2009; **27**: 485–517.

5 Toy D, Kugler D, Wolfson M, *et al.* Interleukin 17 signals through a heteromeric receptor complex. *J Immunol* 2006; **177**: 36–9.

6 Wright JF, Bennett F, Li B, *et al.* The human IL-17F/IL-17A heterodimeric cytokine signals through the IL-17RA/IL-17RC receptor complex. *J Immunol* 2008; **181**: 2799–805.

7 Oppmann B, Lesley R, Blom B, *et al.* Novel p19 protein engages IL-12p40 to form a cytokine, IL-23: with biological activities similar as well as distinct from IL-12. *Immunity* 2000; **13**: 715–25.

8 Langrish CL, Chen Y, Blumenschein WM, *et al.* IL-23 drives a pathogenic T cell population that induces autoimmune inflammation. *J Exp Med* 2005; **201**: 233–40.

9 Weaver CT, Harrington LE, Mangan PR, *et al.* Th17: an effector CD4 T cell lineage with regulatory T cell ties. *Immunity* 2006; **24**: 677–88.

10 McGeachy MJ, Bak-Jensen KS, Chen Y, *et al.* TGF-β and IL-6 drive the production of IL-17 and IL-10 by T

cells and restrain TH17 cell-mediated pathology. *Nat Immunol* 2007; **8**: 1390–7.

11 Busse WW, Lemanske RF, Jr. Asthma. *New Engl J Med* 2001; **344**: 350–62.

12 Umetsu DT, McIntire JJ, Akbari O, *et al.* Asthma: an epidemic of dysregulated. *Immunity Nat Immunol* 2002; **3**: 715–20.

13 Herrick CA, Bottomly K. To respond or not to respond: T cells in allergic asthma. *Nat Rev Immunol* 2003; **3**: 405–12.

14 Hellings PW, Kasran A, Liu Z, *et al.* Interleukin-17 orchestrates the granulocyte influx into airways after allergen inhalation in a mouse model of allergic asthma. *Am J Respir Cell Mol Biol* 2003; **28**: 42–50.

15 Oda N, Canelos PB, Essayan DM, *et al.* Interleukin-17F induces pulmonary neutrophilia and amplifies antigen-induced allergic response. *Am J Respir Crit Care Med* 2005; **171**: 12–18.

16 Molet S, Hamid Q, Davoine F, *et al.* IL-17 is increased in asthmatic airways and induces human bronchial fibroblasts to produce cytokines. *J Allergy Clin Immunol* 2001; **108**: 430–8.

17 Iwakura Y, Nakae S, Saijo S, *et al.* The roles of IL-17A in inflammatory immune responses and host defense against pathogens. *Immunol Rev* 2008; **266**: 55–79.

18 Jatakanon A, Uasuf C, Maziak W, *et al.* Neutrophilic inflammation in severe persistent asthma. *Am J Respir Crit Care Med* 1999; **160**: 1532–9.

19 Louis R, Lau LC, Bron AO, *et al.* The relationship between airways inflammation and asthma severity. *Am J Respir Crit Care Med* 2000; **161**: 9–16.

20 McKinley L, Alcorn JF, Peterson A, *et al.* TH17 cells mediate steroid-resistant airway inflammation and airway hyperresponsiveness in mice. *J Immunol* 2008; **181**: 4089–97.

21 Schnyder-Candrian S, Togbe D, Couillin I, *et al.* Interleukin-17 is a negative regulator of established allergic asthma. *J Exp Med* 2006; **203**: 2715–25.

22 Wakashin H, Hirose K, Maezawa Y, *et al.* IL-23 and Th17 cells enhance Th2 cell-mediated eosinophilic airway inflammation in mice. *Am J Respir Crit Care Med* 2008; **178**: 1023–32.

23 Haworth O, Cernadas M, Yang R, *et al.* Resolvin E1 regulates interleukin 23: interferon-γ and lipoxin A4 to promote the resolution of allergic airway inflammation. *Nat Immunol* 2008; **9**: 873–9.

24 Nakae S, Komiyama Y, Nambu A, *et al.* Antigen-specific T cell sensitization is impaired in IL-17-deficient mice, causing suppression of allergic cellular and humoral responses. *Immunity* 2002; **17**: 375–87.

25 Pichavant M, Goya S, Meyer EH, *et al.* Ozone exposure in a mouse model induces airway hyperreactivity that requires the presence of natural killer T cells and IL-17. *J Exp Med* 2008; **205**: 385–93.

26 Yang XO, Chang SH, Park H, *et al.* Regulation of inflammatory responses by IL-17F. *J Exp Med* 2008; **205**: 1063–75.

28 Leonard WJ Spolski R. Interleukin-21: a modulator of lymphoid proliferation, apoptosis and differentiation. *Nat Rev Immunol* 2005; **5**: 688–98.

27 Mehta DS, Wurster AL, Grusby MJ. Biology of IL-21 and the IL-21 receptor. *Immunol Rev* 2004; **202**: 84–95.

29 Nurieva R, Yang XO, Martinez G, *et al.* Essential autocrine regulation by IL-21 in the generation of inflammatory T cells. *Nature* 2007; **448**: 480–3.

30 Zhou L, Ivanov II, Spolski R, *et al.* IL-6 programs Th-17 cell differentiation by promoting sequential engagement of the IL-21 and IL-23 pathways. *Nat Immunol* 2007; **8**: 967–74.

31 Korn T, Bettelli E, Gao W, *et al.* IL-21 initiates an alternative pathway to induce proinflammatory Th17 cells. *Nature* 2008; **448**: 484–7.

32 Suto A, Kashiwakuma D, Kagami S-I, *et al.* Development and characterization of IL-21-producing CD4$^+$ T cells. *J Exp Med* 2008; **205**: 1369–79.

33 Zheng Y, Danilenko DM, Valdez P, *et al.* Interleukin-22: a Th17 cytokine, mediates IL-23-induced dermal inflammation and acanthosis. *Nature* 2007; **445**: 648–51.

34 Suto A, Nakajima H, Hirose K, *et al.* Interleukin-21 prevents antigen-induced IgE production by inhibiting germline Cε transcription of IL-4-stimulated B cells. *Blood* 2002; **100**: 4565–73.

35 Hoeck J, Woisetschlager M. STAT6 mediates eotaxin-1 expression in IL-4 or TNF-α-induced fibroblasts. *J Immunol* 2001; **166**: 4507–15.

36 Barry MA, Hargadon B, Shelley M, *et al.* Evidence of a role of tumor necrosis factor α in refractory asthma. *N Engl J Med* 2006; **354**: 697–708.

37 Acosta-Rodriguez EV, Rivino L, Geginat J, *et al.* Surface phenotype and antigenic specificity of human interleukin 17-producing T helper memory cells. *Nat Immunol* 2007; **8**: 639–46.

38 LeibundGut-Landmann S, Gross O, Robinson MJ, *et al.* Syk- and CARD9-dependent coupling of innate immunity to the induction of T helper cells that produce interleukin 17. *Nat Immunol* 2007; **8**: 630–8.

39 Fort MM, Cheung J, Yen D, *et al.* IL-25: a novel molecule that induces IL-4: IL-5: and IL-13 and Th2-associated pathologies *in vivo*. *Immunity* 2001; **15**: 985–95.

40 Hurst SD, Muchamuel T, Gorman DM, *et al.* New IL-17 family members promote Th1 or Th2 responses in the lung: *In vivo* function of the novel cytokine IL-25. *J Immunol* 2002; **169**: 443–53.

41 Pan G, French D, Mao W, *et al.* Forced expression of murine IL-17E induces growth retardation, jaundice, a Th2-biased response, and multiorgan inflammation in mice. *J Immunol* 2001; **167**: 6559–67.

42 Lee J, Ho WH, Maruoka M, *et al*. IL-17E, a novel proinflammatory ligand for the IL-17 receptor homolog IL-17Rh1. *J Biol Chem* 2001; **276**: 1660–4.

43 Ikeda K, Nakajima H, Suzuki K, *et al*. Mast cells produce interleukin-25 upon FcεRI-mediated activation. *Blood* 2003; **101**: 3594–6.

44 Angkasekwinai P, Park H, Wang YH, *et al*. Interleukin 25 promotes the initiation of proallergic type 2 responses. *J Exp Med* 2007; **204**: 1509–17.

45 Wang YH, Angkasekwinai P, Lu N, *et al*. IL-25 augments type 2 immune responses by enhancing the expansion and functions of TSLP-DC-activated Th2 memory cells. *J Exp Med* 2007; **204**: 1837–47.

46 Tamachi T, Maezawa Y, Ikeda K, *et al*. IL-25 enhances allergic airway inflammation by amplifying a Th2 cell-dependent pathway in mice. *J Allergy Clin Immunol* 2006; **118**: 606–14.

47 Ballantyne SJ, Barlow JL, Jolin HE, *et al*. Blocking IL-25 prevents airway hyperresponsiveness in allergic asthma. *J Allergy Clin Immunol* 2007; **120**: 1324–31.

48 Letuve S, Lajoie-Kadoch S, Audusseau S, *et al*. IL-17E upregulates the expression of proinflammatory cytokines in lung fibroblasts. *J Allergy Clin Immunol* 2006; **117**: 590–6.

49 Terashima A, Watarai H, Inoue S, *et al*. A novel subset of mouse NKT cells bearing the IL-17 receptor B responds to IL-25 and contributes to airway hyperreactivity. *J Exp Med* 2008; **205**: 2727–33.

50 Claudio E, Sønder SU, Saret S, *et al*. The adaptor protein CIKS/Act1 is essential for IL-25-mediated allergic airway inflammation. *J Immunol* 2009; **182**: 1617–30.

51 Burton JD, Bamford RN, Peters C, *et al*. A, lymphokine, provisionally designated interleukin T, and produced by a human adult T-cell leukemia line, stimulates T-cell proliferation and the induction of lymphokine-activated killer cells. *Proc Natl Acad Sci USA* 1994; **91**: 4935–9.

52 Carson WE, Giri JG, Lindemann MJ, *et al*. Interleukin (IL) 15 is a novel cytokine that activates human natural killer cells via components of the IL-2 receptor. *J Exp Med* 1994; **180**: 1395–403

53 Fehniger TA, Caligiuri MA. Interleukin 15: biology and relevance to human disease. *Blood* 2001; **97**: 14–32.

54 Bamford RN, Battiata AP, Burton JD, *et al*. Interleukin (IL) 15/IL-T production by the adult T-cell leukemia cell line HuT-102 is associated with a human T-cell lymphotrophic virus type I region/IL-15 fusion message that lacks many upstream AUGs that normally attenuates IL-15 mRNA, translation. *Proc Natl Acad Sci USA* 1996; **93**: 2897–902.

55 Rochman Y, Spolski R, Leonard WJ. New insights into the regulation of T cells by γc family cytokines. *Nat Rev Immunol* 2009; **9**: 480–90.

56 Zhang X, Sun S, Hwang I, *et al*. Potent and selective stimulation of memory-phenotype CD8+ T cells *in vivo* by IL-15. *Immunity* 1998; **8**: 591–9.

57 Kennedy MK, Glaccum M, Brown SN, *et al*. Reversible defects in natural killer and memory CD8 T cell lineages in interleukin 15-deficient mice. *J Exp Med* 2000; **191**: 771–80.

58 Lodolce JP, Boone DL, Chai S, *et al*. IL-15 receptor maintains lymphoid homeostasis by supporting lymphocyte homing and proliferation. *Immunity* 1998; **9**: 669–76.

59 Ishimitsu R, Nishimura H, Yajima T, *et al*. Overexpression of IL-15 *in vivo* enhances Tc1 response, which inhibits allergic inflammation in a murine model of asthma. *J Immunol* 2001; **166**: 1991–2001.

60 Aoi N, Masuda T, Murakami D, *et al*. IL-15 prevents allergic rhinitis through reactivation of antigen-specific CD8+ cells. *J Allergy Clin Immunol* 2006; **117**: 1359–66.

61 Rückert R, Brandt K, Braun A, *et al*. Blocking IL-15 prevents the induction of allergen-specific T cells and allergic inflammation *in vivo*. *J Immunol* 2005; **174**: 5507–15.

62 Komai-Koma M, McKay A, Thomson L, *et al*. Immunoregulatory cytokines in asthma: IL-15 and IL-13 in induced sputum. *Clin Exp Allergy* 2001; **31**: 1441-1448.

63 Muro S, Taha R, Tsicopoulos A, *et al*. Expression of IL-15 in inflammatory pulmonary diseases. *J Allergy Clin Immunol* 2001; **108**: 970–5.

64 Kurz T, Strauch K, Dietrich H, *et al*. Multilocus haplotype analyses reveal association between 5 novel IL-15 polymorphisms and asthma. *J Allergy Clin Immunol* 2004; **113**: 896–901.

65 Christensen U, Haagerup A, Binderup HG, *et al*. Family based association analysis of the IL-2 and IL-15 genes in allergic disorders. *Eur J Hum Genet* 2006; **14**: 227–235.

66 Pinto LA, Depner M, Steudemann L, *et al*. IL-15 gene variants are not associated with asthma and atopy. *Allergy* 2009; **64**: 643–6.

16 Thymic stromal lymphopoietin

Kazuhiko Arima[1] and Yong-Jun Liu[2]

[1]Department of Biomolecular Sciences, Division of Medical Biochemistry, Saga Medical School, Saga, Japan

[2]Department of Immunology and Center for Cancer Immunology Research, The University of Texas M. D. Anderson Cancer Center, Houston, TX, USA

Introduction

Thymic stromal lymphopoietin (TSLP) was originally identified as a lymphocyte growth-promoting factor in mice. Recent evidence has demonstrated that TSLP is a critical factor for allergic inflammation by serving as a link between epithelial cells and immune responses. Numerous studies have documented constitutive and upregulated expression of TSLP in multiple cell types under various pathophysiologic settings, particularly epithelial cells in allergic diseases. However, the precise signal transduction mechanism of TSLP has not yet been fully elucidated. In this chapter, we will focus on the role of TSLP in the context of allergic inflammation. To learn more about the role of TSLP in the development and homeostasis of lymphocytes and in the generation of regulatory T cells, we recommend two recent review articles [1,2].

TSLP and TSLP receptor

Thymic stromal lymphopoietin is an interleukin 7 (IL-7)-like four-helix bundle cytokine that was first isolated from a mouse thymic stromal cell line and shown to support B-cell development in the absence of IL-7 [3,4]. Mouse and human TSLP share a poor amino acid homology of 43% [4–6]. The human TSLP (hTSLP) gene was mapped to chromosome 5q22.1, which is adjacent to one of the reported asthma susceptible loci, 5q23–31, where Th2 cytokine genes are clustered [7].

Although epithelial cells appear to be the major source of TSLP [6,8], other cell types, such as fibroblasts, smooth muscle cells, mast cells and basophils, also have the potential to produce TSLP [8,9].

The TSLP receptor (TSLPR) is a heterodimeric receptor complex comprising the TSLPR and the IL-7Rα chains [6,10–13] (Figure 16.1). The TSLPR chain is most closely related to the IL-2Rγ chain (γ_c). The extracellular portion of the TSLPR chain is predicted to be composed of two immunoglobulin-like folds that may form a cytokine recognition homology (CRH) domain. It contains a WSXWS-like motif, a signature for type I cytokine receptor [14]. The intracellular portion of the TSLPR chain harbors a "Box 1" motif and a single tyrosine residue, both of which are involved in signal transduction upon TSLP binding [15,16]. TSLP binds to the TSLPR chain with a low affinity, but does not show any affinity to the IL-7Rα chain alone [12,13]. However, the combination of TSLPR and IL-7Rα chains results in high-affinity binding to TSLP and transduces STAT3 and STAT5 activation upon TSLP binding [6,11].

TSLP in allergic inflammation

TSLP induces innate allergic immune responses by activating myeloid dendritic cells, mast cells, and natural killer T cells

Following the identification of TSLP and TSLPR, hTSLP was found to dramatically and uniquely

Inflammation and Allergy Drug Design, First Edition. Edited by Kenji Izuhara, Stephen T. Holgate, Marsha Wills-Karp.
© 2011 Blackwell Publishing Ltd. Published 2011 by Blackwell Publishing Ltd.

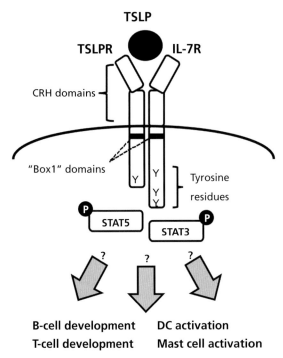

TSLP

TSLPR **IL-7R**

CRH domains

"Box1" domains

Tyrosine residues

STAT5 STAT3

? ? ?

B-cell development **DC activation**
T-cell development **Mast cell activation**

Figure 16.1 TSLP and TSLP receptor structure and function. The functional TSLP receptor complex consists of the TSLPR and IL-7Rα chains. The extracellular domains of these chains comprise the cytokine recognition homology (CRH) domains. The intracellular domains of both receptor chains contain "Box1" domains and tyrosine residues that are involved in signal transduction, including STAT3 and STAT5 activation.

Table 16.1 Myeloid dendritic cell (mDC) maturation triggered by different activators.

	TSLP	CD40L	TLRLs
CD80/CD86	Up	Up	Up
MHC class II	Up	Up	Up
Survival	Up	Up	Up
IL-1 α/β	–	++	++
IL-6	–	++	++
IL-12	–	++	++
IFNs	–	++	++
IP-10	–	++	++
Eotaxin 2	++	–	–
IL-8	++	++	++
TARC	++	–	+
MDC	++	+	+

Thymic stromal lymphopoietin (TSLP) induces mDC maturation that is uncoupled from interleukin 12 (IL-12) production. It upregulates major histocompatibility complex (MHC) class II and multiple co-stimulatory molecules, promotes cell survival, and induces secretion of chemokines (but not production of pro-inflammatory cytokines) such as IL-12. These phenotypic properties instruct DCs to promote T helper 2 (Th2) responses.

activate CD11c+ myeloid dendritic cells (mDCs) [6]. The ability of mDCs to respond to TSLP is consistent with the finding that mDCs express the highest levels of both TSLPR mRNA and protein among all human hematopoietic cell types [6,8,17]. Dendritic cells (DCs) can be activated by many distinct classes of agents and promote T-cell proliferation and differentiation [18]. Like other mDCs, activators, including CD40L and TLR ligands (TLRLs) such as lipopolysaccharide (LPS), poly(I:C) and R848, TSLP strongly upregulates the expression of major histocompatibility complex (MHC) class II, CD54, CD80, CD83, CD86, and DC-LAMP on human mDCs [8]. However, unlike CD40L and TLRLs, TSLP does not stimulate mDCs to produce the Th1-polarizing cytokines IL-12 and type I interferons (IFNs) or the proinflammatory cytokines tumor necrosis factor (TNF), IL-1β, and

IL-6 (Table 16.1) [8]. Instead, TSLP causes mDCs to produce large amounts of the chemokines IL-8 and eotaxin 2 (CCL24), which attract neutrophils and eosinophils, followed by production of thymus and activation-regulated chemokine (TARC) (CCL17) and macrophage-derived chemokine (MDC) (CCL22), which attract Th2 cells. A more recent study showed that hTSLP potently activates mast cells to produce the cytokines IL-5, IL-6, IL-13, and GM-CSF, along with the chemokines IL-8 and I-309 (CCL1) in the presence of IL-1β and TNF [19]. Another study showed that mouse TSLP (mTSLP) potentially activates natural killer T (NKT) cells to produce IL-13 in a mouse model of asthma [20]. These studies collectively suggest that TSLP produced by epithelial cells rapidly induces an innate phase of allergic inflammatory responses by activating mDCs, mast cells and NKT cells to produce Th2 cytokines, chemokines, and proinflammatory cytokines (Figure 16.2). The role of TSLP in the triggering of an early innate phase of allergic inflammation is supported by *in vivo* observations that TSLP can induce skin inflammation

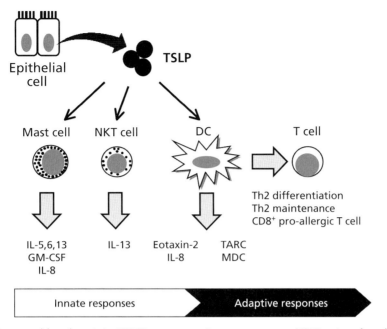

Figure 16.2 Thymic stromal lymphopoietin (TSLP)-induced allergic immune responses. Damaged epithelial cells produce TSLP, which activates mast cells, natural killer T (NKT) cells, and dendritic cells (DCs) to produce various cytokines and chemokines to induce innate immune responses. TSLP-activated myeloid DCs (mDCs) promote adaptive allergic immune responses of both CD4⁺ and CD8⁺ T cells. GM-CSF, granulocyte–macrophage colony-stimulating factor.

consisting of dermal infiltrates of mast cells and eosinophils without IgE production in T-cell-deficient mice [21] and moderate airway inflammation in B- and T-cell-deficient mice [22].

TSLP triggers adaptive allergic immune responses via mDCs

TSLP-DCs induce inflammatory Th2 cells
When co-cultured with allogeneic CD4⁺ T cells *in vitro*, TSLP-activated mDCs (TSLP-DCs) induce a unique type of Th2 cells that produces the classic Th2 cytokines IL-4, IL-5, and IL-13 with large amounts of TNF but little or no IL-10 [8]. Although not typically considered a Th2 cytokine, TNF is prominent in asthmatic airways, and genotypes that correlate with increased TNF secretion are associated with an increased risk of asthma [23], suggesting that TNF plays an important role in the development of asthma and allergic inflammation. IL-10, initially classified as a Th2 cytokine, counteracts inflammation [24] and is produced at decreased levels in bronchoalveolar lavage

fluid from atopic patients compared with normal subjects [25]. Recent studies show that IL-10 derived from DCs or T cells prevents airway hypersensitivity after allergen exposure [26,27]. Thus, decreased IL-10 production by TSLP-DCs agrees with these observations for establishing allergic inflammation. Because of their unique profile of cytokine production, we propose that Th2 cells induced by TSLP-DCs be called inflammatory Th2 cells, in contrast to the conventional Th2 cells. The pathogenic T cells involved in allergic diseases such as atopic dermatitis and asthma are likely to be inflammatory Th2 cells.

TSLP-DCs express a Th2-polarizing molecule, OX40L
To delineate the molecular mechanism by which TSLP-DCs induce TNF-producing inflammatory Th2 cells, a gene expression analysis was performed on immature human mDCs that were unstimulated or stimulated by TSLP, poly(I:C), or CD40L [28,29]. This analysis showed that TSLP selectively induces human mDCs to express the TNF superfamily protein

OX40L (TNFSF4) [28]. The expression of OX40L by TSLP-DCs is critical for the induction of inflammatory Th2 cells, as blocking OX40L with neutralizing antibodies (Abs) inhibits the production of Th2 cytokines and TNF, and enhances the production of IL-10 by the CD4+ T cells. Consistent with these results, treating naïve T cells with recombinant OX40L promotes the production of TNF but inhibits the production of IL-10. It was demonstrated that OX40L signaling in T cells directly induces Th2 lineage commitment by inducing NFATc1, which triggers IL-4 production followed by IL-4-dependent GATA-3 transcription [30].

TSLP-DCs provide a permissive condition for Th2 development

One of the key features of TSLP-DCs is their expression of all the major co-stimulatory molecules and OX40L, that is uncoupled from IL-12 production. In the presence of exogenous IL-12, TSLP-DCs or recombinant OX40L lose the ability to induce Th2 differentiation [28]. We thus conclude that TSLP-DCs create a Th2-permissive microenvironment by upregulating OX40L without inducing the production of Th1-polarizing cytokines. The dominance of IL-12 over OX40L may provide a molecular explanation for the hygiene hypothesis, which proposes that microbial infections triggering Th1 responses may decrease the subsequent development of Th2-driven atopy. Historically, two models have been proposed to explain how Th2 development is initiated: (i) Th2 differentiation requires a positive Th2-polarizing signal and (ii) Th2 development is initiated by a default mechanism in the absence of IL-12 (Figure 16.3) [31]. Our findings suggest that these two models are not mutually exclusive and that Th2 differentiation requires a positive-polarizing signal, such as OX40L, as well as a default mechanism (the absence of IL-12).

TSLP-DCs maintain Th2 memory cells

Recent studies have suggested that Th2 memory cells are the principal cell population responsible for the maintenance of chronic allergic inflammation and the rapid relapse of acute allergic inflammation upon re-exposure to allergens [32]. At the sites of allergic inflammation, DCs are in close contact with epithelial cells and function not only in priming Th2-mediated immune responses, but also in sustaining the allergic inflammation by maintaining the allergen-specific Th2 memory cells. TSLP-DCs can induce a robust expansion of human Th2 memory cells while maintaining their central memory phenotype and Th2 commitment through an IL-7- and IL-15-independent mechanism, demonstrating that TSLP contributes to the maintenance and relapse of Th2-mediated allergic diseases by expanding Th2 memory cells [29]. The immediate production of IL-5 by Th2 memory cells upon activation *in situ* may contribute to the recruitment and survival of eosinophils, which augments allergic inflammation [33].

TSLP-DCs induce proallergic CD8+ T cells

Activation of CD4+ T cells is a hallmark of allergic inflammation and plays an important role in this response. However, there is now broader evidence that CD8+ T cells, once regarded solely as potent cytotoxic effectors in antiviral and antitumoral immunity, also participate in allergic inflammation and secrete Th2 cytokines [34]. TSLP-DCs induce the activation and

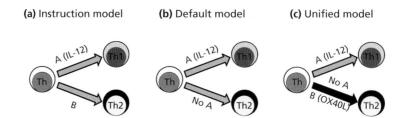

Figure 16.3 Models for the regulation of T helper 1 (Th1) and Th2 differentiation. (a) Instruction model. Th1/2 differentiation depends on respective signals A (interleukin 12 [IL-12]) and B (unknown). (b) Default model. Th1 differentiation requires the Th1-polarizing signal A, but Th2 differentiation occurs spontaneously in the absence of the Th1-polarizing signal A (no A). (c) Unified model. Th1/2 differentiation depends on respective signals A (IL-12) and B (OX40L). However, the Th1-polarizing signal A is dominant over the Th2-polarizing signal B. The Th2-polarizing signal B can induce a Th2 response only in the absence of Th1-polarizing signals.

differentiation of CD8[+] T cells into IL-5- and IL-13-producing T cells, without inducing a strong cytolytic function [35]. Additional stimulation of TSLP-DCs by CD40L induces the differentiation of CD8[+] T cells into effectors that produce both Th1 (IFN-γ) and Th2 (IL-5 and IL-13) cytokines and exhibit potent cytolytic activity. These data support the role of TSLP as an initial trigger of allergic T-cell responses by activating not only CD4[+] T cells but also CD8[+] T cells. CD40L-expressing cells may act in combination with TSLP to amplify and sustain proallergic responses and cause tissue damage by promoting the generation of IFN-γ-producing cytotoxic effectors [35].

The association of TSLP with human allergic diseases

Thymic stromal lymphopoietin mRNA is highly expressed by human primary skin keratinocytes, bronchial epithelial cells, smooth muscle cells, and lung fibroblasts but not by most hematopoietic cells except mast cells [8]. TSLP protein is undetectable in normal skin or nonlesional skin in patients with atopic dermatitis, but it is highly expressed in acute and chronic atopic dermatitis lesions [8]. In atopic skin, TSLP production is a feature of fully differentiated keratinocytes (Figure 16.4). Furthermore, TSLP

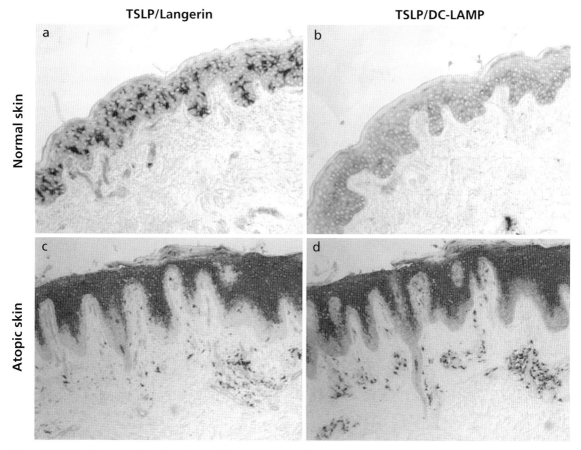

Figure 16.4 Thymic stromal lymphopoietin (TSLP) expression in atopic dermatitis associated with Langerhans cell migration and activation. (a) Normal skin contains Langerin[+] Langerhans cells in epidermis but does not express TSLP. (b) Normal skin does not contain DC-LAMP[+]-activated dendritic cells (DCs) in epidermis and dermis. (c) In a skin lesion of atopic dermatitis, high expression of TSLP (dark grey in epidermis) is associated with the migration of Langerhans cells from epidermis to dermis. (d) The expression of TSLP in a skin lesion of atopic dermatitis is associated with the appearance of DC-LAMP[+]-activated DCs in dermis.

expression in patients with atopic dermatitis is associated with Langerhans cell migration and activation *in situ*, suggesting that TSLP contributes to the activation of these cells, which could migrate into the draining lymph nodes and prime allergen-specific Th2 responses [18]. A recent study showed that TSLP protein expression is upregulated in skin lesions from patients with Netherton syndrome, a severe genetic skin disease with a constant atopic manifestation caused by mutations in the *SPINK5* gene, suggesting a common role of TSLP in the pathogenesis of dermatitis with atopic characteristics [36]. TSLP expression is also increased in asthmatic airways examined by *in situ* hybridization and correlates with both the expression of Th2-attracting chemokines and disease severity, thus providing the first link between TSLP and human asthma [37]. More recently, studies showed that TSLP is highly upregulated in nasal epithelial cells of allergic rhinitis patients [38] and conjunctival epithelial cells of vernal keratoconjunctivitis and atopic keratoconjunctivitis patients [39], further suggesting a common role of TSLP in human allergic diseases.

TSLP function in animal models

Atopic dermatitis

Mice engineered to overexpress TSLP in the skin (under the control of the keratin 5 promoter) develop atopic dermatitis characterized by eczematous skin lesions containing inflammatory cell infiltrates, a dramatic increase in circulating Th2 cells, and elevated serum IgE levels [21]. This study also suggested that TSLP might directly activate DCs in mice. In another study, mice lacking the retinoid X receptor (RXR) selectively in epidermal keratinocytes also develop atopic dermatitis [40]. Detailed analysis revealed that the RXR-deficient keratinocytes overexpress TSLP. The authors established transgenic mice overexpressing TSLP in the skin (under the keratin 14 promoter) and found that they develop atopic dermatitis, confirming the link between TSLP, and the development of atopic dermatitis. More recently, it was demonstrated that keratinocytes from Spink5-deficient mice induce TSLP expression and atopic dermatitis-like lesions when transplanted to nude mice. Spink5 is a serine protease inhibitor and its loss leads to overproduction of kallikrein 5, which binds to protease

activated receptor 2 (PAR-2) to activate nuclear factor (NF)-κB and MAPK pathways, resulting in production of TSLP [36]. Another recent study demonstrated that intradermal injection of anti-TSLP Abs blocks the development of allergic skin inflammation after cutaneous antigen challenge of ovalbumin-immunized mice [41].

Asthma

Mice lacking TSLPR fail to develop asthma in response to inhaled antigen [22,42]. In complementary studies, lung-specific expression of a TSLP transgene in mice induces allergic airway inflammation (asthma) characterized by a massive infiltration of leukocytes (including Th2 cells), goblet cell hyperplasia, and subepithelial fibrosis, as well as by increased serum IgE, levels [22]. Although TSLP can induce a moderate airway inflammation independent of T and B cells as mentioned above, the full development of TSLP-mediated asthma-like symptoms depends on antigenic stimulation and CD4+ T cells [43]. In addition, the lung-specific TSLP transgenic mice do not have asthma-like airway inflammation if STAT6 is deficient or if the function of IL-4 and IL-13 is simultaneously blocked with anti-IL-4Rα Abs, indicating that Th2 responses downstream of TSLP are critical components of asthma pathogenesis [44]. Administration of TSLP protein directly into mouse airways causes asthmatic inflammation, which can be blocked by administration of neutralizing Abs to OX40L [45]. This study also showed that in a rhesus monkey model of dust mite-induced asthma there are elevated expression levels of both TSLP and OX40L in the lung. Treatment with anti-OX40L Abs reduces the number of infiltrating cells and levels of the Th2 cytokines IL-5 and IL-13 in the lung, indicating that OX40L is an essential molecule for the induction of allergic inflammation triggered by TSLP [45].

Intestinal parasite infection

In addition to the allergic Th2 immune responses, TSLP has also been demonstrated to play a key role in the development of a protective Th2 immunity in the gut, which is critical for controlling parasite infection as well as maintaining mucosal immune homeostasis by limiting Th1 or Th17 immune responses [46]. During infection by the parasite *Trichuris*, intestinal epithelial cells deficient in IKK-β fail to produce TSLP, leading to impaired protective Th2 responses and uncontrolled Th1 and Th17 inflammatory responses. Most strikingly, TSLPR-knockout mice fail to mount effective Th2 immunity upon *Trichuris* infection, exhibit a high worm burden and take more time to resolve the infection, showing an essential function of TSLP in establishing protective Th2 immune responses against parasites in the gut mucosa [47].

TSLP production is controlled by NF-κB pathway

Thymic stromal lymphopoietin expression is widely observed among allergic diseases. Transcription of TSLP appears to be regulated by the NF-κB pathway, which is triggered by multiple stimuli, such as inflammatory cytokines (TNF and IL-1) and multiple TLRLs (TLR2, -3, -8, and -9) [19,48,49], and is further modulated by various cytokines [49–51]. Induction of TSLP by poly(I:C) in keratinocytes is synergistically upregulated by Th2 cytokines or type I IFNs and downregulated by IFN-γ, TGF-β, or IL-17 [51]. TSLP production is even induced upon physical injury of normal keratinocytes or loss of epidermal integrity [19,52]. It has also been reported that the nuclear receptors RXR, retinoic acid receptor (RAR), and vitamin D receptor (VDR) are involved in the repression of TSLP, transcription in mouse keratinocytes [40,53]. Recent exciting findings that papain [54] and kallikrein 5 [36] activate PAR-2 to induce TSLP expression in bronchial epithelial cells and keratinocytes, respectively, agree well with the previous findings that administration of house dust mite extract, which has protease activity, to nonhuman primate airway induces TSLP expression by bronchial epithelial cells [45] while papain induces TSLP expression by basophils [9]. Protease-mediated PAR-2 stimulation induces NF-κB pathway activation [55]. In humans, a single nucleotide polymorphism (SNP) within the *TSLP* promoter has been identified to potentially affect its transcriptional activity by altering an AP-1 binding sequence, and found to be associated with asthma susceptibility [56]. Further association studies of this SNP will be required to determine whether TSLP genetic polymorphisms significantly contribute to other forms of allergic disease in humans.

TSLP signal transduction in human primary mDCs

Upon binding with TSLP, the TSLP receptor complex generates intracellular signaling. Earlier studies demonstrated that TSLP induces STAT3 and STAT5 phosphorylation, resulting in transcription of STAT-responsive genes, such as *CIS* [6,10,11]. However, the precise kinase responsible for TSLP-mediated STAT phosphorylation has remained controversial [10,11,16]. It was demonstrated that JAK family kinases are not activated by mTSLP [10,11]. The "Box 1" motif and the tyrosine residue in the cytoplasmic domain of TSLPR have been shown to be critical for the TSLP signals [15].

The pleiotropic function of TSLP in human mDCs apparently cannot be explained by activation of STAT3 and STAT5 alone, which is ubiquitous in many cytokine signaling pathways. We recently performed a large-scale isolation of human primary mDCs to study cellular signaling triggered by TSLP [57] (Figure 16.5). In mDCs we found that hTSLP induces robust and sustained (<1 h) phosphorylation of JAK1 and JAK2, while hIL-7 induces transient (<5 min) phosphorylation of JAK1. Consequently, hTSLP induces broad and sustained (>2 h) phosphorylation of STAT1, STAT3, STAT4, STAT5, and STAT6. Direct STAT6 activation by TSLP seems to be the mechanism responsible for inducing TARC production [57]. In addition, hTSLP induces phosphorylation of AKT, and the MAPKs ERK and JNK, all are sensitive to JAK inhibitors. hTSLP also induces a slow but robust NF-κB activation, as revealed by sustained nuclear localization of p50, p52, and RelB.

How is OX40L selectively upregulated by TSLP-DCs? The promoter region of OX40L has two potential NF-κB binding elements. We found that TSLP induces a predominant and persistent nuclear translocation of the NF-κB molecule p50, which is not prolonged when induced by CD40L or TLRLs. Indeed, the OX40L promoter preferentially binds to p50 [57]. In a promoter-reporter assay, we also demonstrated that p50 plus RelB activates the OX40L promoter. These data suggest that predominant p50 activation triggered by TSLP is the determinant for selective upregulation of OX40L.

We further explored the molecular mechanisms of lack of IL-12 production in spite of DC maturation by

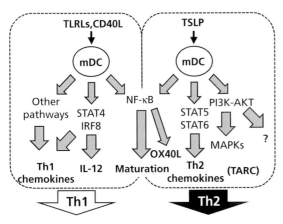

Figure 16.5 Distinct signal codes generate functional plasticity of dendritic cells (DCs). Myeloid DC (mDC) activators, such as TLRLs and CD40L, induce DC maturation and interleukin 12 (IL-12) production, thus promoting T helper 1 (Th1) responses. This IL-12 production is granted by expression and activation of STAT4 and IRF8. By contrast, TSLP induces DC maturation that is uncoupled from IL-12 production due to lack of the induction of STAT4 and IRF8 protein expression. TSLP robustly activates other STATs, including STAT6, leading to production of TARC, a Th2-attracting chemokine. Furthermore, TSLP uniquely induces OX40L expression by mDCs owing to its unique activation of the NF-κB pathway. Collectively, TSLP-activated mDCs induce Th2 responses.

TSLP. Unlike other DC activators that are capable of inducing expression of STAT4 and IRF8, transcription factors required for IL-12 production, TSLP fails to induce protein expression of these molecules (TSLP has the capacity to activate STAT4, but STAT4 protein expression is very low). DC maturation is contributed by NF-κB, activation triggered by most DC activators, as well as TSLP. STAT4 and IRF8 do not mediate DC maturation but are essential in IL-12 production [57].

Summary

We reviewed recent progress regarding roles of TSLP in the pathogenesis of allergic inflammation. Although cell types responding to TSLP, and mechanisms of TSLP signal transduction appear to be diverse among different species, the major cell type responsive to hTSLP is mDC. TSLP represents the factor that activates mDCs without inducing either Th1-polarizing

cytokines or proinflammatory cytokines. This sterile/aseptic way of activating DCs is in contrast to the way microbial components, such as TLRLs, activate DCs, and may explain the uniqueness of TSLP-DC function.

In inflammatory settings, such as atopic dermatitis, epithelial cells markedly increase TSLP expression. The increased local expression of TSLP leads to enhanced DC maturation and activation. The TSLP-activated DCs migrate to the draining lymph nodes, where they prime CD4+ and CD8+ T cells to produce Th2 inflammatory cytokines. Additional cells (eosinophils, neutrophils, and mast cells) are attracted to the site owing to the production of chemokines by the activated DCs and contribute to the subsequent pathology. This innate cell activation initiates the onset of allergic diseases, and the subsequent adaptive immunity-mediated disease process will shape the disease pathology. In this model, lymphocytes, especially CD4+ T cells, may act to amplify the existing pathology at the site of inflammation.

Important questions concerning the actual spatial and temporal role of TSLP in inflammatory responses *in vivo* and whether blockade of TSLP will be efficacious in the treatment of allergic inflammatory diseases remain. In addition to TSLP's critical role in disease initiation—to trigger naïve innate cells and Th2 responses—TSLP may also be involved in disease progression. The production of TSLP by activated mast cells and activation of mast cells by TSLP indicate TSLP's role in the progression of allergic diseases [8,19]. Recently, the existence of a mutually amplifying loop between TSLP and IL-13 in allergy was suggested, illuminating the critical involvement of TSLP in both the initiation and progression of allergic diseases [58]. The findings that anti-TSLP therapy is beneficial in the resolution of allergic symptoms [41,59] provides some promise that TSLP will be a therapeutic target for the treatment of allergic inflammatory disorders.

Acknowledgment

We thank Ms. Melissa J. Wentz for manuscript preparation and Drs. Shino Hanabuchi, Lu Ning, Yui-Hsi Wang, Tomoki Ito, and Norihiko Watanabe for helpful suggestions. Y.-J. L. is supported by M. D. Anderson Cancer Center Foundation and NIAID (AI061645 and U19 AI071130).

References

1 Ziegler SF, Liu YJ. Thymic stromal lymphopoietin in normal and pathogenic T cell development and function. *Nat Immunol* 2006; **7**: 709–14.

2 Liu YJ, Soumelis V, Watanabe N, *et al.* TSLP: an epithelial cell cytokine that regulates T-cell differentiation by conditioning dendritic cell maturation. *Ann Rev Immunol* 2007; **25**: 193–219.

3 Friend SL, Hosier S, Nelson A, *et al.* A thymic stromal cell line supports *in vitro* development of surface IgM⁺ B cells and produces a novel growth factor affecting B, and T, lineage cells. *Exp Hematol* 1994; **22**: 321–8.

4 Sims JE, Williams DE, Morrissey PJ, *et al.* Molecular cloning and biological characterization of a novel murine lymphoid growth factor. *J Exp Med* 2000; **192**: 671–80.

5 Quentmeier H, Drexler HG, Fleckenstein D, *et al.* Cloning of human thymic stromal lymphopoietin (TSLP) and signaling mechanisms leading to proliferation. *Leukemia* 2001; **15**: 1286–92.

6 Reche PA, Soumelis V, Gorman DM, *et al.* Human thymic stromal lymphopoietin preferentially stimulates myeloid cells. *J Immunol* 2001; **167**: 336–43.

7 The Collaborative Study on the Genetics of Asthma (CSGA). A genome-wide search for asthma susceptibility loci in ethnically diverse populations. *Nat Genet* 1997; **15**: 389–92.

8 Soumelis V, Reche PA, Kanzler H, *et al.* Human epithelial cells trigger dendritic cell mediated allergic inflammation by producing TSLP. *Nat Immunol* 2002; **3**: 673–80.

9 Sokol CL, Barton GM, Farr AG, Medzhitov R. A mechanism for the initiation of allergen-induced T helper type 2 responses. *Nat Immunol* 2008; **9**: 310–18.

10 Levin SD, Koelling RM, Friend SL, *et al.* Thymic stromal lymphopoietin: a cytokine that promotes the development of IgM⁺ B cells *in vitro* and signals via a novel mechanism. *J Immunol* 1999; **162**: 677–83.

11 Isaksen DE, Baumann H, Trobridge PA, *et al.* Requirement for STAT5 in thymic stromal lymphopoietin-mediated signal transduction. *J Immunol* 1999; **163**: 5971–7.

12 Park LS, Martin U, Garka K, *et al.* Cloning of the murine thymic stromal lymphopoietin (TSLP) receptor: Formation of a functional heteromeric complex requires interleukin 7 receptor. *J Exp Med* 2000; **192**: 659–70.

13 Pandey A, Ozaki K, Baumann H, *et al.* Cloning of a receptor subunit required for signaling by thymic stromal lymphopoietin. *Nat Immunol* 2000; **1**: 59–64.

14 Bazan JF. Structural design and molecular evolution of a cytokine receptor superfamily. *Proc Natl Acad Sci USA* 1990; **87**: 6934–8.

15 Isaksen DE, Baumann H, Zhou B, *et al.* Uncoupling of proliferation and STAT5 activation in thymic stromal lymphopoietin-mediated signal transduction. *J Immunol* 2002; **168**: 3288–94.

16 Carpino N, Thierfelder WE, Chang MS, *et al.* Absence of an essential role for thymic stromal lymphopoietin receptor in murine B-cell development. *Mol Cell Biol* 2004; **24**: 2584–92.

17 Lu N, Wang YH, Wang YH, *et al.* TSLP and IL-7 use two different mechanisms to regulate human CD4⁺ T cell homeostasis. *J Exp Med* 2009; **206**: 2111–19.

18 Banchereau J, Briere F, Caux C, *et al.* Immunobiology of dendritic cells. *Ann Rev Immunol* 2000; **18**: 767–811.

19 Allakhverdi Z, Comeau MR, Jessup HK, *et al.* Thymic stromal lymphopoietin is released by human epithelial cells in response to microbes, trauma, or inflammation and potently activates mast cells. *J Exp Med* 2007; **204**: 253–8.

20 Nagata Y, Kamijuku H, Taniguchi M, *et al.* Differential role of thymic stromal lymphopoietin in the induction of airway hyperreactivity and Th2 immune response in antigen-induced asthma with respect to natural killer T cell function. *Int Arch Allergy Immunol* 2007; **144**: 305–14.

21 Yoo J, Omori M, Gyarmati D, *et al.* Spontaneous atopic dermatitis in mice expressing an inducible thymic stromal lymphopoietin transgene specifically in the skin. *J Exp Med* 2005; **202**: 541–9.

22 Zhou B, Comeau MR, De Smedt T, *et al.* Thymic stromal lymphopoietin as a key initiator of allergic airway inflammation in mice. *Nat Immunol* 2005; **6**: 1047–53.

23 Moffatt MF, Cookson WO. Tumour necrosis factor haplotypes and asthma. *Hum Mol Genet* 1997; **6**: 551–4.

24 O'Garra A. Cytokines induce the development of functionally heterogeneous T helper cell subsets. *Immunity* 1998; **8**: 275–83.

25 Borish L, Aarons A, Rumbyrt J, *et al.* Interleukin-10 regulation in normal subjects and patients with asthma. *J Allergy Clin Immunol* 1996; **97**: 1288–96.

26 Akbari O, DeKruyff RH, Umetsu DT. Pulmonary dendritic cells producing IL-10 mediate tolerance induced by respiratory exposure to antigen. *Nat Immunol* 2001; **2**: 725–31.

27 Kearley J, Barker JE, Robinson DS, Lloyd CM. Resolution of airway inflammation and hyperreactivity after *in vivo* transfer of CD4⁺CD25⁺ regulatory T cells is interleukin 10 dependent. *J Exp Med* 2005; **202**: 1539–47.

28 Ito T, Wang YH, Duramad O, *et al.* TSLP-activated dendritic cells induce an inflammatory T helper type 2 cell response through OX40 ligand. *J Exp Med* 2005; **202**: 1213–23.

29 Wang YH, Ito T, Wang YH, *et al.* Maintenance and polarization of human T_H2 central memory T cells by thymic stromal lymphopoietin-activated dendritic cells. *Immunity* 2006; **24**: 827–38.

30 So T, Song J, Sugie K, *et al.* Signals from OX40 regulate nuclear factor of activated T cells c1 and T cell helper 2 lineage commitment. *Proc Natl Acad Sci USA* 2006; **103**: 3740–5.

31 Kapsenberg ML. Dendritic-cell control of pathogen-driven T-cell polarization. *Nat Rev Immunol* 2003; **3**: 984–93.

32 Epstein MM. Targeting memory Th2 cells for the treatment of allergic asthma. *Pharmacol Ther* 2006; **109**: 107–36.

33 Wang YH, Angkasekwinai P, Lu N, *et al.* 2007; IL-25 augments type 2 immune responses by enhancing the expansion and functions of TSLP-DC-activated Th2 memory cells. *J Exp Med.* 2007; **204**: 1837–47.

34 Betts RJ, Kemeny DM. CD8⁺ T cells in asthma: friend or foe? *Pharmacol Ther* 2009; **121**: 123–31.

35 Gilliet M, Soumelis V, Watanabe N, *et al.* Human dendritic cells activated by TSLP, and CD40L induce proallergic cytotoxic T cells. *J Exp Med* 2003; **197**: 1059–63.

36 Briot A, Deraison C, Lacroix M, *et al.* Kallikrein 5 induces atopic dermatitis-like lesions through PAR2-mediated thymic stromal lymphopoietin expression in Netherton syndrome. *J Exp Med* 2009; **206**: 1135–47.

37 Ying S, O'Connor B, Ratoff J, *et al.* Thymic stromal lymphopoietin expression is increased in asthmatic airways and correlates with expression of Th2-attracting chemokines and disease severity. *J Immunol* 2005; **174**: 8183–90.

38 Mou Z, Xia J, Tan Y, *et al.* Overexpression of thymic stromal lymphopoietin in allergic rhinitis. *Acta Otolaryngol* 2009; **129**: 297–301.

39 Matsuda A, Ebihara N, Yokoi N, *et al.* Functional role of thymic stromal lymphopoietin in chronic allergic keratoconjunctivitis. *Invest Ophthalmol Vis Sci* 2010; **51**: 151–5.

40 Li M, Messaddeq N, Teletin M, *et al.* Retinoid X receptor ablation in adult mouse keratinocytes generates an atopic dermatitis triggered by thymic stromal lymphopoietin. *Proc Natl Acad Sci USA* 2005; **102**: 14795–800.

41 He R, Oyoshi MK, Garibyan L, *et al.* TSLP acts on infiltrating effector T cells to drive allergic skin inflammation. *Proc Natl Acad Sci USA* 2008; **105**: 11875–880.

42 Al-Shami A, Spolski R, Kelly J, *et al.* A role for TSLP in the development of inflammation in an asthma model. *J Exp Med* 2005; **202**: 829–39.

43 Headley MB, Zhou B, Shih WX, *et al.* TSLP conditions the lung immune environment for the generation of pathogenic innate and antigen-specific adaptive immune responses. *J Immunol* 2009; **182**: 1641–7.

44 Zhou B, Headley MB, Aye T, *et al.* Reversal of thymic stromal lymphopoietin-induced airway inflammation through inhibition of Th2 responses. *J Immunol* 2008; **181**: 6557–62.

45 Seshasayee D, Lee WP, Zhou M, *et al. In vivo* blockade of OX40 ligand inhibits thymic stromal lymphopoietin driven atopic inflammation. *J Clin Invest* 2007; **117**: 3868–78.

46 Zaph C, Troy AE, Taylor BC, *et al.* Epithelial-cell-intrinsic IKK-β expression regulates intestinal immune homeostasis. *Nature* 2007; **446**: 552–6.

47 Taylor BC, Zaph C, Troy AE, *et al.* TSLP regulates intestinal immunity and inflammation in mouse models of helminth infection and colitis. *J Exp Med* 2009; **206**: 655–67.

48 Lee HC, Ziegler SF. Inducible expression of the proallergic cytokine thymic stromal lymphopoietin in airway epithelial cells is controlled by NFκB. *Proc Natl Acad Sci USA* 2007; **104**: 914–19.

49 Bogiatzi SI, Fernandez I, Bichet JC, *et al.* Cutting edge: Pro-inflammatory and Th2 cytokines synergize to induce thymic stromal lymphopoietin production by human skin keratinocytes. *J Immunol* 2007; **178**: 3373–7.

50 Kato A, Favoreto S, Jr., Avila PC, Schleimer RP. TLR3- and Th2 cytokine-dependent production of thymic stromal lymphopoietin in human airway epithelial cells. *J Immunol* 2007; **179**: 1080–7.

51 Kinoshita H, Takai T, Le TA, *et al.* Cytokine milieu modulates release of thymic stromal lymphopoietin from human keratinocytes stimulated with double-stranded RNA. *J Allergy Clin Immunol* 2009; **123**: 179–86.

52 Demehri S, Liu Z, Lee J, *et al.* Notch-deficient skin induces a lethal systemic B-lymphoproliferative disorder by secreting TSLP, a sentinel for epidermal integrity. *PLoS Biol* 2008; **6**: e123.

53 Li M, Hener P, Zhang Z, *et al.* Topical vitamin D3 and low-calcemic analogs induce thymic stromal lymphopoietin in mouse keratinocytes and trigger an atopic dermatitis. *Proc Natl Acad Sci USA* 2006; **103**: 11736–41.

54 Kouzaki H, O'Grady SM, Lawrence CB, Kita H. Proteases induce production of thymic stromal lymphopoietin by airway epithelial cells through protease-activated receptor-2. *J Immunol* 2009; **183**: 1427–34.

55 Kanke T, Macfarlane SR, Seatter MJ, *et al.* Proteinase-activated receptor-2-mediated activation of stress-activated protein kinases and inhibitory kappa B kinases in NCTC 2544; keratinocytes. *J Biol Chem* 2001; **276**: 31657–66.

56 Harada M, Hirota T, Jodo AI, *et al.* Functional analysis of the thymic stromal lymphopoietin variants in human bronchial epithelial cells. *Am J Respir Cell Mol Biol* 2009; **40**: 368–74.

57 Arima K, Watanabe N, Hanabuchi S, *et al.* Distinct signal codes generate dendritic cells functional plasticity. *Sci Signal* 2010; **3**: ra4.

58 Miyata M, Nakamura Y, Shimokawa N, *et al.* TSLP is a critical mediator of IL-13-driven allergic inflammation. *Eur J Immunol* 2009; **39**: 3078–83.

59 Miyata M, Hatsushika K, Ando T, *et al.* 2008; Mast cell regulation of epithelial TSLP expression plays an important role in the development of allergic rhinitis. *Eur J Immunol* **38**: 1487–92.

17 Interleukin 10

Whitney W. Stevens, Larry Borish, and John W. Steinke
Asthma and Allergic Disease Center, Carter Immunology Center, University of Virginia Health Systems, Charlottesville, VA, USA

Overview of the biology of interleukin 10

Interleukin 10 (IL-10) is an immunoregulatory cytokine with multiple biologic effects on many different cell types. It was originally cloned and defined as a product of T helper (Th) 2 lymphocytes that inhibits the function and production of interferon (IFN)-γ by Th1 lymphocytes (and then termed cytokine synthesis inhibitor factor) [1,2]. It has since been discovered to have a more extensive pattern of expression and range of biologic activities. IL-10 not only inhibits the production of IFN-γ by Th1 lymphocytes [3], but it also inhibits the secretion of IL-4 and IL-5 by Th2 lymphocytes [4]; IFN-γ and tumor necrosis factor (TNF)-α by natural killer (NK) cells [5]; IL-1β, IL-6, CXCL8 (IL-8), IL-12, and TNF-α by mononuclear phagocytes [6–8]; and other cytokines by many cell types. IL-10 primarily inhibits cytokine production by T lymphocytes by inhibiting the function of antigen-presenting cells (APCs) [6,9,10]. Thus, IL-10 inhibits major histocompatibility complex (MHC) class II expression (signal 1) on many APCs including dendritic cells (DCs), mononuclear phagocytes, and B lymphocytes [6]. IL-10 inhibits the surface expression of co-stimulatory molecules CD80 and CD86 on DCs and other APCs (signal 2) thereby eliminating the ability of that APC to provide the accessory signals necessary for Th cell activation [11]. Other direct actions of IL-10 on APCs include inhibition of their expression of CD23 (low-affinity IgE receptor; FcεRII), and intracellular adhesion molecule (ICAM) 1; as well as inhibition of their release of cytokines, such as IL-1, which also contribute to T cell activation (signal 3). This comprehensive inhibition of signals 1–3 is primarily responsible for the inhibition of T cell cytokine production. However, IL-10 also functions directly on T cells to inhibit their cytokine production both directly and also by suppressing their expression of CD28 and inducible T cell co-stimulator (ICOS) [12]. As will be discussed below, the constitutive expression of IL-10 in the respiratory tract and other mucosal surfaces of healthy subjects has a role in the maintenance of tolerance to allergens and otherwise benign bioaerosols [13,14], whereas asthma and allergic rhinitis are associated with diminished IL-10 expression [15]. Diminished IL-10 expression contributes to the milieu in which immune responses to allergens develop.

Interleukin 10 signaling

Interleukin 10 binds to a heterodimer receptor complex composed of molecules of the IL-10 receptor 1 (IL-10R1) and IL-10R2 chains [16,17]. IL-10 specifically binds to the IL-10R1 chain, which leads to recruitment of the IL-10R2 subunit (Figure 17.1). IL-10R1 is uniquely involved in IL-10 binding, while IL-10R2 is a common subunit shared with other

Inflammation and Allergy Drug Design, First Edition. Edited by Kenji Izuhara, Stephen T. Holgate, Marsha Wills-Karp.
© 2011 Blackwell Publishing Ltd. Published 2011 by Blackwell Publishing Ltd.

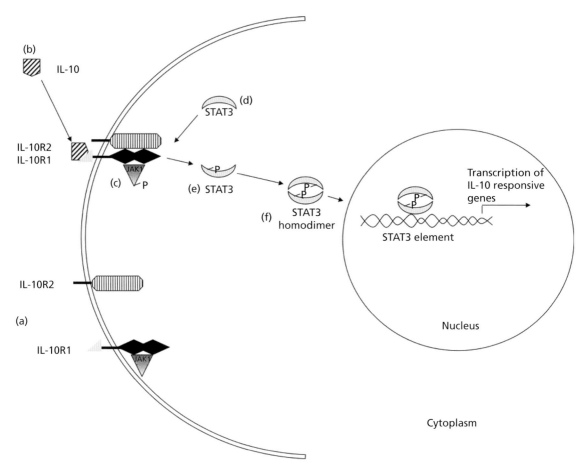

Figure 17.1 Interleukin 10 (IL-10) signaling pathway. (a) In the unbound state IL-10R1 and IL-10R2 are found as monomers. (b) IL-10 binds to the IL-10R1 subunit allowing recruitment of IL-10R2. (c) Association of IL-10R2 phosphorylates the intracellular domain of IL-10R1, leading to Jak1 phosphorylation. (d) STAT3 is recruited to the IL-10 receptor complex. (e) STAT3 becomes phosphorylated and dissociates from the IL-10 receptor complex. (f) STAT3 forms a homodimer and migrates to the nucleus activating IL-10 responsive genes.

members of the IL-10 superfamily, including IL-19, IL-20, IL-22, IL-24, IL-26, IL-28, and IL-29. Upon binding of IL-10, signaling is initiated through activation of Janus kinase 1 (JAK1), which is bound to IL-10R1. Association of IL-10R2 leads to phosphorylation of tyrosine residues on the intracellular domain of the IL-10R1 chain [18]. The phosphorylated IL-10R1 tyrosine residues serve as a docking site for the latent cytosolic transcription factor signal transducers and activators of transcription 3 (STAT3). Following binding of STAT3, JAK1 phosphorylates tyrosine residues in STAT3 allowing the formation of STAT3 homodimers. The STAT3 homodimers dissoci-

ate from the receptor and translocate to the nucleus where they bind to promoters of IL-10-responsive genes [18]. There have been reports of STAT1 and STAT5 activation by IL-10 and association of Tyk2 with the IL-10R2 chain. In murine studies where Tyk2 was knocked out, there were no effects on IL-10 activity [19], whereas studies in which STAT3 has been deleted have demonstrated that the majority of IL-10 activities can be attributed to STAT3 activation [20,21]. The differences in reported STAT activation may be attributed to binding of Tyk2 and subsequent activation of STAT1 and STAT5 to IL-10R2, which, as noted, is a receptor subunit for other IL-10 family members. IL-10 additionally activates PI-3 kinase and its downstream effectors AKT and p70 S6 kinase, thus promoting cell survival of myeloid precursors [22,23].

Sources of interleukin 10

Immature DCs, mononuclear phagocytes, and B cells are the major sources of IL-10 in humans [4]. In contrast to the initial observation that IL-10 is exclusively a Th2 product, in humans the primary T cell source for IL-10 is regulatory T lymphocytes.

Dendritic cells/M2 macrophages

There are numerous studies documenting IL-10 production by innate immune cells such as macrophages [24], DCs [25,26], natural killer cells [27], and eosinophils [28,29]. Such diversity of cell populations able to secrete IL-10 emphasizes the importance of this cytokine in regulating the immune response to prevent excessive inflammation and damage to the host. Macrophages can be subdivided based upon their secretion profile of various soluble factors including IL-10 [30]. M1 macrophages are typically proinflammatory, in large part owing to their ability to secrete high levels of IL-12, TNF-α, and nitric oxide (NO) instead of IL-10. In contrast, M2a macrophages, which develop following an alternate pathway of activation involving IL-4 or IL-13, produce IL-10 and arginase instead of NO, and proinflammatory innate cytokines [31]. While M2a macrophages can inhibit T-cell proliferation, albeit in an IL-10-independent manner [32], it is hypothesized that this macrophage subset, owing to their production of arginase, may play a larger role in the suppression of Th2-type responses as well as in tissue remodeling and repair following injury [33,34]. Type II-activated, or M2b, macrophages comprise another subset of macrophages noted for their secretion of high levels of IL-10, but not IL-12, following activation by immune complexes and signaling via Toll-like receptors [35,36]. These cells are distinguished from M2a macrophages because of their inability to produce arginase, yet they retain the ability to secrete other, proinflammatory, cytokines. M2b macrophages, thus, can play a dual role in regulating an inflammatory response, with studies demonstrating their tendency to promote a Th2-type response as well as to prevent mortality in a traditionally lethal murine model of LPS-induced toxemia [37–39].

The importance of macrophages in an allergic response has been explored with studies showing an enhanced recruitment of this cell population into the airways of allergic individuals following allergen challenge [40]. Additionally, the adoptive transfer of macrophages from nonallergic rat donors into macrophage-depleted recipients attenuates the development of airway hyperreactivity [41]. In addition to evidence that alveolar macrophages from human asthmatics produce less IL-10 than those in nonasthmatic controls [15], such findings suggest that by producing IL-10, M2a and M2b macrophage subsets may be important in regulating the degree of tissue inflammation and injury observed during an allergic response.

Interleukin 10 production by CD4[+] lymphocytes: regulatory T lymphocyte families: nTreg, iTreg, and Th3 cells

As previously noted, IL-10 was originally identified as a Th2 lymphocyte product. While this remains accurate, its production by effector T lymphocytes, especially in humans, is more wide ranging, including its production by Th1 and, likely, Th17 lymphocytes. Production of IL-10 by effector lymphocytes may contribute to a modified, less inflammatory phenotype, for example the modified Th2-like lymphocytes that drive reduced IgE and greater IgG4 production [42,43]. However, it is now apparent that the primary source of IL-10 by CD4[+] T lymphocytes is derived from cells having regulatory function.

In addition to traditional T-helper subclasses, much progress has been made in the past several years in identifying and clarifying the characteristics of several families of regulatory T lymphocytes (Table 17.1) [44]. These include IL-10-producing lymphocytes, termed inducible regulatory T cells, thymic-derived CD25[+] natural regulatory T cells, and TGF-β-producing Th3 cells. Thymus-derived natural Treg (nTreg) cells are characterized by their constitutive expression of IL-2 receptor α chains (CD25) and the transcription factor master regulator Foxp3. Although they secrete IL-10, membrane TGF-β appears to be primarily responsible

Table 17.1 Regulatory T cells.

Cell	Phenotype
Modified Th1 lymphocytes	IFN-γ⁺, IL-10⁺
	Associated with modulated inflammatory responses
Modified Th2 lymphocytes	IL-4⁺, IL-5⁺, IL-10⁺
	Associated with humoral immune response to allergens with increased IgG (IgG4) and diminished IgE
Natural (n)Treg	CD25⁺, FOXP3⁺, membrane
	TGF-β⁺ Mediate tolerance to self antigens presented in thymus
Inducible (i)Treg	±CD25⁺
	Induced regulatory responses to antigens presented in periphery; develop in response to allergen immunotherapy
Th3 lymphocytes	TGF-β⁺, IL-10⁺
	Associated with GI mucosal immunity; IgA-specific immune responses

for mediating their immune suppression, which is contact dependent. nTreg cells are produced in response to thymic expression of self antigens and are thereby important for the prevention of autoimmunity. nTreg cells are unlikely to be involved in tolerance to antigens not presented in the thymus (e.g., in either tolerance to allergens in healthy subjects or in the immune benefits associated with allergen immunotherapy). In contrast to thymus-derived nTreg cells, an additional, less well-characterized class of inducible regulatory T cells (iTreg) has been described, which can develop in the periphery. These iTreg cells are differentiated from preexisting T effector lymphocytes or possibly from circulating naïve Th0 cells, and are characterized by their prominent production of IL-10. iTreg expression of Foxp3 and CD25 is controversial, but does appear to occur. For example, it is unclear whether CD25 expression reflects the constitutive expression of this component of the IL-2 receptor, the signature characteristic of nTreg cells, or the derivation of iTregs from activated effector T cells that are transiently expressing CD25. The induction of IL-10-producing iTreg

cells plays a key role in reducing allergen-specific T-cell responsiveness after immunotherapy, as will be discussed later [45,46]. Finally, Th3 cells are primarily gut-derived CD4⁺ T cells that secrete high concentrations of both IL-10 and TGF-β to generate mucosal tolerance. Reflecting this prominent production of TGF-β, in addition to tolerance, they are also relevant in secretory IgA production.

CD8 lymphocytes

Similar to specific CD4⁺ T cells, subsets of CD8⁺ T cells are also capable of producing IL-10. One such population includes modified "Tc2" type effector CD8⁺ T cells that produce higher levels of IL-10, IL-4, and IL-5 than IFN-γ, and thus help promote the development of a Th2 cytokine signature and not a Th1-type immune response [47,48].

Several subclasses of regulatory CD8⁺ T cells can produce IL-10 [49]. There is literature supporting a role for IL-10 producing nonantigen-specific CD8⁺CD28⁻ T cells in inhibiting T-cell proliferation and cytotoxicity *in vitro* [50,51]. Intraintestinal TCRα⁺β⁺ CD8α⁺β⁻ T cells can produce IL-10 and are capable of preventing the development of colitis in a murine model of inflammatory bowel disease [52]. Additionally, the production of IL-10 by CD8⁺ CD122⁺ T regulatory cells has been implicated in the suppression of CD8⁺ CD122⁻ T cell proliferation and production of IFN-γ *in vitro* [53,54].

Recently, research on the role of IL-10 and CD8⁺ T cells in a murine model of influenza found IL-10 to be rapidly and transiently produced in the lungs following viral infection, predominantly by conventional activated effector CD8⁺ T cells [55]. IL-10 receptor blockade in this model led to increased pulmonary injury and mortality when compared with unmanipulated IL-10-sufficient controls. This suggests that IL-10 production by cytotoxic T cells might mitigate bystander inflammation without interfering with the requisite cytotoxic response. Failure to modulate cytotoxic responses and bystander injury could contribute to a fatal, overexuberant immune response, such as that which occurred during the 1919 swine flu epidemic. Effector memory CD8⁺ T cells also have the capability to secrete IL-10 as demonstrated in a murine model studying the CD8⁺ T cell modulation of respiratory syncytial virus vaccine-enhanced disease [56]. In this model, it is hypothesized that IL-10 produced by activated memory CD8+ T cells may help attenuate the development of pulmonary eosinophilia and the CD4+ T cell Th2 type response typically observed.

Taken together, there is abundant evidence that various subsets of CD8+ T cells are capable of producing IL-10 and that IL-10 is important in suppressing the degree of inflammation and bystander damage generated by the immune response. Furthermore, it is speculated that CD8+ T cells, with their potent proinflammatory and increasingly recognized anti-inflammatory properties, can regulate their own cytotoxic activity as well as influence their surrounding environment to create a balance between immunoprotection and immunopathology.

Interleukin 10 in allergies/asthma

The pattern of immune responses to allergens observed in nonallergic compared with allergic individuals is complex. Normal individuals are exposed to the same concentrations of allergens as their allergic counterparts living in the same environment. Therefore, remaining healthy requires active systems that prevent the development of inflammation. As previously mentioned, IL-10 [15] and the anti-inflammatory cytokine TGF-β [57,58] are constitutively expressed in the healthy airway, downregulating cellular immunity and allergic inflammation, thereby contributing to a state of immune nonresponsiveness. Diminished secretion of this cytokine promotes the development of a milieu in which allergic inflammation and asthma can develop. Tolerance toward inhaled antigens in normal subjects is mediated in part through the absence of mature antigen-presenting cells in the respiratory tract. Alveolar macrophages and immature DCs produce IL-10 and function to dampen immune hyperresponsiveness. In contrast to the asthmatic lung, the resident alveolar macrophage population of the healthy lung is unable to present allergen to T helper lymphocytes and cannot stimulate cellular activation and proliferation [59,60]. Production of IL-10 by iTreg cells is an additional mechanism for preventing or restoring immune nonresponsiveness to allergens.

Support for a modulating role of IL-10 in human allergic disease is derived from this cytokine's numer-ous additional activities. IL-10 inhibits eosinophil survival in part by decreasing IL-5 release from human T cells and by decreasing CD40 expression. This decrease in CD40 leads to an inability of eosinophils to induce GM-CSF and TNF-α production and contributes to their diminished ability to function as APCs [61,62]. Mast cell development and FcεRI expression is inhibited by IL-10 when acting in conjunction with IL-4 [63]. IL-10 has opposing actions on B cells depending on the developmental state. With uncommitted B cells, IL-10 inhibits IL-4 mediated ε transcript expression, while on committed B cells IL-10 potentiates IgE production. However, regardless of B cell state, IL-10 augments IL-4-induced γ4 transcription and IgG4 production [64–66].

Our understanding of the role that IL-10 plays in immune responses has been gleaned from murine studies where the IL-10 gene has been deleted. Several studies demonstrated that, in the absence of IL-10, more robust Th1 and Th2 responses are observed in response to a variety of stimuli including parasites and allergens [67,68]. These results support the concept that one of the main roles of IL-10 is to suppress the immune response. When sensitized mice are challenged with ovalbumin or *Aspergillus fumigatus* antigen, those that are IL-10 deficient develop heightened eosinophilic airway inflammation accompanied by increased IL-5 and IFN-γ in bronchoalveolar lavage fluids [68–70]. Similarly, when sensitized IL-10-deficient mice are challenged with respiratory syncytial virus, there is an increase in AHR [70] that can be reversed if the mice are reconstituted with CD4+ T cells that have been engineered to overexpress IL-10 [71].

Mechanisms of immunotherapy involving interleukin 10

It is currently in vogue to cite immune deviation from a Th2- toward a Th1-like response as the basis for efficacy of immunotherapy [72]. The one consistent finding observed after IT is diminished responsiveness (tolerance) of the allergen-specific Th2-like cells. This model comes under scrutiny, however, because T cells that produce IFN-γ (Th1-like cells) are a characteristic feature of allergic inflammation that contribute to both the presence and severity of allergic disease [73] and immunotherapy is now increasingly recognized to also induce tolerance of these Th1-like cells.

219

Systemic administration of high-dose allergen in humans undergoing immunotherapy induces production of IL-10 by circulating peripheral blood mononuclear cells and is associated with T-cell hyporesponsiveness and increased IgG4 antibody titers [45,74,75]. A direct role for IL-10 in inducing IgG4 antibody has been demonstrated [76] and, as such, the appearance of allergen-specific IgG4 in association with immunotherapy is consistent with being a marker for such an iTreg (or IL-10-producing "modified" Th2) response. In allergen-specific systems, iTreg cells producing IL-10 have been implicated in the regulation of IgE, and IgG4 antibody production, suppression of T-cell proliferation and cytokine production, and respiratory tolerance. Numerous studies have shown that IL-10 is the predominant cytokine in T-cell cultures from individuals undergoing immunotherapy [45,46,74,77–80]. The protective effect of iTreg cells is evident from studies demonstrating that, following 5 years of immunotherapy, subjects remain nonresponsive even after immunotherapy has been stopped [81].

A prominent role for IL-10-producing activated CD4+ cells was first described in studies involving bee venom immunotherapy (Figure 17.2) [45]. Subsequent investigations with house dust mite immunotherapy extended the importance of IL-10 (and TGF-β) production by CD4+ T cells to inhalant

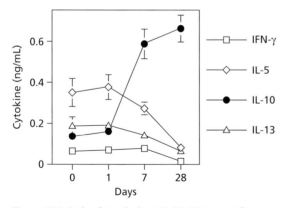

Figure 17.2 Role of interleukin 10 (IL-10) in specific immunotherapy. Peripheral blood mononuclear cells (PBMCs) were obtained from patients undergoing rush immunotherapy to venom and venom-specific secretion of cytokines determined at baseline and at days 1, 7, and 28. Tolerance (diminished production of IL-5, IL-13, and interferon gamma [IFN-γ]) is observed in association with enhanced secretion of IL-10 (from Akdis *et al.*).

allergy and confirmed that this occurred in parallel to the suppression of Th2 proliferative responses and cytokine production [78]. In this study, IL-10 responses in healthy nonatopic individuals who had been exposed to allergen were similar to those in the immunotherapy-treated group, implying the restoration of tolerant T-cell responses in the atopic individual. Other studies have also shown IL-10 production by CD4+ cells without changes in grass pollen-induced T-cell proliferation or Th2 cytokine production following immunotherapy [46]. This area of research remains confused; for example, although a role for CD25 expression has been ascribed to these IL-10-producing cells, it is unclear whether this reflects the constitutive expression of this component of the IL-2 receptor (the signature characteristic of nTreg cells) or (more likely) whether this reflects the activation of effector T cells. However, what is consistent is that each of these studies has found cells capable of making high levels of IL-10 (±TGF-β) consistent with the iTreg cell type, and current concepts therefore focus on the integral role of these IL-10-producing cells in immune tolerance to allergens after immunotherapy.

Influences of asthma and allergy therapeutics on interleukin 10: pharmacologic potential of interleukin 10

Expression of IL-10, as noted, is central to the maintenance of the immune nonresponsiveness to allergens observed in normal subjects and, similarly, induction of IL-10-producing (presumably) iTreg cells is central to the restoration of the healthy state that occurs in association with a successful course of immunotherapy. Induction of IL-10 is also a component of the salubrious benefits observed with many allergy and asthma therapeutics. Theophylline and other phosphodiesterase inhibitors modulate mononuclear phagocytic cell production of TNF-α and other proinflammatory cytokines, and this occurs in association with greatly enhanced IL-10 production [82]. Similarly, inhaled corticosteroids enhance the capability of alveolar macrophages to secrete IL-10 (Figure 17.3) [83] and both leukotriene modifier and corticosteroid administration to asthmatics are associated with increased circulating IL-10 concentrations [84].

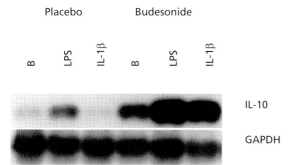

Figure 17.3 Inhaled corticosteroids increase constitutive and inducible interleukin 10 (IL-10) release from alveolar macrophages. Effect of 4 weeks of inhaled budesonide on IL-10 mRNA, expression by alveolar macrophages obtained by bronchoalveolar lavage at baseline (B) and after 24 h of stimulation with lipopolysaccharide (LPS), and IL-1β (from ref. 83).

These observations all suggest the potential utility of direct IL-10 administration as an asthma therapeutic. In theory, exogenously administered IL-10 could reproduce the "immune ignorant" state of nonallergic subjects, would recapitulate one of the most important central mechanisms of immunotherapy, and reflect some of the beneficial mechanisms observed with current asthma therapeutics. Enthusiasm for IL-10 as a therapeutic is tempered by recognition that when generated *in vivo* it is generated in a homeostatically controlled setting where its production and targeting is meticulously regulated. As with other cytokines, the function of IL-10 is determined by which cells are producing it, the stage of the immune response during which it is acting, the nature of the target cell, the different signaling pathways it engages, and other divergent influences. Somehow with immunotherapy this appears to be productively accomplished. However, nontargeted pharmacologic administration of IL-10 must be approached with caution as it is likely to generate a wide range of both pro- and anti-inflammatory effects, many of which may not be beneficial to the recipient.

Acknowledgment

The authors have been supported by National Institutes of Health grants AI057438, AI1090413, and AI50989.

References

1 Fiorentino DF, Bond MW, Mosmann TR. Two types of mouse T helper cell. IV. Th2 clones secrete a factor that inhibits cytokine production by Th1 clones. *J Exp Med* 1989; **170**: 2081–95.

2 Moore KW, Vieira P, Fiorentino DF, Trounstine ML, Khan TA, Mosmann TR. Homology of cytokine synthesis inhibitory factor (IL-10) to the Epstein–Barr virus gene BCRFI. *Science* 1990; **248**: 1230–4.

3 de Waal Malefyt RD, Yssel H, de Vries JE. Direct effects of IL-10 on subsets of human CD4+ T cell clones and resting T cells. Specific inhibition of IL-2 production and proliferation. *J Immunol* 1993; **150**: 4754–65.

4 Del Prete G, De Carli M, Almerigogna F, Giudizi MG, Biagiotti R, Romagnani S. Human IL-10 is produced by both type 1 helper (Th1) and type 2 helper (Th2) T cell clones and inhibits their antigen-specific proliferation and cytokine production. *J Immunol* 1993; **150**: 353–60.

5 D'Andrea A, Aste-Amezaga M, Vaiante NM, Ma X, Kubin M, Trinchieri G. Interleukin 10 (IL-10) inhibits human lymphocyte interferon gamma-production by suppressing natural killer cell stimulatory factor/IL-12 synthesis in accessory cells. *J Exp Med* 1993; **178**: 1041–8.

6 de Waal Malefyt RD, Abrams JS, Bennett B, Figdor CG, de Vries JE. Interleukin 10 (IL-10) inhibits cytokine synthesis by human monocytes: an autoregulatory role of IL-10 produced by monocytes. *J Exp Med* 1991; **174**: 1209–20.

7 Bogdan C, Vodoyotz Y, Nathan C. Macrophage deactivation by interleukin 10. *J Exp Med* 1991; **174**: 1549–55.

8 Ralph P, Nakoinz I, Sampson-Johannes A, *et al.* IL-10: T, lymphocyte inhibitor of human blood cell production of IL-1 and tumor necrosis factor. *J Immunol* 1992; **148**: 808–14.

9 de Waal Malefyt RD, Haanen J, Spits H, *et al.* Interleukin 10 (IL-10) and viral IL-10 strongly reduce antigen-specific human T cell proliferation by diminishing the antigen-presenting capacity of monocytes via downregulation of class II major histocompatibility complex expression. *J Exp Med* 1991; **174**: 915–24.

10 Fiorentino DF, Zlotnik A, Mosmann TR, Howard M, O'Garra A. IL-10 acts on the antigen-presenting cell to inhibit cytokine production by Th1 cells. *J Immunol* 1991; **147**: 3815–22.

11 Ding L, Linsley PS, Huang LY, Germain RN, Shevach EM. IL-10 inhibits macrophage co-stimulatory activity by selectively inhibiting the up-regulation of B7 expression. *J Immunol* 1993; **151**: 1224–34.

12 Taylor A, Akdis M, Joss A, *et al.* IL-10 inhibits CD28 and ICOS costimulations of T cells via src homology 2 domain-containing protein tyrosine phosphatase 1. *J Allergy Clin Immunol* 2007; **120**: 76–83.

13 Enk AH, Angeloni VL, Udey MC, Katz SI. Inhibition of Langerhans cell antigen-presenting function by IL-10. A role for IL-10 in induction of tolerance. *J Immunol* 1993; **151**: 2390–8.

14 Becker JC, Czerny C, Brocker EB. Maintenance of clonal anergy by endogenously produced IL-10. *Int Immunol* 1994; **6**: 1605–12.

15 Borish L, Aarons A, Rumbyrt J, Cvietusa P, Negri J, Wenzel S. Interleukin-10 regulation in normal subjects and patients with asthma. *J Allergy Clin Immunol* 1996; **97**: 1288–96.

16 Liu Y, Wei SH, Ho AS, de Waal Malefyt R, Moore KW. Expression cloning and characterization of a human IL-10 receptor. *J Immunol* 1994; **152**: 1821–9.

17 Lutfalla G, Gardiner K, Uze G. A new member of the cytokine receptor gene family maps on chromosome 21 at less than 35 kb from IFNAR. *Genomics* 1993; **16**: 366–73.

18 Weber-Nordt RM, Riley JK, Greenlund AC, Moore KW, Darnell JE, Schreiber RD. Stat3 recruitment by two distinct ligand-induced, tyrosine-phosphorylated docking sites in the interleukin-10 receptor intracellular domain. *J Biol Chem* 1996; **271**: 27954–61.

19 Karaghiosoff M, Neubauer H, Lassnig C, *et al*. Partial impairment of cytokine responses in Tyk2-deficient mice. *Immunity* 2000; **13**: 549–60.

20 Takeda K, Clausen BE, Kaisho T, *et al*. Enhanced Th1 activity and development of chronic enterocolitis in mice devoid of Stat3 in macrophages and neutrophils. *Immunity* 1999; **10**: 39–49.

21 Williams L, Bradley L, Smith A, Foxwell B. Signal transducer and activator of transcription 3 is the dominant mediator of the anti-inflammatory effects of IL-10 in human macrophages. *J Immunol* 2004; **172**: 567–76.

22 Crawley JB, Williams LM, Mander T, Brennan FM, Foxwell BM. Interleukin-10 stimulation of phosphatidylinositol 3-kinase and p70 S6 kinase is required for the proliferative but not the antiinflammatory effects of the cytokine. *J Biol Chem* 1996; **271**: 16357–62.

23 Zhou JH, Broussard SR, Strle K, *et al*. IL-10 inhibits apoptosis of promyeloid cells by activating insulin receptor substrate-2 and phosphatidylinositol 3′-kinase. *J Immunol* 2001; **167**: 4436–42.

24 Mosser DM. The many faces of macrophage activation. *J Leukoc Biol* 2003; **73**: 209–12.

25 Akbari O, DeKruyff RH, Umetsu DT. Pulmonary dendritic cells producing IL-10 mediate tolerance induced by respiratory exposure to antigen. *Nat Immunol* 2001; **2**: 725–31.

26 Ahrens B, Freund T, Rha RD, *et al*. Lipopolysaccharide stimulation of dendritic cells induces interleukin-10 producing allergen-specific T cells *in vitro* but fails to prevent allergic airway disease. *Exp Lung Res* 2009; **35**: 307–23.

27 Deniz G, Erten G, Kucuksezer UC, *et al*. Regulatory NK cells suppress antigen-specific T cell responses. *J Immunol* 2008; **180**: 850–7.

28 Lamkhioued B, Aldebert D, Gounni AS, *et al*. Synthesis of cytokines by eosinophils and their regulation. *Int Arch Allergy Immunol* 1995; **107**(1–3): 122–3.

29 Spencer LA, Szela CT, Perez SA, *et al*. Human eosinophils constitutively express multiple Th1: Th2: and immunoregulatory cytokines that are secreted rapidly and differentially. *J Leukoc Biol* 2009; **85**: 117–23.

30 Edwards JP, Zhang X, Frauwirth KA, Mosser DM. Biochemical and functional characterization of three activated macrophage populations. *J Leukoc Biol* 2006; **80**: 1298–307.

31 Stein M, Keshav S, Harris N, Gordon S. Interleukin 4 potently enhances murine macrophage mannose receptor activity: a marker of alternative immunologic macrophage activation. *J Exp Med* 1992; **176**: 287–92.

32 Schebesch C, Kodelja V, Muller C, *et al*. Alternatively activated macrophages actively inhibit proliferation of peripheral blood lymphocytes and CD4+ T cells *in vitro*. *Immunology* 1997; **92**: 478–86.

33 Gratchev A, Guillot P, Hakiy N, *et al*. Alternatively activated macrophages differentially express fibronectin and its splice variants and the extracellular matrix protein betaIG-H3. *Scand J Immunol* 2001; **53**: 386–92.

34 Pesce JT, Ramalingam TR, Mentink-Kane MM, *et al*. Arginase-1-expressing macrophages suppress Th2 cytokine-driven inflammation and fibrosis. *PLoS Pathog* 2009; **5**: e1000371.

35 Sutterwala FS, Noel GJ, Clynes R, Mosser DM. Selective suppression of interleukin-12 induction after macrophage receptor ligation. *J Exp Med* 1997; **185**: 1977–85.

36 Sutterwala FS, Noel GJ, Salgame P, Mosser DM. Reversal of pro-inflammatory responses by ligating the macrophage Fcgamma receptor type I. *J Exp Med* 1998; **188**: 217–22.

37 Anderson CF, Mosser DM. A novel phenotype for an activated macrophage: the type 2 activated macrophage. *J Leukoc Biol* 2002; **72**: 101–6.

38 Anderson CF, Mosser DM. Cutting edge: biasing immune responses by directing antigen to macrophage Fc gamma receptors. *J Immunol* 2002; **168**: 3697–701.

39 Gerber JS, Mosser DM. Reversing lipopolysaccharide toxicity by ligating the macrophage Fc gamma receptors. *J Immunol* 2001; **166**: 6861–8.

40 Chanez P, Bousquet J, Couret I, *et al*. Increased numbers of hypodense alveolar macrophages in patients with bronchial asthma. *Am Rev Respir Dis* 1991; **144**: 923–30.

41 Careau E, Bissonnette EY. Adoptive transfer of alveolar macrophages abrogates bronchial hyperresponsiveness. *Am J Respir Cell Mol Biol* 2004; **31**: 22–7.

42 Platts-Mills TA, Vaughan JW, Blumenthal K, Pollart Squillace S, Sporik RB. Serum IgG, and IgG4 antibod-

ies to Fel d 1 among children exposed to 20 microg Fel d 1 at home: relevance of a nonallergic modified Th2 response. *Int Arch Allergy Immunol* 2001; **124**: 126–9.

43 Platts-Mills TA, Woodfolk JA, Erwin EA, Aalberse R. Mechanisms of tolerance to inhalant allergens: the relevance of a modified Th2 response to allergens from domestic animals. *Springer Semin Immunopathol* 2004; **25**: 271–9.

44 Sakaguchi S. Regulatory T cells: key controllers of immunologic self-tolerance. *Cell* 2000; **101**: 455–8.

45 Akdis CA, Blesken T, Akdis M, Wuthrich B, Blaser K. Role of interleukin 10 in specific immunotherapy. *J Clin Invest* 1998; **102**: 98–106.

46 Francis JN, Till SJ, Durham SR. Induction of IL-10$^+$CD4$^+$CD25$^+$ T cells by grass pollen immunotherapy. *J Allergy Clin Immunol* 2003; **111**: 1255–61.

47 Li L, Sad S, Kagi D, Mosmann TR. CD8Tc1 and Tc2 cells secrete distinct cytokine patterns *in vitro* and *in vivo* but induce similar inflammatory reactions. *J Immunol* 1997; **158**: 4152–61.

48 Mosmann TR, Li L, Sad S. Functions of CD8 T-cell subsets secreting different cytokine patterns. *Semin Immunol* 1997; **9**: 87–92.

49 Smith TR, Kumar V. Revival of CD8$^+$ Treg-mediated suppression. *Trends Immunol* 2008; **29**: 337–42.

50 Filaci G, Fravega M, Fenoglio D, *et al*. Non-antigen specific CD8$^+$ T suppressor lymphocytes. *Clin Exp Med* 2004; **4**: 86–92.

51 Filaci G, Fravega M, Negrini S, *et al*. Nonantigen specific CD8$^+$ T suppressor lymphocytes originate from CD8$^+$CD28$^-$ T cells and inhibit both T-cell proliferation and CTL function. *Hum Immunol* 2004; **65**: 142–56.

52 Poussier P, Ning T, Banerjee D, Julius M. A unique subset of self-specific intraintestinal T cells maintains gut integrity. *J Exp Med* 2002; **195**: 1491–7.

53 Endharti AT, Rifa IM, Shi Z, *et al*. Cutting edge: CD8$^+$CD122$^+$ regulatory T cells produce IL-10 to suppress IFN-gamma production and proliferation of CD8$^+$ T cells. *J Immunol* 2005; **175**: 7093–7.

54 Noble A, Giorgini A, Leggat JA. Cytokine-induced IL-10-secreting CD8 T cells represent a phenotypically distinct suppressor T-cell lineage. *Blood* 2006; **107**: 4475–83.

55 Sun J, Madan R, Karp CL, Braciale TJ. Effector T cells control lung inflammation during acute influenza virus infection by producing IL-10. *Nat Med* 2009; **15**: 277–84.

56 Stevens WW, Sun J, Castillo JP, Braciale TJ. Pulmonary eosinophilia is attenuated by early responding CD8($^+$) memory T cells in a murine model of RSV vaccine-enhanced disease. *Viral Immunol* 2009; **22**: 243–51.

57 Aubert JD, Dalal BI, Bai TR, Roberts CR, Hayashi S, Hogg JC. Transforming growth factor beta 1 gene expression in human airways. *Thorax* 1994; **49**: 225–32.

58 McCartney-Francis NL, Wahl S. Transforming growth factor beta: a matter of life and death. *J Leukoc Biol* 1994; **55**: 401–9.

59 Spiteri MA, Knight RA, Jeremy JY, Barnes PJ, Chung KF. Alveolar macrophage-induced suppression of peripheral blood mononuclear cell responsiveness is reversed by *in vitro* allergen exposure in bronchial asthma. *Eur Respir J* 1994; **7**: 1431–8.

60 Chelen CJ, Fang Y, Freeman GJ, *et al*. Human alveolar macrophages present antigen ineffectively due to defective expression of B7 co-stimulatory cell surface molecules. *J Clin Invest* 1995; **95**: 1415–21.

61 Bureau F, Seumois G, Jaspar F, *et al*. CD40 engagement enhances eosinophil survival through induction of cellular inhibitor of apoptosis protein 2 expression: Possible involvement in allergic inflammation. *J Allergy Clin Immunol* 2002; **110**: 443–9.

62 Takanaski S, Nonaka R, Xing Z, O'Bryne P, Dolovich J, Jordana M. Interleukin 10 inhibits lipopolysaccharide-induced survival and cytokine production by human peripheral blood eosinophils. *J Exp Med* 1994; **180**: 711–15.

63 Speiran K, Bailey DP, Fernando J, *et al*. Endogenous suppression of mast cell development and survival by IL-4 and IL-10. *J Leukoc Biol* 2009; **85**: 826–36.

64 Rousset F, Garcia E, Defrance T, *et al*. Interleukin 10 is a potent growth and differentiation factor for activated human B lymphocytes. *Proc Natl Acad Sci USA* 1992; **89**: 1890–3.

65 Jeannin P, Lecoanet S, Delneste Y, Gauchat J-F, Bonnefoy J-Y. IgE versus IgG4 production can be differentially regulated by IL-10. *J Immunol* 1998; **160**: 3555–61.

66 Punnonen J, Malefyt RD, Van Vlasselaer P, Gauchat J-F, de Vries JE. IL-10 and viral IL-10 prevent IL-4-induced IgE synthesis by inhibiting the accessory cell function of monocytes. *J Immunol* 1993; **151**: 1280–9.

67 Kuhn R, Lohler J, Rennick DM, Rajeswky K, Muller W. Interleukin-10-deficient mice develop chronic enterocolitis. *Cell* 1993; **75**: 263–74.

68 Grunig G, Corry DB, Leach MW, Seymour BW, Kurup VP, Rennick DM. Interleukin-10 is a natural suppressor of cytokine production and inflammation in a murine model of allergic bronchopulmonary aspergillosis. *J Exp Med* 1997; **185**: 1089–99.

69 Makela MJ, Kanehiro A, Borish L, *et al*. IL-10 is necessary for the expression of airway hyperresponsiveness but not pulmonary inflammation after allergic sensitization. *Proc Natl Acad Sci USA* 2000; **97**: 6007–12.

70 Makela MJ, Kanehiro A, Dakhama A, *et al*. The failure of interleukin-10-deficient mice to develop airway hyper-responsiveness is overcome by respiratory syncytial virus infection in allergen-sensitized/challenged mice. *Am J Respir Crit Care Med* 2002; **165**: 824–31.

71 Oh J, Seroogy CM, Meyer EH, *et al*. CD4 T-helper cells engineered to produce IL-10 prevent allergen-induced airway hyperreactivity and inflammation. *J Allergy Clin Immunol* 2002; **110**: 460–8.

72 Jutel M, Pichler WJ, Skrbic D, Urwyler A, Dahinden C, Muller UR. Bee venom immunotherapy results in decrease of IL-4 and IL-5 and increase of IFN-gamma secretion in specific allergen-stimulated T cell cultures. *J Immunol* 1995; **154**: 4187–94.

73 Hansen G, Berry G, DeKruyff RH, Umtesu DT. Allergen-specific Th1 cells fail to counterbalance Th2 cell-induced airway hyperreactivity but cause severe airway inflammation. *J Clin Invest* 1999; **103**: 175–83.

74 Akdis CA, Blaser K. IL-10-induced anergy in peripheral T cell and reactivation by microenviromental cytokines: two key steps in specific immunotherapy. *FASEB J* 1999; **13**: 603–9.

75 Fellrath J-M, Kettner A, Dufour N, *et al*. Allergen-specific T-cell tolerance induction with allergen-derived long synthetic peptides: Results of a phase I trial. *J Allergy Clin Immunol* 2003; **111**: 854–61.

76 Satoguina JS, Weyand E, Larbi J, Hoerauf A. T regulatory-1 cells induce IgG4 production by B cells: role of IL-10. *J Immunol* 2005; **174**: 4718–26.

77 Gaglani B, Borish L, Bartelson BL, Buchmeier A, Keller L, Nelson HS. Nasal immunotherapy in weed-induced allergic rhinitis. *Ann Allergy Asthma Immunol* 1997; **79**: 259–65.

78 Jutel M, Akdis M, Budak F, *et al*. IL-10 and TGF-β cooperate in the regulatory T cell response to mucosal allergens in normal immunity and specific immunotherapy. *Eur J Immunol* 2003; **33**: 1205–14.

79 Reefer AJ, Carneiro RM, Custis NJ, *et al*. A role for IL-10-mediated HLA-DR7-restricted T cell-dependent events in development of the modified Th2 response to cat allergen. *J Immunol* 2004; **172**: 2763–72.

80 Verhoef A, Alexander C, Kay AB, Larche M. T cell epitope immunotherapy induces a CD4+ T cell population with regulatory activity. *PLoS Med* 2005; **2**: e78.

81 Durham SR, Walker SM, Varga EM, *et al*. Long-term clinical efficacy of grass-pollen immunotherapy. *N Engl J Med* 1999; **341**: 468–75.

82 Mascali JJ, Cvietusa P, Negri J, Borish L. Anti-inflammatory effects of theophylline: modulation of cytokine production. *Ann Allergy Asthma Immunol* 1996; **77**: 34–8.

83 John M, Lim S, Seybold J, *et al*. Inhaled corticosteroids increase interleukin-10 but reduce macrophage inflammatory protein-1alpha, granulocyte–macrophage colony-stimulating factor, and interferon-gamma release from alveolar macrophages in asthma. *Am J Respir Crit Care Med* 1998; **157**: 256–62.

84 Stelmach I, Jerzynska J, Kuna P. A randomized, double-blind trial of the effect of glucocorticoid, antileukotriene and beta-agonist treatment on IL-10 serum levels in children with asthma. *Clin Exp Allergy* 2002; **32**: 264–9.

18 Tumor necrosis factor alpha

Christopher Brightling, Latifa Chachi, Dhan Desai, and Yassine Amrani

Institute of Lung Health, University of Leicester, Leicester, UK

Introduction

Accumulating clinical evidence from the use of anti-tumor necrosis factor (TNF)-α strategies has suggested that TNF-α represents an attractive target in a number of chronic inflammatory diseases. Current studies showed TNF-α blockade has revolutionized the treatment of certain diseases such as rheumatoid arthritis or ankylosing spondylitis, but is also effective in Crohn's disease, psoriasis, ulcerative colitis, juvenile idiopathic arthritis, and Wegener's granulomatosis, among others [1,2]. The initial enthusiasm for TNF-α blockade in these diseases has been somewhat dampened by the appearance of serious adverse effects seen during anti-TNF-α therapies including malignancies and infection-related complications (reactivation of tuberculosis) [3]. In addition, despite targeting the same cytokine, the different anti-TNF-α strategies (see Figure 18.1) that include human (golimumab) or chimeric mouse–human (infliximab) antibodies, fusion protein (etanercept), or PEGylated human fragment–antigen binding (Fab) (certolizumab) have been associated with various clinical outcomes. It is believed that differences in the drug pharmacokinetics, molecular structure and mode of action could explain in part their therapeutic efficacy. For example, etanercept seems to be less efficacious in treating granulomatous diseases than infliximab, while both drugs have comparable efficacy in treating rheumatoid arthritis. Regarding the adverse effects, the risk of tuberculosis seems to be several times greater for infliximab than etanercept. The purpose of this chapter is to describe the experimental studies that have provided the rationale for the use of TNF-α antagonists in lung diseases such as asthma. We will present and discuss the emerging clinical trials that have used anti-TNF-α therapy in asthmatic patients.

General aspects of tumor necrosis factor biology

Tumor necrosis factor alpha is essential in the regulation of the innate immune response, which plays a key role in the immediate host defense against invading micro-organisms before activation of the adaptive immune system [4]. TNF-α is principally produced by macrophages in response to activation of membrane-bound pattern-recognition molecules such as Toll-like receptors, which detect common bacterial cell surface products such as lipopolysaccharides. TNF-α is also produced by several other proinflammatory cells including monocytes, dendritic cells, B cells, CD4+ cells, neutrophils, mast cells and eosinophils and the structural cells, fibroblasts, epithelial cells and smooth muscle cells [5]. TNF-α is initially produced as a biologically active 26 kDa membrane-anchored

Inflammation and Allergy Drug Design, First Edition. Edited by Kenji Izuhara, Stephen T. Holgate, Marsha Wills-Karp.

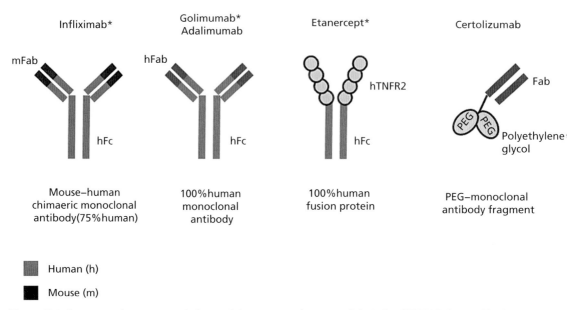

Figure 18.1 Structures of tumor necrosis factor alpha (TNF-α) blockers available in clinical medicine. PEG, PEGylated humanized Fab fragments; hFc, human Fc fragment of the IgG1; hTNFR2, human TNF-α receptor 2. *Indicates the antagonists that have been used in clinical trials in asthmatic patients.

precursor protein (membrane TNF-α [mTNF-α]) [6], which is subsequently cleaved by TNF-α-converting enzyme (TACE) [7] to release the 17kDa free protein. These proteins form biologically active homotrimers [8] that act on the ubiquitously expressed TNF-α receptors 1 and 2 (TNFR1 and TNFR2) [9]. It is important to mention that TNFR2 is mostly activated by membrane-bound TNF-α (mTNF-α) while TNFR1 is activated by soluble TNF-α. This receptor–ligand interaction causes intracellular signaling without internalization of the complex, leading to phosphorylation of IκBα and thus activation of the nuclear factor-κB (NF-κB) (p50–p65) heterodimer, which then interacts with the DNA chromatin structure to increase transcription of proinflammatory genes such as interleukin (IL)-1β, IL-6, IL-8, and TNF-α itself.

Upregulation of tumor necrosis factor alpha in allergic asthma

Elevated levels of TNF-α have been found in the sputum of patients with asthma [10,11]. Observations using mast cells or sensitized tissues showing that production of TNF-α is an IgE-dependent phenomenon

[12–14] strongly suggest the implication of TNF-α in allergic asthma. Indeed, increased TNF-α levels have been detected in the bronchoalveolar lavage (BAL) fluid of symptomatic asthmatic patients [15] or in patients exposed to allergen [16] or even lipopolysaccharide (LPS) [17]. Consistent with this, increased TNF-α amounts have been also reported in the airways following local allergen challenge [18]. BAL leukocytes from patients with ongoing bronchial asthma also spontaneously release high levels of TNF-α [19]. The concept that TNF-α may be of particular relevance in severe refractory asthma is supported by a study by Howarth *et al.*, who reported that TNF-α protein in the BAL, TNF-α protein and mRNA expression in bronchial biopsies were significantly increased in severe asthmatics compared with those with mild disease [20]. We found that increased expression of mTNF-α and TNFR1 on peripheral blood assessed by flow cytometry was only noted in patients with severe disease [21]. Thus, upregulation of TNF-α is a feature associated with severe refractory disease, suggesting that this phenotype may be particularly responsive to anti-TNF-α therapies. Considering the clinical benefit conferred by omalizumab, the humanized monoclonal anti-IgE antibody, in severe asthmatics [22–24], one can speculate that the therapeutic action conferred by omalizumab may involve, at least in part, the inhibition of IgE-dependent secretion of TNF-α by mast cells.

Tumor necrosis factor alpha blockade in experimental and human asthma

Animal studies

Lessons learned from preclinical studies using knockout and transgenic animals
The harmful effects of TNF-α in lungs was in part supported in reports where this cytokine was specifically overexpressed in the airways using transgenic mice in which the TNF-α gene was placed under the control of surfactant protein C promoter. Three studies clearly demonstrated that increasing levels of TNF-α in the airways was associated with many clinical features associated with asthma, chronic obstructive pulmonary disease (COPD) or idiopathic pulmonary fibrosis (IPF) such as lung inflammation, emphysema, and pulmonary fibrosis [25–27]. Other studies performed in mice lacking one component of the gene encoding for TNF signaling pathways have confirmed the putative role of TNF-α in asthma. Mice deficient in TNF receptors (known as TNFR1 or TNFR2) revealed that both TNF-α receptors were involved in toluene diisocyante (TDI)-induced asthmatic reactions including airway hyperresponsiveness, airway inflammation, and dendritic cell migration [28]. A similar finding was described in a murine model of allergic asthma (i.e., mice sensitized and challenged with ovalbumin) where mice lacking TNFR1, but not TNFR2, displayed a reduced airway hyperresponsiveness (AHR) to methacholine following allergen challenge [29]. Interestingly, allergen-dependent infiltration of eosinophils in the peribronchial, perivascular, and peripheral airways was strongly suppressed in the TNFR1-deficient mice. Activation of TNFR2, in contrast, was found to negatively regulate allergen-dependent AHR in part via the activation of γδ T cells [30]. In mice lacking the TNF-α gene, it was found that TNF-α was indeed instrumental in the development of the allergic rhinitis by regulating the generation of allergic-specific IgE, Th2-type cytokines and the recruitment of eosinophil to the inflammatory sites [31]. Another study using TNF-α knockout mice revealed that the implication of TNF-α in experimen-

tal asthma was clearly dependent on the absence of the adjuvant aluminum hydroxide during the sensitization phase, a protocol which elicits IgE- and mast cell-dependent pathways [32]. In this model, the authors made the remarkable finding that TNF-α and both TNFRs participate in antigen-induced bronchial hyperresponsiveness and allergic inflammation. The role of the IgE–mast cell axis in TNF-α pathogenic role in asthma was confirmed by the same group in a later study using mast cell-deficient mice. These mice were protected against allergen-induced airway inflammation and AHR, responses that were restored when mice were engrafted with bone marrow-derived mast cells [33]. These studies could explain the failure of one previous study to demonstrate any role of TNF-α in allergic inflammation in mice sensitized to ovalbumin in the presence of adjuvant aluminum hydroxide [34]. These different studies strongly support the implication of TNF-α and TNFRs in the pathogenesis of allergic rhinitis and asthma as well as occupational asthma. Both antigen-induced airway inflammation and hyperresponsiveness appear to be dependent on TNF-α, with mast cells being a clinically significant source of this cytokine in the airways.

Lessons learned from preclinical studies using anti-TNF-α blocking strategies
The first pharmacologic evidence of a role of TNF-α in experimental asthma was provided by Renzetti and colleagues in 1996, who showed the therapeutic benefit of a soluble TNF-α antagonist, called Ro 45-2081, in two different models of allergic asthma, i.e., guinea-pigs and Brown Norway rats sensitized and challenged with ovalbumin [35]. The inhibitor Ro 45-2081 (1–3 mg/kg i.p.), a TNFR2 fusion protein, was found to be as potent as dexamethasone in suppressing allergen-associated airway infiltration of inflammatory cells including eosinophils and neutrophils. Ro 45-2081 also effectively reduced allergen-induced AHR to substance P in sensitized guinea-pigs. Additional studies using monoclonal antibodies provided supporting evidence about the involvement and the potential underlying mechanisms by which TNF-α may contribute to the development of allergic asthma. In an animal model that displays both early and late asthmatic responses, Choi and colleagues showed that a cPLA2 inhibitor (TMFK) and the anti-TNF-α monoclonal antibody MP6.

227

XT22.11 specifically suppressed the late AHR and lung eosinophilia responses induced by ovalbumin while the early responses were unaffected. Because activation of cPLA2 activity in the allergic lungs was dependent on TNF-α, the authors suggested that cPLA2-dependent metabolites were playing an essential role in mediating TNF-α action during the allergic responses in the lungs [36]. Subsequent studies using the anti-TNF-α monoclonal antibodies, including infliximab or etanercept, have led to similar conclusions about the role of TNF-α in asthma [37–41]. The use of etanercept in ovalbumin-sensitized and -challenged guinea-pigs confirmed the implication of TNF-α in the development of AHR, possibly as a consequence of TNF-α downregulating muscarinic M2 receptor in the parasympathetic neurons within the airways. The protective action of etanercept has also been proven in both acute and long models of allergic inflammation

[38]. A recent report that used etanercept indirectly confirmed the implication of TNF-α in the regulation of antigen-induced Th2 cytokines and infiltration of inflammatory cells (eosinophils) in the airways [40]. Antigen-induced AHR assessed by Enhanced Pause (Penh) was somewhat reduced by etanercept but this effect did not reach statistical significance. These anti-TNF-α antibodies are also effective in different animal models of allergic asthma induced by different types of allergen including ovalbumin [37,40,41] or house dust extracts [39]. The main conclusions of these studies suggest that anti-TNF-α antibodies represent effective therapeutic options to treat many features present in human allergic asthma including production of Th2-type cytokines, and infiltration of various inflammatory cells in the airways. Studies that have used anti-TNF-α therapies in experimental asthma are summarized in Table 18.1.

Table 18.1 Summary of antitumor necrosis factor alpha (TNF-α) strategies in experimental asthma.

TNF-α blockers	Experimental model	Outcome	Reference
Ro 45-2081 TNFR1-FcIgG1 fusion protein	Ovalbumin-sensitized and challenged male guinea-pigs and rats	↓ Neut, Eos in the BAL ↓ AHR	Renzetti et al., 1996
MP6-XT22.11 anti-TNF-α monoclonal antibody	Ovalbumin-sensitized and challenged male BALB/C mice	↓ Eos in the BAL ↓ Late AHR	Choi et al., 2005
Etanercept	Ovalbumin-sensitized and challenged female BALB/C mice	↓ Eos in the BAL Ø AHR	Nam et al., 2009
Etanercept	Ovalbumin-sensitized and challenged guinea-pigs	↓ Eos in the BAL, blood, nerves and within ASM ↓ AHR	Nie et al., 2009
Etanercept	ST and LT model of ovalbumin-sensitized and challenged mice	↓ Eos, and IL-5 in the BAL (ST) ↓ Serum IgE(ST) ↓ IL-5 in the BAL (LT)	Hutchinson et al., 2007
Infliximab	Ovalbumin-sensitized and challenged male mice	↓ Eos in the BAL ↓ Cytokines in BAL	Deveci et al., 2008
Rat anti-TNF-α monoclonal antibody	House dust-sensitized and challenged female BALB/C mice	↓ Th2 cytokines ↓ Eos, Neut, and lymphocytes in the BAL ↓ AHR	Kim et al., 2006

Eos, eosinophils; Neut, neutrophils; BAL, bronchoalveolar lavage; AHR, airway hyperresponsiveness; ST, short-term model of asthma; LT, long-term model of asthma; ø, no effect.

Lessons learned from isolated airway preparations

Animal studies demonstrate that TNF-α is undeniably an important mediator in asthma pathogenesis. Not only does TNF-α participate in allergen-induced airway inflammation through the recruitment and/or activation of inflammatory cells, but it also seems to be essential in the development of AHR. The contribution of TNF-α in AHR could be due to a direct modulatory effect on airway smooth muscle (ASM) function. Pharmacodynamic studies using guinea-pig [42] and ovine tracheal airway preparations [43] demonstrated that incubation with TNF-α increased the contractile responses to methacholine. Similarly, murine-isolated tracheal rings incubated with TNF-α became hyperresponsive to additional G-protein-coupled receptor agonists, including carbachol [44,45], bradykinin [46], or serotonin [47]. Only two studies, possibly owing to the difficulty in obtaining and working with human tissues, showed that TNF-α alone or in combination with IL-1β exerted similar effects in human bronchi by enhancing electric field stimulation- or acetylcholine-associated contractile responses [48,49]. It is clear that a better understanding of the cellular and molecular mechanisms by which TNF-α contributes to asthmatic reactions will lead to novel therapeutic options.

Human studies

Promising data provided in the preclinical studies have encouraged the use of anti-TNF-α strategies in human lung diseases such as asthma and COPD [50,51]. Most human studies that have examined the efficacy of anti-TNF-α blocking strategies in asthma have been performed using *etanercept* (a soluble fusion protein combining two p75 TNF receptors with an Fc fragment of human IgG$_1$), although one study used *infliximab* (a chimeric mouse/humanized monoclonal antibody), and a more recent report used *golimumab*, a fully human monoclonal antibody. Details of these clinical trials in asthma are summarized in Table 18.2.

Lessons learned from human clinical trials using anti-TNF-α antibodies

The first evidence describing the therapeutic benefit of anti-TNF-α strategies in asthma patients was derived from an uncontrolled study of etanercept administered for 12 weeks in 15 severe asthmatics (Global Initiative on Asthma [GINA] stage V). In this report, Howarth *et al.* demonstrated a significant improvement in methacholine AHR, a 240 ml improvement in FEV$_1$, and an improvement in the quality of life of patients with asthma [20]. Similar findings were observed in a randomized, placebo-controlled study in which 10 weeks of treatment of 10 severe patients with etanercept led to a similar improvement in PC$_{20}$ and FEV$_1$, as well as an improvement in asthma-related quality of life [21]. One interesting finding reported in this study was the close correlation between the clinical response and the expression of membrane-bound TNF-α (mTNF-α) and TNFR1 on monocytes. The distinct role of soluble TNF-α (sTNF-α) versus mTNF-α in human asthma is essential: TNFR1 is activated by sTNF-α whereas TNFR2 is preferentially activated by mTNF-α [2]. An interesting preclinical study showed that sTNF-α was a key player in the development of asthma pathogenesis [32]. Whether measurement of the membrane-associated form of TNF-α on monocytes or other inflammatory cells could be used as a useful biomarker of clinical responses to anti-TNF-α therapy remains to be explored. These findings also raise the important question of whether anti-TNF-α approaches are effective only in a subgroup of asthma patients (severe cases). Interestingly, etanercept therapy had no effect on the number of sputum eosinophils or neutrophils, but was associated with a profound reduction in histamine concentration in the sputum. One intriguing possible explanation for this apparent lack of effect on airway inflammation by anti-TNF-α in contrast to a marked effect on AHR is that TNF-α derived from mast cells within the ASM bundle may play a critical role in the development of AHR. This hypothesis is based on previous work showing a direct modulation of airway smooth muscle contractility by TNF-α [52]. Similar beneficial effects, albeit less profound, have been reported in the study by Erin *et al.* [53] of moderate asthma. The authors concluded from their randomized placebo-controlled study that infliximab treatment for 6 weeks in these patients failed to improve morning peak flow, but there was an improvement in peak flow variability and a 50% reduction in the number of mild exacerbations encountered. The relatively poor effect on lung function in this study may reflect either the selection of patients with less severe

Table 18.2 Summary of antitumor necrosis factor alpha (TNF)-α in clinical trials in asthma.

Drug/ duration	Number of patients/severity	Design	Outcome	Result	Reference
Golimumab, 24 weeks	309/severe	Randomized, double blinded, placebo controlled, parallelgroup	1. FEV_1, exacerbations 2. AQLQ PEFR	1. FEV_1 unchanged, reduced exacerbations 2. Unfavorable adverse effects	Wenzel *et al.*, 2009
Etanercept, 12 weeks	15/severe	Open-label, uncontrolled	1. ACQ 2. FEV_1, AHR	1. Significant improvement of ACQ FEV_1 and AHR	Howarth *et al.*, 2005
Etanercept, 10 weeks	30/moderate and severe	Randomized, double blinded, placebo controlled, crossover	1. AHR, AQLQ	1. Improved AQLQ FEV_1, AHR	Berry *et al.*, 2008
Etanercept, 12 weeks	39/severe refractory asthma	Randomized, double blinded, placebo controlled, parallel group	1. AQLQ ACQ 2. FEV_1, AHR, PEFR	1. Improved ACQ 2. Improved AHR	Morjaria *et al.*, 2008
Etanercept, 2 weeks	21/mild to moderate	Randomized, double blinded, placebo controlled	1. Pulmonary Eos, AHR and local inflammation	1. Increased TNFR2 in the BAL	Rouhani *et al.*, 2005
Etanercept, 12 weeks	68/severe persistent	Randomized, double blinded, placebo controlled	1. Change in FEV_1% predicted	1. No change in FEV_1% predicted	Holgate *et al.*, 2007
Infliximab, 6 weeks	38/moderate	Randomized, double blinded, placebo controlled, parallel group	1. PEFR 2. Exacerbations	1. Trend towards reduced exacerbations and sputum TNF-α	Erin *et al.*, 2006

FEV1, forced expiratory volume in 1 s; AQLQ, Asthma Quality of Life Questionnaire; AHR, airway hyperresponsiveness; Eos, eosinophils; ACQ, Asthma Control Questionnaire; PEFR, peak expiratory flow rate; BAL, bronchoalveolar lavage; TNFR2, TNF-α receptor 2.

disease or a therapeutic difference between etanercept and infliximab. It is, however, impossible to objectively compare and contrast these two anti-TNF strategies as there have been no head-to-head comparative clinical trials. It is, however, proven from the use of anti-TNF-α strategies in other diseases that etanercept and infliximab both have different clinical and safety profiles, possibly as a consequence of their differences in mechanisms and pharmacokinetics [1]. In an earlier segmental allergen challenge study, etanercept therapy for 2 weeks was associated with increased levels of TNFR2 in the BAL [54]. Considering previous studies using etanercept in asthmatics, no definitive conclusion should be drawn from this study for multiple reasons: (i) TNF-α levels in the airways in baseline conditions were unknown; (ii) in contrast with previous studies that used the same drug, these patients were not treated with corticosteroids; and (iii) most patients used in this study had mild to moderate asthma, but anti-TNF-α therapy seems to be more effective in severe cases of asthma [20,21]. Interestingly, a 12-week etanercept treatment in corticosteroid refractory asthmatics demonstrates a small improvement in asthma control and systemic inflammation evidence by the reduction in serum of both CRP and albumin levels [55]. This small effect of etanercept could be due to the fact that levels of TNF-α in the airways were low in these patients. The other lesson learned from this study is that TNF-α-associated systemic effects could also play a role in asthma progression and/or severity. In a 12-week placebo-controlled study of etanercept in 132 subjects with moderate to severe asthma there was a doubling in PC20, no change in FEV1% predicted, and, importantly, no serious adverse events [56].

Most recently, Wenzel and colleagues [57] reported the largest published study to date on 309 subjects with severe asthma, treated with either placebo or three different doses of golimumab injections (50, 100 and 200 mg), monthly for 1 year in a randomized, double-blinded fashion. The primary endpoints were an improvement from baseline forced expiratory volume in 1 s (FEV_1) and the number of severe asthma exacerbations. Secondary endpoints were change from baseline in Asthma Quality of Life Questionnaire (AQLQ) score, peak expiratory flow (PEF) and rescue medication use. Unfortunately, the study was terminated early at 24 weeks owing to an unfavorable risk–benefit ratio in patients receiving golimumab treatment with no demonstrable efficacy. Of greatest concern was the high number of serious adverse effects in all the golimumab groups, especially in patients receiving oral corticosteroids. This combination of drugs could explain the increased cases of pneumonia, sepsis, reactivation of tuberculosis (TB), and increased rate of malignancy. It is interesting to note that most of the malignancies occurred in patients who failed to present a bronchodilator response, suggesting that genetic factors could represent essential factors in determining the increased susceptibility for malignancies in patients treated with anti-TNF-α therapies. Subgroup analysis in the Wenzel *et al.* study did suggest some benefit provided by anti-TNF-α strategies in certain phenotypes. A similar unfavorable safety profile for infliximab has been reported in a multicenter, randomized, double-blind, placebo-controlled, parallel-group, dose-finding study in patients with COPD [58]. Of note, all 10 infliximab-treated patients who developed malignancies had a 40 pack-year history. Whether cigarette smoke enhances the susceptibility of patients treated with infliximab to malignancies remains to be further explored. This raises an important question of whether anti-TNF-α therapy could be used in severe asthmatic patients with no smoking history and a bronchodilator response to limit the occurrence of adverse effects. Of course, this will need to be achieved with a substantial reduction in treatment-related adverse outcomes.

What have we learned from antitumor necrosis factor alpha therapies?

Figure 18.2 summarizes the mechanisms by which TNF-α contributes to the pathogenesis of severe asthma. Anti-TNF-α therapies in animal models of asthma first revealed the undeniable role of TNF-α in the development of allergic reactions. It was concluded that TNF-α plays a role in the recruitment of inflammatory cells in the airways as well as contributing to allergen-induced AHR, possibly via the alteration of bronchial smooth muscle function. Our studies using airway smooth muscle cells also demonstrated the implication of TNF-α in the development of steroid resistance [59], a main feature of severe asthma. Initial clinical trials using anti-TNF-α therapies (etanercept) on patients with severe asthma gave promising results with an improvement in lung function, AHR, asthma quality-of-life and exacerbation rate. However, enthusiasm for these findings have been somewhat dampened by the possible occurrence of serious adverse effects associated with TNF-α blockade previously reported in other diseases such as infection-related complications and malignancies. This unfavorable risk–benefit ratio was recently confirmed in severe asthma patients treated with the fully human monoclonal antibody golimumab (see Table 18.3). Lessons from other diseases demonstrate that the poor safety profile of golimumab in asthma cannot simply be extrapolated to etanercept, and thus further long-term safety trials are required. Therefore, in contrast to golimumab, etanercept may still present favorable efficacy without significant adverse effects. The potential discrepancies between etanercept and golimumab in terms of clinical efficacy and/or appearance of side-effects are still unknown but could be attributed to multiple factors such as patient characteristics, treatment duration, or the presence of non-asthma-related factors responsible for their refractory asthma. Heterogeneity in response to TNF-α antagonism in clinical trials could therefore be explained by the fact that severe asthma is indeed a heterogeneous condition. *Post hoc* analysis revealed certain phenotypes in the severe asthmatic population could be controlled by anti-TNF-α therapy (patients not taking antidepressants, for example). In addition, despite being on the market for more than 11 years now, we came to realize that the different clinical outcomes seen with these drugs could also result simply from

231

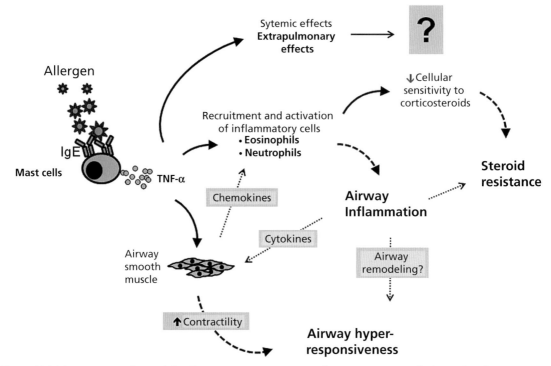

Figure 18.2 Tumor necrosis factor alpha (TNF-α) axis in the pathogenesis of severe asthma: Allergen-induced production of TNF-α via the immunoglobulin E (IgE)-dependent activation of mast cells. Other cellular sources could be involved. Following release, TNF-α contributes to asthma pathogenesis through the regulation of airway inflammation, possibly as a consequence of the recruitment and/or activation of different inflammatory cells. Products released by these activated infiltrated cells could affect the degree of airway hyperresponsiveness in part by acting on airway smooth muscle. A direct action of TNF-α on airway smooth muscle could maintain the inflammatory process via the secretion of a variety of chemokines. TNF-α could play a role in allergen-induced airway hyperresponsiveness by increasing the sensitivity of airway smooth muscle to a variety of contractile antagonists. Additional evidence is clearly needed to assess the importance of TNF-α in the regulation of airway remodeling and its consequence in the impaired lung function seen in asthmatic patients. Evidence from using etanercept therapy also suggests the possible implication of systemic (extrapulmonary) effects in the contribution of TNF-α in asthmatic patients. Corticosteroid resistance often seen in severe asthmatics could be due to TNF-α-induced changes in cellular responsiveness to corticosteroids, as previously reported in airway smooth muscle.

their diverse mechanisms of action and pharmacokinetic properties (reviewed in ref. 2). It is therefore too early to make a negative statement about the therapeutic value of anti-TNF-α therapy in lung diseases. Any decision regarding the future use of anti-TNF-α therapy in severe asthmatics, however, should be carefully based on drug safety, particularly with respect to susceptibility to severe infection, and the potential of solid organ malignancy. A better characterization of the phenotypic markers for severe asthma with the identification and further validation of biomarkers should help in defining the patient population for which anti-TNF-α therapy could be appropriate.

Acknowledgment

The author acknowledges funding from the Wellcome Trust and National Institutes of Health grant HL-06364.

Table 18.3 Adverse effects associated with antitumor necrosis factor alpha (TNF)-α therapies in asthmatic patients.

Transienthemiplegia
  36 h duration
Death (1)
  Septic shock from small bowel pneumatosis in a
  73 year old
Malignancies
  • B lymphoma
  • Melanoma
  • Cervical carcinoma
  • Renal carcinoma
  • Colon cancer
Asthma exacerbations
Respiratory tract infections
  • Pneumonia
Sepsis
Injection site reactions
Antinuclear antibodes (anti-dsDNA)

References

1 Lin J, Ziring D, Desai S, *et al.* TNFalpha blockade in human diseases: an overview of efficacy and safety. *Clin Immunol* 2008; **126**: 13–30.

2 Tracey D, Klareskog L, Sasso EH, Salfeld JG, Tak PP. Tumor necrosis factor antagonist mechanisms of action: a comprehensive review. *Pharmacol Ther* 2008; **117**: 244–79.

3 Wallis RS. Tumour necrosis factor antagonists: structure, function, and tuberculosis risks. *Lancet Infect Dis* 2008; **8**: 601–11.

4 Medzhitov R, Janeway C, Jr. Innate immunity. *N Engl J Med* 2000; **343**: 338–44.

5 Cazzola M, Polosa R. Anti-TNF-alpha and Th1 cytokine-directed therapies for the treatment of asthma. *Curr Opin Allergy Clin Immunol* 2006; **6**: 43–50.

6 Kriegler M, Perez C, DeFay K, Albert I, Lu SD. A novel form of TNF/cachectin is a cell surface cytotoxic transmembrane protein: ramifications for the complex physiology of TNF. *Cell* 1988; **53**: 45–53.

7 Zheng Y, Saftig P, Hartmann D, Blobel C. Evaluation of the contribution of different ADAMs to tumor necrosis factor alpha (TNFalpha) shedding and of the function of the TNFalpha ectodomain in ensuring selective stimulated shedding by the TNFalpha convertase (TACE/ADAM17). *J Biol Chem* 2004; **279**: 42898–906.

8 Smith RA, Baglioni C. The active form of tumor necrosis factor is a trimer. *J Biol Chem* 1987; **262**: 6951–4.

9 Brockhaus M, Schoenfeld HJ, Schlaeger EJ, Hunziker W, Lesslauer W, Loetscher H. Identification of two types of tumor necrosis factor receptors on human cell lines by monoclonal antibodies. *Proc Natl Acad Sci USA* 1990; **87**: 3127–31.

10 Keatings VM, Jatakanon A, Worsdell YM, Barnes PJ. Effects of inhaled and oral glucocorticoids on inflammatory indices in asthma and COPD. *Am J Respir Crit Care Med* 1997; **155**: 542–8.

11 Obase Y, Shimoda T, Mitsuta K, Matsuo N, Matsuse H, Kohno S. Correlation between airway hyperresponsiveness and airway inflammation in a young adult population: eosinophil, ECP, and cytokine levels in induced sputum. *Ann Allergy Asthma Immunol* 2001; **86**: 304–10.

12 Bradding P, Roberts JA, Britten KM, *et al.* Interleukin-4, -5, and -6 and tumor necrosis factor-alpha in normal and asthmatic airways: evidence for the human mast cell as a source of these cytokines. *Am J Respir Cell Mol Biol* 1994; **10**: 471–80.

13 Gordon JR, Galli SJ. Mast cells as a source of both preformed and immunologically inducible TNF-alpha/cachectin. *Nature* 1990; **346**: 274–6.

14 Ohkawara Y, Yamauchi K, Tanno Y, *et al.* Human lung mast cells and pulmonary macrophages produce tumor necrosis factor-alpha in sensitized lung tissue after IgE receptor triggering. *Am J Respir Cell Mol Biol* 1992; **7**: 385–92.

15 Broide DH, Lotz M, Cuomo AJ, Coburn DA, Federman EC, Wasserman SI. Cytokines in symptomatic asthma airways. *J Allergy Clin Immunol* 1992; **89**: 958–67.

16 Gosset P, Tsicopoulos A, Wallaert B, *et al.* Increased secretion of tumor necrosis factor alpha and interleukin-6 by alveolar macrophages consecutive to the development of the late asthmatic reaction. *J Allergy Clin Immunol* 1991; **88**: 561–71.

17 Michel O, Ginanni R, Le Bon B, Content J, Duchateau J, Sergysels R. Inflammatory response to acute inhalation of endotoxin in asthmatic patients. *Am Rev Respir Dis* 1992; **146**: 352–7.

18 Ying S, Robinson DS, Varney V, *et al.* TNF alpha mRNA expression in allergic inflammation. *Clin Exp Allergy* 1991; **21**: 745–50.

19 Cembrzynska-Nowak M, Szklarz E, Inglot AD, Teodorczyk-Injeyan JA. Elevated release of tumor necrosis factor-alpha and interferon-gamma by bronchoalveolar leukocytes from patients with bronchial asthma. *Am Rev Respir Dis* 1993; **147**: 291–5.

20 Howarth PH, Babu KS, Arshad HS, *et al.* Tumour necrosis factor (TNFalpha) as a novel therapeutic target in symptomatic corticosteroid dependent asthma. *Thorax* 2005; **60**: 1012–18.

21 Berry MA, Hargadon B, Shelley M, *et al*. Evidence of a role of tumor necrosis factor alpha in refractory asthma. *N Engl J Med* 2006; **354**: 697–708.

22 Holgate S, Smith N, Massanari M, Jimenez P. Effects of omalizumab on markers of inflammation in patients with allergic asthma. *Allergy* 2009; **64**: 1728–36.

23 Brusselle G, Michils A, Louis R, *et al*. "Real-life" effectiveness of omalizumab in patients with severe persistent allergic asthma: The PERSIST study. *Respir Med* 2009; **103**: 1633–42.

24 Ohta K, Miyamoto T, Amagasaki T, Yamamoto M. Efficacy and safety of omalizumab in an Asian population with moderate-to-severe persistent asthma. *Respirology* 2009; **14**: 1156–65.

25 Lundblad LK, Thompson-Figueroa J, Leclair T, *et al*. Tumor necrosis factor-alpha overexpression in lung disease: a single cause behind a complex phenotype. *Am J Respir Crit Care Med* 2005; **171**: 1363–70.

26 Fujita M, Shannon JM, Irvin CG, *et al*. Overexpression of tumor necrosis factor-alpha produces an increase in lung volumes and pulmonary hypertension. *Am J Physiol Lung Cell Mol Physiol* 2001; **280**: L39–L49.

27 Miyazaki Y, Araki K, Vesin C, *et al*. Expression of a tumor necrosis factor-alpha transgene in murine lung causes lymphocytic and fibrosing alveolitis. A mouse model of progressive pulmonary fibrosis. *J Clin Invest* 1995; **96**: 250–9.

28 Matheson JM, Lemus R, Lange RW, Karol MH, Luster MI. Role of tumor necrosis factor in toluene diisocyanate asthma. *Am J Respir Cell Mol Biol* 2002; **27**: 396–405.

29 Kanehiro A, Lahn M, Makela MJ, *et al*. Requirement for the p75 TNF-alpha receptor 2 in the regulation of airway hyperresponsiveness by gamma delta T cells. *J Immunol* 2002; **169**: 4190–7.

30 Kanehiro A, Lahn M, Makela MJ, *et al*. Tumor necrosis factor-alpha negatively regulates airway hyperresponsiveness through gamma-delta T cells. *Am J Respir Crit Care Med* 2001; **164**: 2229–38.

31 Iwasaki M, Saito K, Takemura M, *et al*. TNF-alpha contributes to the development of allergic rhinitis in mice. *J Allergy Clin Immunol* 2003; **112**: 134–40.

32 Nakae S, Lunderius C, Ho LH, Schafer B, Tsai M, Galli SJ. TNF can contribute to multiple features of ovalbumin-induced allergic inflammation of the airways in mice. *J Allergy Clin Immunol* 2007; **119**: 680–6.

33 Nakae S, Ho LH, Yu M, *et al*. Mast cell-derived TNF contributes to airway hyperreactivity, inflammation, and Th2 cytokine production in an asthma model in mice. *J Allergy Clin Immunol* 2007; **120**: 48–55.

34 Rudmann DG, Moore MW, Tepper JS, *et al*. Modulation of allergic inflammation in mice deficient in TNF receptors. *Am J Physiol Lung Cell Mol Physiol* 2000; **279**: L1047–L1057.

35 Renzetti LM, Paciorek PM, Tannu SA, *et al*. Pharmacological evidence for tumor necrosis factor as a mediator of allergic inflammation in the airways. *J Pharmacol Exp Ther* 1996; **278**: 847–53.

36 Choi IW, Sun K, Kim YS, *et al*. TNF-alpha induces the late-phase airway hyperresponsiveness and airway inflammation through cytosolic phospholipase A(2) activation. *J Allergy Clin Immunol* 2005; **116**: 537–43.

37 Deveci F, Muz MH, Ilhan N, Kirkil G, Turgut T, Akpolat N. Evaluation of the anti-inflammatory effect of infliximab in a mouse model of acute asthma. *Respirology* 2008; **13**: 488–97.

38 Hutchison S, Choo-Kang BS, Bundick RV, *et al*. Tumour necrosis factor-alpha blockade suppresses murine allergic airways inflammation. *Clin Exp Immunol* 2008; **151**: 114–22.

39 Kim J, McKinley L, Natarajan S, *et al*. Anti-tumor necrosis factor-alpha antibody treatment reduces pulmonary inflammation and methacholine hyper-responsiveness in a murine asthma model induced by house dust. *Clin Exp Allergy* 2006; **36**: 122–32.

40 Nam HS, Lee SY, Kim SJ, *et al*. The soluble tumor necrosis factor-alpha receptor suppresses airway inflammation in a murine model of acute asthma. *Yonsei Med J* 2009; **50**: 569–75.

41 Nie Z, Jacoby DB, Fryer AD. Etanercept prevents airway hyperresponsiveness by protecting neuronal M2 muscarinic receptors in antigen-challenged guinea pigs. *Br J Pharmacol* 2009; **156**: 201–10.

42 Pennings HJ, Kramer K, Bast A, Buurman WA, Wouters EF. Tumour necrosis factor-alpha induces hyperreactivity in tracheal smooth muscle of the guinea-pig *in vitro*. *Eur Respir J* 1998; **12**: 45–9.

43 Reynolds A, Holmes M, Scicchitano R. Cytokines enhance airway smooth muscle contractility in response to acetylcholine and neurokinin A. *Respirology* 2000; **5**: 153–60.

44 Chen H, Tliba O, Van Besien CR, Panettieri RA, Jr., Amrani Y. Selected contribution: TNF-{alpha} modulates murine tracheal rings responsiveness to G-protein-coupled receptor agonists and KCl. *J Appl Physiol* 2003; **95**: 864–72.

45 Jain D, Keslacy S, Tliba O, *et al*. Essential role of IFNbeta and CD38 in TNFalpha-induced airway smooth muscle hyper-responsiveness. *Immunobiology* 2008; **213**: 499–509.

46 Zhang Y, Adner M, Cardell LO. Up-regulation of bradykinin receptors in a murine in-vitro model of chronic airway inflammation. *Eur J Pharmacol* 2004; **489**: 117–26.

47 Adner M, Rose AC, Zhang Y, *et al*. An assay to evaluate the long-term effects of inflammatory mediators on murine airway smooth muscle: evidence that TNFalpha

up-regulates 5-HT(2A)-mediated contraction. *Br J Pharmacol* 2002; **137**: 971–82.

48 Anticevich SZ, Hughes JM, Black JL, Armour CL. Induction of human airway hyperresponsiveness by tumour necrosis factor-alpha. *Eur J Pharmacol* 1995; **284**: 221–5.

49 Sukkar MB, Hughes JM, Armour CL, Johnson PR. Tumour necrosis factor-alpha potentiates contraction of human bronchus *in vitro*. *Respirology* 2001; **6**: 199–203.

50 Brightling C, Berry M, Amrani Y. Targeting TNF-alpha: a novel therapeutic approach for asthma. *J Allergy Clin Immunol* 2008; **121**: 5–10; quiz 1–2.

51 Russo C, Polosa R. TNF-alpha as a promising therapeutic target in chronic asthma: a lesson from rheumatoid arthritis. *Clin Sci (Lond)* 2005; **109**: 135–42.

52 Amrani Y. Airway smooth muscle modulation and airway hyper-responsiveness in asthma: new cellular and molecular paradigms. *Exp Rev Clin Immunol* 2006; **2**: 353–64.

53 Erin EM, Leaker BR, Nicholson GC, *et al*. The effects of a monoclonal antibody directed against tumor necrosis factor-alpha in asthma. *Am J Respir Crit Care Med* 2006; **174**: 753–62.

54 Rouhani FN, Meitin CA, Kaler M, Miskinis-Hilligoss D, Stylianou M, Levine SJ. Effect of tumor necrosis factor antagonism on allergen-mediated asthmatic airway inflammation. *Respir Med* 2005; **99**: 1175–82.

55 Morjaria JB, Chauhan AJ, Babu KS, Polosa R, Davies DE, Holgate ST. The role of a soluble TNFalpha receptor fusion protein (etanercept) in corticosteroid refractory asthma: a double blind, randomised, placebo controlled trial. *Thorax* 2008; **63**: 584–91.

56 Holgate S, Noonan MD, Chanez P, *et al*. A randomized, double-blind, placebo controlled trial evaluating the safety of etanercept 25 twice weekly in patients with severe persistent asthma. *Chest* 2007; **132**: 436S.

57 Wenzel SE, Barnes PJ, Bleecker ER, *et al*. A randomized, double-blind, placebo-controlled study of tumor necrosis factor-alpha blockade in severe persistent asthma. *Am J Respir Crit Care Med* 2009; **179**: 549–58.

58 Rennard SI, Fogarty C, Kelsen S, *et al*. The safety and efficacy of infliximab in moderate to severe chronic obstructive pulmonary disease. *Am J Respir Crit Care Med* 2007; **175**: 926–34.

59 Tliba O, Amrani Y. Airway smooth muscle cell as an inflammatory cell: lessons learned from interferon signaling pathways. *Proc Am Thorac Soc* 2008; **5**: 106–12.

19 Profibrotic and angiogenic factors in asthma

Neville Berkman[1] *and Francesca Levi-Schaffer*[2]

[1]Institute of Pulmonary Medicine, Hadassah-Hebrew University Medical Center, Ein Kerem, Jerusalem, Israel

[2]Immunopharmacology Laboratory for Allergy and Asthma Research, Institute for Drug Research, School of Pharmacy, Faculty of Medicine, The Hebrew University of Jerusalem, Jerusalem, Israel

Airway remodeling is a prominent pathophysiologic feature of chronic asthma. It is characterized by changes in tissue structural components, including damage and shedding of airway epithelium, increased number of goblet cells, mucus gland hypertrophy, increased myofibroblast number, subepithelial fibrosis, increased airway smooth muscle (ASM) mass, and neovascularity [1,2]. The poor response to anti-inflammatory treatment seen in patients with refractory asthma may be a consequence of airway remodeling and the subsequent development of fixed airway obstruction [1,2]. Although a cause and effect between remodeling and poor response to treatment is by no means certain, this potential association has given rise to a plethora of research on remodeling in the hope that this will lead to the development of new therapeutic options for refractory asthma. Airway hyperresponsiveness (AHR) is an essential component of asthma and persists even with optimal anti-inflammatory therapy, suggesting that it may mirror airway remodeling. Although smooth muscle hypertrophy has been considered important in AHR, airway fibrosis may also contribute.

In this chapter, we review the major factors contributing to two components of airway remodeling, airway fibrosis, and angiogenesis.

Asthma and airway fibrosis

There is an increase in the number of fibroblasts and in fibroblast activation and differentiation to myofibroblasts in the airways of patients with asthma and in mice chronically exposed to ovalbumin [3,4]. Fibroblast number correlates with thickness of lamina reticularis and with disease severity [5]. There is also increased collagen deposition and extracellular matrix (ECM) deposition in asthmatic airways. The true basement membrane is normal in asthmatics but the subepithelial layer (lamina reticularis) is thickened two- to threefold [6]. Loose collagen fibrils found in normal airways are replaced by dense fibrils. Whether thickening of the lamina reticularis worsens or protects against airway narrowing is unclear [7] and thickness does not necessarily correlate with disease severity [8].

Asthmatic patients have an increased deposition in the airways of collagen I, III, and V, fibronectin, tenascin, hyaluronan, versican, laminin a2/b2, lumican and biglycan but decreased elastin and collagen IV [9,10]. Collagen I is deposited by fibroblasts and ASM in response to transforming growth factor beta (TGF-β) [11].

Extracellular matrix proteins themselves modulate fibroblasts and ASM, and ECM from asthmatics

Inflammation and Allergy Drug Design, First Edition. Edited by Kenji Izuhara, Stephen T. Holgate, Marsha Wills-Karp.

enhances proliferation of nonasthmatic ASM cells [12]. Collagen I and fibronectin enhance proliferation of ASM [13,14] and collagen I enhances inflammatory mediator release [12,13], mediates MMP2 and TIMP expression [15] and confers resistance to the inhibition of proliferation and migration by steroids [16].

Transforming growth factor beta

The TGF-β superfamily comprises over 30 different proteins including BMPs, activins, inhibins and others [17]. TGF-β exists as three different isoforms, TGF-β1, -β2 and -β3. TGF-β is encoded as an inactive precursor, prepro-TGF-β, which is cleaved to yield the 25 kDa mature protein. This then forms a dimer which associates noncovalently with latency-associated peptide (the precursor cleavage product) to form small latent TGF-β. TGF-β is secreted from the cell in the latent form and can then be rapidly sequestered by several binding proteins such as fibronectin, elastin, type IV collagen, decorin, and biglycan [6,18]. The ECM thus acts as a "storage depot" for latent TGF-β. Latent TGF-β is converted to the active form in a controlled manner by serine proteases, thrombospondin, plasmin, reactive oxygen species, and cell-surface integrins [19]. Activation of latent TGF-β is a major mechanism whereby TGF-β is controlled [20].

Transforming growth factor beta signaling is mediated via binding specific transmembrane receptor heterodimers and co-receptors. Type III receptors, betaglycan and endoglin, present TGF-β to the type II receptor, a 70 kDa constitutively active serine/threonine kinase. Following ligand binding, the receptor recruits and phosphorylates the 55 kDa type I receptor, which in turn mediates downstream signaling.

Transforming growth factor beta signal transduction pathways include the SMAD pathway and several nonSMAD pathways. For SMAD signaling, TGF-β receptor binding induces phosphorylation of the C-terminal phosphoserine motif of SMAD2/3. The SMAD2/3 complex then partners with SMAD4 and translocates to the nucleus where they regulate transcription of TGF-β responsive genes. SMAD3-dependent TGF genes include collagens 1, 5, and 6. SMAD3 is required for TGF-β mediated radiation fibrosis and for epithelial–mesenchymal transition (EMT) [21]. SMAD7 serves as an inhibitor of this pathway. NonSMAD pathways of TGF-β signaling include the mitogen-activated protein kinase pathways (Erk 1/2, JNK 1/2/3, and p38), phosphatidylinositol-3 kinase (PI-3K)/AKT pathways, Rho-like GTPase signaling, and others [22,23].

There is evidence that other TGF family members such as activin A may also play a role in asthma [24].

Transforming growth factor beta is critical for normal embryogenesis and tissue repair and plays a key role in mediating immune responses. TGF-β is considered to be the most important mediator of tissue fibrosis, both under physiologic conditions and pathologic states. Aberrant TGF-β expression is present in fibrotic tissue in hepatic, pulmonary, and kidney fibrosis, post-angioplasty restenosis, and progressive systemic sclerosis, as well as in asthmatic airways. Multiple hereditary conditions are associated with aberrant TGF-β regulation such as hereditary hemorrhagic telangiectasia (HHT) and Marfan syndrome. Mice with overexpression or gain-of-function mutations in the TGF-β pathway develop progressive organ fibrosis [25].

Transforming growth factor beta promotes fibroblast proliferation, migration, adhesion, differentiation to myofibroblasts, and survival [26]. TGF-β also enhances fibroblast expression of collagens I, III, and IV; other ECM proteins; and profibrotic factors and cytokines such as platelet-derived growth factor (PDGF) and connective tissue growth factor (CTGF). TGF-β also stimulates proliferation and hypertrophy of ASM [27] and induces synthesis of ECM components such as fibronectin and collagen and mediates expression of MMPs and TIMPs from epithelial and ASM cells [28]. EMT is the process whereby epithelial cells transdifferentiate into cells with a mesenchymal myofibroblastic phenotype. EMT occurs in development and wound healing, metastasis and fibrosis including asthma [29,30]. EMT is TGF-β dependent and mediated via SMAD3 pathways [21].

Transforming growth factor beta is secreted from monocytes, lymphocytes, eosinophils, epithelial cells, fibroblasts and ASM. In asthmatics, eosinophils are considered the major source of TGF-β [31], although this remains controversial [32], and epithelial cells may also be an important source of TGF-β [33]. At least 20 studies have demonstrated increased TGF-β expression in BAL and endobronchial biopsies in asthmatic patients, although some studies have been negative [reviewed in ref. 20]. Several studies in human asthmatics have found an association between TGF-β expression and airway remodeling. Increased levels of TGF-β mRNA and protein are present in bronchial biopsies of patients with moderate to severe asthma [34–38]. TGF-β2 expression from epithelial cells of asthmatic patients is increased and induces expression of the mucin gene *MUC5AC* [39,40].

Polymorphisms of the TGF-β1 gene may be associated with asthma. The C-509T polymorphism in the promoter region of the TGF-β1 is related to airflow obstruction and eosinophilic inflammation but not to airway wall thickness [41]. Others have found that the presence of SNP (+915G/G) in the TGF-β1 gene may be associated with irreversible bronchoconstriction in asthmatics [42].

The role of TGF-β in animal models of airway remodeling has also been evaluated [43–45]. Chronic allergen exposure with OVA in the presence of a neutralizing anti-TGF-β antibody resulted in reduced peribronchial ECM, and collagen deposition, mucus production, and proliferating ASM cells [46,47]. SMAD3-deficient mice exposed to OVA have reduced airway fibrosis and fewer peribronchial myofibroblasts [48]. In contrast to these studies, anti-TGF antibody had no effect on airway remodeling in a house dust mite (HDM) allergen challenge model [43].

Although TGF-β is undoubtedly increased in human and experimental asthma, its primary role may be as a modulator of airway inflammation rather than of fibrosis [49–51]. This effect is mediated primarily through T-regulatory cells and FOXP3, leading to suppression of both Th1 and Th2 responses [52].

Fibroblast growth factor

The fibroblast growth factor (FGF) family of proteins, named FGF1–23, is important for organogenesis and tissue repair [53]. The most extensively evaluated in the context of airway remodeling is FGF2 or basic FGF. FGF2 induces proliferation of fibroblasts, myofibroblasts, ASM, and endothelial cells and potentiates the mitogenic effects of other growth factors such as PDGF. FGF2 enhances responsiveness of ASM to TGF-β, IL-4 and IL-13 [54].

Fibroblast growth factor 2 is stored in basement membranes bound to glycosaminoglycan side chains of heparin sulfate proteoglycans [55]. This provides a source of readily available growth factor. FGF2 is released from ECM by heparinases and other glycosaminoglycan-degrading enzymes. FGF is also a mitogen for endothelial cells and stimulates these cells to produce proteases and plasminogen activators that degrade the vessel basement membrane and allow cells to invade the surrounding matrix [56].

Fibroblast growth factor 2 levels are higher in BAL from asthmatics compared with nonasthmatics, and are further increased following allergen challenge [57]. There is also increased FGF2 protein as detected by immunohistochemistry in bronchial biopsies from asthmatics [58]. In a murine model of allergic airways disease, recombinant FGF2 reduced airway hyperresponsiveness, mucus production and airway inflammation in sensitized animals but the mechanism of this effect is not clear [59].

Platelet-derived growth factor

Human platelet-derived growth factor (PDGF) is a disulfide-linked dimer of two different polypeptide chains, A and B. [60]. It is released from macrophages and mesenchymal cells within the asthmatic airway and enhances activation of eosinophils and secretion of inflammatory and growth factors such as GMCSF from ASM [61]. PDGF expression is no different in bronchial biopsies or BAL of asthmatics compared with nonasthmatics [62]; however, PDGF induces greater proliferation of airway fibroblasts from asthmatics [63], and also induces production of procollagen I from airway fibroblasts. Fibroblasts from severe asthmatics have higher expression of PDGF receptor beta than fibroblasts from mild–moderate asthmatics [64]. PDGF has been shown to enhance airway responsiveness and remodeling in mice exposed to diesel exhaust particulates [65]. In addition, PDGF can modulate MMP–TIMP balance and thereby facilitate migration of ASM cells. The mitogenic effect of IL-13 on mouse, rat, and human lung fibroblasts may be mediated via inducing the release of PDGF-AA. IL-13-induced human lung fibroblast proliferation was attenuated by an anti-PDGF-AA neutralizing antibody, and IL-13 stimulated human lung fibroblasts to secrete PDGF-AA [66].

Endothelin 1

Endothelin 1 (ET-1) expression is increased in the airways of refractory asthmatics [67]. In synergy with other growth factors such as PDGF, ET-1 enhances proliferation of ASM and fibroblasts and collagen production from bronchial fibroblasts obtained from both normal and asthmatic subjects [68]. ET-1 levels in BALF and plasma correlate with pulmonary function tests, suggesting that endothelins may contribute to regulation of bronchial tone [69]. ET-1 also increases airway inflammation via induction of TNF-α, IL-1β, and IL-6 release. Mast cells express both ET-1 as well as ET surface receptors [70]. ET-1 membrane receptor expression is similar in asthmatics and nonasthmatics [71].

Connective tissue growth factor

Connective tissue growth factor (CTGF, CCN2) is likely to be important in remodeling as it mediates many of the cellular effects of TGF-β, including promotion of fibroblast proliferation, ECM production, granulation tissue formation, as well as adhesion and migration of a wide variety of cell types [72,73]. CTGF is clearly upregulated in fibrotic disorders [74], and ASM cells from asthmatic patients produce more CTGF than nonasthmatic cells in response to TGF-β [75]. CTGF also induces ASM to produce fibronectin, collagen I, and VEGF. CTGF co-localizes with VEGF in the ECM, and may serve to anchor VEGF and other effector molecules, thereby facilitating the storage of rapidly available growth factors in the ECM [76].

Epidermal growth factor and EGF-receptor

The epidermal growth factor receptor (EGFR) is a member of the erbB family of tyrosine kinase receptors. Ligand binding to EGFR leads to activation of signal transduction pathways that are involved in regulating cellular proliferation, differentiation and survival [77]. There are several ligands for this receptor in humans, including TGF-α, HB-EGF (heparin-binding epidermal growth factor), and others. EGFR is expressed on fibroblasts and epithelial cells. HB-EGF is a potent mitogen for smooth muscle and promotes a migratory phenotype of ASM and epithelial cells. TGF-α plays an important role in regulation of mucus secretion from airway epithelial cells [51]. Both EGF and EGFR expression are increased in the bronchial epithelium, submucosa, and smooth muscle of asthmatics, and correlate with disease severity [78].

Eotaxins

The eotaxins 1/CCL11, 2/CCL24, and 3/CCL26 belong to the group of CC-chemokines and have chemotactic and activatory effects on eosinophils. Expression is increased in the airways of asthmatic patients and in murine models of asthma [79,80]. We have recently shown that fibroblasts express CCR3, the chemokine receptor that binds the eotaxins. CCL11 enhances fibroblast proliferation, adhesion, and migration but does not induce fibroblast differentiation [81]. Eotaxin 2/CCL24 and eotaxin 3/CCL26 also have profibrogenic effects, although they have different activity profiles [82].

Osteopontin

Osteopontin (OPN) is a 44kDa ECM RGD-containing glycoprotein that has recently been implicated in allergen-induced inflammation and airway remodeling [83,84]. It is produced mainly by epithelial cells, macrophages, T cells, and dendritic cells, and contributes to tissue fibrosis/wound healing via modulation of TGF-β and MMP expression and via enhancement of fibroblast activation [85]. OPN is upregulated in a murine model of allergen-induced airway remodeling and is expressed by eosinophils, T cells, and macrophages [84]. OVA-treated OPN-deficient mice have reduced lung collagen content, subepithelial fibrosis, peribronchial smooth muscle area, mucus-producing cells and inflammatory cell accumulation compared with wild-type mice. These mice had reduced MMP-2 activity and expression of IL-4, IL-12, IL-13, INF-γ, TGF-β1, and VEGF. Lung fibroblasts from OVA-treated OPN$^{-/-}$ mice exhibit reduced proliferation, migration, collagen deposition, and α-SMA expression in comparison with wild-type fibroblasts [86]. Increased OPN expression is also present in bronchial biopsies of asthmatic patients [84]. OPN also promotes angiogenesis *in vitro* and *in vivo* and induces vascular smooth muscle cell migration and proliferation *in vitro* [87]. We have shown that OPN (together with VEGF) accounts for eosinophil-mediated angiogenesis and that OPN-deficient mice have impaired VEGF production [88].

Fibronectin

Extracellular matrix components interact with both structural and inflammatory cells and with mediators in the airway wall and contribute to fibrosis and remodeling. Fibronectin (FN) is a 440 kD dimeric ECM glycoprotein of which two major splice variants exist, *plasma* FN (pFN), and *cellular* FN (cFN). cFN contains additional amino acid sequences termed extra domain-A (EDA) and EDB [89]. Following tissue injury, there is increased expression of EDA-containing FN (EDA-FN) which, together with mechanical stretch and TGF-β, is necessary for differentiation of fibroblasts to a collagen-producing, contractile, α-SMA-expressing myofibroblast phenotype [90]. There is increased expression of EDA-FN in pulmonary fibrosis [91] and EDA-deficient mice treated with bleomycin have attenuated fibrosis. There is also reduced airway fibrosis and collagen content in the airways of OVA-treated EDA-FN-deficient mice, although ASM and inflammation are similar to those in wild-type mice. These mice also have reduced AHR, suggesting that airway fibrosis per se is necessary for development of AHR [92].

Interleukin 4 and interleukin 13

Cytokines derived from Th2 cells are critical mediators of the airway inflammation present in asthma. IL-4 and -13 are also important in the development of airway remodeling. IL-4 and -13 induce subepithelial fibrosis following allergen challenge and promote proliferation of bronchial fibroblasts derived from asthmatic patients [93].

Ovalbumin-challenged mice treated with anti-IL-13 antibodies and IL-13-deficient mice do not develop subepithelial collagen deposition [93,94], while mice with constitutive overexpression of IL-13 do develop subepithelial fibrosis [95]. IL-13 can induce fibroblast differentiation and proliferation and enhance collagen production *in vitro*.

Other mediators

Several additional mediators present in asthmatic airways have important profibrotic effects including GM-CSF, VEGF, NGF, collagen and other ECM components and the tissue metalloproteinases (MMPs) and protease inhibitors (TIMPS). These mediators are covered more fully in other sections of this volume.

Asthma and angiogenesis

Angiogenesis is the growth of new blood vessels from pre-existing ones. It is the predominant mechanism of blood vessel formation for organ growth in the later stages of embryonic development, in postnatal wound repair and cyclically in the female reproductive system [96]. Angiogenesis is also associated with pathologic conditions such as chronic inflammation, fibrosis, and tumor growth [97]. Angiogenesis depends on the balance of positive and negative angiogenic mediators within the vascular microenvironment and requires the functional activities of angiogenic factors, extracellular matrix proteins, adhesion receptors, and proteolytic enzymes [96]. It is therefore a multistep and highly orchestrated process involving not only vessel sprouting but also pericyte detachment, blood vessel dilation, basal membrane and extracellular matrix degradation that allows endothelial cells to migrate into the perivascular space toward angiogenic stimuli, their proliferation and survival, tube and basement membrane formation, pericyte attachment and, finally, blood vessel sprouting.

In normal tissues vascular quiescence is maintained by the dominant influence of endogenous angiogenesis inhibitors over angiogenic stimuli. In contrast, in pathologic situations such as in asthma, angiogenesis might be excessive because of the overproduction of angiogenic factors, downregulation of angiogenesis inhibitors, or both. Numerous inducers of angiogenesis have been identified, including members of the FGF family, vascular permeability factor/vascular endothelial growth factor (VEGF), and others. These factors have been shown to be directly angiogenic or to induce expression of VEGF, or both. In addition, the role of enzymes such as heparanase and MMPs, specifically MMP-2 and -9 must also be considered. Several negative regulators of angiogenesis have now been identified including endostatin, thrombospondin 1 (TSP-1), IFN-α, angiostatin, and TIMPs [98].

In asthmatic patients bronchial blood flow is increased because of an increased number of subepithelial peribronchial blood vessels that are dilated and prone to vascular leakage. New blood vessels can also serve as a source for increased recruitment of inflammatory cells and as a source of nutrients for potentially hypoxic fibrotic tissue. Thus, in asthma, inflammation, fibrosis, and angiogenesis are interactive processes that together perpetuate disease chronicity.

241

Hypervascularity of the airways is physiologically relevant in terms of airflow limitation and AHR, and it has potential to be a significant and even critical pathogenic factor during acute asthma attacks. Increased vascularity in the airways has been recognized not only in patients with severe asthma but also in those with mild forms of the disease [99].

Several factors likely to be produced in the inflamed airways in asthma have now been proposed as possible stimulants of the angiogenic response such as VEGF, PlGF, FGF-2, PDGF, angiogenin, TGF-β, IL-8, MCP-1, TNF-α, ET-1, thrombin, PAF, NO, hemeoxygenase 1, COX2, MMPs, histamine, bradykinin, sulfidopeptide, leukotrienes, and products of the autonomic nervous system. The evidence for a prime angiogenic role in asthma is strongest for VEGF, so we will focus in particular on this factor.

Vascular endothelial growth factor

The most extensively studied mediator in angiogenesis is undoubtedly vascular endothelial growth factor (VEGF). Indeed, VEGF is the most potent direct-acting regulator of angiogenesis, and its expression is increased in chronic inflammation, fibrosis, and cancer. There are at least six VEGF isoforms of variable length, produced by alternate splicing, that differ primarily in their bioavailability, which is conferred by heparin- and heparan sulfate-binding domains. After secretion, $VEGF_{121}$ may diffuse relatively freely in tissues, whereas approximately half of the secreted $VEGF_{165}$ binds to cell-surface heparan sulfate proteoglycans (HSPGs). $VEGF_{189}$ and $VEGF_{206}$ remain almost completely sequestered by HSPGs on the cell surface and in the ECM, making HSPGs a reservoir of VEGF that can be mobilized through proteolysis [97]. The effects of VEGF on endothelial cells are mediated mostly by signals generated by binding to receptor tyrosine kinases (RTKs). Several high-affinity RTKs for VEGF (VEGFRs) have been identified, including VEGFR-1, VEGFR-2, and VEGFR-3. Neuropilin 1 and 2 constitute another class of high-affinity non-RTKs VEGF receptors and can bind certain isoforms of VEGF. Both VEGFR-1 and VEGFR-2 have seven extracellular immunoglobulin-like domains, a single transmembrane region, and a consensus tyrosine kinase sequence. VEGFR-1 binds VEGF, VEGF-B, and placental growth factor with high affinity. VEGFR-1, like VEGFR-2, is expressed mostly on endothelial cells, as well as on other structural and hematopoietic stem cells. VEGFR-2 is the primary receptor transmitting VEGF signals in endothelial cells. VEGF induces proliferation, migration, and tube formation of endothelial cells. It promotes secretion of interstitial collagenase (MMP-1) and von Willebrand factor and the expression of chemokines, as well as leukocyte adhesion molecules, such as intercellular adhesion molecule 1, vascular cell adhesion molecule 1, and E-selectin [100]. VEGF is also a potent survival factor for endothelial cells, and it induces the expression of antiapoptotic proteins, such as survivin in endothelial cells. VEGF also causes vasodilatation through the induction of the endothelial nitric oxide synthase and the subsequent increase in nitric oxide production. Therefore, VEGF acts principally on endothelial cells, even though it can influence other cell types, including hematopoietic stem cells, monocytes, osteoblasts, and neurons, and can also modulate immune cell functions. TGF-β induces VEGF gene expression and secretion in fibroblasts and epithelial cells while IL-5 and GM-CSF have a similar effect on eosinophils. VEGF production is upregulated in endothelial cells by blood and/or tissue hypoxia, mainly through hypoxia-inducible factor transcriptional complex.

The direct contribution of VEGF in allergic responses in asthma has been shown by Lee *et al.* [101] in lung-targeted $VEGF_{165}$ transgenic mice with a Th2-mediated inflammation. Overexpression of VEGF caused predictably marked angiogenesis, edema, and vascular remodeling together with an exaggerated immune response after respiratory allergen challenge and leukocyte infiltration in the lung, overproduction of IL-13, and increases in mucus production, collagen deposition, and smooth muscle hyperplasia. In human asthma, VEGF also seems to have both proangiogenic and immunoregulatory roles [102]. In chronic stable asthmatics, BAL VEGF–albumin ratio, as well as levels of airway VEGF, FGF-2, and angiogenin were higher than in healthy controls or those with chronic bronchitis [103]. Expression of VEGF and its receptors VEGFR-1 and VEGFR-2 inversely correlated with airway function, vascularity and VEGF/VEGF receptor gene expression in airway biopsies in mild asthmatics receiving β-agonists only [104]. VEGF *m*RNA expression correlated with vascularity and AHR and inversely correlated with FEV_1. A more recent study found that BAL from atopic mild asthmatics had increased angiogenic activity [105]. The sputum of children with acute asthma showed an increase in VEGF, and angiogenin, which was proportional to disease severity [106]. In another study in mild asthmatics, an increase in smaller vessel size and BAL VEGF was detected in addition to increased VEGF, and R1 and R2 staining per vessel [107].

Nerve growth factor

Nerve growth factor (NGF), the most important neurotrophic agent, is locally produced in the airways. This production is enhanced in asthmatics in bronchial epithelium, smooth muscle cells and infiltrating inflammatory cells in the submucosa, and in the BALF [108]. NGF has demonstrated angiogenic activity in a quail chorioallantoic membrane (CAM) model, increasing the rate of angiogenesis in a dose-dependent fashion [109]. In a mouse model of allergic asthma NGF-positive cells were detected in the inflammatory infiltrate of the airways, with increased NGF, levels in serum and BAL [110]. In humans, both eosinophils and mast cells store and produce NGF [111].

Angiopoietin 1

Angiopoietin 1 (ANG1) is a primary angiogenic growth factor and is also likely to be involved in the pathogenesis of chronic asthma [112]. In airway biopsies and BALF from subjects with mild to moderate asthma, ANG1 expression (and VEGF), was elevated compared with normal subjects. This increase correlated with the number of vessels [113]. Recently, considerable attentions have been devoted to the physiologic roles of ANG1 and -2 as regulatory factors of VEGF. ANG1 has been shown to induce the migration and sprouting of endothelial cells, and coexpression of ANG1 and VEGF enhances angiogenesis. In the presence of high levels of VEGF, ANG2 also promotes rapid increase in capillary diameter, remodeling of the basal lamina, proliferation and migration of endothelial cells, and stimulates sprouting of new blood vessels. Thus, VEGF and ANG1 and -2 may play complementary and coordinated roles in airway angiogenesis and microvascular remodeling [114].

Endothelin 1

Endothelin 1 (ET-1) expression is increased in asthmatic airways (see above). In addition to its profibrotic effects, ET-1 is also a vasoactive peptide and mediates angiogenesis *in vivo*. ET-1 upregulates VEGF and induces endothelial cell proliferation [115]. Using the CAM assay, ET-1 mediates an angiogenic response via the ET_A receptor and a VEGF receptor [116]. ET-1 promotes HUVEC proliferation, migration, and invasion in a dose-dependent manner mainly through the ET_B receptor. ET-1 also enhances HUVEC differentiation into cord vascular-like structures and stimulates MMP-2 production. Finally, ET-1 stimulates neovascularization *in vivo* in concert with VEGF [117]. ET-1 functions as an antiapoptotic factor for endothelial cells and VSMC; it might also contribute to endothelial cell integrity by acting as a survival factor for newly formed blood vessels [118].

Endothelin 1 also acts as a lymphangiogenic mediator promoting outgrowth of lymphatic vessels *in vivo* [119]. ET-1 is also able to upregulate the expression of VEGF-C, VEGFR-3, and VEGF-A, and to stimulate hypoxia-inducible factor (HIF)-1α.

Angiogenin

Angiogenin (ANG) promotes angiogenesis and levels are increased in BALF and in ASM cultured from subjects with mild or moderate asthma. ANG levels also correlated with measures of angiogenesis [105,120]. Moreover, increased vascularity of the bronchial mucosa in asthmatic subjects is closely related to the expression of ANG [58]. Increased ANG and VEGF concentrations are found in induced sputum supernatants in patients with rhinitis and with asthma. Sputum ANG levels were elevated in children with acute asthma exacerbations and decreased after 6 weeks of therapy [106]. Finally, it has recently been shown that human mast cells store and secrete angiogenin in response to a variety of stimuli [121].

Angiostatin

Angiostatin is a 38 kDa plasminogen fragment and a naturally occurring endogenous angiogenesis inhibitor [122]. Human macrophage elastase (MMP-12) plays an important role in inflammatory processes and is involved in the conversion of plasminogen into angiostatin. To date, there are no published data on the role of angiostatin in asthma.

Endostatin

Endostatin is a 20 kDa C-terminal fragment of collagen XVIII that specifically inhibits endothelial proliferation and potently inhibits angiogenesis and tumor growth [123]. An imbalance between VEGF and endostatin levels has been described in induced sputum from asthmatic subjects [104]. In contrast, although BALF from asthmatics has enhanced proangiogenic capacity (attributable to VEGF), anti-angiogenic factors such as endostatin or Ang-2 were not different from nonasthmatics [105]. Similarly, the induction of angiogenesis by ASM from patients with asthma was found to be VEGF dependent with no changes in endostatin [120]. In a mouse model of asthma, recombinant endostatin can prevent the development of some features of asthma, suggesting that these molecules merit further study as potential therapies for asthma [124].

ADAM33

ADAM33 belongs to a large family of disintegrin and metalloprotease molecules and may be an asthma and COPD susceptibility gene [125]. High levels of soluble ADAM33 (sADAM33), which includes the catalytic domain, are present in BALF of asthmatics. sADAM33 promotes angiogenesis, causing rapid induction of endothelial cell differentiation *in vitro* and neovascularization both *ex vivo* and *in vivo*. Furthermore, TGF-β(2) enhances sADAM33 release from cells overexpressing full-length ADAM33. Environmental factors that cause epithelial damage may synergize with ADAM33 in asthma pathogenesis, resulting in a disease-related gain of function. This highlights the potential for interplay between genetic and environmental factors in this complex disease [126].

Eosinophils and angiogenesis

We have recently focused on the contribution of eosinophils to angiogenesis in the context of asthma.

Eosinophils present in asthmatic airways produce a variety of proangiogenic factors including VEGF, β-FGF, IL-8 and NGF, GM-CSF, and eotaxin. Using a co-culture approach [127], human peripheral blood eosinophils directly promote endothelial cell proliferation, induce endothelial cell VEGF production and enhance endothelial cell responsiveness to VEGF via upregulation of its specific surface receptor. Moreover, eosinophils induce new vessel formation in aorta rings and in CAM models [128]. We have recently found that when eosinophil-derived major basic protein (MBP) is present in subcytotoxic concentrations, it induces endothelial cell proliferation and enhances the promitogenic effect of VEGF without affecting VEGF release. MBP promotes capillarogenesis by endothelial cells seeded on matrigel and sprouting formation in the CAM assay [129].

Osteopontin (OPN), a phosphorylated acidic RGD-containing glycoprotein, has proangiogenic activity in part via enhancing VEGF production and VEGF-stimulated neovascularisation [130]. We found that OPN is expressed in human eosinophils and is increased following GM-CSF and IL-5 activation. Eosinophil-derived OPN contributes to eosinophil-induced angiogenesis as found in endothelial cell proliferation and tube-like formation assays. Recombinant OPN promotes eosinophil chemotaxis *in vitro* by integrin binding. Soluble OPN is increased in the bronchoalveolar lavage fluid from mild asthmatic subjects and correlates with eosinophil counts. We have recently found that eosinophils upregulate VEGF release *in vitro* when subjected to hypoxic conditions, which may be an important trigger for angiogenesis in the asthmatic airway [131].

Therapeutic implications

Glucocorticosteroids continue to be the most effective antiasthmatic drugs available. Although very effective in reducing airway inflammation, the efficacy of corticosteroids in attenuating fibrosis is controversial. Steroids reduce TGF-β1 and -β2 in fetal lung fibroblasts [132], block TGF-β induced collagen synthesis, reduce phospho-SMAD2 expression and increase SMAD7 [133]. *In vitro*, steroids have little effect on ASM ECM production [63,134]. In asthmatic patients treated with corticosteroids, some studies have found changes in basement membrane thickness while others have not [135–137].

The efficacy of steroids on reducing airway vascularity in asthma is more convincing. Budesonide reduced VEGF secretion in human airway and alveolar epithelial cells while fluticasone reduced VEGF expression in the bronchial mucosa of asthmatic patients [138]. Inhaled corticosteroids (ICS) reduced the number of blood vessels and VEGF-positive cells in bronchial biopsies from asthmatic patients and VEGF levels in sputum [139]. In another study, inhaled fluticasone 2000 μg/day for 3 months decreased airway vessel number by 30%, VEGF staining by 40%, and angiogenic sprouting by 25% [140].

Long-acting $β_2$-agonists enhance the effects of ICS, and may thereby contribute to the antiangiogenic effect of steroids [141]. Montelukast, a leukotriene receptor antagonist, inhibited OVA-induced smooth muscle hyperplasia and subepithelial fibrosis in mice [142].

The apparent lack of efficacy of corticosteroid therapy in attenuating airway remodeling, particularly fibrosis and smooth muscle hyperplasia, has led to attempts to develop new therapeutic alternatives.

The importance of TGF-β in fibrogenesis makes blocking the activity of this cytokine an obvious target for new drug development. Potential approaches to blocking TGF-β include blocking TGF-β production or activity using neutralizing antibodies, the use of soluble TGF-β receptors or inhibition of latent TGF-β activation such as by using anti-$α_vβ_6$ antibodies. An attractive alternate approach is blocking TGF-β receptor activation by small molecule serine/threonine kinase inhibitors or the use of nucleic acid inhibitors (antisense, siRNA). Several small molecular inhibitors of the type I TGF-β receptor have been identified which selectively inhibit aspects of fibrosis such as collagen-1 induction [143,144].

Transforming growth factor beta is, however, also pivotal in maintaining immune tolerance and attenuation of its activity may therefore potentially be harmful. A more selective approach to blocking the activity of TGF-β by using pathway-specific inhibitors makes better physiologic sense and may be safer. Possible approaches include blocking SMAD or other intracellular signal transduction pathways using synthetic SMAD-interacting peptides [145] or endogenous inhibitors such as SMAD7. BMP-7 attenuates TGF-β-induced EMT, and fibrosis and IL-7 inhib-

its TGF-β induction of SMAD7 [146]. Inhibition of SMAD3 is a particularly attractive target; this strategy will block EMT, induction of collagen synthesis and recruitment of fibroblasts [146]. IFN-α inhibits SMAD3 by phosphorylation of STAT1, which competes with SMAD3 for limited amounts of CBP/p300 thereby inhibiting TGF-β-stimulated collagen gene transcription. 1,25-dihydroxyvitamin D3 has been shown to decrease SMAD3 and TGF expression in the kidney [147].

Halofuginone inhibits collagen synthesis via inhibition of SMAD2 and SMAD3 phosphorylation and induction of SMAD7 expression. Halofuginone prevented development of radiation-induced and dermal fibrosis and reduced skin fibrosis in some patients with scleroderma [148].

Both natural (15-deoxyprostaglandin) and synthetic ligands (GW7845) for the peroxisome proliferator-activated receptor gamma (PPAR-γ) inhibit induced CTGF production. PPAR-γ physically interacts with SMAD3 and PPAR-γ ligands prevent TGF-β induced production of fibronectin [11]. Ciglitazone, a synthetic PPAR-γ agonist, reduced mucus gland hyperplasia, basement membrane thickness, collagen, and TGF-β levels in a mouse model of asthma [149]. This agent also reduces eosinophil and IL-4, -5, and -13 levels in murine airways and inhibits smooth muscle proliferation. PPAR-γ expression is increased in the airways of asthmatics [150] and this may act as a negative feedback pathway to quench inflammation and remodeling.

Another potential means of blocking TGF-β activity is by blocking recruitment of coactivator or intracellular downstream molecules such as CTGF. CTGF, antisense, and neutralizing antibodies block the effect of TGF-β on fibroblast collagen production and proliferation. Protein kinase C inhibitors suppress CTGF levels, and in animal models the use of CTGF antagonists prevents or reverses development of tissue fibrosis [151].

The human pregnancy hormone relaxin has also been shown to inhibit TGF-β-induced collagen, fibronectin and MMP-1 expression in human lung fibroblasts [152].

The use of cytokines or anticytokines may be of value in attenuating airway fibrosis and remodeling. Interferon (IFN)-γ gene transfer reversed airway inflammation and hyperresponsiveness in mice, but IFN-γ has no effect in humans [153,154]. Anti-IL-5 attenuates subepithelial fibrosis in OVA-treated mice, and mice that are IL-5Ra deficient were protected from increased subepithelial matrix deposition. IL-5-deficient mice have reduced airway collagen, ASM, and mucus production, although other studies did not observe differences in remodeling [155]. In a small study using anti-IL-5 in mild atopic asthmatics, there was reduced tenascin, lumican, and procollagen III deposition in the subepithelial tissue [38].

In chronic OVA exposure, anti-IL-13 Abs and IL-13-deficient mice are protected against some features of remodeling, such as subepithelial collagen deposition and mucus production, and have reduced airway hyperresponsiveness. This effect is only observed if IL-13 blocking precedes challenge [33].

Attenuation of angiogenesis has been evaluated in the context of cancer therapies. Recognition of the VEGF pathway as a key regulator of angiogenesis has led to the development of various therapeutic strategies designed to either stimulate or inhibit VEGF production [97]. In an animal model of allergic asthma, VEGF was necessary for Th2 inflammation and to augment antigen sensitization by acting on pulmonary dendritic cells [101]. Specific VEGF neutralization reduces not only angiogenesis but also some features of inflammation. Neutralizing monoclonal anti-VEGF, antibodies such as bevacizumab are used in cancer therapy although its effect in airway disease has not been evaluated. Inhibiting VEGF receptors may be even more effective than blocking the ligand as the number of VEGF receptors in tissue is relatively low. The use of angiostatic agents such as angiostatin or endostatin may be a potential therapeutic approach to reduce angiogenesis and even bring about recovery from tissue remodeling. Other compounds have been described to be inhibitors of angiogenesis. For example, fumagallin and its synthetic analog inhibit endothelial cell proliferation *in vitro* and angiogenesis in experimental models [156]. Rapamycin inhibits angiogenesis *in vivo* [157]. This activity has been related to the inhibition of endothelial cell proliferation after VEGF stimulation. Everolimus is a rapamycin analog more selective for endothelial cells and with more favorable pharmacokinetic properties. Because of the importance of MMP in angiogenesis, major efforts are currently being made to find a way to inhibit these proteinases in an attempt to reduce angiogenesis. Neovastat, an antiangiogenic drug used in the field of cancer treatment, effectively suppressed

airway inflammation and airway hyperresponsiveness in a mouse model of asthma. These effects were associated with a decrease in MMP-9 activity [158]. Endothelin 1 induces both fibrosis and angiogenesis. Both bosentan, a mixed ET_A/ET_B receptor antagonist, and selective ET_A receptor antagonists inhibit angiogenesis. Endothelin (ET) receptor antagonists are efficacious for the treatment of pulmonary arterial hypertension. Thus, ET receptor blockers are a potentially attractive treatment option in asthma. ET_A receptor antagonists decreased eosinophil number in BALF and neutrophil infiltration into the lungs in a model of lung inflammation after antigen challenge in sensitized mice [159].

Although many of the mediators mentioned in this review may be potential targets for new drug development aimed at preventing fibrosis and angiogenesis in asthma, effective antiremodeling therapy would ideally also reverse existing structural changes. An approach that targets mediators with multiple effects on inflammation and remodeling such as TGF-β1, IL-13, or osteopontin may be more effective but potentially more toxic, whereas a more selective approach such as targeting EDA-fibronectin or angiostatin may prove both efficacious and safe.

Acknowledgment

We would like to thank Alon Hur Nissim Ben Efraim, MSc, for assistance in preparing the chapter.

References

1 Davies DE, Wicks J, Powell RM, *et al*. Airway remodeling in asthma: new insights. *J Allergy Clin Immunol* 2003; **111**: 215–25.

2 Homer RJ, Elias JA. Airway remodeling in asthma: therapeutic implications of mechanisms. *Physiology (Bethesda)* 2005; **20**: 28–35.

3 Homer RJ, Elias JA. Consequences of long-term inflammation. Airway remodeling. *Clin Chest Med* 2000; **21**: 331–43.

4 McMillan SJ, Lloyd CM. Prolonged allergen challenge in mice leads to persistent airway remodeling. *Clin Exp Allergy* 2004; **34**: 497–507.

5 Benayoun L, Druilhe A, Dombret MC, *et al*. Airway structural alterations selectively associated with severe asthma. *Am J Respir Crit Care Med* 2003; **167**: 1360–8.

6 Boxall C, Holgate ST, Davies DE. The contribution of transforming growth factor-β and epidermal growth factor signalling to airway remodeling in chronic asthma. *Eur Respir J* 2006; **27**: 208–29.

7 Pare PD, Roberts CR, Bai TR, Wiggs BJ. The functional consequences of airway remodeling in asthma. *Monaldi Arch Chest Dis* 1997; **52**: 589–96.

8 Chu HW, Halliday JL, Martin RJ, *et al*. Collagen deposition in large airways may not differentiate severe asthma from milder forms of the disease. *Am J Respir Crit Care Med* 1998; **158**: 1936–44.

9 Roberts CR, Burke AK. Remodeling of the extracellular matrix in asthma: proteoglycan synthesis and degradation. *Can Resp J* 1998; **5**: 48–50.

10 Huang J, Olivenstein R, Taha R, Hamid Q, Ludwing M. Enhanced proteoglycan deposition in the airway wall of atopic asthmatics. *Am J Respir Crit Care Med* 1999; **160**: 725–9.

11 Johnson PR, Burgess JK, Ge Q, *et al*. Connective tissue growth factor induces extracellular matrix in asthmatic airway smooth muscle. *Am J Respir Crit Care Med* 2006; **173**: 32–41.

12 Chan V, Burgess JK, Ratoff JC, *et al*. Extracellular matrix regulated enhanced eotaxin expression in asthmatic airway smooth muscle cells. *Am J Respir Crit Care Med* 2006; **174**: 379–85.

13 Hirst SJ, Twort CH, Lee TH. Differential effects of extracellular matrix proteins on human airway smooth muscle cell proliferation and phenotype. *Am J Respir Cell Mol Biol* 2000; **23**: 335–44.

14 Dekkers BG, Schaafsma D, Nelemans SA, Zaagsma J, Meurs H. Extracellular matrix proteins differentially regulate airway smooth muscle phenotype and function. *Am J Physiol Lung Cell Mol Physiol* 2007; **292**: L1405–L1413.

15 Henderson N, Markwick LJ, Elshaw SR, Freyer AM, Knox AJ, Johnson SR. Collagen 1 and thrombin activate MMP-2 by MMP-14 dependent and independent pathways: applications for airway smooth muscle migration. *Am J Physiol Lung Cell Mol Physiol* 2007; **292**: L1030–L1038.

16 Bonacci JV, Schuliga M, Harris T, Stewart AG. Collagen impairs glucocorticoid actions in airway smooth muscle through integrin signaling. *Br J Pharmacol* 2006; **149**: 365–73.

17 Miyazono K, Kusanagi K, Inoue H. Divergence and convergence of TGF-beta/BMP signaling. *J Cell Physiol* 2001; **187**: 265–76.

18 Miyazono K, Ichijo H, Heldin Ch. Transforming growth factor-beta; latent forms, binding proteins and receptors. *GRF* 1993; **8**: 11–22.

19 Khalil N. TGF-beta; from latent to active. *Microbes Infect* 1999; **1**: 1255–63.

20 Bossé Y, Rola-Pleszczynski M. Controversy surrounding the increased expression of TGF-β1 in asthma. *Respir Res* 2007; **8**: 66.

21 Roberts AB, Tian F, Dacosta Byfield S, *et al*. Smad3 is key to TGF-β-mediated epithelial to mesenchymal transition, fibrosis, tumor suppression and metastasis. *Cytokine Growth Factor Rev* 2006; **17**: 19–27.

22 Shi Y, Massague J. Mechanisins of TGF-beta signaling from cell membrane to the nucleus. *Cell* 2003; **113**: 685–700.

23 Guo X, Wang XF. Signaling cross-talk between TGF-beta/BMP and other pathways. *Cell Res* 2009; **19**: 71–88.

24 Kariyawasam HH, Pegorier S, Barkans J, *et al*. Activin and transforming growth factor-β signaling pathways are activated after allergen challenge in mild asthma. *J Allergy Clin Immunol* 2009; **124**: 454–62.

25 Sime PJ, Xing Z, Graham FL, Csaky KG, Gauldie J. Adenovector-mediated gene transfer of active transforming growth factor-beta 1 induces prolonged severe fibrosis in rat lung. *J Clin Invest* 1997; **100**: 768–76.

26 Evans RA, Tian YC, Steadman R, Phillips AO. TGF-beta-1 mediated fibroblast-myofibroblast terminal differentiation—the role of Smad proteins. *Exp Cell Res* 2003; **282**: 90–100.

27 Goldsmith AM, Bentley JK, Zhou L, *et al*. Transforming growth factor- beta induces airway smooth muscle hypertrophy. *Am J Respir Cell Mol Biol* 2006; **34**: 247–254.

28 Duvernelle C, Freund V, Frossard N. Transforming growth factor-beta and its role in asthma. *Pulm Pharmacol Ther* 2003; **16**: 181–96.

29 Kalluri R, Neilson EG. Epithelial mesenchymal transition and its implications for fibrosis. *J Clin Invest* 2003; **112**: 1776–84.

30 Hackett TL, Warner SM, Stefanowicz D, *et al*. Induction of epithelial-mesenchymal transition in primary airway epithelial cells from patients with asthma by transforming growth factor-β1. *Am J Respir Crit Care Med* 2009; **180**: 122–33.

31 Elovic AE, Ohyama H, Sauty A, *et al*. IL-4 dependent regulation of TGF, alfa and TGF beta 1 expression in human eosinophils. *J Immunol* 1998; **160**: 6121–7.

32 Humbles AA, Lloyd CM, McMillan SJ, *et al*. A critical role for eosinophils in allergic airways remodeling. *Science* 2004; **305**: 1776–9.

33 Fattouh R, Jordana M. TGF-β, eosinophils and IL-13 in allergic airway remodeling: A critical appraisal with therapeutic considerations. *Inflamm Allergy Drug Targets* 2008; **7**: 224–36.

34 Minshall EM, Leung DY, Martin RJ, *et al*. Eosinophil-associated TGF-beta1 mRNA, expression and airways

fibrosis in bronchial asthma. *Am J Respir Cell Mol Biol* 1997; **17**: 326–33.

35 Ohno I, Nitta Y, Yamauchi K, *et al.* Transforming growth factor beta 1 (TGF-beta1) gene expression by eosinophils in asthmatic airway inflammation. *Am J Respir Cell Mol Biol* 1996; **15**: 404–9.

36 Redington AE, Madden J, Frew AJ, *et al.* Transforming growth factor-beta 1 in asthma/Measurement in bronchoalveolar lavage fluid. *Am J Respir Crit Care Med* 1997; **156**: 642–7.

37 Vignola AM, Chanez P, Chiappara G, *et al.* Transforming growth factor-beta expression in mucosal biopsies in asthma and chronic bronchitis. *Am J Respir Crit Care Med* 1997; **156**: 591–9.

38 Flood-Page P, Menzies-Gow A, Phipps S, *et al.* Anti-IL-5 treatment reduces deposition of ECM proteins in the bronchial subepithelial basement membrane of mild atopic asthmatics. *J Clin Invest* 2003; **112**: 1029–36.

39 Balzar S, Chu HM, Silkoff P, *et al.* Increased TGF-beta 2 in severe asthma with eosinophilia. *J Allergy Clin Immunol* 2005; **115**: 110–17.

40 Chu HW, Balzar S, Seedorf GJ. Transforming growth factor-beta2 induces bronchial epithelial mucin expression in asthma. *Am J Pathol* 2004; **165**: 1097–106.

41 Ueda T, Niimi A, Matsumoto H, *et al.* TGFB1 promoter polymorphism C-509T, and pathophysiology of asthma. *J Allergy Clin Immunol* 2008; **121**: 659–64.

42 Liebhart J, Polak M, Dabrowski A, *et al.* The G/G genotype of transforming growth factor beta 1 (TGF beta 1) single nucleotide polymorphism coincident with other host and environmental factors is associated with irreversible bronchoconstriction in asthmatics. *Int J Immunogenet* 2008; **35**: 417–22.

43 Fattouh R, Midence NG, Arias K, *et al.* Transforming growth factor-beta regulated house dust mite- induced allergic airway inflammation but not airway remodeling. *Am J Respir Crit Care Med* 2008; **177**: 593–603.

44 Kelly MM, Leigh R, Bonniaud P, *et al.* Epithelial expression of profibrotic mediators in a model of allergen induced airway remodeling. *Am J Respir Cell Mol Biol* 2005; **32**: 99–107.

45 Karnar RK, Herbert C, Foster PS. Expression of growth factors by airway epithelial cells in a model of chronic asthma; regulation and relationship to subepithelial fibrosis. *Clin Exp Allergy* 2004; **34**: 567–75.

46 McMillan SJ, Xanthou G, Lloyd CM. Manipulation of allergen induced airway remodeling by treatment with anti TGF-beta antibody: effect on the Smad signaling pathway. *J Immunol* 2005; **174**: 5774–80.

47 Alcorn JF, Rinaldi LM, Jaffie EF, *et al.* Transforming growth factor beta1 suppresses airway hyperresponsiveness in allergy disease. *Am J Respir Crit Care Med* 2007; **176**: 974–982.

48 Le AV, Cho JY, Miller M, McElwain S, Golgotiu K, Broide DH. Inhibition of allergen induced airway remodeling in Smad 3 deficient mice. *J Immunol* 2007; **178**: 7310–16.

49 Letterio JJ, Roberts AB. Regulation of immune responses by TGF-beta. *Ann Rev Immunol* 1998; **16**: 137–161.

50 Scherf W, Burdach S, Hansen G. Reduced expression of transforming growth factor beta 1 exacerbates pathology in an experimental asthma model. *Eur J Immunol* 2005; **35**: 198–206.

51 Barnes PJ. The cytokine network in asthma and chronic obstructive pulmonary disease. *J Clin Invest* 2008; **118**: 3546–56.

52 Wan YY, Flavell RA. Regulatory T cells, transforming growth factor-beta and immune suppression. *Proc Am Thorac Soc* 2007; **4**: 271–6.

53 Eswarakumar VP, Lax I, Schlessinger J. Cellular signaling by fibroblast growth factor receptors. *Cytokine Growth Factor Rev* 2005; **16**: 139–49.

54 Bosse Y, Thompson C, Stankova J, Rola-Pleszczynki M. Fibroblast growth factor 2 and transforming growth factor beta1 in human bronchial smooth muscle cell proliferation. *Am J Respir Cell Moll Biol* 2006; **34**: 746–53.

55 Nugent MA, Iozzo RV. Fibroblast growth factor 2. *Int J Biochem Cell Biol* 2000; **32**: 115–20.

56 Cross MJ, Claesson-Welsh L. FGF and VEGF function in angiogenesis: signaling pathways, biological responses and therapeutic inhibition. *Trends Pharmacol Sci* 2001; **22**: 201–7.

57 Redington AE, Roche WR, Madden J, *et al.* Basic fibroblast growth factor in asthma; measurement in bronchoalveolar lavage fluid basally and following allergen challenge. *J Allergy Clin Immunol* 2001; **107**: 384–7.

58 Hoshino M, Takahashi M, Aoike N. Expression of vascular endothelial growth factor basic fibroblast growth factor and angiogenin immunoreactivity in asthmatic airways and its relationship to angiogenesis. *J Allergy Clin Immunol* 2001; **107**: 295–301.

59 Jeon SG, Lee CG, Oh MH, *et al.* Recombinant basic fibroblast growth factor inhibits the airway hyperresponsiveness, mucus production and lung inflammation induced by an allergen challenge. *J Allergy Clin Immunol* 2007; **119**: 831–7.

60 Fredriksson L, Li H, Eriksson U. The PDGF family: Four gene products from five dimeric isoforms. *Cytokine Growth Factor Rev* 2004; **15**: 197–204.

61 Bach MK, Brashler JR, Stout BK, *et al.* Activation of human eosinophils by platelet-derived growth factor. *Int Arch Allergy Immunol* 1992; **97**: 121–9.

62 Chanez P, Vignola M, Stenger R, Vic P, Michel FB, Bousquet J. Platelet derived growth factor in asthma. *Allergy* 1995; **50**: 878–83.

63 Dube J, Chakir J, Laviolette M, *et al. In vitro* procollagen synthesis and proliferative phenotype of bronchial fibroblasts from normal and asthmatic subjects. *Lab Invest* 1998; **78**: 297–307.

64 Lewis CC, Chu HW, Westcott JY, *et al.* Airway fibroblasts exhibit a synthetic phenotype in severe asthma. *J Allergy Clin Immunol* 2005; **115**: 534–40.

65 Yamashita N, Sekine K, Miyasaka T, *et al.* Platelet-derived growth factor is involved in the augmentation of airway responsiveness through remodeling of airways in diesel exhaust particulate-treated mice. *J Allergy Clin Immunol* 2001; **107**: 135–42.

66 Ingram JL, Rice AB, Geisenhoffer K, Madtes DK, Bonner JC. IL-13 and IL-1beta promote lung fibroblast growth through coordinated up-regulation of PDGF-AA and PDGF-R alpha. *FASEB J* 2004; **18**: 1132–4.

67 Pegorier S, Arouche N, Dombret MC, Aubier M, Pretolani M. Augmented epithelial endothelin-1 expression in refractory asthma. *J Allergy Clin Immunol* 2007; **120**: 1301–7.

68 Yahiaoui L, Villeneuve A, Valderrama-Carvajal H, Burke F, Fixman ED. Endothelin-1 regulates proliferative responses, both alone and synergistically with PDGF, in rat tracheal smooth muscle cells. *Cell Physiol Biochem* 2006; **17**: 37–46.

69 Gawlik R, Jastrzebski D, Ziora D, Jarzab J. Concentration of endothelin in plasma and BALF fluid from asthmatic patients. *J Physiol Pharmacol* 2006; **57** (Suppl 4): 103–10.

70 Ehrenreich H, Burd PR, Rottem M, *et al.* Endothelins belong to the assortment of mast cell-derived and mast cell-bound cytokines. *New Biol* 1992; **4**: 147–56.

71 Knott PG, D'Aprile AC, Henry PJ, Hay DW, Goldie RG. Receptors for endothelin-1 in asthmatic human peripheral lung. *Br J Pharmacol* 1995; **114**: 1–3.

72 Leask A, Holmes A, Abraham DJ. Connective tissue growth factor: A new and important player on the pathogenesis of fibrosis. *Curr Rhematol Rep* 2002; **4**: 136–42.

73 Xie S, Sukar MB, Issa R, Oltanns U, Nicholson AG, Chung KF. Regulation of TGF beta 1 induced connective tissue growth factor expression in airway smooth muscle cells. *Am J Physiol Luang Cell Mol Physiol* 2005; **288**: L68–L76.

74 Brigstock DR. Connective tissue growth factor (CCN2: CTGF) and organ fibrosis: lessons from transgenic animals. *J Cell Commun Signal* 2010; **4**: 1–4.

75 Burgess JK, Johnson PR, Ge Q, *et al.* Expression of connective tissue growth factor in asthmatic airway smooth muscle cells. *Am J Respir Crit Care Med* 2003; **167**: 71–7.

76 Burgess JK. The role of the extracellular matrix and specific growth factors in the regulation of inflammation and remodeling in asthma. *Pharmacol Therap* 2009; **122**: 19–29.

77 Herbst RS. Review of epidermal growth factor receptor biology. *Int J Radiat Oncol Biol Phys* 2004; **59**: 21–6.

78 Amishima M, Munakata M, Nasuhara Y, *et al.* Expression of epidermal growth factor and epidermal growth factor receptor immunoreactivity in the asthmatic human airway. *Am J Respir Crit Care Med* 1998; **157**: 1907–12.

79 Jose PJ, Griffiths-Johnson DA, Collins PD, *et al.* Eotaxin: a potent eosinophil chemoattractant cytokine detected in a guinea-pig model of allergic airways inflammation. *J Exp Med* 1994; **179**: 881–7.

80 Berkman N, Ohnona S, Chung FK, Breuer R. Eotaxin-3 but eotaxin gene expression is upregulated in asthmatics 24 hours after allergen challenge. *Am J Resp Cell Mol Biol* 2001; **24**: 682–7.

81 Puxeddu I, Bader R, Piliponsky AM Reich R, Levi-Schaffer F, Berkman N. The CC chemokine eotaxin/CCL11 has a selective profibrogenic effect on human lung fibroblasts. *J Allergy Clin Immunol* 2006; **117**: 103–10.

82 Kohan M, Puxeddu I, Reich R, Levi-Schaffer F, Berkman N. Eotaxin-2/CCL24 and eotaxin-3/CCL26 exert differential profibrogenic effects on human lung fibroblasts. *Ann Allergy Asthma Immunol* 2010; **104**: 66–72.

83 Xanthou G, Alisaffi T, Semitekolou M, *et al.* Osteopontin has a crucial role in allergic airway disease through regulation of dendritic cell subsets. *Nature Med* 2007; **13**: 570–8.

84 Kohan M, Bader R, Puxeddu I, Levi-Schaffer F, Breuer R, Berkman N. Enhanced osteopontin expression in a murine model of allergen-induced airway remodelling. *Clin Exp Allergy* 2007; **37**: 1444–54.

85 Lenga Y, Koh A, Perera AS, McCulloch CA, Sodek J, Zohar R. Osteopontin expression is required for myofibroblast differentiation. *Circ Res* 2008; **102**: 319–27.

86 Kohan M, Breuer R, Berkman N. Osteopontin induces airway remodeling and lung fibroblast activation in a murine model of asthma. *Am J Resp Cell Mol Biol* 2009; **41**: 290–6.

87 Leali D, Dell'Era P, Stabile H, *et al.* Osteopontin (Eta-1) and fibroblast growth factor-2 cross-talk in angiogenesis. *J Immunol* 2003; **71**: 1085–93.

88 Puxeddu I, Berkman N, Ribatti D, *et al.* Osteopontin is expressed and functional in human eosinophils. *Allergy* 2010; **65**: 168–74.

89 White ES, Baralle FE, Muro AF. New insights into form and function of fibronectin splice variants. *J Pathol* 2008; **216**: 1–14.

90 Gabbiani G. The myofibroblast in wound healing and fibrocontractive diseases. *J Pathol* 2003; **200**: 500–3.

91 Muro AF, Moretti FA, Moore BB, *et al.* An essential role for fibronectin extra type III domain A in

pulmonary fibrosis. *Am J Respir Crit Care Med* 2008; **177**: 638–45.

92 Kohan M, Muro AF, Bader R, Berkman N. The extra domain-A of fibronectin is essential for allergen-induced airway fibrosis and hyperresponsiveness in mice. *J Allergy Clin Immunol* 2011; **127**: 439–46.

93 Leigh R, Ellis R, Wattie JN, *et al*. Type 2 cytokines in the pathogenesis of sustained airway dysfunction and airway remodeling in mice. *Am J Respir Crit Care Med* 2004; **169**: 860–7.

94 Yang G, Volk A, Petley T, *et al*. Anti IL-13 monoclonal antibody inhibits airway responsiveness, inflammation and airway remodeling. *Cytokine* 2004; **28**: 224–32.

95 Zhu Z, Homer RJ, Wang Z, *et al*. Pulmonary expression of interleukin-13 causes inflammation, mucus hypersecretion, subepithelial fibrosis, physiological abnormalities and eotaxin production. *J Clin Invest* 1999; **103**: 779–88.

96 Risau W. Mechanisms of angiogenesis. *Nature* 1997; **386**: 671–4.

97 Folkman J. Angiogenesis in cancer, vascular, rheumatoid and other disease. *Nat Med* 1995; **1**: 27–31.

98 Folkman J. Endogenous angiogenesis inhibitors. *Acta Pathol Micro Immunol Scand* 2004; **112**: 496–507.

99 Li X, Wilson JW. Increased vascularity of the bronchial mucosa in mild asthma. *Am J Respir Crit Care Med* 1997; **156**: 229–33.

100 Leung DW, Cachianes G, Kuang WJ, Goeddel DV, Ferrara N. Vascular endothelial growth factor is a secreted angiogenic mitogen. *Science* 1989; **246**: 1306–9.

101 Lee CG, Link H, Baluk P, *et al*. Vascular endothelial growth factor (VEGF) induces remodeling and enhances TH2-mediated sensitization and inflammation in the lung. *Nat Med* 2004; **10**: 1095–103.

102 Walters EH, Soltani A, Reid DW, Ward C. Vascular remodelling in asthma. *Curr Opin Allergy Clin Immunol* 2008; **8**: 39–43.

103 Demoly P, Maly FE, Mautino G, *et al*. VEGF levels in asthmatic airways do not correlate with plasma extravasation. *Clin Exp Allergy* 1999; **29**: 1390–4.

104 Asai K, Kanazawa H, Otani K, Shiraishi S, Hirata K, Yoshikawa J. Imbalance between vascular endothelial growth factor and endostatin levels in induced sputum from asthmatic subjects. *J Allergy Clin Immunol* 2002; **110**: 571–5.

105 Simcock DE, Kanabar V, Clarke GW, O'Connor BJ, Lee Th, Hirst SJ. Proangiogenic activity in bronchoalveolar lavage fluid from patients with asthma. *Am J Respir Crit Care Med* 2007; **176**: 146–53.

106 Abdel-Rahman AM, el-Sahrigy SA, Bakr SI. A comparative study of two angiogenic factors: vascular endothelial growth factor and angiogenin in induced sputum from asthmatic children in acute attack. *Chest* 2006; **129**: 266–71.

107 Feltis BN, Wignarajah D, Reid DW, Ward C, Harding R, Walters EH. Effects of inhaled fluticasone on angiogenesis and vascular endothelial growth factor in asthma. *Thorax* 2007; **62**: 314–19.

108 Olgart Hoglund C, de Blay F, Oster JP, Duvernelle C, Kassel O, Pauli G, Frossard N. Nerve growth factor levels and localisation in human asthmatic bronchi. *Eur Respir J* 2002; **20**: 1110–16.

109 Lazarovici P, Gazit A, Staniszewska I, Marcinkiewicz C, Lelkes PI. 2006; Nerve growth factor (NGF) promotes angiogenesis in the quail chorioallantoic membrane. *Endothelium* 13: 51–9.

110 Braun A, Appel E, Baruch R, *et al*. Role of nerve growth factor in a mouse model of allergic airway inflammation and asthma. *Eur J Immunol* 1998; **28**: 3240–51.

111 Solomon A, Aloe L, Pe'er J, Frucht-Pery J, Bonini S, Levi-Schaffer F. Nerve growth factor is preformed in and activates human peripheral blood eosinophils. *J Allergy Clin Immunol* 1998; **102**: 454–60.

112 Makinde T, Murphy RF, Agrawal DK. Immunomodulatory role of vascular endothelial growth factor and angiopoietin-1 in airway remodeling. *Curr Mol Med* 2006; **6**: 831–41.

113 Feltis BN, Wignarajah D, Zheng L, Ward C, Reid D, Harding R, Walters EH. Increased vascular endothelial growth factor and receptors: relationship to angiogenesis in asthma. *Am J Respir Crit Care Med* 2006; **173**: 1201–7.

114 Kanazawa H, Nomura S, Asai K. Roles of angiopoietin-1 and angiopoietin-2 on airway microvascular permeability in asthmatic patients. *Chest* 2007; **131**: 1035–41.

115 Alagappan VK, Willems-Widyastuti A, Seynhaeve AL, *et al*. Vasoactive peptides upregulate mRNA, expression and secretion of vascular endothelial growth factor in human airway smooth muscle cells. *Cell Biochem Biophys* 2007; **47**: 109–18.

116 Cruz A, Parnot C, Ribatti D, Corvol P, Gasc JM. Endothelin-1: a regulator of angiogenesis in the chick chorioallantoic membrane. *J Vasc Res* 2001; **38**: 536–45.

117 Salani D, Taraboletti G, Rosano L, *et al*. Endothelin-1 induces an angiogenic phenotype in cultured endothelial cells and stimulates neovascularization *in vivo*. *Am J Pathol* 2000; **157**: 1703–11.

118 Shichiri M, Kato H, Marumo F, Hirata Y. Endothelin-1 as an autocrine/paracrine apoptosis survival factor for endothelial cells. *Hypertension* 1997; **30**: 1198–203.

119 Spinella F, Garrafa E, Di Castro V, *et al*. Endothelin-1 stimulates lymphatic endothelial cells and lymphatic vessels to grow and invade. *Cancer Res* 2009; **69**: 2669–76.

120 Simcock DE, Kanabar V, Clarke GW, *et al*. Induction of angiogenesis by airway smooth muscle from patients

with asthma. *Am J Respir Crit Care Med* 2008; **178**: 460–8.

121 Kulka M, Fukuishi N, Metcalfe DD. Human mast cells synthesize and release angiogenin, a member of the ribonuclease A (RNase A) superfamily. *J Leukoc Biol* 2009; **86**: 1217–26.

122 O'Reilly MS, Holmgren L, Shing Y, *et al*. Angiostatin: a novel angiogenesis inhibitor that mediates the suppression of metastases by a Lewis lung carcinoma. *Cell* 1994; **79**: 315–28.

123 O'Reilly MS, Boehm T, Shing Y, *et al*. Endostatin: an endogenous inhibitor of angiogenesis and tumor growth. *Cell* 1997; **88**: 277–85.

124 Suzaki Y, Hamada K, Sho M, *et al*. A potent antiangiogenic factor, endostatin prevents the development of asthma in a murine model. *J Allergy Clin Immunol* 2005; **116**: 1220–7.

125 Van Eerdewegh P, Little RD, Dupuis J, *et al*. Association of the ADAM33 gene with asthma and bronchial hyperresponsiveness. *Nature* 2002; **418**: 426–30.

126 Puxeddu I, Pang YY, Harvey A, *et al*. The soluble form of a disintegrin and metalloprotease 33 promotes angiogenesis: implications for airway remodeling in asthma. *J Allergy Clin Immunol* 2008; **121**: 1400–6.

127 Puxeddu I, Alian A, Piliponsky AM, Ribatti D, Panet A, Levi-Schaffer F. Human peripheral blood eosinophils induce angiogenesis. *Int J Biochem Cell Biol* 2005; **37**: 628–36.

128 Puxeddu I, Ribatti D, Crivellato E, Levi-Schaffer F. Mast cells and eosinophils: a novel link between inflammation and angiogenesis in allergic diseases. *J Allergy Clin Immunol* 2005; **116**: 531–6.

129 Puxeddu I, Berkman N, Ben Efraim N, *et al*. The role of eosinophil major basic protein in angiogenesis. *Allergy* 2009; **64**: 368–74.

130 Chakraborty G, Jain S, Kundu GC. Osteopontin promotes vascular endothelial growth factor-dependent breast tumor growth and angiogenesis via autocrine and paracrine mechanisms. *Cancer Res* 2008; **68**: 152–61.

131 Nissim Ben Efraim AH, Eliashar R, Levi-Schaffer F. Hypoxia modulates human eosinophil function. *Clin Mol Allergy* 2010; **8**: 10.

132 Wen FQ, Kohyama T, Skold CM, *et al*. Glucocorticoids modulate TGF beta production. *Inflammation* 2002; **26**: 279–90.

133 Meisler N, Keefer KA, Ehrlich HP, Yager DR, Myers-Parrelli J, Cutroneo KR. Dexamethasone abrogates the fibrogenic effect of transforming growth factor beta in rat granuloma and granulation tissue fibroblasts. *J Invest Dermatol* 1997; **108**: 285–9.

134 Johnson PR, Black JL, Carlin S, Ge Q, Underwood PA. The production of extracellular matrix proteins by

human passively sensitized airway smooth muscle cells in culture: the effect of beclomethasone. *Am J Respir Crit Care Med* 2000; **162**: 2145–51.

135 Olivieri D, Chetta A, Del Donno M. Effect of short term treatment with low-dose inhaled fluticasone propionate on airway inflammation and remodeling in mild asthma; a placebo-controlled study. *Am J Respir Crit Care Med* 1997; **155**: 1864–971.

136 Sont JK, Willems LN, Bel EH, *et al*. Clinical control and histopathological outcome of asthma when using airway hyperresponsiveness as an additional guide to long-term treatment. *Am J Respir Crit Care Med* 1999; **159**: 1043–51.

137 Lundgren R, Soderberg M, Horstedt P Stenling R. Morphological studies of bronchial biopsies from asthmatics before and after ten years of treatment with inhaled steroids. *Eur Respir J* 1988; **1**: 883–9.

138 Chetta A, Zanini A, Foresi A. Vascular endothelial growth factor up-regulation and bronchial wall remodelling in asthma. *Clin Exp Allergy* 2005; **35**: 1437–42.

139 Asai K, Kanazawa H, Kamoi H, Shiraishi S, Hirata K, Yoshikawa J. Increased levels of vascular endothelial growth factor in induced sputum in asthmatic patients. *Clin Exp Allergy* 2003; **33**: 595–9.

140 Feltis BN, Wignarajah D, Reid DW, Ward C, Harding R, Walters EH. Effects of inhaled fluticasone on angiogenesis and vascular endothelial growth factor in asthma. *Thorax* 2007; **62**: 314–19.

141 Orsida C, Ward C, Li X, *et al*. Effect of a long acting beta-2 agonist over three months on airway wall vascular remodelling in asthma. *Am J Respir Crit Care Med* 2001; **164**: 117–121.

142 Henderson WR Jr, Chiang GK, Tien YT, Chi EY. Reversal of allergen-induced airway remodeling by CysLT1 receptor blockade. *Am J Respir Crit Care Med* 2006; **173**: 718–28.

143 Laping NJ, Grygielko E, Mathur A. Inhibition of transforming growth factor (TGF) beta 1-induced extracellular matrix with a novel inhibitor of the TGF-beta type I receptor kinase activity; SB-431542; *Mol Pharmacol* 2002; **62**: 58–64.

144 DaCosta BS, Major C, Laping NJ, Roberts AB. SB–505124; is a selective inhibitor of transforming growth factor- beta type I receptors ALK4: ALK5. *Mol Pharmacol* 2006; **65**: 744–52.

145 Cui Q, Lim SK, Zhao B, Hoffman FM. Selective inhibition of TGF-beta responsive genes by Smad-interacting peptide aptamers from FoxH1: Lef1 and CBP. *Oncogene* 2005; **24**: 3864–74.

146 Flanders K. Smad3 as a mediator of the fibrotic response. *Int J Exp Path* 2004; **85**: 47–64.

147 Aschenbrenner JK, Sollinger HW, Becker BN, Hullett DA. 1,25-(OH)(2)D(3) alters the transforming growth

factor beta signaling pathway in renal tissue. *J Surg Res* 2001; **100**: 171–5.

148 Pines M, Snyder D, Yarkoni S, Nagler A. Halofuginone to treat fibrosis in chronic graft-versus-host disease and scleroderma. *Biol Bld Marrow Transpl* 2003; **9**: 417–25.

149 Honda K, Marquillies P, Capron M, Dombrowicz D. Peroxisome proliferator-activated receptor gamma is expressed in airways and inhibits features of airway remodeling in a mouse asthma model. *J Allergy Clin Immunol* 2004; **113**: 882–8.

150 Benayoun L, Letuve S, Druilhe A. Regulation of peroxisome proliferator-activated receptor gamma expression in human asthmatic airways relationship with proliferation, apoptosis and airway remodeling. *Am J Respir Crit Care Med* 2001; **164**: 1487–94.

151 Brigstock DR. Strategies for blocking the fibrogenic actions of connective tissue growth factor (CCN2): from pharmacological inhibition in-vitro to targeted siRNA, therapy in-vivo. *J Cell Commun Signal* 2009; **3**: 5–18.

152 Unemori EN, Pickford LB, Salles AL. Relaxin induced an extracellular matrix degrading, phenotype in human lung fibroblasts *in vitro* and inhibits lung fibrosis in a murine model *in vivo*. *J Clin Invest* 1996; **98**: 2739–45.

153 Behera AK, Kumar M, Lockey RF, Mohapatra SS. Adenovirus-mediated interferon gamma gene therapy for allergic asthma involvement of interleukin 12 and STAT4 signaling. *Hum Gene Ther* 2002; **13**: 1697–709.

154 Boguniewicz M, Martin RJ, Martin D. The effects of nebulized recombinant interferon-gamma in asthmatic airways. *J Allergy Clin Immunol* 1995; **95**: 133–5.

155 Cho JY, Miller M, Baeck KJ, *et al.* Inhibition of airway remodeling in IL-5 deficient mice. *J Clin Invest* 2004; **113**: 551–60.

156 Ingber D, Fujita T, Kishimoto S, *et al.* Synthetic analogues of fumagillin that inhibit angiogenesis and suppress tumour growth. *Nature* 1990; **348**: 555–7.

157 Guba M, von Breitenbuch P, Steinbauer M, *et al.* Rapamycin inhibits primary and metastatic tumor growth by antiangiogenesis: involvement of vascular endothelial growth factor. *Nat Med* 2002; **8**: 128–35.

158 Lee SY, Paik SY, Chung SM. Neovastat (AE-941) inhibits the airway inflammation and hyperresponsiveness in a murine model of asthma. *J Microbiol* 2005; **43**: 11–16.

159 Fujitani Y, Trifilieff A, Tsuyuki S, Coyle AJ, Bertrand C. Endothelin receptor antagonists inhibit antigen-induced lung inflammation in mice. *Am J Respir Crit Care Med* 1997; **155**: 1890–4.

20 Chemokines

Luis M. Teran and Juan R. Velazquez
National Institute of Respiratory Diseases, Mexico City, Mexico

Introduction

Allergic diseases, including asthma, allergic rhinitis, and atopic dermatitis, are characterized by inflammation with pronounced infiltration of T helper type 2 (Th2) cells, lymphocytes, mast cells, and eosinophils. Activation of these cells within the airway leads to the release of proinflammatory mediators, which in turn cause vascular leakage, bronchial smooth muscle contraction, inflammatory cell infiltration, mucus hypersecretion, airway hyperresponsiveness and, ultimately, airway remodeling. The molecular mechanisms that regulate the allergic inflammatory process are not fully understood. However, cytokines such as interleukin 4 (IL-4), IL-5, and IL-13 play a critical role in differentiating Th2 cells from uncommitted Th0 cells; promoting IgE production; differentiating mast cells; and the growth, migration and activation of eosinophils, which lead to pathologic abnormalities in allergic diseases [1]. Chemokines are important for the recruitment of both immune and structural cells to the lung and in directing leukocytes into different compartments within the lung tissue.

Chemokines

The term chemokine was used for first time in 1992 to describe a group of 8–10 kDa chemotactic cytokines that have the ability to bind heparin with high affinity.

Chemokines constitute a family of structurally related cytokines, which, based on the position of two conserved cysteine residues, have been grouped into four subfamilies: CCL, CXCL, CX3CL, and CL chemokines [2]. To date the chemokines comprises a family of almost 50 cytokines (Figure 20.1). A first generation of chemokines was discovered mainly on the basis of their chemotactic properties, most of which direct the migration of leukocytes through the body, under both physiologic and inflammatory conditions. However, it was soon demonstrated that in addition to their chemotactic properties, they can induce cell activation and degranulation, stimulate the respiratory burst in leukocytes, modulate endothelial cell adhesion, increase vascular permeability, and increase cellular proliferation. Furthermore, chemokines can stimulate several processes including myelopoiesis, tumor growth, angiogenesis, immunomodulation, and morphogenesis.

Chemokines in allergic inflammation

Leukocyte recruitment is a feature of allergic inflammation. Recruitment of these cells from the peripheral blood into the allergic inflammatory site involves a series of events that include adhesion to endothelial cells, diapedesis, and subsequent chemotactic movements. In this multistep model of leukocyte extravasation, chemokines are important as they direct

Inflammation and Allergy Drug Design, First Edition. Edited by Kenji Izuhara, Stephen T. Holgate, Marsha Wills-Karp.
© 2011 Blackwell Publishing Ltd. Published 2011 by Blackwell Publishing Ltd.

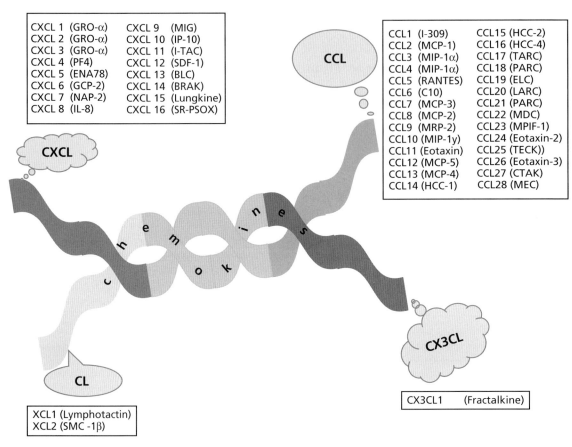

Figure 20.1 Based on the position of two conserved cysteine residues, chemokines have been grouped into four subfamilies: CCL, CXCL, CX3CL, and CL chemokines (former nomenclature of chemokines is given in brackets).

leukocytes into different compartments within the tissue (Figure 20.2). In 1988, Schall *et al.* described RANTES (CCL5), a cytokine chemotactic for monocytes and lymphocytes [3], which was subsequently found to exert potent eosinophil chemotactic activity [4]. This was relevant as these cells are considered to cause tissue damage, leading to disruption of the bronchial epithelium, enhanced bronchial hyperresponsiveness, and obstruction of the airway. In 1993, Meurer *et al.* first demonstrated that the intradermal injection of human RANTES (hRANTES) in dogs induced the recruitment of eosinophils and monocytes at the injection site, with cell infiltration peaking 16–24 h after hRANTES injection [5]. Subsequently, Beck *et al.* reported similar findings in humans [6]; however, they observed that eosinophil recruitment occurred more rapidly in allergic patients than in

nonallergic patients at the CCL5 injection site: by 30 min significant eosinophil infiltrate was seen, reaching near-maximum levels by 6 h in allergic patients, whereas no eosinophil infiltrate was observed in nonallergic patients at both 30 min and 6 h. At 24 h eosinophil numbers were similar in both allergic and nonallergic subjects. To elucidate the role of CCL5, our group undertook a series of endobronchial allergen challenge studies in mild asthmatics and demonstrated that, 4–6 h after challenge, eosinophil recruitment takes place predominantly in the bronchial submucosa and migrates into the airway lining fluid 24 h after challenge [7]. Interestingly, levels of CCL5 peak at 4 h in bronchoalveolar lavage (BAL) fluid and returned to baseline values at 24 h [8]. Following the discovery of CCL5, novel eosinophil chemokines were discovered including CCL7

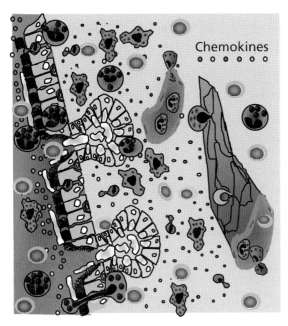

Figure 20.2 Hypothetical model of cell recruitment in asthmatic airways by the chemokines.

(MCP-3), CCL8 (MCP-2), CCL11 (eotaxin), CCL13 (MCP-4), CCL24 (eotaxin-2) and CCL26 (eotaxin-3) [9–13]. CCL11, CCL13, and CCL24 attract eosinophil specifically whereas CCL7, CCL8, and CCL13 attract monocytes and lymphocytes, in addition to eosinophils. There are now many data indicating that these eosinophil-activating chemokines can influence the allergic inflammatory process, and their role in asthma has already been reviewed [14].

Between 1996 and 1997, a second generation of chemokines emerged largely on account of developments in bioinformatics and expressed sequence tag (EST) databases [15,16]. These chemokines include CCL17 (TARC), CCL18 (PARC), CCL19 (ELC), CCL 20 (LARC), and CCL22 (MDC), most of which are expressed constitutively but selectively in some specific cell types and are assumed to orchestrate the homeostatic trafficking of lymphocytes and the organization of lymphoid tissues [15,16]. Lymphocytes are involved in initiating and maintaining airway inflammation and obstruction in asthma. Activated CD4+ T cells producing IL-4, IL-5, and IL-13 have been identified in BAL and bronchial biopsies of both atopic and nonatopic asthmatic patients, and they increase during late asthmatic responses [17]. Most of the

lymphocyte-activating chemokines mentioned above have been associated with the allergic inflammatory process. For example, CD4 T naïve cells derived from asthmatic patients release increased concentrations of both CCL17 and CCL22 [18] and both have been detected in BAL fluid derived from asthmatic patients [19,20]. Moreover, allergen challenge increases further the levels of both CCL17 and CCL22 into the airway epithelial lining fluid [20]. CCL18 is another lymphocyte-activating chemokine (PARC), which is preferentially expressed in the lung and induced by Th2 cytokines. *In vitro* studies conducted by Nadai *et al.* showed that PBMC from asthmatics allergic to house dust mite release CCL18 in culture 48 and 72 h after dermatophagoides pteronyssinus stimulation [21]. Increased levels of CCL18 have also been found in the BAL fluid of asthmatics, and treating patients with inhaled corticosteroids reduces significantly CCL18 release [21]. In this study, chemotaxis assays showed that CCL18 attracts not only Th2 cells but also basophils. Using microarray technology, Kin *et al.* have shown increased CCL18 expression in the sputum of asthmatics [22].

Over the last 5 years a number of studies have extensively investigated the role of chemokines in both mast cell trafficking and airway smooth muscle cell (ASMC) activation. This is relevant as both cell types play an important role in allergic inflammation: mast cells release a plethora of autacoid mediators, proteases, and cytokines upon immunologic and nonimmunologic stimuli, whereas ASMCs have the ability to proliferate within the airways of asthmatic patients. Interestingly, mast cells have been found to localize to the airway smooth muscle (ASM) bundle of asthmatic patients, suggesting that they may migrate toward the ASM bundle under the influence of ASM-derived chemotaxins. ASMCs release a number of chemokines including CCL11, CCL19 (ELC), CXCL8 (IL-8), CXCL10 (IP-10), and CXCL12 (SDF-1α) [23]. In support of this hypothesis, both mast cells and ASM have been found to express several chemokine receptors [24–26].

CC chemokine receptors in the allergic inflammatory process

Chemokines exert their effects through over 20 distinct G protein-coupled seven-transmembrane receptors which belong to the subfamily of class A rhodopsin-like receptors and take up almost 5% of the human genome. Chemokine receptors can bind multiple ligands, for example, CCR2 can bind CCL2, CCL7, CCL8, and CCL13. Upon ligation of the chemokine to the extracellular portion of the chemokine receptor, the intracellular domain binds and activates the heterotrimeric G protein. In response, the $G\alpha_i$ subunit exchanges GDP for GTP, resulting in the dissociation of the heterotrimeric complex into the $G\alpha_I$- and the $\beta\gamma$-subunits. Downstream signaling triggers integrin activation, which enables firm adhesion of leukocytes to endothelial cells. Focal actin polymerization of the leading edge of the cell leads to forward extension. At the rear end of the cell, focal activation of myosin II, and formation and contraction of myosin–actin complexes retracts the cell, allowing migration in the direction of the chemotactic gradient. Chemokine receptors (CCRs) have been classified into subfamilies including CCR, CXCR, CX$_3$CR, and XCR chemokines receptors (Table 20.1).

CC chemokine receptors

CCR1

CCR1 is expressed on macrophages, eosinophils, basophils, and dendritic cells. The ligands for this receptor include CCL3 (MIP1-α), CCL5 CCL7, CCL13, CCL14, CCL15 (HCC-1), CCL16 (HCC-2), and CCL23 (MIPF-1). It has been proposed that CCR1 plays a central role in airway remodeling [27]. This hypothesis is supported by a study conducted in a murine model of asthma with genetic deletion of CCR1, which showed reduced airway remodeling after an intrapulmonary allergen challenge [27]. Interestingly, these mice were found to exhibit high levels of interferon (IFN)-γ and low levels of IL-4, IL-13, CCL6, CCL11, and CCL22. Increased CCR1 expression in the airways of asthmatics has been reported by two separate groups that localized this receptor to mast cells and ASMC [28,29]. Joubert et al. showed that ASMC stimulated with CCR1 ligands induce calcium mobilization. The demonstration that CCR1 ligands

Table 20.1 Chemokine receptors.

Family	Receptors	Chemokine ligands	Cell types
CCR	CCR1	CCL3, CCL5, CCL7, CCL13, CCL14, CCL15, CCL16	Mn, Tmem, NK, Eos, MC
	CCR2	CCL2, CCL7, CCL8, CCL13	Mn, Bas, Tmem, DC, N
	CCR3	CCL5, CCL7, CCL11, CCL24, CCL26	Eos, Bas, T, MC, EpC
	CCR4	CCL17, CCL22	Eos, Bas, Th2, Treg, NK, MC
	CCR5	CCL3, CCL4, CCL5, CCL8	DC, Mn, Th1, Treg, NK, Eos
	CCR6	CCL20	B, DC, Tmem
	CCR7	CCL19, CCL21	B, DC, Tnaïve, Treg, NK, fib
	CCR8	CCL1	Mn, T
	CCR9	CCL25	Tmem
	CCR10	CCL27, CCL28	Tmem
CXCR	CXCR1	CXCL6, CXCL7, CXCL8	N, Mn, MC, T
	CXCR2	CXCL1, CXCL2, CXCL3, CXCL5, CXCL6, CXCL7, CXCL8	N, Mn, MC
	CXCR3	CXCL9, CXCL10, CXCL11	Th1, Nk, DC, MC
	CXCR4	CXCL12	N, B, DC, Mn, Eo, Ba, T, NK, C
	CXCR5	CXCL13	B, fol T
CX3CR	CX3CR1	CX3CL1	Mn, Th1, NK, N
XCR	XCR1	XCL1, XCL2	NK, T

B, B cells; Bas, basophil; DC, dendritic cells; EpC, epithelial cells; Eos, eosinophils; Fib, fibrocytes; fol T, follicular T lymphocyte; MC, mast cell; MN, monocyte; N, neutrophil; NK, natural killer cell; T, T cell; Tnaïve, naïve T cell; Tmem, memory T cell.

are released into the airways of asthmatic patients [8] supports the hypothesis that CCR1 activation may occur during the allergic asthmatic reaction.

CCR2

This is a high-affinity receptor for the macrophage chemotactic protein family of chemokines including CCL-2 (MCP-1), CCL-7, CCL-8, and CCL-13. The CCR2 receptor is present in mononuclear cells, basophils, memory T cells, and DCs. Using a murine model of asthma, Campbell *et al.* showed that CCR2$^{-/-}$ mice exhibit an attenuated airway hyperreactive response to either allergen challenge or direct instillation of CCL2 [30], suggesting that CCR2 may be involved in the airway hyperreactivity process. In this last study, authors found that instillation of CCL-2 into the airways induced prolonged airway hyperresponse in mice, which was associated with mast cell degradation as a consequence of leukotriene C$_4$ release. Moreover, CCR2$^{-/-}$ mice showed a decreased mononuclear cell influx into the airways, suggesting that CCR2 not only mediates airway hyperreactivity but also regulates mononuclear cell infiltration.

CCR3

CCR3 plays a central role in allergic inflammation. This receptor is highly expressed on eosinophils and, to a lesser extent, on other cell types including airway epithelial cells, CD4$^+$ T lymphocytes, and basophils. The chemokine ligands for CCR3 include CCL5, CCL7, CCL8, CCL11, CCL13, CCL24, and CCL26. CCR3 mediates eosinophil recruitment, but its role in airway hyperreactivity is contradictory. Using a systemic ovalbumin (OVA)/alum sensitization followed by respiratory OVA challenge to mimic the asthmatic response [31], Humbles *et al.* found a reduction in lung eosinophils in CCR3$^{-/-}$ mice. The eosinophils appeared to be able to migrate through the endothelial cells, but not the endothelial basement membrane, suggesting that in this model CCR3-binding chemokines are not essential for rolling, adhesion, and transmigration through endothelium, but important for migration into the lung parenchyma. Interestingly, this reduction in eosinophil recruitment was accompanied by a marked increase in BHR. In contrast, Ma *et al.*, using epicutaneous OVA sensitization,

were able to significantly reduce BAL eosinophils, with a parallel decrease in BHR [32]. CCR3 ligands such as CCL5, CCL7, CCL13, CCL24, and CCL26 have been detected in the lungs of asthmatics [14], suggesting that, once these chemokines are released locally, they may activate and recruit eosinophils into the airways of asthmatics. Using murine models of asthma, Lukas [33] proposed a mechanism for migration in response to chemokines, where migration from blood into the lung tissue is regulated by CCL3, CCL7, and CCL22 (MDC), produced by macrophages in the lung interstitium.

CCR6

CCR6 is expressed on human peripheral blood memory CD45RO$^+$ T cells, B cells, and certain dendritic cell subsets. CCL20 is the ligand for CCR6. The interaction ligand/receptor results in firm arrest of memory T cells on activated endothelial cells [34]. In a murine model of asthma, CCR6$^{-/-}$ animals showed reduced airway inflammatory responses with lower production of IL-5 [35]. In humans, CCR6 is expressed on a higher proportion of CD3$^+$ T cells from BAL [36]. Thomas *et al.* showed that CCR6 is expressed on virtually all CD4$^+$ BAL T cells pre challenge and they are markedly decreased following antigen challenge, suggesting that these receptors are internalized following encounter with ligand in the airways [37]. In a separate study CCR6 was found to be expressed in a high proportion of CD4$^+$ T cells derived from nasal mucosal tissue and CCL20 levels were elevated in BAL fluid derived from asthmatics following endobronchial allergen provocation [38]. Moreover, chemotaxis assays showed that CCR6$^+$ cells migrate in response to CCL20. Taken together, these observations suggest that CCR6 may be important in the regulation of T-cell recruitment to tissue.

CCR4/CCR8

CCR4 and CCR8 are expressed on Th2 lymphocytes. However, the role of both chemokines in the recruitment of these cells into the asthmatic airways is not fully understood. CCR4 binds both CCL17 and CCL22 whereas CCR8 ligand binds CCL1. Using immunohistochemistry and reverse transcription polymerase chain reaction (RT-PCR), Panina-Bordignon *et al.* [39] reported that over 90% of T cells infiltrating the bronchial biopsies of allergen-challenged asthmatics produce IL-4 and express CCR4. They also reported that CCR8 was expressed on approximately 28% of infiltrating CCR4+ IL-4+ T cells, whereas no T cells were CCR3+. This later finding contends with the study conducted by Morgan *et al.*, who used single-cell flow cytometry to demonstrate that IL-4-expressing blood and BAL fluid T cells express CCR3 and CCR4, with 10-fold and twofold differences in expression, respectively, in both asthmatic and control patients [40]. The demonstration that the CCR4 and CCR8 ligands, CCL1, CCL17, and CCL22, are released in high concentration into the asthmatic airways [19,20,41] suggests that they may activate and recruit Th2 lymphocytes during the allergic asthmatic reaction.

Other chemokine receptors

The role of the chemokine receptors CXCR, XCR, and CX3CR in allergic inflammation has been investigated less extensively. Of these chemokine receptors, only those that have been studied most will be discussed below.

CXCR1

CXCR1 is the classic receptor for both CXCL8 (IL-8) and CXCL6 (GCP-2), which is strongly expressed by neutrophils, with weaker expression on monocytes and dendritic cells. However, Francis *et al.* demonstrated that a proportion of CD4+ T lymphocytes (9.8%), derived from atopic patients, express CXCR1 [42]. Similarly, they identified enhanced CXCR1 expression on both freshly isolated peripheral blood cells and nasal CD4 cells. Moreover, using endobronchial allergen challenge, authors detected increased levels of CXCL8 in BAL fluid after allergen challenge compared with the baseline lavage [42]. We have previously used a similar approach to investigate CXCL8 release, and detected increased levels of CXCL8 both at the allergen- and saline challenge sites compared with the baseline lavage in asthmatics [43]. In the former study, authors did not perform saline control lavage in asthmatics, which explains the increased levels of CXCL8. In a separate study we have found that CXCL8 plays a major role in virus exacerbations of asthma [44].

CXCR3

CXCR3 is expressed mainly in activated T cells and NK cells. Three ligands have been identified for this receptor including CXCL9 (Mig), CXCL10 (IP-10), and CXCL1 (ITAC), all of which are induced by IFN-γ. Therefore, these chemokines are considered to promote a Th1 response. Interestingly, CXCR3 ligands appears to antagonize eotaxin-activated CCR3 [45]. Using endobronchial segmental allergen challenge in atopic asthmatics, Thomas *et al.* [37] showed CXCR3 expression on virtually all CD4(+) BAL T cells prechallenge. However, this receptor was markedly decreased on CD4(+) BAL T following Ag challenge, suggesting that CXCR3 was internalized following encounter with ligand in the airway [37]. These data provide evidence for the involvement of CXCR3 in the recruitment of inflammatory T cells into the airways during the allergic asthmatic response. Brightling *et al.* have shown that human lung mast cells express CXCR3, and have proposed that these cells may migrate in response to the production of CXCL10 by ASMC [25].

CXCR4

CXCL12, formerly known as stromal cell-derived factor 1 (SDF-1), is the main ligand for CXCR4. CXCL12 is a chemokine with two isoforms: SDF-1α is an 89 amino acid protein (the predominant form of SDF-1), and SDF-1β, which contains a four amino acid extension at the carboxyl terminus. A third form of SDF (SDF-1γ) was identified in rat; the former is identical to SDF-1β, except for the insertion of 30 additional amino acids at the carboxyl terminus. When CXCL12 binds to the chemokine receptor CXCR4, it attracts a variety of cells including resting T lymphocytes, monocytes, CD34+ stem cells, and mature eosinophils [46]. Gonzalo *et al.* showed that the CXCL12/CXCR4 axis plays a pivotal role in the allergic airway response in a mouse model of allergic airway inflammation; in this study, authors proposed that CXCL12 contribute to lung inflammation and airway hyperresponsiveness [47]. Moreover, treating allergic mice with the CXCR4 antagonist AMD3100 reduced airway hyperresponsiveness, peribronchial eosinophilia, and inflammatory responses [48]. Hoshino *et al.* reported increased CXCL12 immunoreactivity in bronchial biopsies derived from asthmatic patients and proposed that the CXCL12/CXCR4 axis could play a role in airway remodeling via angiogenesis [49].

Chemokine receptor antagonist

Several chemokine receptors have been identified as potential drug targets to reduce cell infiltration. Most of the chemokine receptor antagonists identified so far possess basic regions characterized by the presence of piperidine, piperazine, spiropiperidine, pyrrolidine, guanidine, quaternary nitrogen, or bicyclam groups. Piperidine-containing compounds represent one of the most common templates for G protein-coupled receptors (GPCRs). Indeed, the presence of piperidine confers to several small molecules either potent antagonist or agonist features on several receptors, including those for chemokines, somatostatin, C5a, tachykinin, neuropeptide Y, and cholecystokinin [50].

A number of studies have proposed to target several chemokines receptors including CCR1, CCR2, CCR3, CCR6, CCR4, CCR8, and CXCR4 among others. For example, mice treated with the CXCR4 antagonist AMD3100 showed reduced airway hyperreactivity, airway eosinophilia, and inflammatory responses [49]. The finding that CCR6-deficient mice had reduced airway resistance, fewer eosinophils within the airways, lower levels of IL-5 in the lung, and reduced serum levels of IgE [35] places this receptor as a potential drug target. On the other hand, using neutralizing antibodies to MCP-1, several groups have shown reduced airway inflammation in murine models of asthma [26,51] and proposed CCR2 as a good candidate for therapeutic intervention. To date, however, CCR3 is the chemokine receptor to which many antagonists have been developed, owing to the fact that it is expressed on many cell types that are involved in the allergic inflammatory process including eosinophils, Th2 cells, basophils, and mast cells. Small-molecule inhibitors for CCR3 include UCB35625, SB-297006, and SB-328437 and they have been proved to be effective in inhibiting eosinophil recruitment in allergen models of asthma [52,53]. The A-122058 antagonist compound is effective in reducing eosinophil numbers after CCL11 intraperitoneal injection in mice [54].

Antagonists for other chemokine receptors include BX471 (CCR1 antagonist; Berlex Inc., Montville, NJ, USA), SCHC (CCR5 antagonist; Schering-Plough, Kenilworth, NJ, USA), AMD3100 (CXCR4 antagonist; AnorMED Inc., Langley, BC, Canada), E913 (CCR5 antagonist; ONO Pharmaceutical Co., Ltd., Osaka, Japan), TAK779 (CCR5 antagonist; Takeda Pharmaceutical Co., Ltd., Osaka, Japan), AMD3389 (CXCR4 antagonist; AnorMED), and Cyclam (CXCR4 antagonist; AnorMED), among others. Many of these chemokine receptor antagonists are making the transition from lead compounds to clinical candidates and although there has been no clinical success, these compounds have been invaluable in generating information on allergic disease, which may allow for the production of successful therapeutics in the future.

References

1 Nakajima H, Takatsu K. Role of cytokines in allergic airway inflammation. *Int Arch Allergy Immunol* 2007; **142**: 265–73.

2 Zlotnik A, Yoshie O. Chemokines: a new classification system and their role in immunity. *Immunity* 2000; **12**: 121–7.

3 Schall TJ, Jongstra J, Dyer BJ, *et al*. A human T cell-specific molecule is a member of a new gene family. *J Immunol* 1988; **141**: 1018–25.

4 Kameyoshi Y, Dörschner A, Mallet AI, Christophers E, Schröder JM. Cytokine RANTES released by thrombin-stimulated platelets is a potent attractant for human eosinophils. *J Exp Med* 1992; **176**: 587–92.

5 Meurer R, Van Riper G, Feeney W, *et al*. Formation of eosinophilic and monocytic intradermal inflammatory sites in the dog by injection of human RANTES but not human monocyte chemoattractant protein 1: human macrophage inflammatory protein 1 alpha, or human interleukin 8. *J Exp Med* 1993; **178**: 1913–21.

6 Beck LA, Dalke S, Leiferman KM, *et al*. Cutaneous injection of RANTES causes eosinophil recruitment: comparison of nonallergic and allergic human subjects. *J Immunol* 1997; **159**: 2962–72.

7 Teran LM, Noso N, Carroll M, Davies DE, Holgate S, Schröder JM. Eosinophil recruitment following allergen challenge is associated with the release of the chemokine RANTES into asthmatic airways. *J Immunol* 1996; **157**: 1806–12.

8 Holgate ST, Bodey KS, Janezic A, Frew AJ, Kaplan AP, Teran LM. Release of RANTES, MIP-1 alpha, and

MCP-1 into asthmatic airways following endobronchial allergen challenge. *Am J Respir Crit Care Med* 1997; **156**: 1377–83.

9 Jose PJ, Griffiths-Johnson DA, Collins PD, *et al*. Eotaxin: a potent eosinophil chemoattractant cytokine detected in a guinea pig model of allergic airways inflammation. *J Exp Med* 1994; **179**: 881–7.

10 White JR, Imburgia C, Dul E, *et al*. Cloning and functional characterization of a novel human CC chemokine that binds to the CCR3 receptor and activates human eosinophils. *J Leukoc Biol* 1997; **62**: 667–75.

11 Shinkai A, Yoshisue H, Koike M, *et al*. A novel human CC chemokine, eotaxin-3, which is expressed in IL-4-stimulated vascular endothelial cells, exhibits potent activity toward eosinophils. *J Immunol* 1999; **163**: 1602–10.

12 Van Damme J, Proost P, Lenaerts JP, Opdenakker G. Structural and functional identification of two human, tumor-derived monocyte chemotactic proteins (MCP-2 and MCP-3) belonging to the chemokine family. *J Exp Med* 1992; **176**: 59–65.

13 Garcia-Zepeda EA, Combadiere C, Rothenberg ME, *et al*. Human monocyte chemoattractant protein (MCP)-4 is a novel CC chemokine with activities on monocytes, eosinophils, and basophils induced in allergic and nonallergic inflammation that signals through the CC chemokine receptors (CCR)-2 and -3. *J Immunol* 1996; **157**: 5613–26.

14 Teran LM. Chemokines in asthma. *Immunol Today* **21**: 235–41.

15 Yoshie O, Imai T, Nomiyama H. Novel lymphocyte-specific CC chemokines and their receptors. *J Leukoc Biol* 1997; **62**: 634–44. Review.

16 Chang MS, McNinch J, Elias CG, *et al*. Molecular cloning and functional characterization of a novel CC chemokine, stimulated T cell chemotactic protein (STCP-1) that specifically acts on activated T lymphocytes. *J Biol Chem* 1997; **272**: 25229–37.

17 Robinson DS, Hamid Q, Ying S, *et al*. Predominant TH2-like bronchoalveolar T-lymphocyte population in atopic asthma. *N Engl J Med* 1992; **326**: 298–304.

18 Hirata H, Arima M, Cheng G, *et al*. Chemokines and their receptors as potential targets for the treatment of asthma. *J Clin Immunol* 2003; **23**: 34–45.

19 Lezcano-Meza D, Negrete-Garcia MC, Dante-Escobedo M, Teran LM. The monocyte-derived chemokine is released in the bronchoalveolar lavage fluid of steady-state asthmatics. *Allergy* 2003; **58**: 1125–30.

20 Bochner BS, Hudson SA, Xiao HQ, Liu MC. Release of both CCR4-active and CXCR3-active chemokines during human allergic pulmonary late-phase reactions. *J Allergy Clin Immunol* 2003; **112**: 930–4.

21 de Nadaï P, Charbonnier AS, Chenivesse C, *et al*. PARC involvement of CCL18 in allergic asthma. *J Immunol* 2006; **176**: 6286–93.

22 Kim HB, Kim CK, Iijima K, Kobayashi T, Kita H. Protein microarray analysis in patients with asthma: elevation of the chemokine PARC/CCL18 in sputum. *Chest* 2009; **135**: 295–302.

23 Sutcliffe A, Kaur D, Page S, *et al*. Mast cell migration to Th2 stimulated airway smooth muscle asthmatics. *Thorax* 2006; **61**: 657–62.

24 Brightling CE, Kaur D, Berger P, Morgan AJ, Wardlaw AJ, Bradding P. Differential expression of CCR3 and CXCR3 by human lung and bone marrow-derived mast cells: implications for tissue mast cell migration. *J Leukoc Biol* 2005; **77**: 759–66.

25 Brightling C, Ammit AJ, Kaur D, *et al*. The CXCL10/CXCR3 axis mediates human lung mast cell migration to asthmatic airway smooth muscle. *Am J Respir Crit Care Med* 2005; **171**: 1103–8.

26 Saunders R, Sutcliffe A, Kaur D, *et al*. Airway smooth muscle chemokine receptor expression and function in asthma. *Clin Exp Allergy* 2009; **39**: 1684–92.

27 Blease K, Mehrad B, Standiford TJ, *et al*. Airway remodeling is absent in CCR1–/– mice during chronic fungal allergic airway disease. *J Immunol* 2000; **165**: 1564–72.

28 Amin K, Janson C, Harvima I, Venge P, Nilsson G. CC chemokine receptors CCR1 and CCR4 are expressed on airway mast cells in allergic asthma. *J Allergy Clin Immunol* 2005; **116**: 1383–6.

29 Joubert P, Lajoie-Kadoch S, Welman M, *et al*. Expression and regulation of CCR1 by airway smooth muscle cells in asthma. *J Immunol* 2008; **180**: 1268–75.

30 Campbell EM, Charo IF, Kunkel SL, *et al*. Monocyte chemoattractant protein-1 mediates cockroach allergen-induced bronchial hyperreactivity in normal but not CCR2–/– mice: the role of mast cells. *J Immunol* 1999; **163**: 2160–7.

31 Humbles AA, Lu B, Friend DS, *et al*. The murine CCR3 receptor regulates both the role of eosinophils and mast cells in allergen-induced airway inflammation and hyperresponsiveness. *Proc Natl Acad Sci USA* 2002; **99**: 1479–84.

32 Ma W, Bryce PJ, Humbles AA, *et al*. CCR3 is essential for skin eosinophilia and airway hyperresponsiveness in a murine model of allergic skin inflammation. *J Clin Invest* 2002; **109**: 621–8.

33 Lukacs NW. Role of chemokines in the pathogenesis of asthma. *Nat Rev Immunol* 2001; **1**: 108–16.

34 Fitzhugh DJ, Naik S, Gonzalez E, Caughman SW, Hwang ST. CC chemokine receptor 6 (CCR6) is a marker for memory T cells that arrest on activated human dermal microvascular endothelium under shear stress. *J Invest Dermatol* 2000; **115**: 332.

35 Lundy SK, Lira SA, Smit JJ, Cook DN, Berlin AA, Lukacs NW. Attenuation of allergen-induced responses in CCR6–/– mice is dependent upon altered pulmonary T lymphocyte activation. *J Immunol* 2005; **174**: 2054–60.

36 Kallinich T, Schmidt S, Hamelmann E, *et al*. Chemokine-receptor expression on T cells in lung compartments of challenged asthmatic patients. *Clin Exp Allergy* 2005; **35**: 26–33.

37 Thomas SY, Banerji A, Medoff BD, Lilly CM, Luster AD. Multiple chemokine receptors, including CCR6 and CXCR3: regulate antigen-induced T cell homing to the human asthmatic airway. *J Immunol* 2007; **179**: 1901–12.

38 Francis JN, Sabroe I, Lloyd CM, Durham SR, Till SJ. Elevated CCR6+ CD4+ T lymphocytes in tissue compared with blood and induction of CCL20 during the asthmatic late response. *Clin Exp Immunol* 2008; **152**: 440–7.

39 Panina-Bordignon P, Papi A, Mariani M, *et al*. The C-C chemokine receptors CCR4 and CCR8 identify airway T cells of allergen-challenged atopic asthmatics. *J Clin Invest* 2001; **107**: 1357–64.

40 Morgan AJ, Symon FA, Berry MA, Pavord ID, Corrigan CJ, Wardlaw AJ. IL-4-expressing bronchoalveolar T cells from asthmatic and healthy subjects preferentially express CCR 3 and CCR 4. *J Allergy Clin Immunol* 2005; **116**: 594–600.

41 Montes-Vizuet R, Vega-Miranda A, Valencia-Maqueda E, Negrete-Garcia MC, Velasquez JR, Teran LM. CC chemokine ligand 1 is released into the airways of atopic asthmatics. *Eur Respir J* 2006; **28**: 59–67.

42 Francis JN, Jacobson MR, Lloyd CM, Sabroe I, Durham SR, Till SJ. CXCR1+CD4+ T cells in human allergic disease. *J Immunol* 2004; **172**: 268–73.

43 Teran LM, Carroll MP, Frew AJ, *et al*. Leukocyte recruitment after local endobronchial allergen challenge in asthma. Relationship to procedure and to airway interleukin-8 release. *Am J Respir Crit Care Med* 1996; **154**: 469–76.

44 Teran LM, Johnston SL, Schröder JM, Church MK, Holgate ST. Role of nasal interleukin-8 in neutrophil recruitment and activation in children with virus-induced asthma. *Am J Respir Crit Care Med* 1997; **155**: 1362–6.

45 Loetscher P, Pellegrino A, Gong JH, *et al*. The ligands of CXC chemokine receptor 3: I-TAC, Mig, and IP10: are natural antagonists for CCR3. *J Biol Chem* 2001; **276**: 2986–91.

46 McQuibban GA, Butler GS, Gong JH, *et al*. Matrix metalloproteinase activity inactivates the CXC chemokine stromal cell-derived factor-1. *J Biol Chem* 2001; **276**: 43503–8.

47 Gonzalo JA, Lloyd CM, Peled A, Delaney T, Coyle AJ, Gutierrez-Ramos JC. Critical involvement of the chemotactic axis CXCR4/stromal cell-derived factor-1 alpha in the inflammatory component of allergic airway disease. *J Immunol* 2000; **165**: 499–508.

48 Lukacs NW, Berlin A, Schols D, Skerlj RT, Bridger GJ. AMD3100: a CxCR4 antagonist, attenuates allergic lung inflammation and airway hyperreactivity. *Am J Pathol* 2002; **160**: 1353–60.

49 Hoshino M, Aoike N, Takahashi M, Nakamura Y, Nakagawa T. Increased immunoreactivity of stromal cell-derived factor-1 and angiogenesis in asthma. *Eur Respir J* 2003; **21**: 804–9.

50 Onuffer JJ, Horuk R. Chemokines, chemokine receptors and small-molecule antagonists: recent developments. *Trends Pharmacol Sci* 2002; **23**: 459–67.

51 Gonzalo JA, Lloyd CM, Kremer L, *et al*. Eosinophil recruitment to the lung in a murine model of allergic inflammation. The role of T cells, chemokines, and adhesion receptors. *J Clin Invest* 1996; **98**: 2332–45.

52 Sabroe I, Peck MJ, Van Keulen BJ, *et al*. A small molecule antagonist of chemokine receptors CCR1 and CCR3. Potent inhibition of eosinophil function and CCR3-mediated HIV-1 entry. *J Biol Chem* 2000; **275**: 25985–92.

53 White JR, Lee JM, Dede K, *et al*. Identification of potent, selective nonpeptide CC chemokine receptor-3 antagonist that inhibits eotaxin-, eotaxin-2-, and monocyte chemotactic protein-4-induced eosinophil migration. *J Biol Chem* 2000; **275**: 36626–31.

54 Warrior U, McKeegan EM, Rottinghaus SM, *et al*. Identification and characterization of novel antagonists of the CCR3 receptor. *J Biomol Screen* 2003; **8**: 324–31.

21 Epithelial growth factors

Yasuhiro Gon[1] and Shu Hashimoto[2]
[1]Division of General Medicine, Department of Internal Medicine, Nihon University School of Medicine, Tokyo, Japan
[2]Division of Respiratory Medicine, Department of Internal Medicine, Nihon University School of Medicine, Tokyo, Japan

Introduction

Asthma and chronic obstructive pulmonary disease (COPD) are chronic inflammatory diseases of the lungs characterized by persistent airway inflammation, structural remodeling of the airway wall, and airflow obstruction. Asthma is characterized by an inflammation of the airway wall, with an abnormal accumulation of basophils, eosinophils, lymphocytes, mast cells, macrophages, dendritic cells, and myofibroblasts. Airway inflammation results in a peculiar type of lymphocytic infiltration in which T helper 2 (Th2) lymphocytes secrete cytokines that orchestrate cellular inflammation and promote airway hyperresponsiveness [1,2]. To date, COPD is characterized by an airflow limitation that is not fully reversible. The airflow limitation is, in most cases, both progressive and associated with an abnormal inflammatory response of the lungs to noxious particles or gases [3]. Airway remodeling results in alterations in the airway epithelium, lamina propria, and submucosa, leading to a thickening of the airway wall [4]. The consequences of airway remodeling in asthma include incompletely reversible airway narrowing, bronchial hyperresponsiveness, airway edema, and mucus hypersecretion; these effects may predispose subjects with asthma to exacerbations and even death due to airway obstruction. Airway remodeling is an ongoing repair process in reaction to inflammation, and several epithelial growth factors and cytokines have been reported to be overexpressed in airway epithelial tissues of those with asthma and COPD alike [5,6]. Among these growth factors, epidermal growth factor (EGF) and its receptor (EGFR) are, together, one of the most important factors in the pathogenesis of airway remodeling [7]. As the details become clearer regarding the roles of EGFR pathways in the repair process of damaged airway epithelia and in the regulation of mucus production, EGFR is drawing greater attention as an important target for the treatment of airway remodeling in patients with asthma and COPD. In the present review, we focus on the EGFR signaling pathway, with a particular emphasis on mucin production and secretion, epithelial wound healing and regeneration, and the stability of the airway barrier.

Epidermal growth factors and their receptors

Epidermal growth factor was discovered by the scientists Stanley Cohen and Rita Levi-Montalcini, who were awarded a Nobel Prize in Medicine in 1986 [8,9]. They created the basis for the biology of EGF, including the understanding of EGF and its receptor, EGFR. This receptor is a 170 kDa membrane glycoprotein that is activated by multiple ligands, including EGF, transforming growth factor alpha (TGF-α), heparin-binding EGF, amphiregulin, β-cellulin, and

Inflammation and Allergy Drug Design, First Edition. Edited by Kenji Izuhara, Stephen T. Holgate, Marsha Wills-Karp.
© 2011 Blackwell Publishing Ltd. Published 2011 by Blackwell Publishing Ltd.

epiregulin, all of which are synthesized as transmembrane precursors that are added to the cell surface and cleaved by proteases to release the mature soluble growth factor. Amphiregulin, epiregulin, EGF, and TGF-α only bind and activate EGFRs (also known as ErbB-1 and HER1), and together they are referred to as group one of the EGF family. Group two is composed of neuregulins, which bind ErbB-3 and -4. Group three consists of heparin-binding EGF, betacellulin, and epiregulin, which bind both EGFR and ErbB-4. ErbB-2 does not bind ligands directly but is the preferred heterodimerization partner for all other ErbB members [10,11]. A recent study suggested that mucin 4 (MUC4) and sialomucin complex can act as an intramembrane ligand for ErbB-2 via an EGF-like domain present in the transmembrane subunit. MUC4 was cloned from tracheobronchial mucosa complementary DNA (cDNA) [12]. Interestingly, MUC4 expression has been reported to be high in all types of airway epithelial cells [13].

Epidermal growth factor signal and lung development

Epidermal growth factors are widely known to be involved in virtually all aspects of lung development. During the initial stages of lung bud morphogenesis and the subsequent formation of the bronchial tree, the activation of EGFR signaling in the epithelium by EGFR ligands is critical. One study demonstrated the important role of EGFR signaling on lung morphogenesis by analyzing the developmental phenotype of lungs in mice with an inactivated EGFR gene [14]; neonatal EGFR-deficient mice often show evidence of lung immaturity, which can result in visible respiratory distress. The lungs of these mutant mice had impaired branching and deficient alveolization and septation, resulting in a 50% reduction in alveolar volume and, thus, a markedly reduced surface area for gas exchange. Signal transduction through the EGFR plays a major role in lung development, and its inactivation leads to respiratory dysfunction.

In experiments on the primary roles of EGFR ligands on lung development, it is difficult to interpret the results of the studies using EGFR ligand-deficient mice because of the complications of functional redundancy. For example, heparin-binding EGF knockout mice and tumor necrosis factor alpha (TNF-α)

converting enzyme (TACE)-deficient mice displayed indistinguishable cardiac valve defects and abnormal lung development [15]. In contrast, EGF, TGF-α, and amphiregulin deficiency has a negligible effect on the development of the heart and lungs [16,17]. Crossbreeding experiments between various genotypes have also revealed the importance of partial functional redundancy between these ligands.

An EGFR mutant lacking a portion of the intracytoplasmic domain (EGF-R-M) under control of the human surfactant protein C (SP-C) promoter has been made [18]. Transcripts of the SP-C–EGF-R-M transgene were detected in distal bronchiolar and type II cells by *in situ* hybridization. Lung fibrosis was not detected and airspace hypoplasia was significantly corrected in bi-transgenic mice derived from the breeding of SP-C–TGF-α and SP-C–EGF-R-M mice. A correction of lung pathology in the bi-transgenic mice occurred without altering the level of human TGF-α (hTGF-α) mRNA using this approach [18].

Expression of the epidermal growth factor family and its receptors in airway diseases

The EGFR pathway has emerged as a key target in non-small-cell lung cancer [19]. During the last decade there has been an explosion of knowledge regarding the biologic and clinical significance of EGFR for lung cancer [19]. However, the pathologic significance of EGFR for other lung diseases, excluding cancer, has not been determined. In the case of asthma, a previous report demonstrated that EGFR expression increased markedly in areas of epithelial damage in bronchial biopsies from the airways of patients with asthma, but not in similar areas in control subjects [5]. Another study demonstrated that bronchial epithelial expression of EGFR, ErbB-3 and MUC5AC are augmented in current smokers with and without COPD, suggesting that ErbB receptor heterodimerization may be an important determinant of epithelial responses to cigarette smoke [6].

A model of growth factor imbalance in asthma has been proposed by Holgate *et al.* [20]. They report that epithelial expression of EGFR is increased in the damaged airways of those both with and without asthma. Unlike the normal bronchial epithelium, where elevated EGFR expression was observed only in areas of structural damage, in patients with asthma they found a striking disease-related overexpression of EGFR, in both damaged and morphologically intact epithelia, the extent of which correlates with sub-basement membrane (SBM) collagen thickness [12]. Further contrasting with normal epithelia, EGFR immunostaining of the epithelia from those with asthma occurs throughout the epithelial layer, which is indicative of widespread functional changes [12]. This was confirmed by another study, in which bronchial tissue from patients with asthma was examined post mortem or taken from surgical resections [21]. In this study, researchers evaluated the expression of EGF and EGFR on airway specimens from seven patients with asthma and eight control subjects. Their results demonstrated that clear EGF immunoreactivities were widely observed on bronchial epithelium, glands, and smooth muscle in the airways of those with asthma. In the controls, the bronchial epithelia and the bronchial glands partially expressed faint EGF immunoreactivities. For EGFR, clear immunoreactivities were also observed on bronchial epithelium, glands, smooth muscle, and basement membranes in the airways of patients with asthma. In the control airways, only a part of the bronchial epithelium and smooth muscle weakly expressed EGFR immunoreactivity [21]. As we will discuss later, because EGFR plays an important role in epithelial repair, one explanation for the high level of EGFR expression in the epithelium of individuals with asthma is that their airway epithelium may be repeating injury and repair in a much wider area than we thought. Another possibility is that the epithelial cells may be suspended in a repair phenotype and be functionally undeveloped.

In the airways of patients with asthma, under stable conditions, there is no evidence of epithelial hyperproliferation, despite EGFR upregulation. Rather, structural changes are found in the mesenchyme, as shown by deposition of interstitial collagens and other matrix proteins in sub-basement lamina. In these patients, although EGF levels appear normal, high levels of TGF-β1 have been detected in airway tissue and bronchoalveolar lavage fluid [22,23]. The suppression of epithelial proliferation and the stimulation of matrix deposition suggest a predominance of TGF-β over the EGF effects, as though airways are being held in a "repair default." The process of "remodeling" the airways, as seen in adult asthma, has many similarities with airway "modeling" observed during branching morphogenesis in the developing fetal lung and the structural changes seen early during the development of asthma in infancy. Similarities that exist between organ morphogenesis and wound healing have led to a new concept of chronic inflammation, namely one that is supported by structural components through activation of the epithelial mesenchymal trophic unit (EMTU) [22].

A new paradigm for persistent asthma is that of a damaged epithelium that repairs incompletely. The consequence of this is a chronic wound scenario characterized by the secretion of a range of secondary growth factors by epithelial cells and underlying fibroblasts capable of driving structural changes linked to airway remodeling [1]. Recently, we reported the concentrations of EGF and amphiregulin in sputum samples obtained from patients with asthma during an acute attack and during the subsequent recovery phase [24]. We found that the sputum EGF levels in these patients increased during an acute attack and remained elevated during the recovery phase. In contrast, the sputum concentrations of amphiregulin and tryptase were only transiently elevated during the acute attack [24].

Interleukin-8 synthesis via epidermal growth factor receptor signaling

Neutrophils have been considered to play important roles in chronic airway diseases such as cystic fibrosis (CF), COPD, and severe asthma [25]. Interleukin 8 (IL-8) is a chemokine that is expressed in many cell types, including airway epithelial cells. Airway epithelium produces IL-8 in response to various stimuli, such as the influenza virus, double-stranded RNA (dsRNA), osmotic stress, and bacterial wall components such as lipothecoid acid, peptidoglycan, liposaccharide, and lipid A [26–29].

A recent finding is that the synthesis and secretion of IL-8 is also dependent, at least in part, on EGFR activation. The treatment of EGF or TGF-α, two EGFRs, has been reported to increase IL-8 production in airway epithelial cells [30]. In addition, another study demonstrated that cigarette smoke induces the production of IL-8 mediated through the activated EGFR, and this effect was prevented by the selective EGFR tyrosine kinase inhibitor AG1478 [31]. The study also demonstrated that the EGFR-dependent

IL-8 secretion in response to cigarette smoke was the result of TGF-α shedding from airway epithelial cells. Nakanaga et al. [32] found that TACE is responsible for the synthesis and release of IL-8 from airway epithelial cells in response to bacterial lipopolysaccharide (LPS) via a Duox1–TACE–TGF-α–EGFR signaling pathway on the surface of airway epithelial cells. Neutrophil elastase also induces IL-8 production in airway epithelial cells through similar surface signaling [33].

Interleukin 8 has been found to be an important neutrophil chemoattractant in the sputum of patients with chronic inflammatory diseases, including CF, bronchiectasis and chronic bronchitis [34]. Therefore, IL-8 is considered to be substantially involved in the pathogenesis of chronic airway inflammation. Another function of IL-8 is its role in angiogenesis [35]. Angiogenesis is a multistep process which includes endothelial cell proliferation and migration resulting from degradation of the extracellular matrix by matrix metalloproteinases (MMPs) and capillary tube formation [36]. Although the series of phenomena in angiogenesis is mediated by various angiogenic factors, IL-8, as well as vascular endothelial growth factor (VEGF), which is the most well-known angiogenic factor, has also been found to directly enhance endothelial cell survival, proliferation and MMP production, and to regulate angiogenesis.

Epithelial wound repair via epithelial growth factor receptor signaling

The important role of EGFR activation in epithelial repair has been demonstrated in various cell types in vitro, including keratinocytes [37], mammary epithelial cells [38], and alveolar epithelial cells [39]. An in vitro mechanical wound repair model using airway epithelial cells revealed that EGF accelerated the repair of scrape-wounded monolayers of airway epithelial cells and that the EGFR-selective inhibitor, tyrphostin AG1478, inhibited both EGF-stimulated and basal wound closure [5].

A previous study demonstrated that administration of aerosolized EGF plus platelet-derived growth factor (PDGF) for 2 weeks enhanced the repair of sheep tracheal epithelia after cotton smoke injury in vivo [40]. It was suggested that cell proliferation and differentiation were responsible for epithelial regeneration, but the exact cellular mechanisms were not identified. Kim et al. [41] hypothesized that EGF accelerates wound closure in airway epithelial cells independently of cell proliferation. Culturing guinea-pig airway epithelial cells in vitro, they found that EGF accelerated the closure of small wounds in confluent epithelial monolayers over 24 hours and that EGF elicited the migration of airway epithelial cells, suggesting that early events in EGF-mediated wound closure involve cell migration [41]. In a study using cultured human airway epithelial cells, it was demonstrated that EGF-induced epithelial repair occurred within 18 hours and that cell proliferation did not occur at this time, establishing that EGF promotes airway epithelial repair via cell migration in this model. However, it is likely that cell proliferation is implicated in the repair of larger wounds in the airway epithelium [42].

Role of epithelial growth factors in epithelial barrier function

The airway epithelial barrier is often disrupted in patients with asthma, with evidence of shedding of ciliated cells [43,44]. During the airway sensitization phase and the attack of allergic asthma, causative allergens must cross the airway epithelium to interact with antigen-presenting cells and mast cells. However, the mechanism by which the allergens cross the airway lining has not been completely determined.

The tight junction belongs to the category of epithelial cell junctional complexes that are important for the development of an intact barrier [45]. These junctional complexes also include focal adhesions composed mainly of integrin molecules: the adherens junction composed of E-cadherin, and the gap junctions composed of connexins. The tight junction is located at the most apical region of the lateral membrane in epithelial cell sheets. Tight junctions are composed of transmembrane and cytosolic proteins, such as claudins, occludin, and zonula occludens, which seal the intercellular space between adjacent cells to create a primary barrier against the diffusion of fluid, electrolytes, macromolecules, and pathogens via the paracellular pathway [46,47]. Therefore, the tight junction is essential for the barrier function of the epithelium by restricting paracellular diffusion.

The FcεRI-activated release of tryptase from allergen-activated mast cells in the airway lumen contributes to the late phase of the allergen response by stimulating epithelial cells to release metalloproteinase-9 and thus open up tight junctions, promoting allergen penetration into the submucosa. It is possible that the stimulated epithelial cells release trypsin, another stimulus of proteinase-activated receptor 2 (PAR-2) [48]. Alternatively, the epithelial cells could be activated by airborne proteases from molds, mites, or pollens. Various allergens, including a cysteine protease (Der p 1) and a serine peptidase (Der p 9) from the house dust mite *Dermatophagoides pteronyssinus,* have been shown to facilitate the transepithelial delivery of allergens by disrupting tight junctions with their serine protease activity. Der p 1 is one of the most common aeroallergens associated with atopic asthma [49,50]. A number of recent studies have implicated the cysteine protease activity of Der p 1 in the pathogenesis of asthma [51,52]. Der p 1 led to a cleavage of the tight junction adhesion protein occludin [53]. This cleavage was attenuated by antipain, but not by inhibitors of serine, aspartic, or MMPs. Putative Der p 1 cleavage sites were found in peptides from an extracellular domain of occludin and in the tight junction adhesion protein claudin 1. Tight junction breakdown increased epithelial permeability non-specifically, allowing Der p 1 to cross the epithelial barrier. Thus, transepithelial movement of Der p 1 to dendritic antigen-presenting cells via the paracellular pathway may be promoted by the allergen's own proteolytic activity. These results suggest that the opening of tight junctions by environmental proteinases may be the initial step in the development of asthma to a variety of allergens.

Viral infection is a common cause of the exacerbation of asthma. Human rhinovirus (HRV) causes the majority of common colds, and possibly also asthma exacerbations. A previous study reported that HRV disrupts the barrier function of the airway epithelium and induces dissociation of ZO-1 from the cell membrane both *in vitro* and *in vivo* [54]. The effect on barrier function appears to depend on viral replication. An inadequate repair response and inability to restore cell–cell contacts after damaging stimuli may be responsible for the damaged and activated phenotype of the bronchial epithelium because the tight junction maintains epithelial cell polarity. This is suggested by the increased expression of EGFR

and TGF-β at sites of ciliated cell detachment, as described above.

Another important molecule for the maintenance of epithelial integrity is E-cadherin, an adhesion molecule that mediates intercellular contact through homophilic interactions [55]. E-cadherin is predominantly located in adherens junctions and is linked to the actin cytoskeleton via β-catenin [56]. An epithelial damage and an inadequate repair may result in loss of E-cadherin membrane expression and intercellular contacts. It has recently been demonstrated that E-cadherin membrane expression is reduced in the airway epithelia obtained from bronchial biopsies of patients with asthma [57]. E-cadherin is known to negatively regulate multiple signaling pathways. Interestingly, a loss of E-cadherin expression has been demonstrated to increase the activity of EGFR [58]. These observations support the idea that overexpression of EGFR on epithelial cells in those with asthma may be seen as a reflection of a repair phenotype, as stated above.

Mucus secretion and epithelial growth factor receptor signaling

Over the past several years, an intense effort has been aimed at elucidating the cellular and molecular mechanisms contributing to the process of airway remodeling. Increasing evidence has revealed potentially important roles of EGFR in several aspects of airway remodeling. As described above, EGFR and its ligands are upregulated in the epithelium of individuals with asthma, and induction of this system correlates with goblet cell hyperplasia [59,60]. With an understanding of the mechanisms that regulate the EGFR and its ligands in mediating mucus hypersecretion by airway epithelial cells, this subject has become an active area of research, with attempts being made to understand airway remodeling in individuals with asthma. Goblet-cell hyperplasia is an important feature of chronic airway diseases such as asthma and COPD. Excessive secretion of mucus by hyperplastic goblet cells causes airway mucus impaction and contributes to morbidity and mortality in patients with asthma [61]. Nineteen different mucin genes have been identified. Among these, MUC5AC is a predominant component of the mucus produced by airway epithelial cells [62], and its production is known to be regulated by the EGFR signaling pathway [63,64]. Human rhinovirus, respiratory syncytial virus, influenza virus, and parainfluenza virus are particularly common pathogens that induce the hypersecretion of mucus and exacerbation of asthma [65,66].

It is widely assumed that dsRNA is generated by viral RNA polymerases as an intermediary in genome replication of RNA viruses. TLR3 recognizes dsRNA and activates genes that increase inflammatory cytokines important for protection against virus infection [67]. Therefore, TLR3 has been assumed to play a central role in the host response to infection by viruses [67]. A recent study has demonstrated that dsRNA synergistically increased MUC5AC gene induction by TGF-α in both NCI-H292 and normal human bronchial epithelial cells [68]. MEK1/2 inhibitors significantly inhibited MUC5AC production [69]. A previous report indicated that EGFR activation induced the expression of MKP3, which is one of the negative regulators of Erk1/2, while co-stimulation with a synthetic dsRNA poly(I:C) inhibited MKP3 upregulation dose dependently [68]. Thus, the synergistic effect of dsRNA on MUC5AC production may be a result of enhanced activation of extracellular signal-regulated kinase through the inhibition of MKP3 by poly(I:C). Another study also demonstrated that rhinoviruses directly induce mucin production though a TLR3-mediated pathway that is partly dependent on TRIF and is negatively regulated by MYD88. This TLR3-mediated mucin-inducing pathway further leads to an increase of TGF-α and AREG (amphiregulin) production, and the subsequent activation of EGFR through an autocrine–paracrine mechanism [65].

Conclusion

On the basis of the effects of EGFR on the airway described above, EGFR may become a new therapeutic target in chronic airway inflammatory diseases. Because EGFR and its ligands are essential for mucus hypersecretion by airway epithelial cells, a treatment targeting EGFR would be beneficial for controlling hypersecretion in patients with asthma and COPD. On the other hand, inhibitors of EGFR would potentially also suppress EGFR-mediated signals needed for the sufficient repair of a damaged epithelium, and to differentiate between a damaged or fully mature epithelium with complete barrier function. Therefore, it is predicted that blocking of all EGFR-mediated signaling would produce a range of side-effects. To take advantage of EGFR as a therapeutic target for the treatment of asthma and COPD, understanding the distinct signaling pathway which regulates the oversecretion of mucus, as well as any other beneficial effects of EGFR, would be indispensable in the development of new drugs.

References

1 Holgate ST, Davies DE. Rethinking the pathogenesis of asthma. *Immunity* 2009; **31**: 362–7.

2 Barnes PJ. The cytokine network in asthma and chronic obstructive pulmonary disease. *J Clin Invest* 2008; **118**: 3546–56.

3 Barnes PJ. Chronic obstructive pulmonary disease. *N Engl J Med* 2000; **343**: 269–80.

4 Davies DE, Wicks J, Powell RM, Puddicombe SM, Holgate ST. Airway remodeling in asthma: new insights. *J Allergy Clin Immunol* 2003; **111**: 215–25; quiz 26.

5 Puddicombe SM, Polosa R, Richter A, *et al.* Involvement of the epidermal growth factor receptor in epithelial repair in asthma. *FASEB J* 2000; **14**: 1362–74.

6 O'Donnell RA, Richter A, Ward J, *et al.* Expression of ErbB receptors and mucins in the airways of long term current smokers. *Thorax* 2004; **59**: 1032–40.

7 Davies DE, Polosa R, Puddicombe SM, Richter A, Holgate ST. The epidermal growth factor receptor and its ligand family: their potential role in repair and remodelling in asthma. *Allergy* 1999; **54**: 771–83.

8 Cohen S, Levi-Montalcini R, Hamburger V. A Nerve growth-stimulating factor isolated from sarcom as 37 and 180. *Proc Natl Acad Sci USA* 1954; **40**: 1014–18.

9 Levi-Montalcini R, Hamburger V. Selective growth stimulating effects of mouse sarcoma on the sensory and sympathetic nervous system of the chick embryo. *J Exp Zool* 1951; **116**: 321–61.

10 Baselga J, Swain SM. Novel anticancer targets: revisiting ERBB2 and discovering ERBB3. *Nat Rev Cancer* 2009; **9**: 463–75.

11 Burgess AW. EGFR family: structure physiology signalling and therapeutic targets. *Growth Factors* 2008; **26**: 263–74.

12 Chaturvedi P, Singh AP, Batra SK. Structure, evolution, and biology of the MUC4 mucin. *FASEB J* 2008; **22**: 966–81.

13 Hattrup CL, Gendler SJ. Structure and function of the cell surface (tethered) mucins. *Annu Rev Physiol* 2008; **70**: 431–57.

14 Miettinen PJ, Warburton D, Bu D, *et al.* Impaired lung branching morphogenesis in the absence of functional EGF receptor. *Dev Biol* 1997; **186**: 224–36.

15 Jackson LF, Qiu TH, Sunnarborg SW, *et al.* Defective valvulogenesis in HB-EGF and TACE-null mice is associated with aberrant BMP signaling. *EMBO J* 2003; **22**: 2704–16.

16 Mann GB, Fowler KJ, Gabriel A, Nice EC, Williams RL, Dunn AR. Mice with a null mutation of the TGF alpha gene have abnormal skin architecture, wavy hair, and curly whiskers and often develop corneal inflammation. *Cell* 1993; **73**: 249–61.

17 Nam KT, Varro A, Coffey RJ, Goldenring JR. Potentiation of oxyntic atrophy-induced gastric metaplasia in amphiregulin-deficient mice. *Gastroenterology* 2007; **132**: 1804–19.

18 Hardie WD, Kerlakian CB, Bruno MD, *et al.* Reversal of lung lesions in transgenic transforming growth factor alpha mice by expression of mutant epidermal growth factor receptor. *Am J Respir Cell Mol Biol* 1996; **15**: 499–508.

19 Sharma SV, Bell DW, Settleman J, Haber DA. Epidermal growth factor receptor mutations in lung cancer. *Nat Rev Cancer* 2007; **7**: 169–81.

20 Holgate ST, Lackie PM, Davies DE, Roche WR, Walls AF. The bronchial epithelium as a key regulator of airway inflammation and remodelling in asthma. *Clin Exp Allergy* 1999; **29** (Suppl 2): 90–5.

21 Amishima M, Munakata M, Nasuhara Y, *et al.* Expression of epidermal growth factor and epidermal growth factor receptor immunoreactivity in the asthmatic human airway. *Am J Respir Crit Care Med* 1998; **157**: 1907–12.

22 Holgate ST, Davies DE, Lackie PM, Wilson SJ, Puddicombe SM, Lordan JL. Epithelial–mesenchymal interactions in the pathogenesis of asthma. *J Allergy Clin Immunol* 2000; **105**: 193–204.

23 Chu HW, Trudeau JB, Balzar S, Wenzel SE. Peripheral blood and airway tissue expression of transforming growth factor beta by neutrophils in asthmatic subjects and normal control subjects. *J Allergy Clin Immunol* 2000; **106**: 1115–23.

24 Enomoto Y, Orihara K, Takamasu T, *et al.* Tissue remodeling induced by hypersecreted epidermal growth factor and amphiregulin in the airway after an acute asthma attack. *J Allergy Clin Immunol* 2009; **124**: 913–20, e1–7.

25 Watt AP, Schock BC, Ennis M. Neutrophils and eosinophils: clinical implications of their appearance, presence and disappearance in asthma and COPD. *Curr Drug Targets Inflamm Allergy* 2005; **4**: 415–23.

26 Hashimoto S, Matsumoto K, Gon Y, Nakayama T, Takeshita I, Horie T. Hyperosmolarity-induced interleukin-8 expression in human bronchial epithelial

cells through p38 mitogen-activated protein kinase. *Am J Respir Crit Care Med* 1999; **159**: 634–40.

27 Takizawa H. Bronchial epithelial cells in allergic reactions. *Curr Drug Targets Inflamm Allergy* 2005; **4**: 305–11.

28 Kujime K, Hashimoto S, Gon Y, Shimizu K, Horie T. p38 mitogen-activated protein kinase and c-jun-NH2-terminal kinase regulate RANTES production by influenza virus-infected human bronchial epithelial cells. *J Immunol* 2000; **164**: 3222–8.

29 Gon Y, Asai Y, Hashimoto S, *et al.* A20 inhibits toll-like receptor 2- and 4-mediated interleukin-8 synthesis in airway epithelial cells. *Am J Respir Cell Mol Biol* 2004; **31**: 330–6.

30 Subauste MC, Proud D. Effects of tumor necrosis factor-alpha, epidermal growth factor and transforming growth factor-alpha on interleukin-8 production by, and human rhinovirus replication in, bronchial epithelial cells. *Int Immunopharmacol* 2001; **1**: 1229–34.

31 Richter A, O'Donnell RA, Powell RM, *et al.* Autocrine ligands for the epidermal growth factor receptor mediate interleukin-8 release from bronchial epithelial cells in response to cigarette smoke. *Am J Respir Cell Mol Biol* 2002; **27**: 85–90.

32 Nakanaga T, Nadel JA, Ueki IF, Koff JL, Shao MX. Regulation of interleukin-8 via an airway epithelial signaling cascade. *Am J Physiol Lung Cell Mol Physiol* 2007; **292**: L1289–96.

33 Kuwahara I, Lillehoj EP, Lu W, *et al.* Neutrophil elastase induces IL-8 gene transcription and protein release through p38/NF-κB activation via EGFR transactivation in a lung epithelial cell line. *Am J Physiol Lung Cell Mol Physiol* 2006; **291**: L407–16.

34 Richman-Eisenstat JB, Jorens PG, Hebert CA, Ueki I, Nadel JA. Interleukin-8: an important chemoattractant in sputum of patients with chronic inflammatory airway diseases. *Am J Physiol* 1993; **264**: L413–18.

35 Petzelbauer P, Watson CA, Pfau SE, Pober JS. IL-8 and angiogenesis: evidence that human endothelial cells lack receptors and do not respond to IL-8 *in vitro*. *Cytokine* 1995; **7**: 267–72.

36 Eble JA, Niland S. The extracellular matrix of blood vessels. *Curr Pharm Des* 2009; **15**: 1385–400.

37 Stoll S, Garner W, Elder J. Heparin-binding ligands mediate autocrine epidermal growth factor receptor activation in skin organ culture. *J Clin Invest* 1997; **100**: 1271–81.

38 Matthay MA, Thiery JP, Lafont F, Stampfer F, Boyer B. Transient effect of epidermal growth factor on the motility of an immortalized mammary epithelial cell line. *J Cell Sci* 1993; **106** (Pt 3): 869–78.

39 Kheradmand F, Folkesson HG, Shum L, Derynk R, Pytela R, Matthay MA. Transforming growth

factor-alpha enhances alveolar epithelial cell repair in a new *in vitro* model. *Am J Physiol* 1994; **267**: L728–38.

40 Barrow RE, Wang CZ, Evans MJ, Herndon DN. Growth factors accelerate epithelial repair in sheep trachea. *Lung* 1993; **171**: 335–44.

41 Kim JS, McKinnis VS, Nawrocki A, White SR. Stimulation of migration and wound repair of guinea-pig airway epithelial cells in response to epidermal growth factor. *Am J Respir Cell Mol Biol* 1998; **18**: 66–74.

42 White SR, Dorscheid DR, Rabe KF, Wojcik KR, Hamann KJ. Role of very late adhesion integrins in mediating repair of human airway epithelial cell monolayers after mechanical injury. *Am J Respir Cell Mol Biol* 1999; **20**: 787–96.

43 Holgate ST. Epithelium dysfunction in asthma. *J Allergy Clin Immunol* 2007; **120**: 1233–44; quiz 45–6.

44 Swindle EJ, Collins JE, Davies DE. Breakdown in epithelial barrier function in patients with asthma: identification of novel therapeutic approaches. *J Allergy Clin Immunol* 2009; **124**: 23–34; quiz 5–6.

45 Tsukita S, Furuse M, Itoh M. Multifunctional strands in tight junctions. *Nat Rev Mol Cell Biol* 2001; **2**: 285–93.

46 Balkovetz DF, Katz J. Bacterial invasion by a paracellular route: divide and conquer. *Microbes Infect* 2003; **5**: 613–19.

47 Gonzalez-Mariscal L, Betanzos A, Nava P, Jaramillo BE. Tight junction proteins. *Prog Biophys Mol Biol* 2003; **81**: 1–44.

48 Jacob C, Yang PC, Darmoul D, *et al*. Mast cell tryptase controls paracellular permeability of the intestine. Role of protease-activated receptor 2 and beta-arrestins. *J Biol Chem* 2005; **280**: 31936–48.

49 Platts-Mills TA. House dust mites. *N Engl Reg Allergy Proc* 1985; **6**: 158–9.

50 Platts-Mills TA, Vervloet D, Thomas WR, Aalberse RC, Chapman MD. Indoor allergens and asthma: report of the Third International Workshop. *J Allergy Clin Immunol* 1997; **100**: S2–24.

51 Kalsheker NA, Deam S, Chambers L, Sreedharan S, Brocklehurst K, Lomas DA. The house dust mite allergen Der p1 catalytically inactivates alpha 1-antitrypsin by specific reactive centre loop cleavage: a mechanism that promotes airway inflammation and asthma. *Biochem Biophys Res Commun* 1996; **221**: 59–61.

52 Hewitt CR, Brown AP, Hart BJ, Pritchard DI. A major house dust mite allergen disrupts the immunoglobulin E network by selectively cleaving CD23: innate protection by antiproteases. *J Exp Med* 1995; **182**: 1537–44.

53 Wan H, Winton HL, Soeller C, *et al*. Der p 1 facilitates transepithelial allergen delivery by disruption of tight junctions. *J Clin Invest* 1999; **104**: 123–33.

54 Sajjan U, Wang Q, Zhao Y, Gruenert DC, Hershenson MB. Rhinovirus disrupts the barrier function of polar-ized airway epithelial cells. *Am J Respir Crit Care Med* 2008; **178**: 1271–81.

55 Takeichi M. Cadherins: a molecular family important in selective cell–cell adhesion. *Annu Rev Biochem* 1990; **59**: 237–52.

56 Ozawa M, Baribault H, Kemler R. The cytoplasmic domain of the cell adhesion molecule uvomorulin associates with three independent proteins structurally related in different species. *EMBO J* 1989; **8**: 1711–17.

57 Trautmann A, Kruger K, Akdis M, *et al*. Apoptosis and loss of adhesion of bronchial epithelial cells in asthma. *Int Arch Allergy Immunol* 2005; **138**: 142–50.

58 Qian X, Karpova T, Sheppard AM, McNally J, Lowy DR. E-cadherin-mediated adhesion inhibits ligand-dependent activation of diverse receptor tyrosine kinases. *EMBO J* 2004; **23**: 1739–48.

59 Burgel PR, Nadel JA. Roles of epidermal growth factor receptor activation in epithelial cell repair and mucin production in airway epithelium. *Thorax* 2004; **59**: 992–6.

60 Morcillo EJ, Cortijo J. Mucus and MUC in asthma. *Curr Opin Pulm Med* 2006; **12**: 1–6.

61 Rogers DF. Physiology of airway mucus secretion and pathophysiology of hypersecretion. *Respir Care* 2007; **52**: 1134–46; discussion 46–9.

62 Williams OW, Sharafkhaneh A, Kim V, Dickey BF, Evans CM. Airway mucus: from production to secretion. *Am J Respir Cell Mol Biol* 2006; **34**: 527–36.

63 Takeyama K, Dabbagh K, Jeong Shim J, Dao-Pick T, Ueki IF, Nadel JA. Oxidative stress causes mucin synthesis via transactivation of epidermal growth factor receptor: role of neutrophils. *J Immunol* 2000; **164**: 1546–52.

64 Takeyama K, Fahy JV, Nadel JA. Relationship of epidermal growth factor receptors to goblet cell production in human bronchi. *Am J Respir Crit Care Med* 2001; **163**: 511–16.

65 Zhu L, Lee PK, Lee WM, Zhao Y, Yu D, Chen Y. Rhinovirus-induced major airway mucin production involves a novel TLR3-EGFR-dependent pathway. *Am J Respir Cell Mol Biol* 2009; **40**: 610–19.

66 He SH, Zheng J, Duan MK. Induction of mucin secretion from human bronchial tissue and epithelial cells by rhinovirus and lipopolysaccharide. *Acta Pharmacol Sin* 2004; **25**: 1176–81.

67 Takeuchi O, Akira S. Recognition of viruses by innate immunity. *Immunol Rev* 2007; **220**: 214–24.

68 Tadaki H, Arakawa H, Mizuno T, *et al*. Double-stranded RNA and TGF-alpha promote MUC5AC induction in respiratory cells. *J Immunol* 2009; **182**: 293–300.

69 Song KS, Lee WJ, Chung KC, *et al*. Interleukin-1 beta and tumor necrosis factor-alpha induce MUC5AC overexpression through a mechanism involving ERK/p38 mitogen-activated protein kinases-MSK1-CREB activation in human airway epithelial cells. *J Biol Chem* 2003; **278**: 23243–50.

Part III
Other mediators contributing to the pathogenesis of allergic diseases in the respiratory tract

22 Prostanoids

Sarah A. Maher, Deborah L. Clarke, and Maria G. Belvisi
Department of Pharmacology and Toxicology, Imperial College, London, UK

Introduction to prostanoids

Prostanoids were first identified in 1936 by Ulf von Euler, who injected semen into animals and found that it lowered blood pressure. The biologically active components were named "prostaglandins" because they were apparently produced in the prostate gland [1]. More than 20 years later, in 1957, the first prostaglandins (PGE_1 and $PGF_{2\alpha}$) were purified [2]. Over the following years, it became apparent that prostanoids represent a large and diverse family of lipid mediators, which are found ubiquitously in almost every tissue in mammals.

The term prostanoid is a name that collectively represents thromboxane (Tx), prostacyclin and prostaglandins, examples of which are prostacyclin (PGI_2), PGD_2, PGE_2, $PGF_{2\alpha}$, and TxA_2. They are 20 carbon cyclooxygenase (COX) products of arachidonic acid metabolism, which mediate a wide variety of effects in the body, including contraction and relaxation of smooth muscle, ion transport, modulation of neurotransmitter release, and control of body temperature. They also regulate apoptosis, cell differentiation, and oncogenesis. Other prostaglandin-like derivatives such as isoprostanes, produced by a free radical-catalyzed mechanism, are not discussed in this chapter.

Synthesis of prostanoids

Prostaglandins and thromboxane are derived from metabolism of arachidonic acid by COX-1 (constitutively expressed) and COX-2 (inducible), and from subsequent metabolism by prostaglandin synthase enzymes (Figure 22.1). Arachidonic acid is liberated from the membrane by phospholipase A_2 and oxidized by COX enzymes into PGG_2. This is then followed by a reduction by COX to an unstable endoperoxidase PGH_2. This endoperoxidase acts as a substrate for a variety of synthase enzymes responsible for producing the bioactive prostaglandins: PGI_2, PGD_2, PGE_2, $PGF_{2\alpha}$ and TxA_2. The end product that is formed is dependent on the different supply of enzymes in different cell types; for example, PGI_2 synthase is expressed abundantly in vascular smooth muscle cells and PGE_2 isomerase is the most abundant enzyme in human airway smooth muscle cells (HASM) – hence PGI_2 and PGE_2 are the major COX products of vascular and HASM cells, respectively [3,4].

Prostanoids and their receptors

Prostanoids were originally thought to be hydrophobic and to enter the cell by perturbing lipid fluidity to mediate their actions. It became apparent, however, through comparisons in the potencies of various prostanoids and their synthetic analogs on various tissues by bioassay, that each prostanoid had a specific site of action. Work carried out on lung and platelets [5,6] led to a proposal to classify the prostanoid receptors [7]. They recognized that a receptor exists for PGD_2, PGE_2, $PGF_{2\alpha}$, PGI_2 and TXA_2, and accordingly named them DP, EP, FP, IP and TP, respectively, according

Inflammation and Allergy Drug Design, First Edition. Edited by Kenji Izuhara, Stephen T. Holgate, Marsha Wills-Karp.
© 2011 Blackwell Publishing Ltd. Published 2011 by Blackwell Publishing Ltd.

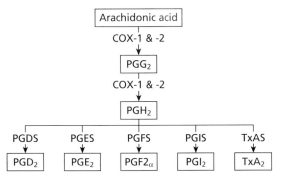

Figure 22.1 Biosynthesis of prostaglandins. Arachidonic acid is metabolized by COX-1 or -2 to PGH$_2$, the common precursor for the prostaglandin synthase enzymes. The prostanoids TxA$_2$, PGD$_2$, PGE$_2$, PGI$_2$, and PGF2$_\alpha$ are produced by their individual synthase enzymes TxAS, PGDS, PGES, PGIS, and PGFS, respectively.

to the prostanoid that had the highest affinity at the receptor type. The PGE$_2$ receptor, EP, can be further classified into four distinct subtypes (EP$_1$ to EP$_4$) [8,9]. Furthermore, the PGD$_2$ class of receptors is composed of DP1 and DP2. DP2 is also known as CRTh2 (chemoattractant receptor-homologous molecule expressed on T helper type II cells) [10,11]. However, all the prostanoids can activate the various receptor subtypes to some degree [12]. The prostanoid receptors are seven transmembrane G-protein coupled rhodopsin-like proteins acting through different types of G proteins and signaling cascades, allowing the prostanoids to produce their diverse range of physiologic effects (Figure 22.2). In general, IP, EP$_2$, EP$_4$, and DP receptors activate G$_s$, stimulating cyclic adenosine monophosphate (cAMP) production by adenylyl cyclase. TP, EP$_1$, and FP receptors mediate contractile-type responses by activating the G protein G$_q$ and increasing intracellular Ca^{2+}. Finally, EP$_3$ is generally thought to be inhibitory, and it inhibits adenylyl cyclase and increased cAMP via G$_i$. However, these guidelines are not always true, and receptor signaling can depend on the existence of splice variants, the cell and tissue type, or changes in disease [13].

PGE$_2$ is the most studied of the prostanoids and has the most diverse physiologic effects. The EP receptors were originally classified by their ability to relax and constrict smooth muscle, as well as by the receptor pharmacology [14]. The existence of multiple receptor subtypes was later confirmed by molecular cloning of these four receptors from both human

tissue [15–18] and mouse tissue [19–22]. Molecular cloning has also revealed splice variants of the EP$_3$ receptor, providing further variation for the actions of PGE$_2$ through these EP receptors [15].

Through knockout mouse studies, a wide range of phenotypes dependent on the EP receptors have been identified. Prostanoids and the EP receptors have been shown to play a key role in aspects of central nervous system function. Fever represents a component of the acute-phase immunologic challenge, and can be inhibited by non-steroidal anti-inflammatory drugs (NSAIDs), such as aspirin. For this reason, it was hypothesized that the EP receptors played a role in fever generation, and the receptor involved was later identified as the EP$_3$ receptor through knockout mouse studies [23]. EP$_3$ and EP$_1$ have been found to play a role in hyperalgesia [24,25]; the EP$_4$ receptor is involved in facilitating the closure of the ductus arteriosus during development [26], and both the EP$_4$ and EP$_2$ receptors have been shown to play a role in arthritic inflammation [27]. Prostanoids, particularly PGE$_2$, are thought to play a major role in inflammation, and from knockout mouse studies it has been revealed that these actions can be pro- or anti-inflammatory, depending on the expression in relevant tissues.

The role of prostanoids in airway inflammatory diseases

A wealth of literature surrounds the role of prostanoids in airway inflammatory diseases, and it appears that a fine balance exists between the pro- and anti-inflammatory effects of these endogenous mediators. It is now known that NSAIDs exert their effects via inhibition of the COX enzymes, and thus the production of prostanoids. As mentioned previously, prostanoids and their receptors mediate fever [23], edema and pain [28,29], hyperalgesia [24,25], and arthritic inflammation [27], which can be treated with aspirin. However, in airway inflammatory diseases such as asthma, NSAIDs are contra-indicated, and, in a subset of patients with asthma, aspirin, or other non-selective NSAIDs, can induce bronchoconstriction and acute asthma [30]. Therefore, in contrast to the joint, for example, prostaglandins in the lung are on balance protective and beneficial.

The mechanism of aspirin-induced asthma remains controversial. Some researchers suggest that, by

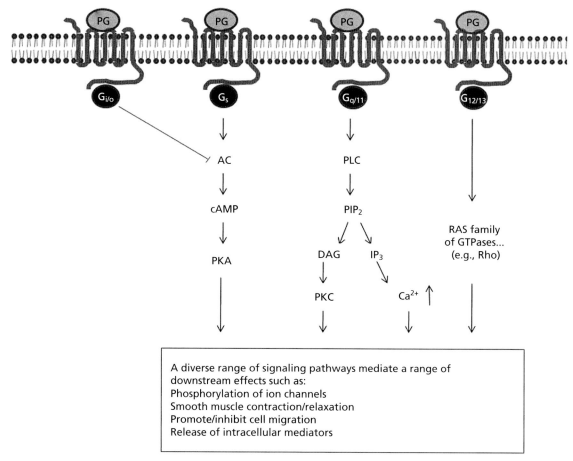

Figure 22.2 Signaling pathways of the prostanoid receptors. The EP_1, TP, and FP receptors predominantly couple to G_q, the EP_2, EP_4, DP, and IP to G_s, and the EP_3 receptor to G_i. Activation of G_q leads to the activation of phospholipase C and an increase in calcium/protein kinase C. G_s causes the activation of adenylyl cyclase and an increase in cAMP. G_i inhibits adenylyl cyclase thereby decreasing cAMP. Prostanoids are known to mediate a range of effects via these G proteins; however, the pathways mediating specific effects are largely unknown.

inhibiting COX and the production of prostanoids, a higher proportion of arachidonic acid (the precursor) is shunted into the leukotriene pathway, making more arachidonic acid available to the enzyme 5-lipoxygenase (5-LO). This, therefore, results in an increase in the production of the bronchoconstrictor agents, leukotrienes. Studies have shown that leukotriene E_4 (LTE_4) is increased in the urine of individuals with asthma after aspirin administration [31], and anti-leukotrienes have been implicated in the treatment of aspirin-sensitive asthma [32]. However, lipoxygenase products are not increased in blood from aspirin-sensitive patients with asthma [33], and, furthermore,

aspirin-tolerant patients do not have an increase in leukotrienes when the COX pathway is inhibited [34]. An alternative hypothesis has also been proposed by Mitchell and Belvisi [35], which suggests that, in aspirin-sensitive patients, COX-2 predominates and is modified biochemically by aspirin. This has been supported by a study by Holtzman *et al.* [36], which illustrates COX-2 being modified by aspirin to form alternative products. The normal production of prostanoids is therefore altered and thus facilitates the production of 5-LO products via COX-2. It has been shown that endothelial cells expressing COX-2 produced 15-HETE in the presence of aspirin. This was then metabolized by 5-LO, forming a group of metabolites known as the 15-epilipoxins [37]. However, the effect these 15-epilipoxins have on airway function is unclear.

In addition to these two hypotheses proposed above, it could also be suggested that prostanoids have a protective role in the airways and that they prevent the release of mediators from airway cells [38–40]. By inhibiting the production of prostanoids, the protective effect is removed and asthmatic symptoms are exacerbated. It has been found that COX-2 selective drugs are safe for aspirin-sensitive individuals with asthma [41–44], which has been supported more recently by research suggesting that COX-1, and not COX-2, regulates airway contractile function. This would support the previous evidence that inhibition of COX-2 does not induce aspirin-sensitive asthma, and that the adverse effect of NSAIDs in asthmatics is mediated by inhibition of COX-1 [45].

Despite conflicting theories as to the mechanism of aspirin-sensitive asthma, the fact that inhibiting the production of prostanoids can lead to bronchoconstriction and acute asthma suggests a role for prostanoids in the control of airway smooth muscle. It is clear that prostanoids and prostanoid receptors have important functions in both the control of airway smooth muscle contraction/relaxation and inflammation. The section below will discuss the bronchoprotective/bronchoconstrictor effects of prostanoids, as well as the pro- and anti-inflammatory effects in the airways.

Airway smooth muscle tone and prostanoids

One of the first studies looking at the bronchodilator effects of inhaled prostanoids was investigated by Kawakami and colleagues [46]; they revealed that, in a range of patients (normal, asthmatic, and chronic bronchitis), PGE_2 had a bronchodilator effect. Using *in vitro* preparations of human airways, it has been shown that the concentration–response curves to PGE_2 were biphasic: relaxing smooth muscle at lower concentrations and contracting the muscle at higher concentrations. Furthermore, their study also revealed that $PGF_{2\alpha}$ (FP agonist), 16,16-dimethyl PGE_2 (EP_1 agonist), sulprostone (EP_1/EP_3 agonist), and U46619 (TP agonist) contracted the airway smooth muscle. This contraction was antagonized by a TP receptor

antagonist, suggesting that the contractile response to prostanoids is via the TP receptor [47,48]. In addition, airway contraction to PGD_2 has also been shown to be mediated via the TP receptor [48]. In further studies, PGE_2 has inhibited histamine-induced contraction of human bronchi in a dose-dependent manner [49]. Studies characterizing the different prostanoid receptors involved in the relaxation of human bronchial preparations suggest that IP, EP_2, and DP receptors are involved [49,50]. Norel *et al.* [50] found that PGE_2, misoprostol (EP_2 agonist), and PGI_2 analogs totally reversed the histamine-induced contraction, whereas agonists at the DP receptor (PGD_2 or BW245C) only partially reversed this contraction. The PGE_2 effect could be attenuated by AH6809 (EP_1, EP_2, DP antagonist) but not by a selective EP_4 antagonist. A range of prostanoid receptors have been implicated in the contraction–relaxation responses to PGE_2, and more selective agonists and antagonists may be required to identify the receptors involved.

Studies using guinea-pig tracheal strips have revealed that PGE_2 has the opposite effects in guinea-pig compared with human smooth muscle, and that it causes contraction at lower concentrations and relaxation at higher concentrations. However, despite these contrasting effects, in line with findings in human tissues, the EP_1 and TP receptors have been implicated in the mediation of prostanoid-induced contraction of the guinea-pig trachea [51–53]. A bronchoprotective effect of PGE_2 has also been observed in animal models. One study has found that increasing the levels of endogenous PGE_2, by knocking out the gene controlling the catabolic enzyme for PGE_2, decreased airway responsiveness in mice [54]. Using animal models, it has been suggested that the EP_1 receptor is responsible for the bronchoconstriction, and the EP_2 receptor for the relaxation of airway smooth muscle. In contrast, EP_3 has been reported to inhibit electric field stimulation (EFS)-evoked [^{3}H]acetylcholine release from cholinergic nerves innervating the guinea-pig trachea by interacting with prejunctional prostanoid receptors of the EP_3 subtype [55]. It has been illustrated using EP_1, EP_2, EP_3 and EP_4 knockout mice that, in EP_1 or EP_3 receptor knockout mice, the increase in Penh (an indirect measure of airway constriction) to PGE_2 is reduced. Furthermore, although PGE_2 alone increases Penh, PGE_2 protects against methacholine-induced constriction. In EP_2 knockout mice this protection is lost, suggesting that the EP_2 receptor is involved in bronchodilation [56,57]. In parallel, Fortner *et al.* [58] found that PGE_2 causes relaxation in wild-type mice, and that in EP_2 knockout mice the relaxant effect is significantly decreased [58]. Further evidence for the role of EP_2 in bronchodilation was shown by Nials *et al.* [59], who demonstrated that an EP_2 selective agonist, AH13205, relaxed guinea-pig airways.

The receptors responsible for PGE_2-induced relaxation and contraction of airway smooth muscle have been previously investigated, as described in this section. However, much of the work was carried out with agonists and antagonists that are not particularly selective, and little or no research investigating

the receptor involved in the relaxation in guinea-pigs has been done. More recently, selective ligands have been developed for prostanoid receptors, as the use of these selective compounds will enable researchers to further dissect out the receptors involved (Table 22.1). The development of prostanoid-receptor knockout mice has benefited this area of research; however, it is unknown whether different receptors may be involved in different species, and, furthermore, knocking out one prostanoid receptor could possibly impact on the functionality or expression of another receptor. In addition, the receptors involved in the control of airway smooth muscle in the disease state may be different to those of a normal state. It has been indicated in a study by Tanaka *et al.* [60] that the

Table 22.1 Characteristics of the prostanoids receptors; agonist, antagonists, signaling pathways, and expression.

Receptor subtype	Natural ligand	Agonist	Antagonist	Signaling pathway	Expression
EP_1	PGE_2	Iloprost, sulprostone, 17-phenyl-trinor PGE_2, ONO-DI-004	SC51322, SC51089, AH6809, GW848687X, ONO-8711	G_q?	High levels in kidney, stomach, adrenal tissue
EP_2		Butaprost, AH13205, ONO-AE1–259	AH6809	G_s	Low levels in uterus, lung, spleen
EP_3		Sulprostone, SC46275, ONO-AE-249	L-826266, ONO-AE3–240	G_i (also possibly G_q and G_s)	High levels in many tissues; kidney, uterus, adrenal gland, stomach
EP_4		ONO-AE1–329	GW627368X ONO-AE3–208	G_s	Small intestines, lung, kidney, spleen, adrenal gland, and thymus
FP	$PGF_{2\alpha}$	Fluprostenol	AL8810	G_q	Kidney, uterus, placenta
IP	PGI_2	Iloprost, cicaprost	RO3244794, RO1138452	G_s (also G_i and G_q)	Heart, aorta, lung, kidney, liver
TP	TxA_2	I-BOP, U46619	SQ,29548, S-145, Ramatroban	G_q (isoforms can couple to other G-proteins)	Vascular/airway smooth muscle, platelets, placenta, small intestines, thymus, brain, endothelial cells
DP	PGD_2	BW245C, 15d-PGJ_2	BWA868C (partial agonist), AH6809	G_s	Low levels in most tissues
CRTh2/DP2		15d-PGJ_2	Ramatroban	G_i	Th2 cells, basophils, eosinophils

EP$_2$ and EP$_4$ receptors are involved in the inhibition of ovalbumin-induced bronchoconstriction. ONO-AE1-259 (EP$_2$ agonist) and ONO-AE1-329 (EP$_4$ agonist) mimicked the inhibition of ovalbumin-induced bronchoconstriction observed with PGE$_2$ (EP$_{1-4}$ agonist) in the guinea-pig [60]. However, further studies would be needed to support these initial findings to confirm the role of PGE$_2$ in the control of airway smooth muscle.

Airway inflammation and prostanoids

As described above, complete blockade of prostanoids is contra-indicated as this can induce symptoms of asthma, suggesting that prostanoids possess both detrimental and beneficial effects. This section will discuss the pro- and anti-inflammatory roles of prostanoids and their receptors.

PGD$_2$ has been implicated in airway inflammatory diseases for many years. In 1985, PGD$_2$ was shown to be released during acute allergic bronchospasm in man [61,62], and, subsequently, it was illustrated that inhalation of aerosolized PGD$_2$ enhanced eosinophilic and lymphocytic airway inflammation in sensitized mice following allergen challenge [63]. Furthermore, PGD$_2$ enhances leukotriene C$_4$ (LTC$_4$) synthesis by eosinophils during allergic inflammation *in vivo* [64]. PGD$_2$ has been shown to exert proinflammatory effects via the CRTh2 receptor by stimulating chemotaxis of eosinophils [10,11,65–68], Th2 cells [63,69], and basophils [10,70]. Inhibitors of CRTh2 have therapeutic potential in the treatment of airway inflammatory diseases, and it has been found that antagonism of the CRTh2 receptor attenuates asthma pathology in mice [71,72]. However, after allergen exposure, the inflammation was not attenuated in the airways of CRTh2-deficient mice [73,74]. Inhibitors of CRTh2 for the treatment of asthma are being trialled by several pharmaceutical companies.

Additionally, PGD$_2$ also mediates some proinflammatory effects in the airways via the DP receptor. An increase in ovalbumin-induced airway inflammation was observed in wild types compared with DP$^{-/-}$ mice [75]. In addition, PGD$_2$ has been found to mediate inhibition of eosinophil apoptosis via the DP receptor [66]. In genetic studies in humans, polymorphisms in the gene encoding the DP receptor have been linked with susceptibility to asthma [76–78].

In contrast to the proinflammatory evidence above, a small number of studies have found that PGD$_2$ possesses anti-inflammatory properties via the DP receptor, and that it can inhibit activation/migration of eosinophils, basophils, dendritic cells, and fibroblasts [10,11,66,70,79,80].

Although the majority of the studies above suggest that PGD$_2$ is proinflammatory in the airways, the fact that NSAIDs are not effective treatments for asthma would suggest that other prostanoids are having beneficial effects that mask the PGD$_2$-driven component. For example, the activation of the IP receptor by its endogenous prostanoid PGI$_2$ has been found to inhibit inflammation [81]. In a study by Takahashi *et al.* [81], IP-receptor-deficient mice demonstrated an increased allergic response in the airways. Furthermore, in a more recent study, PGI$_2$–IP signaling has been shown to be anti-inflammatory by inhibiting the recruitment of Th2 cells to the airways [82]. In addition, Nagao *et al.* [83] suggested that PGI$_2$ plays an inhibitory role in the development of allergen-induced airway remodeling; moreover, PGI$_2$ has also been found to have an inhibitory role on IgE production, Th2 cytokine production, and inflammatory infiltrates associated with allergic asthma.

The prostanoid PGE$_2$ has received the most interest in relation to inflammatory diseases. It is commonly considered to be a proinflammatory mediator involved in the pathogenesis of several inflammatory disease states, including UVB-mediated cutaneous inflammation and rheumatoid arthritis [84,85]. In such diseases, there is a correlation between disease progression and levels of PGE$_2$ in the tissue; furthermore, COX inhibitors can reduce the progression of the disease. In contrast to these inflammatory diseases, PGE$_2$ in the lung is normally much higher than in plasma, and evidence suggests that increased levels of PGE$_2$ in the lung may be therapeutically beneficial [86].

Using a range of cell-based assays, researchers have demonstrated that PGE$_2$ possesses a range of anti-inflammatory properties, and suggest that these effects may be mediated via the EP$_2$ and/or the EP$_4$ receptor. A study by Kay *et al.* [39] revealed that PGE$_2$ inhibits mast cell degranulation via the EP$_2$ receptor. Furthermore, PGE$_2$ has been found to inhibit the release of various cytokines and chemokines from human airway smooth muscle cells and macrophages via the EP$_2$/EP$_4$ receptors [38,87,88]. In fibroblasts,

PGE$_2$ inhibits collagen proliferation and protects against cigarette-induced apoptosis via the EP$_2$ receptor [89,90]. Additionally, PGE$_2$ suppresses Th1 and Th2 polarization via the EP$_2$ and/or EP$_4$ receptors [91]. Eosinophil trafficking can be inhibited by activation of the EP$_2$ receptor [92]. In contrast, PGE$_2$ has been found to act as a chemoattractant for mouse mast cells via the EP$_3$ receptor [93]. The EP$_3$ receptor has been implicated also in PGE$_2$-induced degranulation of mast cells, contrary to the anti-inflammatory effects described above [94].

In these cell-based assay systems, PGE$_2$ has been found to be predominantly anti-inflammatory, exerting its effects via the EP$_2$ and EP$_4$ receptors. The latter study demonstrating PGE$_2$ as a chemoattractant [93] would suggest that PGE$_2$ has some proinflammatory properties, but through a different receptor.

From *in vivo* models, PGE$_2$ has been found to be anti-inflammatory in a rat ovalbumin model [95]. In contrast to the data described in human cell-based assays, Kunikata *et al.* [96] found that the activation of the EP$_3$ receptor suppressed inflammation, and that the EP$_3$ knockout mice had an increased inflammatory response compared with the wild types. This would suggest that the EP$_3$ receptor could be involved in the anti-inflammatory effects of PGE$_2$. Additionally, PGE$_2$ acting via the EP$_4$ subtype signals to promote immune inflammation through Th$_1$ cell differentiation and Th$_{17}$ cell expansion [97]. The majority of studies linking PGE$_2$ with an anti-inflammatory effect have been performed in human cell-based assays. As such, the limited numbers of *in vivo* studies suggest that more research would be needed to further investigate the receptors involved in the anti-inflammatory effects of PGE$_2$. As described earlier, the improved range of pharmacologically selective agonists and antagonists that are now available will enable the researcher to dissect further the receptors involved in these processes.

Prostanoids as a therapy for airway inflammatory diseases

Despite discrepancies as to the receptors responsible for the bronchodilator and anti-inflammatory effects of PGE$_2$, there is clear evidence that PGE$_2$ is beneficial to the lungs. In addition to the *in vitro* and *in vivo* studies described above, the beneficial potential of PGE$_2$ as a therapy has long been recognized. In 1973, Kawakami *et al.* [46] found that inhaled PGE$_2$ was a bronchodilator in normal subjects and in patients with asthma and chronic bronchitis. This was supported in subsequent studies demonstrating that inhaled PGE$_2$ could act as a bronchodilator agent in both normal subjects [98] and in individuals with exercise-induced asthma [99]. In addition to the bronchodilator effects, PGE$_2$ has been found to attenuate an allergen-induced fall in FEV$_1$, methacholine-induced airway hyperresponsiveness, and increases in sputum eosinophils [100,101].

Despite the benefits of inhaled PGE$_2$, the development of prostanoid agonists for the treatment of airway inflammatory diseases has been hindered as prostanoids induce irritancy of the upper airway, resulting in a reflex cough. PGE$_2$ has been found to excite airway afferent nerves [102,103]; this concurs with the transient cough observed in both normal individuals and patients with asthma during studies of inhaled PGE$_2$ [46,99–101,104]. It has recently been identified that the EP$_3$ receptor is responsible for the PGE$_2$-induced sensory nerve activation and cough, using an *in vitro* isolated vagus nerve preparation, knockout mice, and a guinea-pig *in vivo* model of cough [105]. If the receptors responsible for the beneficial effects are indeed EP$_2$ and/or EP$_4$, as suggested by human cell-based assay data, an agonist could be developed for airway inflammatory diseases that targets these receptors only, without causing cough via the EP$_3$ receptor.

Acknowledgment

The research was funded by project grants from the Medical Research Council (MRC), UK (G0800195 and G0502019).

References

1 von Euler US. On the specific vaso-dilating and plain muscle stimulating substances from accessory genital glands in man and certain animals (prostaglandin and vesiglandin). *J Physiol* 1936; **88**: 213–34.

2 Bergstrom S, Sjovall J. The isolation of prostaglandin. *Acta Chemica Scandinavica* 1957; **11**: 1086.

3 Stanford SJ, Pepper JR, Mitchell JA. Release of GM-CSF and G-CSF by human arterial and venous smooth muscle cells: differential regulation by COX-2. *Br J Pharmacol* 2000; **129**: 835–8.

4 Belvisi MG, Saunders MA, Haddad el-B, *et al*. Induction of cyclo-oxygenase-2 by cytokines in human cultured airway smooth muscle cells: novel inflammatory role of this cell type. *Br J Pharmacol* 1997; **120**: 910–16.

5 Gardiner PJ, Collier HO. Specific receptors for prostaglandins in airways. *Prostaglandins* 1980; **19**: 819–41.

6 Andersen NH, Eggerman TL, Harker LA, *et al*. On the multiplicity of platelet prostaglandin receptors. I. Evaluation of competitive antagonism by aggregometry. *Prostaglandins* 1980; **19**: 711–35.

7 Kennedy I, Coleman RA, Humphrey PP, *et al*. Studies on the characterisation of prostanoid receptors: a proposed classification. *Prostaglandins* 1982; **24**: 667–689.

8 Coleman RA, Smith WL, Narumiya S. International Union of Pharmacology classification of prostanoid receptors: properties, distribution, and structure of the receptors and their subtypes. *Pharmacol Rev* 1994; **46**: 205–29.

9 Narumiya S, Sugimoto Y, Ushikubi F. Prostanoid receptors: structures, properties and functions. *Physiological Reviews* 1999; **79**: 1193–226.

10 Hirai H, Tanaka K, Yoshie O, *et al*. Prostaglandin D2 selectively induces chemotaxis in T-helper type 2 cells, eosinophils, and basophils via seven-transmembrane receptor CRTH2. *J Exper Med* 2001; **193**: 225–61.

11 Monneret G, Gravel S, Diamond M, *et al*. Prostaglandin D2 is a potent chemoattractant for human eosinophils that acts via a novel DP receptor. *Blood* 2001; **98**: 1942–8.

12 Breyer RM, Bagdassarian CK, Myers SA, *et al*. Prostanoid receptors: subtypes and signaling 1. *Annu Rev Pharmacol Toxicol* 2001; **41**: 661–90.

13 Bos CL, Richel DJ, Ritsema T, *et al*. Prostanoids and prostanoid receptors in signal transduction. *Int J Biochem Cell Biol* 2004; **36**: 1187–205.

14 Gardiner PJ. Characterization of prostanoid relaxant/inhibitory receptors (psi) using a highly selective agonist, TR4979. *Br J Pharmacol* 1986; **87**: 45–56.

15 Adam M, Boie Y, Rushmore TH, *et al*. Cloning and expression of three isoforms of the human EP3 prostanoid receptor. *FEBS Lett* 1994; **338**: 170–4.

16 Bastien L, Sawyer N, Grygorczyk R, *et al*. Cloning, functional expression, and characterization of the human prostaglandin E2 receptor EP2 subtype. *J Biol Chem* 1994; **269**: 11873–7.

17 Funk CD, Furci L, FitzGerald GA, *et al*. Cloning and expression of a cDNA for the human prostaglandin E receptor EP1 subtype. *J Biol Chem* 1993; **268**: 26767–72.

18 Regan JW, Bailey TJ, Pepperl DJ, *et al*. Cloning of a novel human prostaglandin receptor with characteristics of the pharmacologically defined EP2 subtype. *Mol Pharmacol* 1994; **46**: 213–20.

19 Honda A, Sugimoto Y, Namba T, *et al*. Cloning and expression of a cDNA for mouse prostaglandin E receptor EP2 subtype. *J Biol Chem* 1993; **268**: 7759–62.

20 Katsuyama M, Nishigaki N, Sugimoto Y, *et al*. The mouse prostaglandin E receptor EP2 subtype: cloning, expression, and Northern blot analysis. *FEBS Lett* 1995; **372**: 151–6.

21 Sugimoto Y, Namba T, Honda A, *et al*. Cloning and expression of a cDNA for mouse prostaglandin E receptor EP3 subtype. *J Biol Chem* 1992; **267**: 6463–6.

22 Watabe A, Sugimoto Y, Honda A, *et al*. Cloning and expression of cDNA for a mouse EP1 subtype of prostaglandin E receptor. *J Biol Chem* 1993; **268**: 20175–8.

23 Ushikubi F, Segi E, Sugimoto Y, *et al*. Impaired febrile response in mice lacking the prostaglandin E receptor subtype EP3. *Nature* 1998; **395**: 281–4.

24 Moriyama T, Higashi T, Togashi K, *et al*. Sensitization of TRPV1 by EP1 and IP reveals peripheral nociceptive mechanism of prostaglandins. *Mol Pain* 2005; **1**: 3.

25 Ueno A, Matsumoto H, Naraba H, *et al*. Major roles of prostanoid receptors IP and EP3 in endotoxin-induced enhancement of pain perception. *Biochem Pharmacol* 2001; **62**: 157–60.

26 Segi E, Sugimoto Y, Yamasaki A, *et al*. Patent ductus arteriosus and neonatal death in prostaglandin receptor EP4-deficient mice. *Biochem Biophys Res Comm* 1998; **246**: 7–12.

27 Honda T, Segi-Nishida E, Miyachi Y, *et al*. Prostacyclin-IP signaling and prostaglandin E2-EP2/EP4 signaling both mediate joint inflammation in mouse collagen-induced arthritis. *J Exp Med* 2006; **203**: 325–35.

28 Murata T, Ushikubi F, Matsuoka T, *et al*. Altered pain perception and inflammatory response in mice lacking prostacyclin receptor. *Nature* 1997; **388**: 678–82.

29 Ueno A, Naraba H, Ikeda Y, *et al*. Intrinsic prostacyclin contributes to exudation induced by bradykinin or carrageenin: a study on the paw edema induced in IP-receptor-deficient mice. *Life Sci* 2000; **66**: L155–60.

30 Kowalski ML. Aspirin-sensitive rhinosinusitis and asthma. *Clin Allergy Immunol* 2007; **19**: 147–75.

31 Christie PE, Tagari P, Ford-Hutchinson AW, *et al*. Urinary leukotriene E4 concentrations increase after aspirin challenge in aspirin-sensitive asthmatic subjects. *Am Rev Respir Dis* 1991; **143**: 1025–9.

32 Dahlen B. Treatment of aspirin-intolerant asthma with antileukotrienes. *Am J Respir Crit Care Med* 2000; **161**: 137–41.

33 Gray PA, Warner TD, Vojnovic I, *et al*. Effects of non-steroidal anti-inflammatory drugs on cyclo-oxygenase

and lipoxygenase activity in whole blood from aspirin-sensitive asthmatics vs healthy donors. *Br J Pharmacol* 2002; **137**: 1031–8.

34 Dahlen B, Dahlen SE. Leukotrienes as mediators of airway obstruction and inflammation in asthma. *Clin Exp Allergy* 1995; **25**: 50–4.

35 Mitchell JA, Belvisi MG. Too many COX (cyclooxygenase) spoil the broth: aspirin-sensitive asthma and 5-lypoxygenase. *Thorax* 1997; **52**: 933–5.

36 Holtzman MJ, Turk J, Shornick LP. Identification of a pharmacologically distinct prostaglandin H synthase in cultured epithelial cells. *J Biol Chem* 1992; **267**: 21438–45.

37 Claria J, Serhan CN. Aspirin triggers previously undescribed bioactive eicosanoids by human endothelial cell–leukocyte interactions. *Proc Natl Acad Sci USA* 1995; **92**: 9475–9.

38 Clarke DL, Belvisi MG, Catley MC, *et al*. Identification in human airways smooth muscle cells of the prostanoid receptor and signalling pathway through which PGE2 inhibits the release of GM-CSF. *Br J Pharmacol* 2004; **141**: 1141–50.

39 Kay LJ, Yeo WW, Peachell PT. Prostaglandin E2 activates EP2 receptors to inhibit human lung mast cell degranulation. *Br J Pharmacol* 2006; **147**: 707–13.

40 Pavord ID, Tattersfield AE. Bronchoprotective role for endogenous prostaglandin E2. *Lancet* 1995; **345**: 436–8.

41 Gyllfors P, Bochenek G, Overholt J, *et al*. Biochemical and clinical evidence that aspirin-intolerant asthmatic subjects tolerate the cyclooxygenase 2-selective analgetic drug celecoxib. *J Allergy Clin Immunol* 2003; **111**: 1116–21.

42 Martin-Garcia C, Hinojosa M, Berges P, *et al*. Celecoxib, a highly selective COX-2 inhibitor, is safe in aspirin-induced asthma patients. *J Invest Allergol Clin Immunol* 2003; **13**: 20–5.

43 Stevenson DD, Simon RA. Lack of cross-reactivity between rofecoxib and aspirin in aspirin-sensitive patients with asthma. *J Allergy Clin Immunol* 2001; **108**: 47–51.

44 Woessner KM, Simon RA, Stevenson DD. The safety of celecoxib in patients with aspirin-sensitive asthma. *Arthritis Rheum* 2002; **46**: 2201–6.

45 Harrington LS, Lucas R, McMaster SK, *et al*. COX-1, and not COX-2 activity, regulates airway function: relevance to aspirin-sensitive asthma. *FASEB J* 2008; **22**: 4005–10.

46 Kawakami Y, Uchiyama K, Irie T, *et al*. Evaluation of aerosols of prostaglandins E1 and E2 as bronchodilators. *Eur J Clin Pharmacol* 1973; **6**: 127–32.

47 Armour CL, Johnson PRA, Alfredson ML, *et al*. Characterization of contractile prostanoid receptors on human airway smooth muscle. *Eur J Pharmacol* 1989; **165**: 215–22.

48 Coleman RA, Sheldrick R. Prostanoid-induced contraction of human bronchial smooth muscle is mediated by TP-receptors. *Br J Pharmacol* 1989; **96**: 688–92.

49 Knight DA, Stewart GA, Thompson PJ. Prostaglandin E2, but not prostacyclin inhibits histamine-induced contraction of human bronchial smooth muscle. *Eur J Pharmacol* 1995; **272**: 13–19.

50 Norel X, Walch L, Labat C, *et al*. Prostanoid receptors involved in the relaxation of human bronchial preparations. *Br J Pharmacol* 1999; **126**: 867–72.

51 Coleman RA, Kennedy I, Sheldrick RL. AH6809, a prostanoid EP$_1$ receptor blocking drug. *Br J Pharmacol* 1985; **85**: 273P.

52 Francis HP, Morris TG, Thompson AM, *et al*. The thromboxane receptor antagonist BAY u3405 reverses prostaglandin D2 (PGD2)-induced bronchoconstriction in the anaesthetised guinea pig. *Ann N Y Acad Sci* 1991; **629**: 399–401.

53 McKenniff M, Rodger IW, Norman P, *et al*. Characterisation of receptors mediating the contractile effects of prostanoids in guinea-pig and human airways. *Eur J Pharmacol* 1988; **153**: 149–59.

54 Hartney JM, Coggins KG, Tilley SL, *et al*. Prostaglandin E2 protects lower airways against bronchoconstriction. *Am J Physiol Lung Cell Mol Physiol* 2006; **290**: L105–13.

55 Clarke DL, Giembycz MA, Patel HJ, *et al*. E-ring 8-isoprostanes inhibit ACh release from parasympathetic nerves innervating guinea-pig trachea through agonism of prostanoid receptors of the EP3-subtype. *Br J Pharmacol* 2004; **141**: 600–9.

56 Sheller JR, Mitchell D, Meyrick B, *et al*. EP2 receptor mediates bronchodilation by PGE2 in mice. *J Appl Physiol* 2000; **88**: 2214–18.

57 Tilley SL, Hartney JM, Erikson CJ, *et al*. Receptors and pathways mediating the effects of prostaglandin E2 on airway tone. *Am J Physiol Lung Cell Mol Physiol* 2003; **284**: L599–606.

58 Fortner CN, Breyer RM, Paul RJ. EP2 receptors mediate airway relaxation to substance P, ATP, and PGE2. *Am J Physiol Lung Cell Mol Physiol* 2001; **281**: L469–74.

59 Nials AT, Vardey CJ, Denyer LH, *et al*. AH13205, a selective prostanoid EP2-receptor agonist. *Cardiovasc Drug Rev* 1993; **11**: 165–79.

60 Tanaka H, Kanako S, Abe S. Prostaglandin E2 receptor selective agonists E-prostanoid 2 and E-prostanoid 4 may have therapeutic effects on ovalbumin-induced bronchoconstriction. *Chest* 2005; **128**: 3717–23.

61 Murray JJ, Tonnel AB, Brash AR, *et al*. Prostaglandin D2 is released during acute allergic bronchospasm in man. *Trans Assoc Am Phys* 1985; **98**: 275–80.

62 Murray JJ, Tonnel AB, Brash AR, *et al.* Release of prostaglandin D2 into human airways during acute antigen challenge. *N Engl J Med* 1986; **315**: 800–4.

63 Honda K, Arima M, Cheng G, *et al.* Prostaglandin D2 reinforces Th2 type inflammatory responses of airways to low-dose antigen through bronchial expression of macrophage-derived chemokine. *J Exp Med* 2003; **198**: 533–43.

64 Mesquita-Santos FP, Vieira-de-Abreu A, Calheiros AS, *et al.* Cutting edge: prostaglandin D2 enhances leukotriene C4 synthesis by eosinophils during allergic inflammation: synergistic *in vivo* role of endogenous eotaxin. *J Immunol* 2006; **176**: 1326–30.

65 Almishri W, Cossette C, Rokach J, *et al.* Effects of prostaglandin D2: 15-Deoxy-{Delta}12,14-prostaglandin J2, and selective DP1 and DP2 receptor agonists on pulmonary infiltration of eosinophils in brown Norway rats. *J Pharmacol Exp Ther* 2005; **313**: 64–9.

66 Gervais FG, Cruz RPG, Chateauneuf A, *et al.* Selective modulation of chemokinesis, degranulation, and apoptosis in eosinophils through the PGD2 receptors CRTH2 and DP. *J Allergy Clin Immunol* 2001; **108**: 982–8.

67 Shiraishi Y, Asano K, Nakajima T, *et al.* Prostaglandin D2-induced eosinophilic airway inflammation is mediated by CRTH2 receptor. *J Pharmacol Exp Ther* 2005; **312**: 954–60.

68 Sugimoto H, Shichijo M, Iino T, *et al.* An orally bioavailable small molecule antagonist of CRTH2, ramatroban (BAY u3405), inhibits prostaglandin D2-induced eosinophil migration *in vitro*. *J Pharmacol Exp Ther* 2003; **305**: 347–52.

69 Xue L, Gyles SL, Wettey FR, *et al.* Prostaglandin D2 causes preferential induction of proinflammatory Th2 cytokine production through an action on chemoattractant receptor-like molecule expressed on Th2 cells. *J Immunol* 2005; **175**: 6531–6.

70 Yoshimura-Uchiyama C, Iikura M, Yamaguchi M, *et al.* Differential modulation of human basophil functions through prostaglandin D2 receptors DP and chemoattractant receptor-homologous molecule expressed on Th2 cells/DP2. *Clin Exp Allergy* 2004; **34**: 1283–90.

71 Uller L, Mathiesen JM, Alenmyr L, *et al.* Antagonism of the prostaglandin D2 receptor CRTH2 attenuates asthma pathology in mouse eosinophilic airway inflammation. *Resp Res* 2007; **8**: 16.

72 Lukacs NW, Berlin AA, Franz-Bacon K, *et al.* CRTH2 antagonism significantly ameliorates airway hyperreactivity and downregulates inflammation-induced genes in a mouse model of airway inflammation. *Am J Physiol Lung Cell Mol Physiol* 2008; **295**: L767–79.

73 Shiraishi Y, Asano K, Niimi K, *et al.* Cyclooxygenase-2/prostaglandin D2/CRTH2 pathway mediates double-stranded RNA-induced enhancement of allergic airway inflammation. *J Immunol* 2008; **180**: 541–9.

74 Chevalier E, Stock J, Fisher T, *et al.* Cutting edge: chemoattractant receptor-homologous molecule expressed on Th2 cells plays a restricting role on IL-5 production and eosinophil recruitment. *J Immunol* 2005; **175**: 2056–60.

75 Matsuoka T, Hirata M, Tanaka H, *et al.* Prostaglandin D2 as a mediator of allergic asthma. *Science* 2000; **287**: 2013–17.

76 Oguma T, Palmer LJ, Birben E, *et al.* Role of prostanoid DP receptor variants in susceptibility to asthma. *N Engl J Med* 2004; **351**: 1752–63.

77 Sanz C, Isidoro-Garcia M, Davila I, *et al.* Promoter genetic variants of prostanoid DP receptor (PTGDR) gene in patients with asthma. *Allergy* 2006; **61**: 543–8.

78 Zhu G, Vestbo J, Lenney W, *et al.* Association of PTGDR gene polymorphisms with asthma in two caucasian populations. *Genes Immun* 2007; **8**: 398–403.

79 Angeli V, Staumont D, Charbonnier AS, *et al.* Activation of the D prostanoid receptor 1 regulates immune and skin allergic responses. *J Immunol* 2004; **172**: 3822–9.

80 Hammad H, Jan de Heer H, Soullie T, *et al.* Prostaglandin D2 inhibits airway dendritic cell migration and function in steady state conditions by selective activation of the D prostanoid receptor 1. *J Immunol* 2003; **171**: 3936–40.

81 Takahashi Y, Tokuoka S, Masuda T, *et al.* Augmentation of allergic inflammation in prostanoid IP receptor deficient mice. *Br J Pharmacol* 2002; **137**: 315–22.

82 Jaffar Z, Ferrini ME, Buford MC, *et al.* Prostaglandin I2-IP Signaling blocks allergic pulmonary inflammation by preventing recruitment of CD4+ Th2 cells into the airways in a mouse model of asthma. *J Immunol* 2007; **179**: 6193–203.

83 Nagao K, Tanaka H, Komai M, *et al.* Role of prostaglandin I2 in airway remodeling induced by repeated allergen challenge in mice. *Am J Respir Cell Mol Biol* 2003; **29**: 314–20.

84 McCoy JM, Wicks JR, Audoly LP. The role of prostaglandin E2 receptors in the pathogenesis of rheumatoid arthritis. *J Clin Invest* 2002; **110**: 651–8.

85 Wilgus TA, Parrett ML, Ross MS, *et al.* Inhibition of ultraviolet light B-induced cutaneous inflammation by a specific cyclooxygenase-2 inhibitor. *Adv Exp Med Biol* 2002; **507**: 85–92.

86 Vancheri C, Mastruzzo C, Sortino MA, *et al.* The lung as a privileged site for the beneficial actions of PGE2. *Trends Immunol* 2004; **25**: 40–6.

87 Ratcliffe MJ, Walding A, Shelton PA, *et al.* Activation of E-prostanoid4 and E-prostanoid2 receptors inhibits TNF-α release from human alveolar macrophages. *Eur Respir J* 2007; **29**: 986–94.

88 Takayama K, Garcia-Cardena G, Sukhova GK, et al. Prostaglandin E2 suppresses chemokine production in human macrophages through the EP4 receptor. *J Biol Chem* 2002; **277**: 44147–54.

89 Huang S, Wettlaufer SH, Hogaboam C, et al. Prostaglandin E2 inhibits collagen expression and proliferation in patient-derived normal lung fibroblasts via E prostanoid 2 receptor and cAMP signaling. *Am J Physiol Lung Cell Mol Physiol* 2007; **292**: L405–13.

90 Sugiura H, Liu X, Togo S, et al. Prostaglandin E(2) protects human lung fibroblasts from cigarette smoke extract-induced apoptosis via EP(2) receptor activation. *J Cell Physiol* 2007; **210**: 99–110.

91 Okano M, Sugata Y, Fujiwara T, et al. E prostanoid 2 (EP2)/EP4-mediated suppression of antigen-specific human T-cell responses by prostaglandin E2. *Immunology* 2006; **118**: 343–52.

92 Sturm EM, Schratl P, Schuligoi R, et al. Prostaglandin E2 inhibits eosinophil trafficking through E-prostanoid 2 receptors. *J Immunol* 2008; **181**: 7273–83.

93 Weller CL, Collington SJ, Hartnell A, et al. Chemotactic action of prostaglandin E2 on mouse mast cells acting via the PGE2 receptor 3. *Proc Natl Acad Sci USA* 2007; **104**: 11712–17.

94 Nguyen M, Solle M, Audoly LP, et al. Receptors and signaling mechanisms required for prostaglandin E2-mediated regulation of mast cell degranulation and IL-6 production. *J Immunol* 2002; **169**: 4586–93.

95 Martin JG, Suzuki M, Maghni K, et al. The immunomodulatory actions of prostaglandin E2 on allergic airway responses in the rat. *J Immunol* 2002; **169**: 3963–9.

96 Kunikata T, Yamane H, Segi E, et al. Suppression of allergic inflammation by the prostaglandin E receptor subtype EP3. *Nat Immunol* 2005; **6**: 524–31.

97 Yao C, Sakata D, Esaki Y, et al. Prostaglandin E2-EP4 signaling promotes immune inflammation through Th1 cell differentiation and Th17 cell expansion. *Nat Med* 2009; **15**: 633–40.

98 Walters EH, Bevan C, Parrish RW, et al. Time-dependent effect of prostaglandin E2 inhalation on airway responses to bronchoconstrictor agents in normal subjects. *Thorax* 1982; **37**: 438–42.

99 Melillo E, Woolley KL, Manning PJ. Effect of inhaled PGE2 on exercise-induced bronchoconstriction in asthmatic subjects. *Am J Respir Crit Care Med* 1994; **149**: 1138–41.

100 Gauvreau GM, Watson RM, O'Byrne PM. Protective effects of inhaled PGE2 on allergen-induced airway responses and airway inflammation. *Am J Respir Crit Care Med* 1999; **159**: 31–6.

101 Pavord ID, Wong CS, Williams J, et al. Effect of inhaled prostaglandin E2 on allergen-induced asthma. *Am Rev Respir Dis* 1993; **148**: 87–90.

102 Coleridge HM, Coleridge JC, Ginzel KH. Stimulation of 'irritant' receptors and afferent C-fibres in the lungs by prostaglandins. *Nature* 1976; **264**: 451–3.

103 Mohammed SP, Higenbottam TW, Adcock JJ. Effects of aerosol-applied capsaicin, histamine and prostaglandin E2 on airway sensory receptors of anaesthetized cats. *J Physiol* 1993; **469**: 51–66.

104 Costello JF, Dunlop LS, Gardiner PJ. Characteristics of prostaglandin induced cough in man. *Br J Clin Pharmacol* 1985; **20**: 355–9.

105 Maher SA, Birrell MA, Belvisi MG. Prostaglandin E2 mediates cough via the EP3 receptor: implications for future disease therapy. *Am J Respir Crit Care Med* 2009; **180**: 923–8.

23 Leukotrienes

Katsuhide Okunishi and Marc Peters-Golden
Division of Pulmonary and Critical Care Medicine, Department of Internal
Medicine, University of Michigan Health System, Ann Arbor, MI, USA

Introduction

Leukotrienes are potent lipid mediators that contribute to multiple aspects of asthma pathophysiology [1]. Airway inflammation is a central feature of asthma, and the dominant therapeutic paradigm for control of this disease consists of suppression of airway inflammation with inhaled corticosteroids (ICS) [2]. However, the leukotriene pathway is relatively steroid resistant [3], which suggests the possibility that its control by alternate means may facilitate asthma disease management.

Cysteinyl leukotriene receptor 1 antagonists (LTRAs) were first marketed in 1995, and are now well accepted worldwide for their efficacy and safety in the treatment of asthma. However, their limitations are also quite evident. In this chapter, we summarize the biologic effects of leukotrienes in asthma, review recent advances in our understanding of leukotriene receptors, and consider possible new targets in the leukotriene pathway that offer the potential to achieve better control of asthma in the future.

Leukotriene biosynthesis

Leukotriene biosynthesis is triggered by stimuli such as antigens, cytokines, immune complexes, and microbes that promote the translocation of the enzymes cytosolic phospholipase A_2 (cPLA$_2$) and

5-lipoxygenase (5-LO) to the perinuclear region of leukocytes [4]. cPLA$_2$ cleaves the polyunsaturated fatty acid arachidonic acid from perinuclear membrane glycerophospholipids, and arachidonic acid is then oxygenated by 5-LO in concert with 5-LO activating protein (FLAP) to yield the unstable precursor LTA$_4$ [5]. Oxygenation of arachidonic acid by other enzymes gives rise to alternate bioactive arachidonate metabolites such as the prostaglandins, the role of which in asthma is considered in Chapter 22. The necessity of FLAP is thought to involve its ability to bind and selectively transfer arachidonic acid to 5-LO. Once generated, LTA$_4$ can be conjugated with reduced glutathione by LTC$_4$ synthase (LTC$_4$S) to form LTC$_4$, or hydrolyzed by LTA$_4$ hydrolase (LTA$_4$H) to form LTB$_4$ (Figure 23.1). Both LTB$_4$ and LTC$_4$ are transported to the extracellular space by transporters such as ATP-binding cassette (ABC) transporters or multi-drug resistant proteins (MRPs) [6]. After its export, LTC$_4$ is rapidly converted to LTD$_4$, and then to LTE$_4$ [4]. Leukotrienes C$_4$, D$_4$, and E$_4$ are collectively termed "cysteinyl leukotrienes" (cysLTs).

As implied by their original designation, *leukotrienes* are predominantly produced by leukocytes because only leukocytes express high levels of 5-LO and FLAP [1]. However, the specific profile of leukotrienes produced depends on the cell type [1] (see Table 23.1). Neutrophils produce exclusively LTB$_4$, whereas eosinophils, mast cells, and basophils mainly produce cysLTs. Macrophages and dendritic cells

Inflammation and Allergy Drug Design, First Edition. Edited by Kenji Izuhara, Stephen T. Holgate, Marsha Wills-Karp.
© 2011 Blackwell Publishing Ltd. Published 2011 by Blackwell Publishing Ltd.

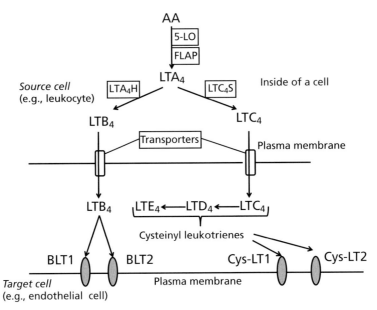

Figure 23.1 Leukotriene synthesis. Arachidonic acid is converted first to LTA$_4$ by 5-LO, then to LTB$_4$ by LTA$_4$H or to LTC$_4$ by LTC$_4$S. After it has been exported from the cell, LTC$_4$ is rapidly converted to LTD$_4$ and LTE$_4$ sequentially. LTB$_4$ and cysteinyl leukotrienes exhibit their biologic effects after binding to their specific receptors, BLT(1 or 2) and CysLT (1 or 2), respectively.

synthesize both LTB$_4$ and cysLTs. Even non-leukocyte cell types can meaningfully contribute to overall tissue leukotriene biosynthesis [7] because of their substantial expression of distal LTA$_4$-metabolizing enzymes LTA$_4$H and LTC$_4$S. Via a process termed "transcellular biosynthesis," cells such as endothelial cells can convert LTA$_4$ derived from a donor cell (e.g. a neutrophil) to, for example, LTC$_4$ [4].

Many factors can influence the output of the leukotriene biosynthetic pathway, and the reader is referred to more comprehensive reviews of pathway regulation (see, for example, references 2–5). Two important forms of regulation warrant brief mention here. First, polymorphisms in the genes encoding 5-LO, FLAP, LTC$_4$S, and LTA$_4$H are recognized [8]; these gene variants may be associated with altered function of the respective proteins, and could for this reason influence responses to antileukotriene drugs (see section on CysLT1 antagonists). Second, transcription of genes encoding leukotriene biosynthetic proteins can be modulated by a variety of relevant substances, including cytokines, adipokines, growth factors, sex hormones, and endotoxin. A feature that is particularly germane to allergic diseases is the ten-dency of many Th2 cytokines to enhance leukotriene biosynthesis.

Leukotriene actions

Table 23.1 summarizes leukotriene receptor expression in different cell types. In the following sections, we will review the actions of cysLTs and LTB$_4$ through their specific G protein-coupled receptors.

Biology of and receptors for cysLTs

In 1979, a mixture of cysLTs were identified to account for the contractile bioactivity previously known as slow-reacting substance of anaphylaxis (SRS-A), which for decades had been implicated in asthmatic bronchoconstriction [9]. It is now well recognized that cysLTs participate in many aspects of asthma beyond bronchoconstriction, and can directly activate almost all the cell types that are involved in the pathogenesis of asthma, except perhaps CD8$^+$ T cells and neutrophils (Table 23.1). The first cysLT receptor to be molecularly identified was the type 1

Table 23.1 Leukotriene synthesis and receptor expression.

| Type of cell | Leukotriene production[1] | | Expression and functions of receptor[2] | | | | | |
| | LTB$_4$ | cysLTs | BLT1 | | CysLT1 | | CysLT2 | |
			Expression	Function	Expression	Function	Expression	Function
Neutrophil	+++	–	+	Migration ↑	±	?	±	?
				Apoptosis ↓				
				Microbial killing ↑				
				Phagocytosis ↑				
				Cytokine production ↑				
Macrophage or monocyte	++	++	+	Phagocytosis ↑	+	Phagocytosis ↑	+	
				Microbial killing ↑		Microbial killing ↑[3]		
				Cytokine generation ↑		Cytokine generation ↑		
Dendritic cell	++	+	+	Migration ↑	+	Migration ↑	?	
						Antigen presentation ↑		
						Modulation of cytokine production		
Eosinophil	–	+++	+	Migration ↑	+	Migration ↑	+	
						Adhesion ↑		
						Survival ↑		
						Activation ↑		
Basophil	–	+++	+	?	+	Activation ↑	+	
Mast cell	+	+++	+	?	+	Cytokine production ↑	+	
B cell	–	–	?	–	+	IgG and E production ↑	?	
CD4 T cell	–	–	+	Migration ↑	+	Migration ↑	?	
				Cytokine production ↑				
CD8 T cell	–	–	+	Migration ↑	?	?	?	

(*Continued*)

Table 23.1 (*Continued*)

| Type of cell | Leukotriene production[1] | | Expression and functions of receptor[2] | | | | | |
| | LTB$_4$ | cysLTs | BLT1 | | CysLT1 | | CysLT2 | |
			Expression	Function	Expression	Function	Expression	Function
Hematopoietic progenitor cell	–	–	?	?	+	Migration ↑	?	?
Epithelial cell	+[4]	+	?	?	+	TGF-β production ↑		
						Goblet cell degranulation ↑	+	?
Airway smooth muscle cell				Proliferation		Contraction ↑		
	?	?	+	Migration	+	Migration ↑	?	
						Migration ↑		
Fibroblast	+	+	+	?	+	Collagen production ↑	?	
						Proliferation ↑		
Fibrocyte	?	+	?	?	+	Migration ↑	+	
						Proliferation ↑		
Endothelial cell	?	+	+	NO and MCP-1 production	+	?	+	Vasodilation ↑
								Activation ↑

↓, Suppression or decrease; ↑, enhancement or increase.
[1]Relative synthetic capacity of leukotrienes by leukocytes are expressed by the number of plus (+) signs; a minus sign (–) denotes no or eligible synthetic capacity.
[2]Receptor expression is classified as positive (+), negative (–), minimal (±) or not determined yet (?).
[3]LTB$_4$ has a more potent microbial killing ability than LTC$_4$.
[4]Structural cells produce leukotrienes mainly through transcellular biosynthesis; they can produce a much smaller amount of leukotrienes than leukocytes alone. So, we are not aiming to express relative synthetic capacity for structural cells.

receptor, termed CysLT1 [10], followed shortly thereafter by the identification of CysLT2 [11]. Binding studies of the individual cysLTs to these two receptors indicate that LTD$_4$ has the highest affinity for both CysLT1 and CysLT2, whereas LTE$_4$ has very low affinity for both receptors. Very recent reports indicate the presence of other receptors for cysLTs, including specific receptors for LTE$_4$ [12] and the orphan receptor GPR17 [13]. Here, we will summarize current knowledge regarding each cysLT receptor and its role in asthma.

CysLT1
More is known about CysLT1 than any other cysLT receptor. It is expressed on a variety of both immune-competent cells and structural cells (Table 23.1), and results with both CysLT1-deficient mice and CysLT1 antagonists suggest that many of the features of

asthma (eosinophilic airway inflammation, bronchoconstriction, edema, goblet cell hyperplasia, and structural remodeling of the airway) are mediated by CysLT1 signaling [1]. The cysLTs–CysLT1 pathway is also implicated in the pathogenesis of allergic rhinitis [14].

Through CysLT1, cysLTs activate immune-competent cells important for the development of asthma, such as dendritic cells, CD4$^+$ T cells, and eosinophils, resulting in Th2-biased immune responses (reviewed in ref. 1). CysLT-induced migration of CD34$^+$ hematopoietic progenitor cells from the bone marrow into the circulation system occurs via CysLT1 as well [15]. On the other hand, CysLT1 is minimally expressed on either CD8$^+$ T cells or neutrophils [1], paralleling the generally observed lack of direct effects of cysLTs on these cells.

Among structural cells, CysLT1 is expressed on smooth muscle cells [16], fibroblasts [17], fibrocytes [18], endothelial cells [1], and epithelial cells [19]. CysLTs elicit potent airway smooth muscle cell contraction [16] and migration [20] through CysLT1. LTD$_4$–CysLT1 signaling enhances collagen production by [1], and migration of [21], human lung fibroblasts. A recent article demonstrated that CysLT1 signaling enhances and contributes to migration and proliferation of murine and human fibrocytes, bone marrow-derived fibroblast precursors that are the subject of increasing interest [18]. Finally, cysLTs increase transforming growth factor (TGF)-β production by human airway epithelial cells [22] and antigen-induced goblet cell degranulation in the rat nasal epithelium [23] in a CysLT1-dependent manner.

Just as expression of leukotriene biosynthetic proteins can be regulated by a variety of inflammatory molecules such as cytokines, cysLT receptors can as well. In particular, CysLT1 has been found to be transcriptionally upregulated *in vitro* by the Th2 cytokine IL-13 [24], and its expression was reported to be upregulated in nasal inflammatory cells obtained from patients with aspirin-sensitive asthma [25].

CysLT2

CysLT2 is co-expressed with CysLT1 in many cell types, including endothelium, eosinophils, mast cells, and macrophages (Table 23.1). Although its role in immunocompetent cells remains unclear, distinct proinflammatory actions not shared by CysLT1 have been described [26]. However, a more clear and important functional role of CysLT2 in mediating vascular permeability [27] and endothelial cell activation is emerging [28]. One study with CysLT2-deficient mice suggested its potential to contribute to the development of pulmonary fibrosis [27]. A novel perspective on the function of CysLT2 stems from the interesting finding that CysLT1 and CysLT2 heterodimerize and that CysLT2 downregulates both expression and functional responses of CysLT1 in human mast cells [29]. A major gap in our understanding of CysLT2 functionality is the lack of specific antagonists targeting this receptor, and the development of such agents will be indispensable to clarify the actual role of CysLT2 in asthma and other allergic conditions.

Other receptors for cysLTs: GPR17 and P2Y$_{12}$

Certain reported actions of cysLTs cannot be explained by their ligation of either CysLT1 or CysLT2 [12]. Moreover, the bronchoconstrictor activity of LTE$_4$, previously shown to be equipotent with that of LTC$_4$ and LTD$_4$ [30], is inconsistent with its low affinity to both CysLT1 and CysLT2. These results indicate that there may be other cysLT receptors, including receptors specific for LTE$_4$. Two candidates that have emerged also share the ability to bind nucleotides.

GPR17 is a dual uracil nucleotide–cysLT receptor [13]. Although the biologic role of this receptor remains unclear, a recent report suggests that GPR17 may negatively regulate both the expression and the function of CysLT1 in bone marrow-derived macrophages [31], an action similar to that observed for CysLT2 [28]. Further studies will be necessary to clarify the role of this receptor in cysLT biology.

Recently, LTE$_4$ was identified by *in silico* and *in vitro* approaches as a ligand for P2Y$_{12}$ [32], which is the target of clinically well-accepted antiplatelet thienopyridine derivatives such as clopidogrel and ticlopidine [33]. This was confirmed *in vivo* by the demonstration that enhancement of eosinophilic lung inflammation by LTE$_4$ inhalation in a mouse model of asthma was potently suppressed by treatment with P2Y$_{12}$ antagonist clopidogrel or in P2Y$_{12}$ knockout mice, but not in CysLT1/CyLT2 double-knockout mice [34]. Although the P2Y$_{12}$-expressing target cells for LTE$_4$ remain to be defined, platelets seem to be critical for LTE$_4$-exaggerated eosinophilic lung inflammation because depletion of platelets completely abolished the effect of LTE$_4$ [34]. However, that clopidogrel failed to attenuate LTE$_4$-induced vascular permeability [12] suggests the possible existence of an LTE$_4$ receptor other than P2Y$_{12}$. These new findings concerning alternate cysLT receptors provide possible explanations for the incomplete efficacy of currently available CysLT1 antagonists [35], and have implications for the relationship between CysLT1 receptor antagonist therapy and Churg–Strauss syndrome (CSS); both of these points are considered later in this chapter.

Biology of and receptors for LTB$_4$

There are two known receptors for LTB$_4$, the high-affinity B leukotriene 1 (BLT1) receptor [36] and the lower affinity BLT2 receptor [37]. The former is expressed mainly in leukocytes (Table 23.1), whereas the latter is expressed ubiquitously [38]. Recently, another oxygenated lipid, 12 (S)-hydroxyheptadeca-5Z, 8E, 10E-trienoic acid, was identified as a natural ligand for BLT2, whose affinity for this receptor exceeds that of LTB$_4$ [39]. As no clear biologic effects or role of BLT2 signaling are appreciated at this time, we will limit our consideration to LTB$_4$–BLT1 signaling.

LTB$_4$ was originally described as a potent chemoattractant for neutrophils [40], and may participate in severe asthma or asthma exacerbations. However, it is now recognized as both a chemoattractant and a general activator for eosinophils, macrophages [38], CD4$^+$ T cells [41], and dendritic cells [42], and all of these actions appear to be mediated by BLT1. Of great interest is the fact that LTB$_4$ also enhances migration of CD8$^+$ T cells [41], which lack CysLT1, and are now recognized as important players in the pathogenesis of asthma [43]. The importance of BLT1 in the development of allergic airway inflammation has been established also with BLT1-deficient mice [44].

Among structural cells, airway smooth muscle cells express BLT1, and LTB$_4$ enhances proliferation and migration of human airway smooth muscle cells through BLT1 [45]. Effects of LTB$_4$ on epithelial cells and fibroblasts remain unclear.

Antileukotriene drugs

Currently, three CysLT1 receptor antagonists (montelukast, Merck and Co. Inc., Whitehouse Station, NJ, USA; zafirlukast, AstraZeneca, Wilmington, DE, USA; and pranlukast, Ono Pharmaceuticals, Trenton,

NJ, USA) and one 5-LO inhibitor (zileuton, Abbott Laboratories, now Cornerstone Therapeutics, Cary, NC, USA) are clinically available. However, pranlukast is available only in Japan and zileuton only in the USA; montelukast is the agent most widely available and most actively marketed. Although these drugs are clearly superior to a placebo at improving lung function and decreasing asthmatic symptoms and exacerbations [2], their overall efficacy has not lived up to the high expectations that surrounded their development. Specific limitations include the fact that they are generally inferior to inhaled corticosteroids in anti-inflammatory and clinical effects [2], and that a substantial subset of patients (~50%) is non-responsive [35]. Reflecting these limitations, the 2007 National Institutes of Health (NIH) Expert Panel Report 3 classified leukotriene modifiers as "alternate" treatment options, but not as "first line" therapy for asthma [2]. On the other hand, these drugs have proven to be genuinely useful in certain clinical situations as either add-on or first-line agents. Examples of the former include patients with aspirin-exacerbated respiratory disease, and examples of the latter include patients who either cannot use inhaler devices or are unwilling to use or cannot tolerate ICS. Additional interest in the therapeutic potential of leukotriene blockade derives from the facts that (1) neither leukotriene synthesis nor receptor expression [3] appears to be inhibited by corticosteroids, and (2) anti-leukotriene agents have demonstrated a remarkable capacity to prevent [46] or even reverse [47] the airway remodeling observed in a mouse model of chronic allergic asthma, whereas corticosteroids lack this ability in the mouse model, and ICS fail to prevent progressive loss of lung function in children with chronic asthma [48]. Data such as these motivate a desire to enhance the efficacy of leukotriene pathway blockade to achieve better outcomes in patients with asthma. Here, we will further consider limitations of the currently available leukotriene modifiers as well as possible opportunities to target this pathway via alternate strategies for future drug development.

Currently available drugs

CysLT1 antagonists

CysLT1 antagonists, also called LTRAs, were developed and marketed more than a decade ago, and substantial worldwide experience with these agents has been accumulated. Their efficacy and safety in the treatment of asthma have recently been reviewed [49], and we will consider the most pertinent limitations in both categories.

Limited efficacy The efficacy of LTRAs in clinical usage is modest and inferior to ICS [2]. The proportion of non-responders to LTRAs [35] exceeds that observed for other classes of medication.

There are three possible explanations that might account for unresponsiveness to LTRAs in a given patient. The first is that the patient may fail to overproduce cysLTs to a degree sufficient to contribute meaningfully to disease pathogenesis. This could reflect polymorphisms in genes encoding 5-LO, FLAP, or LTC_4S that result in loss of function of these proteins. Indeed, it is reported that increased cysLT production is not seen in all patients with asthma [50], and that these patients could be divided into high and low leukotriene-producing groups following allergen challenge, with sensitivity to zileuton being seen only in the high leukotriene-producing subset [51]. Similarly, therapeutic efficacy of antileukotriene drugs has been associated with the presence of gene variants of 5-LO and LTC_4S (see ref. 8 for further review).

The second reason is that CysLT1 expression or function may be insufficient to provide a robust therapeutic target. Theoretically, this could reflect genetic or non-genetic loss-of-function alterations in CysLT1 itself or in its coupled G proteins or downstream signaling partners. Alternatively, it could reflect functional inhibition of CysLT1 by other cysLT receptors, such as CysLT2 [28] or GPR17 [30].

The third possible reason hinges on the importance to asthma pathogenesis of either cysLT receptors other than CysLT1 (e.g. CysLT2, GPR17, or $P2Y_{12}$) or alternate 5-LO products such as LTB_4 and its receptor BLT1.

LTRAs and Churg–Strauss syndrome

Churg–Strauss syndrome is a rare but life-threatening granulomatous and eosinophilic vasculitis that occurs preferentially in patients with pre-existing asthma. Soon after the introduction of LTRAs, a number of case reports and case series were published of patients who developed CSS after starting treatment with each of the LTRAs [52]. An NIH expert panel concluded that, for a variety of reasons, LTRAs could not be

causally linked to CSS [52]. By contrast, a more recent analysis argued, instead, that a causal relationship between LTRA and CSS could not be excluded and, indeed, must be seriously considered [53]. The recent identification of a putative receptor for LTE_4 important in driving eosinophilic disease [34] and the observation that deletion or pharmacologic blockade of CysLT1 actually augmented LTE_4-induced vascular permeability [12] provide a possible mechanism by which LTRA therapy could induce CSS. The relevance of such a mechanism in humans remains to be determined.

5-LO inhibitor (zileuton)

A drug that directly targets 5-LO (or FLAP), and therefore inhibits the biosynthesis of all 5-LO metabolites, is highly appealing for the treatment of asthma as it would surmount two key limitations of LTRAs. First, by inhibiting the generation of all cysLTs, it obviates the limitations inherent in targeting any single specific cysLT receptor in isolation, as well as the potential complexities stemming from possible cross-talk between cysLT receptors. Second, it has the potential to interfere with the asthmagenic actions of not only cysLTs, but also of LTB_4 and another 5-LO metabolite not previously mentioned, 5-oxo-eicosatetraenoic acid [54]. However, the efficacy of zileuton may be limited by its incomplete (26–86%) inhibition of leukotriene synthesis [55], and it remains unknown whether zileuton is superior to LTRAs in the treatment of asthma [56]. Furthermore, zileuton—the only marketed inhibitor of leukotriene biosynthesis—has not been widely used because of the initial need to take it four times daily (a controlled-release tablet can now be used twice daily), and the requirement for liver function test monitoring because of possible hepatocellular injury [57].

Optimizing antileukotriene therapy: future directions

Table 23.2 lists the possible targets within the leukotriene pathway for new drug development, along with their anticipated beneficial effects and side-effects.

Although data from the murine allergic asthma model support the potential efficacy of targeting the $cPLA_2$ enzyme [58], such an approach should be viewed with caution because such upstream inhibition also suppresses production of prostaglandins,

Table 23.2 Targets for new drugs in the future.

Targets for inhibition	Purpose	Anticipated[1]		Previous reports
		Results	Side-effects	
cPLA$_2$	Inhibition of arachidonic acid release	Leukotriene synthesis ↓	Prostaglandin synthesis ↓	Human: N [66], mouse: Y [58]
Transporters	Inhibition of export	Leukotriene export ↓	Export of other mediators such as prostaglandins ↓	N/A
FLAP	Inhibition of 5-LO metabolism	Leukotriene synthesis ↓	Infection ↑ (?)	Mouse: Y [67]
LTC$_4$S	Inhibition of LTC$_4$S	cysLT synthesis ↓	LTB$_4$ synthesis ↑ (shunting)	Mouse: Y [68]
P2Y$_{12}$	Inhibition of LTE$_4$ signaling	LTE$_4$ signaling ↓	Bleeding tendency	Mouse: Y [34]
CysLT2	Inhibition of cysLT2 signaling	CysLT2 signaling ↓	CysLT1 signaling ↑	N/A
BLT1	Inhibition of BLT1 signaling	LTB$_4$-BLT1 signaling ↓	Infection ↑ (?)	Human: N [61], Mouse: Y [69]

↓, Suppression or decrease; ↑, enhancement or increase.

Y, previous papers demonstrated this inhibitor effective or beneficial in the treatment of asthma or in a mouse model of asthma; N, previous papers did not demonstrate the beneficial effect of the inhibitor in human asthmatics or in a mouse model of asthma; N/A, no previous paper is applicable to this inhibitor.

which mediate cardioprotective actions. Moreover, one of the major prostaglandins of most tissues, PGE$_2$, protects against both inflammation and bronchoconstriction in asthma [59], especially in aspirin-induced asthma [16], and its inhibition may be harmful in asthma.

If cysLTs are the only 5-LO products important in the pathogenesis of asthma and allergic diseases, optimal therapeutic targeting can be accomplished by focusing on their synthesis and receptors. Unless a role for CysLT2 in asthma is identified, targeting this receptor does not seem fruitful; moreover, if it actually suppresses CysLT1 and/or LTE$_4$ receptor function in humans *in vivo*, as it can do *in vitro*, antagonizing CysLT2 could unmask excessive responses mediated by these other receptors. Although CysLT1 antagonism is clearly beneficial, the possibility that it may likewise unmask excessive LTE$_4$ receptor signaling has already been mentioned. However, dual blockade of CysLT1 and LTE$_4$ receptor(s) is an attractive strategy that would overcome such a concern. If P2Y$_{12}$ is

indeed confirmed to be an important LTE$_4$ receptor in humans, this approach could be implemented today with existing LTRAs and clopidogrel; additional superior P2Y$_{12}$ antagonists are under development [60]. The other attractive strategy for comprehensive inhibition of cysLTs is to target the LTC$_4$S enzyme itself.

If 5-LO products other than cysLTs contribute to disease expression in certain patients, blockade of cysLT synthesis or receptors would be insufficient for optimal control. Complete blockade of the leukotriene pathway could be achieved with 5-LO inhibitors or FLAP inhibitors that are more potent and more user-friendly than zileuton. This approach has the additional potential benefit that it may shunt arachidonic acid toward enhanced PGE$_2$ synthesis, which itself may be bronchoprotective. It should be noted that a BLT1 antagonist by itself was not efficacious in allergen-challenged humans with asthma [61]. It is worth noting that LTB$_4$–BLT1 signaling is an attractive target in other conditions, such as chronic obstructive pulmonary disease and athero-sclerosis [62], and this approach may suppress not only asthma, but also the progression of atherosclero-sis, which can accompany asthma [63]. On the other hand, one risk of potently inhibiting LTB_4 biosyn-thesis or BLT1 is reducing innate immunity against microbial pathogens [64]; indeed, increased infectious exacerbations necessitated the discontinuation of a clinical trial of a BLT1 antagonist in cystic fibrosis [65]. However, it is unlikely that this would pose as much a risk in individuals with asthma.

References

1 Peters-Golden M, Henderson WR, Jr. Leukotrienes. *N Engl J Med* 2007; **357**: 1841–54.
2 National Institutes of Health; National Heart, Lung, and Blood Institute. National Asthma Education and Prevention Program. Expert Panel Report 3: guidelines for the diagnosis and management of asthma, 2007. No. 07-4051. Available from: http://www.nhlbi.nih.gov/guidelines/asthma/asthgdln.htm.
3 Negri J, Early SB, Steinke JW, *et al.* Corticosteroids as inhibitors of cysteinyl leukotriene metabolic and sig-naling pathway. *J Allergy Clin Immunol* 2008; **121**: 1232–7.
4 Murphy RC, Gijon MA. Biosynthesis and metabolism of leukotrienes. *Biochem J* 2007; **405**: 379–95.
5 Peters-Golden M, Brock TG. 5-Lipoxygenase and FLAP. *Prostaglandins Leukot Essent Fatty Acids* 2003; **69**: 99–109.
6 van de Ven R, Scheffer GL, Scheper RJ, *et al.* The ABC of dendritic cell development and function. *Trends Immunol* 2009; **30**: 421–9.
7 Fabre JE, Goulet JL, Riche E, *et al.* Transcellular bio-synthesis contributes to the production of leukotrienes during inflammatory responses *in vivo. J Clin Invest* 2002; **109**: 1373–80.
8 Tantisira KG, Drazen JM. Genetics and pharmacogenet-ics of the leukotriene pathway. *J Allergy Clin Immunol* 2009; **124**: 422–7.
9 Murphy RC, Hammarstrom S, Samuelsson B. Leukotriene C: a slow-reacting substance from murine mastocytome cells. *Proc Natl Acad Sci USA* 1979; **76**: 4275–9.
10 Lynch KR, O'Neill GP, Liu Q, *et al.* Characterization of the human cysteinyl leukotriene CysLT1 receptor. *Nature* 1999; **399**: 789–93.
11 Heise CE, O'Dowd BF, Figueroa DJ, *et al.* Characterization of the human cysteinyl leukotriene 2 receptor. *J Biol Chem* 2000; **275**: 30531–6.
12 Maekawa A, Kanaoka Y, Xing W, *et al.* Functional recognition of a distinct receptor preferential for leu-kotriene E_4 in mice lacking the cysteinyl leukotriene 1 and 2 receptors. *Proc Natl Acad Sci USA* 2008; **105**: 16695–700.
13 Ciana P, Fumagalli M, Trincavelli ML, *et al.* The orphan receptor GPR17 identified as a new dual uracil nucleotides/cysteinyl-leukotrienes receptor. *EMBO J* 2006; **25**: 4615–27.
14 Peters-Golden M, Gleason MM, Togias A. Cysteinyl leu-kotrienes: multi-functional mediators in allergic rhinitis. *Clin Exp Allergy* 2006; **36**: 689–703.
15 Bautz F, Denzlinger C, Kanz L, *et al.* Chemotaxis and transendothelial migration of CD34(+) hematopoietic progenitor cells induced by the inflammatory mediator leukotriene D4 are mediated by the 7-transmembrane receptor CysLT1. *Blood* 2001; **97**: 3433–40.
16 Holgate ST, Peters-Golden M, Panettieri RA, *et al.* Roles of cysteinyl leukotrienes in airway inflammation, smooth muscle function, and remodeling. *J Allergy Clin Immunol* 2003; **111**: S18–34.
17 James AJ, Penrose JF, Cazaly AM, *et al.* Human bron-chial fibroblasts express the 5-lipoxygenase pathway. *Respir Res* 2006; **7**: 102.
18 Vanella KM, McMillan TR, Charbeneau RP, *et al.* Cysteinyl leukotrienes are autocrine and paracrine reg-ulators of fibrocyte function. *J Immunol* 2007; **179**: 7883–90.
19 Jame AJ, Lackie PM, Cazaly AM, *et al.* Human bron-chial epithelial cells express an active and inducible bio-synthetic pathway for leukotriene B_4 and C_4. *Clin Exp Allergy* 2007; **37**: 880–92.
20 Parameswaran K, Cox G, Radford K, *et al.* Cysteinyl leu-kotrienes promote human airway smooth muscle migra-tion. *Am J Respir Crit Care Med* 2002; **166**: 738–42.
21 Kato J, Kohyama T, Okazaki H, *et al.* Leukotriene D4 potentiates fibronectin-induced migration of human lung fibroblasts. *Clin Immunol* 2005; **117**: 177–81.
22 Perng DW, Wu YC, Chang KT, *et al.* Leukotriene C_4 induces TGF-β1 production in airway epithelium via p38 kinase pathway. *Am J Respir Cell Mol Biol* 2006; **34**: 101–7.
23 Shimizu T, Shimizu S, Hattori R, *et al.* A mechanism of antigen-induced goblet cell degranulation in the nasal epithelium of sensitized rats. *J Allergy Clin Immunol* 2003; **112**: 119–25.
24 Thivierge M, Stanková J, Rola-Pleszczynski M. IL-13 and IL-4 up-regulate cysteinyl leukotriene 1 receptor expression in human monocytes and macrophages. *J Immunol* 2001; **167**: 2855–60.
25 Sousa AR, Parikh A, Scadding G, *et al.* Leukotriene-receptor expression on nasal mucosal inflammatory cells in aspirin-sensitive rhinosinusitis. *N Engl J Med* 2002; **347**: 1493–9.

26 Mellor EA, Frank N, Soler D, *et al.* Expression of the type 2 receptor for cysteinyl leukotrienes (CysLT2R) by human mast cells: functional distinction from CysLT1R. *Proc Natl Acad Sci USA* 2003; **100**: 11589–93.

27 Beller TC, Maekawa A, Friend DS, *et al.* Targeted gene disruption reveals the role of the cysteinyl leukotriene 2 receptor in increased vascular permeability and in bleomycin-induced pulmonary fibrosis in mice. *J Biol Chem* 2004; **279**: 46129–34.

28 Uzonyi B, Lotzer K, Jahn S, *et al.* Cysteinyl leukotriene 2 receptor and protease-activated receptor 1 activate strongly correlated early genes in human endothelial cells. *Proc Natl Acad Sci USA* 2006; **103**: 6326–31.

29 Jiang Y, Borrelli LA, Kanaoka Y, *et al.* CysLT2 receptors interact with CysLT1 receptors and down-modulate cysteinyl leukotriene-dependent mitogenic responses of mast cells. *Blood* 2007; **110**: 3263–70.

30 Davidson AB, Lee TH, Scanlon PD, *et al.* Bronchoconstrictor effects of leukotriene E_4 in normal and asthmatic subjects. *Am Rev Respir Dis* 1987; **135**: 333–7.

31 Maekawa A, Balestrieri B, Austen KF, *et al.* GPR17 is negative regulator of the cysteinyl leukotriene 1 receptor response to leukotriene D_4. *Proc Natl Acad Sci USA* 2009; **106**: 11685–90.

32 Nonaka Y, Hiramoto T, Fujita N. Identification of endogenous surrogate ligands for human $P2Y_{12}$ receptors by in silico and *in vitro* methods. *Biochem Biophys Res Commun* 2005; **337**: 281–8.

33 Savi P, Herbert JM. Clopidogrel and ticlopidine: $P2Y_{12}$ adenosine diphosphate-receptor antagonists for the prevention of atherothrombosis. *Semin Thromb Hemost* 2005; **31**: 174–83.

34 Paruchuri S, Tashimo H, Feng C, *et al.* Leukotriene E_4-induced pulmonary inflammation is mediated by the $P2Y_{12}$ receptor. *J Exp Med* 2009; **206**: 2543–55.

35 Barnes N, Thomas M, Price D, *et al.* The national montelukast survey. *J Allergy Clin Immunol* 2005; **115**: 47–54.

36 Yokomizo T, Izumi T, Chang K, *et al.* A G-protein-coupled receptor for leukotriene B_4 that mediates chemotaxis. *Nature* 1997; **387**: 620–4.

37 Yokomizo T, Kato K, Terawaki K, *et al.* A second leukotriene B (4) receptor, BLT2. A new therapeutic target in inflammation and immunological disorders. *J Exp Med* 2000; **192**: 421–32.

38 Tager AM, Luster AD. BLT1 and BLT2: the leukotriene B (4) receptors. *Prostaglandins Leuko Essent Fatty Acids* 2003; **69**: 123–34.

39 Okuno T, Iizuka Y, Okazaki H, *et al.* 12(S)-hydroxyheptadeca-5Z, 8E, 10E-trienoic acid is a natural ligand for leukotriene B_4 receptor 2. *J Exp Med* 2008; **205**: 759–66.

40 Ford-Hutchinson AW, Bray MA, Doig MV, *et al.* Leukotriene B, a potent chemokinetic and aggregating substance released from polymorphonuclear leukocytes. *Nature* 1980; **286**: 264–5.

41 Tager AM, Bromley SK, Medoff BD, *et al.* Leukotriene B_4 receptor BLT1 mediates early effector T cell recruitment. *Nat Immunol* 2003; **4**: 982–90.

42 Miyahara N, Ohnishi H, Matsuda H, *et al.* Leukotriene B_4 receptor 1 expression on dendritic cells is required for the development of Th2 responses and allergen-induced airway hyperresponsiveness. *J Immunol* 2008; **181**: 1170–8.

43 Miyahara N, Swanson BJ, Takeda K, *et al.* Effector CD8+ T cells mediate inflammation and airway hyperresponsiveness. *Nat Med* 2004; **10**: 865–9.

44 Terawaki K, Yokomizo T, Nagase T, *et al.* Absence of leukotriene B_4 receptor 1 confers resistance to airway hyperresponsiveness and Th2-type immune responses. *J Immunol* 2005; **175**: 4217–25.

45 Watanabe S, Yamasaki A, Hashimoto K, *et al.* Expression of functional leukotriene B_4 receptors on human airway smooth muscle cells. *J Allergy Clin Immunol* 2009; **124**: 59–65.

46 Henderson WR Jr, Tang LO, Chu SJ, *et al.* A role for cysteinyl leukotrienes in airway remodeling in a mouse asthma model. *Am J Respir Crit Care Med* 2002; **165**: 108–16.

47 Henderson WR Jr, Chiang GK, Tien YT, *et al.* Reversal of allergen-induced airway remodeling by CysLT1 receptor blockade. *Am J Respir Crit Care Med* 2006; **173**: 718–28.

48 Covar RA, Spahn JD, Murphy JR, *et al.* Progression of asthma measured by lung function in the Childhood Asthma Management Program. *Am J Respir Crit Care Med* 2004; **170**: 234–41.

49 O'Byrne PM, Gauvreau GM, Murphy DM. Efficacy of leukotriene receptor antagonists and synthesis inhibitors in asthma. *J Allergy Clin Immunol* 2009; **124**: 397–403.

50 Kawagishi Y, Mita H, Taniguchi M, *et al.* Leukotriene C_4 synthase promoter polymorphism in Japanese patients with aspirin-induced asthma. *J Allergy Clin Immunol* 2002; **109**: 936–42.

51 Hasday J, Meltzer S, Moore W, *et al.* Anti-inflammatory effects of zileuton in a subpopulation of allergic asthmatics. *Am J Respir Crit Care Med* 2000; **161**: 1229–36.

52 Weller PF, Plaut M, Taggart V, *et al.* The relationship of asthma therapy and Churg–Strauss syndrome: NIH workshop summary report. *J Allergy Clin Immunol* 2001; **108**: 175–83.

53 Nathani N, Little MA, Kunst H, *et al.* Churg–Strauss syndrome and leukotriene antagonist use: a respiratory perspective. *Thorax* 2008; **63**: 883–8.

54 Grant GE, Rokach J, Powell WS. 5-Oxo-ETE and the OXE receptor. *Prostaglandins Other Lipid Mediat* 2009; **89**: 98–104.

55 Dube LM, Swanson LJ, Awni W. Zileuton, a leukotriene synthesis inhibitor in the management of chronic asthma: clinical pharmacokinetics and safety. *Clin Rev Allergy Immunol* 1999; **17**: 213–21.

56 Isarael E, Cohn J, Dube L, Drazen JM. Effect of treatment with zileuton, a 5-lipoxygenase inhibitor, in patients with asthma. A randomized controlled trial. *JAMA* 1996; **275**: 931–6.

57 Product label, ZyfloR (Zileuton Tablets). Abbott Laboratories, now Cornerstone Therapeutics: Cary, NC, USA. Revised November 2005.

58 Malaviya R, Ansell J, Hall L, *et al*. Targeting cytosolic phospholipase A_2 by arachidonyl trifluoromethyl ketone prevents chronic inflammation in mice. *Eur J Pharmacol* 2006; **539**: 195–204.

59 Gauvreau GM, Watson RM, O'Byrne PM. Protective effect of inhaled PGE_2 on allergen-induced airway responses and airway inflammation. *Am J Respir Crit Care Med* 1999; **159**: 31–6.

60 Cattaneo M. New P2Y12 blockers. *J Thromb Haemost* 2009; **7**(Suppl 1): 262–5.

61 Evans DJ, Barnes PJ, Spaethe SM, *et al*. Effect of a leukotriene B_4 receptor antagonist, LY293111, on allergen induced responses in asthma. *Thorax* 1996; **51**: 1178–84.

62 Spanbroek R, Gräbner R, Lötzer K, *et al*. Expanding expression of the 5-lipoxygenase pathway within the arterial wall during human atherogenesis. *Proc Natl Acad Sci USA* 2003; **100**: 1238–43.

63 Bom AT, Pinto AM. Allergic respiratory diseases in the elderly. *Respir Med* 2009; **103**: 1614–22.

64 Peters-Golden M, Canetti C, Mancuso P, *et al*. Leukotrienes: underappreciated mediators of innate immune responses. *J Immunol* 2005; **174**: 589–94.

65 Schmitt-Grohe S, Zielen S. Leukotriene receptor or antagonists in children with cystic fibrosis lung disease: anti-inflammatory and clinical effects. *Paediatr Drugs* 2005; **7**: 353–63.

66 Bowton DL, Dmitrienko AA, Israel E, *et al*. Impact of a soluble phospholipase A_2 inhibitor on inhaled allergen challenge in subjects with asthma. *J Asthma* 2005; **42**: 65–71.

67 Lorrain DS, Bain G, Correa LD, *et al*. Pharmacological characterization of 3-[3-tert-butylsulfanyl-1-[4-(6-methoxy-pyridin-3-yl)-benzyl]-5-(pyridin-2-ylmethoxy)-1H-indol-2-yl]-2,2-dimethyl-propionic acid (AM103), a novel selective five-lipoxygenase-activating protein (FLAP) inhibitor reduces acute and chronic inflammation. *J Pharmacol Exp Ther* 2009; **331**: 1042–50.

68 Kim DC, Hsu FI, Barrett NA, *et al*. Cysteinyl leukotrienes regulate Th2 cell-dependent pulmonary inflammation. *J Immunol* 2006; **176**: 4440–8.

69 Cheraim AB, Xavier-Elas P, de Oliveira SH, *et al*. Leukotriene B_4 is essential for selective eosinophil recruitment following allergen challenge of CD4[+] cells in a model of chronic eosinophilic inflammation. *Life Sci* 2008; **83**: 214–22.

24 Proteases in allergy

Keisuke Oboki and Hirohisa Saito
Department of Allergy and Immunology, National Research Institute for Child
Health and Development, Tokyo, Japan

Introduction

Although only a few drugs targeting proteases are available, various proteases are crucially involved in inflammation and allergic responses. For example, inflammasome has been recently identified as a molecular complex involved in the activation of inflammatory caspases, resulting in the processing of immature proIL-1β and proIL-18 into their mature forms; they are a crucial element in the adjuvant effect and they play an important role in exaggerating an adaptive immune response [1]. Owing to the space limitation, however, only the roles of endogenous proteases, such as mast cell tryptase, and exogenous proteases, such as house dust mite allergens in asthma and allergic diseases, are discussed here in this chapter.

Endogenous proteases

Role of mast cells in asthma

Bronchial asthma is characterized by airway inflammation, airway hyperresponsiveness, and airway remodeling. Airway remodeling is defined as the structural changes in the airways that may affect their functional properties. The structural changes include an increased airway smooth muscle mass, mucous gland hypertrophy, deposition of extracellular matrix components, thickening of the reticular basement membrane, and angiogenesis. Patients with asthma have accelerated loss of lung function over time, and some patients develop progressive fixed airflow obstruction. These features may reflect airway remodeling in severe and chronic asthma. Although the relationship between remodeling and inflammation has not been fully understood, many reports suggest that airway remodeling might be a consequence of repeated injury and persistent inflammation [2].

It has been reported that sustained airway hyperresponsiveness can be uncoupled from inflammatory cell infiltration [3,4], and the observation that profound airway hyperresponsiveness is sustained in asthma irrespective of prolonged treatment with anti-inflammatory corticosteroids supports the finding that persistence of airway hyperresponsiveness is not dependent on sustained inflammatory cell recruitment. Mast cells are known to be the primary responders in allergic reactions, most of which are triggered by cross-linking of a high-affinity immunoglobulin E (IgE) receptor, FcεRI. After activation, mast cells exert their biologic effects by releasing preformed and *de novo* synthesized mediators, such as histamine, leukotrienes, and various cytokines/chemokines. Biogenic amines and lipid mediators cause rapid leakage of plasma from blood vessels, vasodilation, and bronchoconstriction. Cytokines mediate the late-phase reaction characterized by an inflammatory infiltrate composed of eosinophils, basophils, neutrophils, and lymphocytes. Bronchial asthma is a manifestation of immediate hypersensitivity and late-phase reactions in the lower respiratory tract [5].

Airway smooth muscle mass is increased in patients with asthma, particularly in individuals with severe asthma [6]. Mast cells were found to be required for the full development of each of the features of the chronic asthma model, such as enhanced airway responses to methacholine or antigen, chronic inflammation (including infiltration by eosinophils and lymphocytes), airway epithelial goblet cell hyperplasia, enhanced expression of the mucin genes *MUC5AC* and *MUC5B*, and increased pulmonary collagen levels [7]. These studies of chronic asthma models have suggested that early Th2 cytokine-mediated inflammatory events contribute to the initiation of remodeling events—such as an increase in airway smooth muscle mass—and that sustained airway hyperresponsiveness is associated with airway remodeling, which consists of multiple structural changes.

It has been reported that the infiltration of airway smooth muscle by mast cells is associated with the disordered airway function found in asthma [8]. It has been reported also that increased intact and degranulated mast cells were observed in airway smooth muscle and in the submucosal gland of fatal asthma airways, and that they were associated with a greater degree of airway smooth muscle shortening and larger submucosal gland area, respectively [9]. These observations indicate direct interaction between mast cells and airway smooth muscle cells, and between mast cells and the mucous gland.

Among mast cell-producing products, activin A promoted the proliferation of human airway smooth muscle cells [10]. The induction of platelet-derived growth factor (PDGF) and transforming growth factor (TGF)-β1 has been reported in human cord blood-derived mast cells following FcεRI aggregation [11]. It has been demonstrated that PDGF induces proliferation of human cultured airway smooth muscle cells [12]. TGF-β1 is capable of inducing phenotypic modulation of human lung fibroblasts to myofibroblasts [13], and promotes airway smooth muscle cells [14]. A member of the epidermal growth factor (EGF) family, amphiregulin, is secreted by human mast cells following aggregation of FcεRI, and its expression is not inhibited by a corticosteroid. Upregulation of amphiregulin expression is observed in mast cells of patients with asthma, but not normal control subjects. Furthermore, upregulation of amphiregulin in

mast cells significantly correlated with the extent of goblet cell hyperplasia in the mucosa of individuals with bronchial asthma [15]. It has been recently reported that acute asthma attacks are associated with hypersecretion of EGF and amphiregulin in the airway. Thus, recurrent acute attacks may aggravate airway remodeling [16].

Tryptase

Mast cells, leukocytes, and lung structural cells contribute to the pathophysiology of asthma through the production of numerous mediators, including serine proteases. Such proteases include mast cell tryptase and chymase; neutrophil elastase, cathepsin G, and myeloblastin (proteinase 3); bronchial epithelial cell-derived transmembrane protease, serine 11D (human airway trypsin-like protease); cytotoxic T lymphocyte- and natural killer cell-derived granzyme B; and eosinophil serine protease 1 (testisin) [17]. Mast cell neutral proteases (tryptases, chymases, and carboxypeptidase A), which catalyze the cleavage of peptide bonds at neutral pH, are the dominant protein components in secretory granules. Tryptases comprise a group of trypsin-like serine proteases that are highly and selectively expressed in mast cells, and to a lesser extent in basophils. In humans, enzymatically active tryptase is a heparin-stabilized tetrameric endoprotease of 134 kDa with subunits of 31–34 kDa, each with an active enzymatic site. Human mast cell tryptase comprises the products of four gene loci localized in chromosome 16, *TPSAB1*, *TPSB2*, *TPSD1*, and *TPSG1*, and achieves additional diversity through allelic variation. Among them, tryptase β, which is encoded by *TPSAB1* and *TPSB2*, is the predominant protease and protein component of mast cells. Although mature β-tryptase is stored in secretory granules of mast cells, unprocessed α-protryptases are inactive and spontaneously secreted from human mast cells [18]. Tryptase is, therefore, known to be a clinically useful marker of mast cells and their activation. Bonadonna *et al.* [19] recently demonstrated that patients with a serum baseline total tryptase level >11.4 ng/mL who were culled from 379 patients with a previous systemic immediate hypersensitivity reaction to a Hymenoptera sting have an underlying clonal mast cell disorder, suggesting that serum tryptase levels can be used as biomarkers for predicting anaphylactic risk.

The cleavage of a substrate by tryptase leads to its degradation and hence loss of biologic activity. Conversely, cleavage by tryptase is also an activating process, for example the removal of a propeptide. Tryptase degrades fibrinogen (anticoagulant factor) [20], generates bradikinin through the cleavage of high-molecular-weight kininogen and prekallikrein [21], activates the plasminogen activator [22], and cleaves promatrix metalloproteinase 3 (MMP-3) and C3 into mature MMP-3 [23] and C3a [24], respectively. Tryptase degrades high-density lipoproteins [25], type VI collagen [26], fibronectin [27,28], vasoactive intestinal peptide [29], and calcitonin gene-related peptide [30]. Recent studies have provided convincing evidence that tryptase contributes to the pathogenesis of allergic inflammatory disorders, most notably asthma. Among such evidence, mast cell tryptase is involved in the proliferation of airway smooth muscle cells [31], probably via proteolysis of other growth factors such as TGF-β1 on airway smooth muscle cells [32]. Additionally, gelatin [33], pre-elafin (serine protease inhibitor trappin 2) [34], and chemokines [35], and major grass and birch pollen allergens [36], have been identified as novel substrates for tryptase. Very recently, mice lacking mast cell protease 6 (mMCP-6), the ortholog of human tryptase β, have been developed. Using the tryptase knockout mice, various roles of tryptase have begun to be examined [37]. Regarding human tryptase, potent specific non-peptide inhibitor has been developed [38]. Using these novel tools, the biologic function of tryptase will be comprehensively understood in the near future.

Chymase

Chymase is the major enzyme accounting for chymotrypsin-like activity [39]. The enzyme was purified from human skin, and the corresponding gene, CMA1, was cloned and localized to human chromosome 14. Human chymase is a monomer of 30 kDa with endopeptidase activity. Regarding heterogeneity among human mast cells, two types have been recognized; MC_{TC} cells contain tryptase together with chymase and mast cell carboxypeptidase, and MC_T cells contain tryptase but lack the other neutral proteases present in MC_{TC} cells. Although MC_T cells are preferentially present in lung or mucosal tissue, MC_{TC} cells exclusively present in skin or connective

tissue [40]. The biologic role of human chymase in allergic diseases is largely unknown. However, the genetic variance of the chymase gene is reported to be associated with the onset of atopic dermatitis [41]. Also, a chymase inhibitor has been demonstrated to ameliorate skin inflammation and pruritus in a mouse model for atopic dermatitis [42]. Interestingly, human mast chymase has been found recently to cleave pro-IL-18 and to generate biologically active IL-18, like inflammasome caspase 1 [43]. Chymase may act as an adjuvant or a danger signal during antigen presentation. MC_{TC} cells are increased in the lungs of individuals with asthma, and chymase is reported to play a role in the vascular component of airway remodeling in asthma [44]. In this setting, MC_{TC} is reported to be a relevant cellular source of vascular endothelial growth factor.

Conservation and evolution of mast cell proteases

Human mast cells also express carboxypeptidase A3/mast cell carboxypeptidase A (MC-CPA), which is an exopeptidase that preferentially cleaves at C-terminal aliphatic amino acids. Carboxypeptidase A3/MC-CPA is encoded by the CPA3 locus, and is localized to chromosome 3. The tryptase genes seem to be evolutionarily conserved between humans and rodents, but, on the other hand, there are more than six paralogs in rodent chymase. In rats, there are four tryptases (Mcpt-6, -7, Prss34, and Tpsg1) that are localized in chromosome 10, and eight chymases (Mcpt-1, -2, -3, -4, -5, -8, -9, and -10) that are localized in chromosome 15. Rat mast cells also express MC-CPA, which is found on chromosome 2. In mice, four tryptases (mMCP-6, -7, −11, and TMT), six chymases (mMCP-1, -2, -4, -5, -8, and -9), and one MC-CPA have been reported [45,46]. The mMCP-1, -2, −4, -5, −8, and -9 genes are localized on chromosome 14, the mMCP-6, -7, -11 and TMT genes on chromosome 17, and the MC-CPA gene on chromosome 3. In addition to these proteases, cathepsin G and granzyme B are expressed in human and rodent mast cells.

Protease functions in vivo using mouse models

In addition to the above mention of mMCP-6, functions of other proteases have been studied by gene-disrupting mice. mMCP-1 is expressed predominantly by mucosal mast cells, and levels in the bloodstream and intestinal lumen are maximal at the time of worm expulsion in parasitized mice. In experiments in mice infected with *Trichinella spiralis*, the deletion of the mMCP-1 gene is associated with significantly delayed expulsion of the worms [47]. In other experiments, the deletion of mMCP-4, which is expressed by connective tissue-type mast cells (CTMCs), resulted in complete loss of chymotryptic activity in the peritoneum and in ear tissue, indicating that mMCP-4 is the main source of stored chymotrypsin-like protease activity at these sites [48]. mMCP-4-deficient mice fail to cleave promatrix metalloprotease 9 (pro-MMP-9) to its active form *in vivo* [49]. An asthma model using mMCP-4-deficient mice demonstrated an interesting phenotype; mMCP-4 acted as a protective factor for airway inflammation [50]. In a mouse model of ischemia–reperfusion injury of skeletal muscle, mice deficient in mMCP-5, which is expressed by CTMCs, are protected from full injury, suggesting that cytotoxic activity of mMCP-5 is critical for this pathology [51]. In experiments with MC-CPA-deficient mice, the immediate hypersensitivity reaction occurs normally, and peritoneal mast cells develop in normal numbers but fail to mature. Also, MC-CPA-lacking mast cells are devoid of Mcp-5 protein, the mechanism of which remains to be determined [52]. High endothelin 1 (ET-1) levels are associated with morbidity and mortality in patients with sepsis. An MC-CPA-deficient mouse model implicates that MC-CPA-mediated ET-1 cleavage attenuates the harmful effect of ET-1-induced vasoconstriction [53].

Exogenous proteases

House dust mite proteases

House dust mites of two species, *Dermatophagoides farinae* and *Dermatophagoides pteronyssinus*, are major sources of allergens associated with allergic diseases such as asthma in temperate zones [54]. Of these mite species, group 1 and group 2 allergens are identified as major allergens based on the frequency of patients sensitized, the amount of specific IgE, and the content in mite extract [55]. The group 1 allergens, Der f 1 and Der p 1, belong to the papain-like cysteine protease family [56], and exhibit cysteine protease activity [57]. Der f 1 and Der p 1 have 82% amino acid sequence identity with each other.

IgE epitopes of Der f 1 and Der p 1 are dependent on the integrity of the conformational structure, and high cross-reactivity between Der f 1 and Der p 1 has been reported [58].

Wan *et al.* [59] have reported that Der p 1 facilitates transepithelial allergen delivery by disruption of tight junctions of bronchial epithelium, which are the principal components of the epithelial paracellular permeability barrier. As such, the proteolytic activity of Der f 1 and Der p 1 has been proposed to be involved in the pathogenesis of allergies and the sensitization to the production of IgE by reducing physical and biochemical tissue barriers, cleaving various molecules, and modulating the functions of various cells [60,61].

Papain, a cysteine protease contained in papaya or pineapple, is also known to be an allergen, and can induce Th2-type allergic inflammation in exposed animals or humans; the mechanism for which has already been uncovered. It has been recently demonstrated that basophils directly respond to papain (by producing IL-4), thymic stromal lymphopoietin (TSLP), and other Th2-associated cytokines and chemokines [62], and that basophils are essential accessory cells for inducing Th2-type response via IL-4 production and antigen presentation in draining lymph nodes [63]. Basophils may bypass the Th2-type immune response. The effect of other protease allergens remains to be determined; however, this will provide a fascinating theory in protease allergen-related allergic inflammation.

Activation of innate pattern recognition receptors such as Toll-like receptors (TLRs) plays a critical role in helper T type 1 cell differentiation, yet their contribution to the generation of Th2 responses to clinically relevant aeroallergens has remained poorly defined. TLR4 was originally thought to specifically recognize a structure present in the endotoxin molecule; however, it turned out to recognize a variety of molecules other than microbial components. Hammad *et al.* [64] recently reported that house dust mite extract can trigger TLR4 present on the airway structural cell types to produce the innate proallergic cytokines TSLP, granulocyte–macrophage colony-stimulating factor, IL-25, and IL-33. These proallergic cytokines can act as Th2 adjuvants and can enhance the allergen-specific Th2 cell proliferation from naïve T cells. The absence of TLR4 on structural cells, but not on hematopoietic cells, abolished the house dust mite-driven allergic airway inflammation. Phipps *et al.* [65] also found that the diminished house dust mite-stimulated Th2 response found in MyD88$^{-/-}$ and TLR4$^{-/-}$ mice was associated with fewer OX40 ligand-expressing myeloid dendritic cells in the draining lymph nodes during allergic sensitization. Also, house dust mite-specific IL-17 production and airway neutrophilia were attenuated in MyD88$^{-/-}$ but not TLR4$^{-/-}$ mice. They concluded that Th2- and Th17-mediated inflammation generated on inhalational house dust mite exposure in mice is differentially regulated.

Other allergen proteases

Cockroach allergens are strongly associated with asthma in the inner cities of the USA, yet none of the cockroach allergens that have been cloned are proteolytic enzymes. Thus, although mite proteases allergens may act as Th2 adjuvants, a paradoxical effect is that other allergens may elicit strong Th2 responses in the absence of enzyme activity [61]. Cockroach allergens are known to stimulate the airway epithelial cells to produce inflammatory cytokines [66]. Matrix metalloproteinase 9 is released mainly from neutrophils and is abundantly found in the airways of chronic asthma. While house dust allergens mainly stimulate TLR4 present on epithelial cells, German cockroach frass contains a TLR2 ligand, and the cockroach-induced TLR2 activation of neutrophils recruited into the bronchial epithelium leads to release of matrix metalloproteinase 9, which decreases allergic responses to cockroach frass [67].

Compared with house dust mite allergens, sensitization to fungal allergens is less frequent, even though they have some protease activities and the air we breathe is filled with fungal spores such as *Cladosporium*, *Penicillium*, *Alternaria* and *Aspergillus*. Aimanianda *et al.* [68] recently showed that the surface layer on the dormant fungal spores masks their recognition by the immune system and hence prevents immune response.

Protease-activated receptors

Extracellular endogenous proteases, such as mast cell tryptase, as well as exogenous proteases from mites and molds, react with cell surface receptors in the airways to generate leukocyte infiltration and to amplify the response to allergens (Figure 24.1). Serine proteases are well known as enzymes involved in digestion of dietary proteins, blood coagulation, and homeostasis. Recent studies revealed a novel role of serine proteases as signaling molecules acting via protease-activated receptors (PARs), which are 7-transmembrane proteins coupled to G proteins. PARs are widely distributed on the cells of the airways, where they contribute to the inflammation characteristic of allergic diseases. The crucial role of PAR activation during disease progression has been revealed mainly in animal models of different gastrointestinal pathologies; neuroinflammatory and neurodegenerative processes; skin, joint and airway inflammation; or allergic responses. PAR activation modulates functional responses of innate and adaptive immune cells [69]. PAR stimulation of epithelial cells opens tight junctions, causes desquamation, and produces cytokines, chemokines, and growth factors. They degranulate eosinophils and mast cells. Proteases contract bronchial smooth muscle and cause it to proliferate. PARs also promote maturation, proliferation, and collagen production of fibroblast precursors and mature fibroblasts. PAR-2, apparently the most important of the four PARs that have been characterized, is increased on the epithelium of patients with asthma. Trypsin, a product of injured epithelial cells, and mast cell tryptase are considered to be potent activators of PAR-2. Mast cell chymase activates PAR-1. They both amplify IgE production to allergens, degranulate eosinophils, and can generate inflammation, even in the absence of IgE [70,71]. However, PAR-2 involvement in the mast cell tryptase activation is recently reported to be unlikely because PAR-2-specific inhibitor, SLIGKV, had no effect [72]. On the other hand, human mast cells themselves express functional PAR-2 and can be activated by PAR-2 activating peptide, 2-furoyl-LIGRLO-amide, to release cytokines but not preformed granule-associated mediators such as histamine [73].

The recent identification of loss-of-function mutations in the structural protein filaggrin as a widely replicated major risk factor for eczema sheds new light on disease mechanisms in atopic dermatitis and allergic diseases. The filaggrin gene (*FLG*) mutation findings are consistent with a recently proposed unifying hypothesis that offers a mechanistic understanding of eczema pathogenesis synthesizing a heritable

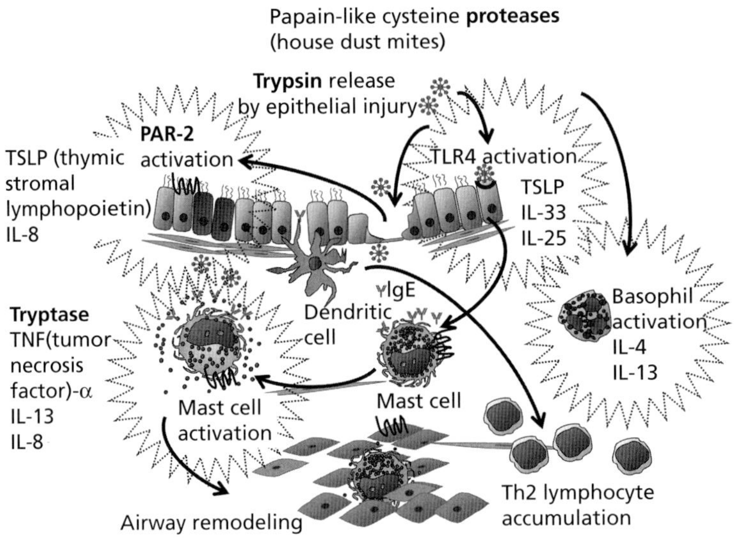

Figure 24.1 Role of proteases in allergic inflammation in the airways. When papain-like cysteine proteases such as Der p 1 allergen are inhaled into the airways, epithelial injury occurs. Epithelial injury results in increased allergen infiltration and release of trypsin protease. Allergen infiltration stimulates mast cells, basophils, dendritic cells and T helper 2 (Th2) lymphocytes to release a variety of proteases and inflammatory mediators/cytokines. Trypsin or tryptase activate protease-activated receptor 2 (PAR-2) to release a variety of proallergic cytokines.

epithelial barrier defect and resultant diminished epidermal defense mechanisms to allergens and microbes, followed by polarized Th2 lymphocyte responses with resultant chronic inflammation, including autoimmune mechanisms. Although compelling evidence from genetic studies on filaggrin implicates perturbed barrier function as a key player in the pathogenesis of eczema in many patients, much is still unknown about the sequence of biologic, physicochemical, and aberrant regulatory events that constitute the transition from an inherited barrier defect to clinical manifestations of inflammatory eczematous lesions and susceptibility to related atopic disorders [74]. *SPINK5* is another susceptible gene for the onset of atopic dermatitis and its complete loss causes an inherited skin disorder called Netherton syndrome. Very recently, by using a skin graft model in nude mice with the epidermis of Spink5$^{-/-}$ embryos, it was revealed that *SPINK5* deficiency results in unregulated kallikrein 5, and then the unregulated kallikrein 5 directly activates PAR-2 [75]. Thus, PAR-2 induces nuclear factor κB-mediated overexpression of a proallergic cytokine, i.e., TSLP, intracellular adhesion molecule 1, tumor necrosis factor α, and IL-8. This proinflammatory

and proallergic pathway is independent of the primary epithelial failure and is activated under basal conditions in Netherton syndrome keratinocytes. These data establish that uncontrolled kallikrein activity can trigger atopic dermatitis-like lesions, independent of the environment and the adaptive immune system, and illustrate the crucial role of protease signaling in skin inflammation. Also, endogenous proteases, matriptase, prostasin, and furin, are implicated in a cascade that activates sodium channel, non-voltage-gated 1 α, leading to epidermal barrier formation and hydration, probably through their involvement in filaggrin processing [76].

Conclusion

It is becoming clear that pathologies regarding asthma, atopic dermatitis and other allergic diseases are associated with abnormal activities of both endogenous and exogenous proteases. Therefore, a deeper knowledge of regulating these proteases could form the basis for development of appropriate treatments for allergic and inflammatory disorders.

References

1 Martinon F, Mayor A, Tschopp J. The inflammasomes: guardians of the body. *Annu Rev Immunol* 2009; **27**: 229–65.

2 Busse W, Elias J, Sheppard D, *et al*. Airway remodeling and repair. *Am J Respir Crit Care Med* 1999; **160**: 1035–42.

3 Kariyawasam HH, Aizen M, Barkans J, *et al*. Remodeling and airway hyperresponsiveness but not cellular inflammation persist after allergen challenge in asthma. *Am J Respir Crit Care Med* 2007; **175**: 896–904.

4 Southam DS, Ellis R, Wattie J, *et al*. Components of airway hyperresponsiveness and their associations with inflammation and remodeling in mice. *J Allergy Clin Immunol* 2007; **119**: 848–54.

5 Boulet LP, Turcotte H, Laviolette M, *et al*. Airway hyperresponsiveness, inflammation, and subepithelial collagen deposition in recently diagnosed versus long-standing mild asthma. Influence of inhaled corticosteroids. *Am J Respir Crit Care Med* 2000; **162**: 1308–13.

6 Carroll N, Elliot J, Morton A, *et al*. The structure of large and small airways in nonfatal and fatal asthma. *Am Rev Respir Dis* 1993; **147**: 405–10.

7 Yu M, Tsai M, Tam SY, *et al*. Mast cells can promote the development of multiple features of chronic asthma in mice. *J Clin Invest* 2006; **116**: 1633–41.

8 Brightling CE, Bradding P, Symon FA, *et al*. Mast-cell infiltration of airway smooth muscle in asthma. *N Engl J Med* 2002; **346**: 1699–705.

9 Chen FH, Samson KT, Miura K, *et al*. Airway remodeling: a comparison between fatal and nonfatal asthma. *J Asthma* 2004; **41**: 631–8.

10 Cho SH, Yao Z, Wang SW, *et al*. Regulation of activin A expression in mast cells and asthma: its effect on the proliferation of human airway smooth muscle cells. *J Immunol* 2003; **170**: 4045–52.

11 Kanbe N, Kurosawa M, Nagata H, *et al*. Cord blood-derived human cultured mast cells produce transforming growth factor β1. *Clin Exp Allergy* 1999; **29**: 105–13.

12 Hirst SJ, Barnes PJ, Twort CH. PDGF isoform-induced proliferation and receptor expression in human cultured airway smooth muscle cells. *Am J Physiol* 1996; **270**: L415–28.

13 Hashimoto S, Gon Y, Takeshita I, *et al*. Transforming growth factor-β1 induces phenotypic modulation of human lung fibroblasts to myofibroblast through a c-Jun-NH2-terminal kinase-dependent pathway. *Am J Respir Crit Care Med* 2001; **163**: 152–7.

14 Woodman L, Siddiqui S, Cruse G, *et al*. Mast cells promote airway smooth muscle cell differentiation via autocrine up-regulation of TGF-β1. *J Immunol* 2008; **181**: 5001–7.

15 Okumura S, Sagara H, Fukuda T, *et al*. FcεRI-mediated amphiregulin production by human mast cells increases mucin gene expression in epithelial cells. *J Allergy Clin Immunol* 2005; **115**: 272–9.

16 Enomoto Y, Orihara K, Takamasu T, *et al*. Tissue remodeling induced by hypersecreted epidermal growth factor and amphiregulin in the airway after an acute asthma attack. *J Allergy Clin Immunol* 2009; **124**: 913–20.

17 Guay C, Laviolette M, Tremblay GM. Targeting serine proteases in asthma. *Curr Top Med Chem* 2006; **6**: 393–402.

18 Schwartz LB, Min HK, Ren S, *et al*. Tryptase precursors are preferentially and spontaneously released, whereas mature tryptase is retained by HMC-1 cells, Mono-Mac-6 cells, and human skin-derived mast cells. *J Immunol* 2003; **170**: 5667–73.

19 Bonadonna P, Perbellini O, Passalacqua G, *et al*. Clonal mast cells disorders in patients with systemic reactions to Hymenoptera stings and increased serum tryptase levels. *J Allergy Clin Immunol* 2009; **123**: 680–6.

20 Schwartz LB, Bradford TR, Littman BH, *et al*. The fibrinogenolytic activity of purified tryptase from human lung mast cells. *J Immunol* 1985; **135**: 2762–7.

21 Imamura T, Dubin A, Moore W, *et al*. Induction of vascular permeability enhancement by human tryptase: dependence on activation of prekallikrein and direct release of bradykinin from kininogens. *Lab Invest* 1996; **74**: 861–70.

22 Stack MS and Johnson DA. Human mast cell tryptase activates single-chain urinary-type plasminogen activator (pro-urokinase). *J Biol Chem* 1994; **269**: 9416–19.

23 Gruber BL, Marchese MJ, Suzuki K, *et al*. Synovial procollagenase activation by human mast cell tryptase dependence upon matrix metalloproteinase 3 activation. *J Clin Invest* 1989; **84**: 1657–62.

24 Schwartz LB, Kawahara MS, Hugli TE, *et al*. Generation of C3a anaphylatoxin from human C3 by human mast cell tryptase. *J Immunol* 1983; **130**: 1891–5.

25 Lee M, Sommerhoff CP, von Eckardstein A, *et al*. Mast cell tryptase degrades HDL and blocks its function as an acceptor of cellular cholesterol. *Arterioscler Thromb Vasc Biol* 2002; **22**: 2086–91.

26 Kielty CM, Lees M, Shuttleworth CA, *et al*. Catabolism of intact type VI collagen microfibrils: susceptibility to degradation by serine proteinases. *Biochem Biophys Res Commun* 1993; **191**: 1230–6.

27 Hallgren J, Spillmann D, Pejler G. Structural requirements and mechanism for heparin-induced activation of a recombinant mouse mast cell tryptase, mouse mast cell protease 6: formation of active tryptase monomers in the presence of low molecular weight heparin, *J Biol Chem* 2001; **276**: 42774–81.

28 Kaminska R, Helisalmi P, Harvima RJ, *et al*. Focal dermal–epidermal separation and fibronectin cleavage

in basement membrane by human mast cell tryptase. *J Invest Dermatol* 1999; **113**: 567–73.

29 Caughey GH, Leidig F, Viro NF, *et al*. Substance P and vasoactive intestinal peptide degradation by mast cell tryptase and chymase. *J Pharmacol Exp Ther* 1988; **244**: 133–7.

30 Tam EK and Caughey GH. Degradation of airway neuropeptides by human lung tryptase. *Am J Respir Cell Mol Biol* 1990; **3**: 27–32.

31 Brown JK, Jones CA, Rooney LA, *et al*. Mast cell tryptase activates extracellular-regulated kinases (p44/p42) in airway smooth-muscle cells: importance of proteolytic events, time course, and role in mediating mitogenesis. *Am J Respir Cell Mol Biol* 2001; **24**: 146–54.

32 Tatler AL, Porte J, Knox A, *et al*. Tryptase activates TGF-β in human airway smooth muscle cells via direct proteolysis. *Biochem Biophys Res Commun* 2008; **370**: 239–42.

33 Fajardo I and Pejler G. Human mast cell β-tryptase is a gelatinase. *J Immunol* 2003; **171**: 1493–9.

34 Guyot N, Zani ML, Berger P, *et al*. Proteolytic susceptibility of the serine protease inhibitor trappin-2 (pre-elafin): evidence for tryptase-mediated generation of elafin. *J Biol Chem* 2005; **386**: 391–9.

35 Pang L, Nie M, Corbett L, *et al*. Mast cell-tryptase selectively cleaves eotaxin and RANTES and abrogates their eosinophil chemotactic activities. *J Immunol* 2006; **176**: 3788–95.

36 Rauter I, Krauth MT, Flicker S, *et al*. Allergen cleavage by effector cell-derived proteases regulates allergic inflammation. *FASEB J* 2006; **20**: 967–9.

37 Shin K, Nigrovic PA, Crish J, *et al*. Mast cells contribute to autoimmune inflammatory arthritis via their tryptase/heparin complexes. *J Immunol* 2009; **182**: 647–56.

38 Costanzo MJ, Yabut SC, Zhang HC, *et al*. Potent, nonpeptide inhibitors of human mast cell tryptase. Synthesis and biological evaluation of novel spirocyclic piperidine amide derivatives. *Bioorg Med Chem Lett* 2008; **18**: 2114–2121.

39 Caughey GH (2007) Mast cell tryptases and chymases in inflammation and host defense. *Immunol Rev* 2007; **217**: 141–54.

40 Irani AM, Schwartz LB. Human mast cell heterogeneity. *Allergy Proc* 1994; **15**: 303–8.

41 Morar N, Willis-Owen SA, Moffatt MF, *et al*. The genetics of atopic dermatitis. *J Allergy Clin Immunol* 2006; **118**: 24–34.

42 Terakawa M, Fujieda Y, Tomimori Y, *et al*. Oral chymase inhibitor SUN13834 ameliorates skin inflammation as well as pruritus in mouse model for atopic dermatitis. *Eur J Pharmacol* 2008; **601**: 186–91.

43 Omoto Y, Tokime K, Yamanaka K, *et al*. Human mast cell chymase cleaves pro-IL-18 and generates a novel and biologically active IL-18 fragment. *J Immunol* 2006; **177**: 8315–19.

44 Zanini A, Chetta A, Saetta M, *et al*. Chymase-positive mast cells play a role in the vascular component of airway remodeling in asthma. *J Allergy Clin Immunol* 2007; **120**: 329–33.

45 Stevens RL, Adachi R. Protease–proteoglycan complexes of mouse and human mast cells and importance of their β-tryptase–heparin complexes in inflammation and innate immunity. *Immunol Rev* 2007; **217**: 155–67.

46 McNeil HP, Adachi R, Stevens RL. Mast cell-restricted tryptases: structure and function in inflammation and pathogen defense. *J Biol Chem* 2007; **282**: 20785–9.

47 Knight PA, Wright SH, Lawrence CE, *et al*. Delayed expulsion of the nematode Trichinella spiralis in mice lacking the mucosal mast cell-specific granule chymase, mouse mast cell protease-1. *J Exp Med* 2000; **192**: 1849–56.

48 Tchougounova E, Pejler G, Abrink M. The chymase, mouse mast cell protease 4, constitutes the major chymotrypsin-like activity in peritoneum and ear tissue. A role for mouse mast cell protease 4 in thrombin regulation and fibronectin turnover. *J Exp Med* 2003; **198**: 423–31.

49 Tchougounova E, Lundequist A, Fajardo I, *et al*. A key role for mast cell chymase in the activation of pro-matrix metalloprotease-9 and pro-matrix metalloprotease-2. *J Biol Chem* 2005; **280**: 9291–6.

50 Waern I, Jonasson S, Hjoberg J, *et al*. Mouse mast cell protease 4 is the major chymase in murine airways and has a protective role in allergic airway inflammation. *J Immunol* 2009; **183**: 6369–76.

51 Abonia JP, Friend DS, Austen WG Jr, *et al*. Mast cell protease 5 mediates ischemia–reperfusion injury of mouse skeletal muscle. *J Immunol* 2005; **174**: 7285–91.

52 Feyerabend TB, Hausser H, Tietz A, *et al*. Loss of histochemical identity in mast cells lacking carboxypeptidase A. *Mol Cell Biol* 2005; **25**: 6199–210.

53 Schneider LA, Schlenner SM, Feyerabend TB, *et al*. Molecular mechanism of mast cell mediated innate defense against endothelin and snake venom sarafotoxin. *J Exp Med* 2007; **204**: 2629–39.

54 Platts-Mills TA, Chapman MD. Dust mites: immunology, allergic disease, and environmental control. *J Allergy Clin Immunol* 1987; **80**: 755–75.

55 Yasueda H, Mita H, Yui Y, Shida T. Comparative analysis of physicochemical and immunochemical properties of the two major allergens from Dermatophagoides pteronyssinus and the corresponding allergens from Dermatophagoides farinae. *Int Arch Allergy Appl Immunol* 1989; **88**: 402–7.

56 Chua KY, Stewart GA, Thomas WR, *et al*. Sequence analysis of cDNA coding for a major house dust mite

allergen Der p 1: homology with cysteine proteases. *J Exp Med* 1988; **167**: 175–82.

57 Takai T, Kato T, Sakata Y, *et al*. Recombinant Der p 1 and Der f 1 exhibit cysteine protease activity but no serine protease activity. *Biochem Biophys Res Commun* 2005; **328**: 944–52.

58 Takai T, Kato T, Yasueda H, *et al*. Analysis of the structure and allergenicity of recombinant pro- and mature Der p 1 and Der f 1: major conformational IgE epitopes blocked by prodomains. *J Allergy Clin Immunol* 2005; **115**: 555–63.

59 Wan H, Winton HL, Soeller C, *et al*. Der p 1 facilitates transepithelial allergen delivery by disruption of tight junctions. *J Clin Invest* 1999; **104**: 123–33.

60 Shakib F, Ghaemmaghami AM, Sewell HF. The molecular basis of allergenicity. *Trends Immunol* 2008; **29**: 633–42.

61 Chapman MD, Wünschmann S, Pomés A. Proteases as Th2 adjuvants. *Curr Allergy Asthma Rep* 2007; **7**: 363–7.

62 Sokol CL, Barton GM, Farr AG, *et al*. A mechanism for the initiation of allergen-induced T helper type 2 responses. *Nat Immunol* 2008; **9**: 310–18.

63 Sokol CL, Chu NQ, Yu S, *et al*. Basophils function as antigen-presenting cells for an allergen-induced T helper type 2 response. *Nat Immunol* 2009; **10**: 713–20.

64 Hammad H, Chieppa M, Perros F, *et al*. House dust mite allergen induces asthma via Toll-like receptor 4 triggering of airway structural cells. *Nat Med* 2009; **15**: 410–16.

65 Phipps S, Lam CE, Kaiko GE, *et al*. Toll/IL-1 signaling is critical for house dust mite-specific helper T cell type 2 and type 17 responses. *Am J Respir Crit Care Med* 2009; **179**: 883–93.

66 Lee KE, Kim JW, Jeong KY, *et al*. Regulation of German cockroach extract-induced IL-8 expression in human airway epithelial cells. *Clin Exp Allergy* 2007; **37**: 1364–73.

67 Page K, Ledford JR, Zhou P, *et al*. A TLR2 agonist in German cockroach frass activates MMP-9 release and is protective against allergic inflammation in mice. *J Immunol* 2009; **183**: 3400–8.

68 Aimanianda V, Bayry J, Bozza S, *et al*. Surface hydrophobin prevents immune recognition of airborne fungal spores. *Nature* 2009; **460**: 1117–21.

69 Shpacovitch V, Feld M, Hollenberg MD, *et al*. Role of protease-activated receptors in inflammatory responses, innate and adaptive immunity. *J Leukoc Biol* 2008; **83**: 1309–22.

70 Reed CE, Kita H. The role of protease activation of inflammation in allergic respiratory diseases. *J Allergy Clin Immunol* 2004; **114**: 997–1008.

71 D'Agostino B, Roviezzo F, De Palma R, *et al*. Activation of protease-activated receptor-2 reduces airways inflammation in experimental allergic asthma. *Clin Exp Allergy* 2007; **37**: 1436–43.

72 Chhabra J, Li YZ, Alkhouri H, Blake AE, *et al*. Histamine and tryptase modulate asthmatic airway smooth muscle GM-CSF and RANTES release. *Eur Respir J* 2007; **29**: 861–70.

73 Carvalho RF, Nilsson G, Harvima IT. Increased mast cell expression of PAR-2 in skin inflammatory diseases and release of IL-8 upon PAR-2 activation. *Exp Dermatol* 2010; **19**: 117–22.

74 O'Regan GM, Sandilands A, McLean WH, *et al*. Filaggrin in atopic dermatitis. *J Allergy Clin Immunol* 2009; **124**: R2–6.

75 Briot A, Deraison C, Lacroix M, *et al*. Kallikrein 5 induces atopic dermatitis-like lesions through PAR2-mediated thymic stromal lymphopoietin expression in Netherton syndrome. *J Exp Med* 2009; **206**: 1135–47.

76 Ovaere P, Lippens S, Vandenabeele P, *et al*. The emerging roles of serine protease cascades in the epidermis. *Trends Biochem Sci* 2009; **34**: 453–63.

25 Toll-like receptors

Jessica L. Allen,[1] *Aurelien Trompette,*[2] *and Christopher L. Karp*[1]

[1]Division of Molecular Immunology, Cincinnati Children's Hospital Research Foundation, and the University of Cincinnati College of Medicine, Cincinnati, OH, USA

[2]University Hospital Center of Lausanne, Lausanne, Switzerland

The molecular identification of long-sought-for receptors that signal the presence of microbial infection and tissue injury revolutionized the study of innate immunity over the last decade, upending paradigms and providing novel mechanistic insights into immune homeostasis as well as widely diverse immunologically driven disease processes [1,2]. Study of the Toll-like receptors (TLRs) has led the way. Several lines of evidence—epidemiologic, genetic, and experimental—have linked exposure to TLR ligands with protection from the development of allergic asthma as well as exacerbation of existing asthma, allergic or not [3]. This chapter will provide an overview of these data linking TLRs and TLR signaling to regulation of the development and expression of allergic asthma, as well as to the molecular substrates of allergenicity itself.

Immune recognition in the innate and adaptive immune systems

Providing protection against the microbial universe and injury constitutes a primary function of the interlinked innate and adaptive immune systems. This overarching function can be broken down into: (a) recognition (of microbes or injury); (b) response (containment or elimination of microbes or injury); and (c) resolution (control of immune response vigor and duration). It is useful to contrast immune recognition in the innate and adaptive immune systems. In the adaptive immune system, recognition occurs via receptors that are clonally distributed on individual B cells (surface immunoglobulins) and T cells (T cell receptors), or secreted by the former (immunoglobulins). Through such receptors, the adaptive immune system is able to engender recognition of essentially any molecular structure. This receptor repertoire, practically infinite, is generated through somatic gene segment rearrangement and somatic mutation. Lymphocytes bearing specific receptors undergo selection during the lifetime of individual organisms. This ability to generate receptors specific for any molecular structure raises the problem of deleterious self-recognition. Avoidance of harmful recognition of self by the adaptive immune system is largely prevented by a variety of mechanisms referred to collectively as "immunologic tolerance," including deletion of developing lymphocytes that carry receptors having an inappropriate affinity for self antigens during lymphocyte development and maturation; alteration of the effector characteristics of mature lymphocytes that recognize self antigen in the absence of activating cues from the innate immune system; and direct suppression of harmfully autoreactive lymphocytes by regulatory lymphocyte populations.

In the innate immune systems, on the other hand, recognition occurs via germ line-encoded, non-rearranging (apart from isoform generation) receptors. As a result, such receptors are relatively few in

Inflammation and Allergy Drug Design, First Edition. Edited by Kenji Izuhara, Stephen T. Holgate, Marsha Wills-Karp.
© 2011 Blackwell Publishing Ltd. Published 2011 by Blackwell Publishing Ltd.

number and are the result of selection over evolutionary time scales. Charles Janeway, in 1989, published a prescient theoretical paper that discussed the likely consequences of these constraints for the process of innate immune recognition, a process that he conceived of in terms of the discrimination of "non-infectious self from infectious non-self" [4]. Given the enormous universe of microbial structures and the high mutation rate of microbes compared with vertebrates, he postulated: (i) that the structures so recognized had to be expressed by large groups of microbes; (ii) that such structures had to be essential to microbial survival and thus constrained from mutational variation; and (iii) that such structures must be distinct from host structures, in order to avoid the harmful consequences of self-recognition. In Janeway's schema, innate immune recognition occurs via pattern recognition receptors (PRRs) whose ligands are pathogen-associated molecular patterns (PAMPs). Even within this schema, the name was misleading—there were clear reasons to postulate that the structures recognized by PRRs are not unique to pathogens (something subsequently borne out experimentally). The TLR family of membrane-bound PRRs that signal the presence of microbial structures conserved across broad classes of microbes, discovered in 1998, fit this schema beautifully. Other families of PRRs were soon discovered and/or delineated within this schema, including cytoplasmic PRRs (e.g., the nucleotide-binding oligomerization domain, leucine-rich repeat and pyrin domain containing proteins [NLRs] and the RIG-I-like helicase receptors [RLRs]) and transmembrane and secreted PRRs belonging to the C-type lectin family (CLRs).

An alternate theoretical model for innate immune recognition, the "danger hypothesis," was elaborated by Polly Matzinger in the 1990s [5]. In this schema, immune recognition is conceived not in terms of discrimination of non-infectious self from infectious non-self, but in terms of the detection of "danger." The presence of microbes or microbial products in normally sterile tissue sites is clearly dangerous. However, non-microbial "danger"—including traumatic tissue injury, tissue ischemia and infarction, and crystal deposition—also leads to innate immune activation, something that suggests the existence of innate immune receptors for structures that are upregulated, solubilized or induced by cellular injury. Given that sterile inflammation can mimic infection-associated inflammation [6], it is not surprising that there appears to be considerable overlap between PRRs for PAMPs and PRRs for injured or altered self ("damage-associated molecular patterns;" DAMPs) [7–9].

Toll-like receptors: basic biology

Toll receptors were first described in *Drosophila*, Toll being first identified as a transmembrane receptor required for dorsal–ventral patterning during larval development [10]. The evident homology between the signaling domains of Toll and the mammalian IL-1 receptor (IL-1R) [11] was found to be mirrored by similarities in the signaling pathways activated by these receptors, something that suggested a possible role for Toll in immunity [12]. Indeed, the Toll pathway was found to be required for resistance to both fungal and Gram-positive bacterial infections in *Drosophila* [13,14].

A mammalian family of Toll homologs, the TLRs, was subsequently identified and cloned. It had been appreciated for decades that Gram-negative sepsis could be experimentally mimicked by injection of a purified constituent of the outer membrane of Gram-negative bacteria ("endotoxin"). Biochemical identification of endotoxin as lipopolysaccharide (LPS), and identification of the critical role of LPS-driven myeloid cell production of proinflammatory mediators in the pathogenesis of endotoxic shock, proceeded in parallel with the search for the host sensor for LPS [15]. The first LPS receptors discovered (including LPS-binding protein—a soluble lipid transferase that facilitates extraction of LPS monomers from the surface of Gram-negative bacteria and from micelles in plasma—and CD14—a soluble or GPI-linked protein that transfers LPS monomers to the cell surface LPS signaling complex) were not themselves signaling proteins. The cloning and functional identification of TLR4, the vertebrate TLR to be identified, ended the long search for the signaling LPS receptor [16–18]. Subsequently, the other vertebrate TLRs have been shown to be essential for recognition of a variety of PAMPs from bacteria, protozoa, fungi and viruses, as well diverse DAMPs (Table 25.1) [19].

The vertebrate TLR family members are type I integral transmembrane proteins characterized by an extracellular leucine-rich repeat (LRR) domain, a conserved pattern of juxtamembrane cysteine residues and

Table 25.1 Toll-like receptors (TLRs) and selected pathogen-associated TLR agonists.

TLR	Ligand
TLR2/TLR1	Triacyl lipopeptides (bacteria, mycobacteria)
TLR2/TLR6	Diacyl lipopeptides (bacteria), Lipoarabinomannan (mycobacteria), phospholipomannan (fungi)
TLR2/TLR10 (human)	Triacyl lipopeptides (bacteria, mycobacteria) [97]
TLR3	dsRNA
TLR4	LPS (bacteria)
TLR5	Flagellin (bacteria)
TLR7	ssRNA (viruses)
TLR8 (human)	ssRNA (viruses)
TLR9	Unmethylated CpG DNA (bacteria, viruses)
TLR11 (mouse)	Profilin (protozoa: *Toxoplasma gondii*)

an intracytoplasmic signaling domain (Toll/IL-1 resistance [TIR]) that is highly conserved across the TLRs as well as in the IL-1R and IL-18R. Crystal structures of several TLRs complexed with their PAMP ligands have recently been published [20–23]. For signaling, TLRs complex as homodimers (e.g., TLR9–TLR9, TLR3–TLR3) or heterodimers (e.g., TLR2–TLR1, TLR2–TLR6). The signaling TLR4 complex involves homodimerization of heterodimers involving the primary LPS-binding member of the complex, the secreted protein MD-2 (TLR4/MD-2-TLR4/MD-2). The TLRs that signal in response to nucleic acids (TLR3, TLR7, TLR8, TLR9) are expressed in intracellular vesicular compartments. TLR1, TLR2, TLR5, TLR6, TLR10, and TLR11 are expressed on the cell surface. Of note, TLR4, the most robust signaling TLR, signals from both the cell surface and endosomal compartments (Figure 25.1) [24].

Although no role has been found for TLRs in mammalian development, the TLRs play a critical role in the activation of mammalian immune responses[19]. Antigen-presenting cells (APCs) are major sites of TLR expression [1]. The various TLRs are differ-

entially expressed on different subsets and maturation stages of dendritic cells [25]. Several TLRs are expressed on B cells [26]. Monocyte/macrophages appear to express all TLRs except for TLR3. Other professional innate immune cells (e.g., mast cells, neutrophils), as well as a variety of parenchymal cell types, including, importantly, airway epithelial cells, also express TLRs. TLR signaling leads to proinflammatory (e.g., TNF, IL-8, IFN-β) and immunoregulatory (e.g., IL-12, IL-10) cytokine production, as well as to upregulation of major histocompatibility complex and co-stimulatory molecule expression on APCs [19]. TLR-driven cytokine production is key to the activation of both innate and adaptive immunity. TLR-driven upregulation of MHC and co-stimulatory molecule expression is essential for the activation of adaptive immune responses. Further, TLRs are directly involved in the activation of antimicrobial activity by both phagocytic and epithelial cells [19]. Recent data have also demonstrated a critical role for TLRs in regulating the development of immune cells. Hematopoietic progenitor cells express TLRs, including TLR4. TLR signaling preferentially drives myelopoiesis, as well as driving lymphoid progenitors to become dendritic cells, providing a means for replenishment of innate immune cells during infection [27].

Toll-like receptor signaling

Ligand-induced TLR dimerization creates a TIR–TIR platform that acts to recruit TIR-containing signaling adapter molecules [MyD88, Mal (TIRAP), TRIF and/or TRAM] through homophilic interactions. In turn, the TLR adapter molecules recruit a variety of kinases and substrates, leading to the activation of distinct signaling pathways that result in the activation of pathway-specific transcription factors. Stimulation through TLRs induces activation of NF-κB, MAPK (p38, ERK) and IRF signaling pathways (Figure 25.1) (reviewed in refs. 28 and 29). Differential association of adapter molecules with specific TLRs provides a mechanistic underpinning for the differing patterns of gene expression resulting from activation of the different TLRs. The fact that TLRs form signaling receptor clusters provides an additional mechanism for the induction of specific signaling pathways, even through the same TLR. For example, CD14

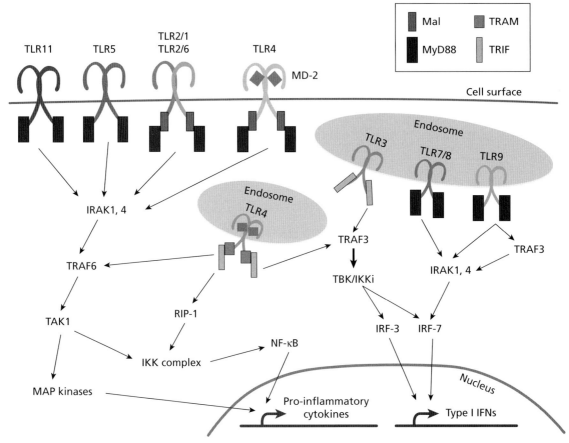

Figure 25.1 Schematic of Toll-like receptor (TLR) signaling. Ligand-induced TLR dimerization creates a TIR–TIR platform that acts to recruit TIR-containing signaling adapter molecules: MyD88 (recruited by all TLRs except for TLR3), Mal (TIRAP; recruited to bridge TLR and MyD88 TIR domains by TRL2 heterodimers and TLR4); TRIF (recruited by TLR3 and TLR4); and TRAM (bridging the TLR4 TIR domain with that in TRIF). TLR1, TLR2, TLR5, TLR6, TLR10, and TLR11 signal from the cell surface; TLR3, TLR7, TLR8, and TLR9 from endosomal compartments. In the case of TLR4, which signals from both the cell surface (via Mal/MyD88) and from endosomal compartments (via TRIF/TRAM), LPS monomers are transferred sequentially from the LPS-binding protein (in plasma) to CD14 to MD-2, the LPS–MD-2 complex being the activating ligand for TLR4. MyD88 recruits IRAK kinases, leading to the activation of NF-κB and MAP kinases (p38 and ERK). TRIF recruits TRAF3 (leading to IRF activation via TBK1/IKKi), as well as TRAF6 and RIP (leading to NF-κB and MAP kinase activation). In plasmacytoid dendritic cells, TLR7- and TLR9-mediated IRF activation occurs via TRAF3 and IRAK kinases.

can dictate TLR4 adapter usage: in the absence of CD14, rough LPS only drives MyD88-dependent activation (and smooth LPS fails to signal entirely) [30,31]. In the case of some TLR2/TLR6 ligands, CD14 appears to be needed for activation of the MyD88 pathway [30]. Similarly, CD36 appears to be an essential co-receptor for signaling of some (but not all) TLR2 ligands [32,33]. TLRs have also been reported to exhibit synergy in signaling with diverse other innate immune receptors, including NLR family members, the CLR dectin 1, and receptors for complement [28,34].

Control of Toll-like receptor signaling

Although activation of proinflammatory responses is critical for both innate and adaptive immunity, excessive or inappropriate inflammation can be harmful or even fatal. As might thereby be expected, TLR pathways are normally kept under tight regulation. Control of TLR expression levels is one clear mechanism of regulation. For example, while airway epithelial cells express TLR4, they normally express little or no MD-2 [35]. This, along with the targeting of both CD14 and MD-2 by inhibitory interactions with surfactant lipids [36], prevents harmful TLR4 activation in response to the low levels of LPS and Gram-negative bacteria that are routinely aspirated. Another mechanism of control is the phenomenon of endotoxin tolerance, the secondary blunting of a subset of microbial product-driven responses. A particular instance of a more general phenomenon of activation-induced macrophage reprogramming, the molecular mechanisms underlying endotoxin tolerance remain controversial [37,38]. Numerous direct, negative regulators of TLR signaling have been identified, including SARM (an inhibitory TIR-containing adapter), RP105, IRAK-M, soluble TLRs, SOCS1, SOCS3, SHP1, ATF3, TAM receptors, and A20 [28,39,40].

Toll-like receptors, atopy, and asthma: epidemiologic and genetic data

The prevalence of allergic (and autoimmune) diseases underwent a rapid rise in westernized environments during the 20th century. Although considerable experimental work has gone into delineating the heritable components of allergic diseases [41], the speed of this shift suggests that important causal variables are likely to be found in environmental changes, or in the interaction of environmental changes with genetic substrates. A useful organizing hypothesis has focused on decreasing early childhood exposure to microbes and/or microbial products. This "hygiene hypothesis" posits that such exposures tend to inhibit the development of allergic (and autoimmune) diseases, most likely through facilitating the generation of robust counter-regulatory responses in the developing immune system [42,43].

Multiple studies have shown that residence on a farm during early life is associated with a lower risk of atopic disease [44–47]. In an attempt to achieve mechanistic insight into these findings, several studies demonstrated an inverse correlation between LPS levels in house dust (in both farming and non-farming households) and the risk of developing allergic disease [48–52]. That said, other large studies were not able to replicate these findings [53–55]. Analysis of the association of genetic polymorphisms in LPS receptor complex members followed a similar pattern. Association—in opposite directions, or the lack of an association—between common alleles in CD14 and atopic disease have been reported in different cohorts in different environments (reviewed in refs. 56 and 57). Of note, recent data from four independent cohorts suggests an informative reason for these apparent discrepancies, one that is rooted in gene–environment interactions. That is, the C allele of the rs2569190 promoter polymorphism in *CD14* appears to provide protection against the development of atopy—but only in the face of high domestic LPS exposure [58–62].

It is worth pointing out that LPS is just an easily measured marker of bacterial product contamination, that CD14 facilitates signaling through both TLR4 and TLR2, and that polymorphisms in the genes encoding both of these TLRs have also been associated with risk for developing atopy and/or asthma in different cohorts [3,56,63]. The actual ligands responsible for driving these environmental effects remain to be defined. It should also be noted that, in addition to an apparent role in inhibiting the developing of allergy and asthma, exposure to LPS has also convincingly been shown to exacerbate established asthma (whether allergic or non-allergic) as well as to induce non-atopic wheezing [48,64–68].

Toll-like receptors and asthma: experimental models

Studies in rodent models have confirmed the ability of LPS exposure to exacerbate the course of established allergic asthma [69]. Such studies have also provided mechanistic insight into the ability of TLR4 signaling to promote or inhibit the development of experimental allergic asthma. Consonant with the hygiene hypothesis, the TLR4 ligand dose appears to be key. Eisenbarth and colleagues reported that airway sensitization with ovalbumin (OVA): (a) along with "very low-dose" LPS (<1 ng/dose) leads to tolerance; (b) along with "low-dose" LPS (100 ng/dose) drives Th2 inflammation in the airway, in a TLR4-dependent fashion; and (c) along with "high-dose" LPS (100 μg/dose) drives Th1 inflammation in the airway, probably with a strong counter-regulatory response as well [70,71]. Thus, LPS exhibits a biphasic effect, promoting allergic airway inflammation at low doses, but inhibiting it at high doses. As the thought at the time was that Th1 differentiation depended on TLR signaling but that Th2 differentiation was independent of such signaling, these data were initially surprising. However, several groups subsequently also showed that, whereas TLR-independent pathways are capable of driving Th2 polarization, TLR4 signaling can play an important role in Th2 polarization and allergic asthma pathogenesis [72–74]. Of interest, experiments employing bone marrow chimeras have indicated an important for TLR4 expression by radioresistant nonhematopoietic cells in these effects, although the results appear to vary by LPS dose and antigen employed (OVA vs. dust mite culture lysates) [75,76].

TLRs besides TLR4 also play important roles in regulating the development of experimental allergic asthma. Similar to low doses of TLR4 ligands, TLR2 ligands can promote Th2 differentiation and allergic inflammation in the lung [77,78]. On the other hand, TLR9 ligands both prevent and ameliorate experimental allergic asthma, exhibiting no facilitation at low doses [79–82]. Signaling through TLR7 and TLR3 has also been shown to suppress allergic asthma in mouse models [83–85].

Toll-like receptors and allergenicity

We recently discovered a more intimate link between TLR signaling and allergic sensitization [86]. House dust mites represent a major source of aeroallergens in the indoor environment [87]. Der p 2 and Der f 2, the major group II allergens of such mites, are secreted by epithelial cells lining the mite gut; human exposure is via inhalation of mite feces [88]. Der p 2 and Der f 2 are highly allergenic, having the highest rates of skin test positivity among defined

dust mite antigens [89]. They are also homologs of MD-2, the eponymous member of the MD-2-related lipid-recognition (ML) family of proteins [90,91], and the LPS-binding member of the TLR4 signaling complex. Given structural homologies between Der p 2 and MD-2 [23,92–94], we asked whether there was functional homology as well. Notably, we found that: (a) Der p 2 interacts directly with the TLR4 signaling complex, facilitating TLR4 signaling in the presence of MD-2 and reconstituting it in the absence of MD-2; (b) Der p 2 similarly facilitates TLR4 signaling in primary antigen-presenting cells, in the presence and absence of MD-2; and (c) Der p 2 has *in vivo* allergenic activity that mirrors its biochemical and functional activity *in vitro*—driving robust Th2 inflammation in the airway in a TLR4-dependent fashion, retaining this functional activity in mice with a genetic deletion in MD-2 [86].

A central question in allergy is why specific, ubiquitous, otherwise apparently innocuous proteins tend to be targeted by (mal)adaptive immune responses in susceptible hosts. Our results strongly suggest that intrinsic adjuvant properties provide the answer in the case of Der p 2. Is this more than a bizarre oddity? In fact, several other ML family members are major allergens, including Lep d 2, Tyr p 2, Gly d 2 and Eur m 2. Mimicry of, and functional interactions with, the TLR4 complex may thus underlie the allergenicity of several major aeroallergens. Of interest, another house dust mite allergen, Der p 7, was recently shown to have a fold similar to that in LPS-binding protein, and to bind a bacterially derived lipopeptides [95]—suggesting that direct mimicry of TLR complex proteins may have broader applicability as a mechanism underlying allergenicity. More broadly, more than 50% of defined major allergens are lipid-binding proteins. Quite diverse protein families are represented, including, apart from the ML family, secretoglobins (e.g., Fel d 1), pathogenesis-related 10 family proteins (e.g., Bet v 1), lipocalins (e.g., Can f 1), non-specific lipid transfer proteins (e.g., Pru p 3), 2S albumins (e.g., Ara h 9), and apolipophorins (e.g., Der p 14). It is likely that intrinsic adjuvant activity provided by these proteins and their associated lipid cargo is central to the immunogenicity and/or allergenicity of these proteins.

Even more broadly, evidence from numerous studies suggests that direct, if inadvertent, interactions with innate immune activation pathways that evolved to signal the presence of microbial infection has considerable generality as a molecular substrate of allergenicity. In addition to the effects of bound lipids on innate immune activation, relevant adjuvant activity appears to be provided by carbohydrate epitopes on glycoprotein allergens and allergen-associated protease activity (reviewed in ref. 96). Better molecular insight into the critical ligands, receptors and signaling pathways involved in pathophysiologic interactions of allergens with the innate immune system has promise for leading to novel therapeutic and preventive approaches to atopy and asthma.

Acknowledgment

The authors were supported in part by grants from the American Asthma Foundation and the National Institute of Allergy and Infectious Diseases to C. Karp.

References

1 Iwasaki A, Medzhitov R. Regulation of adaptive immunity by the innate immune system. *Science* 2010; **327**: 291–5.

2 Kawai T, Akira S. The roles of TLRs, RLRs and NLRs in pathogen recognition. *Int Immunol* 2009; **21**: 317–37.

3 Williams LK, Ownby DR, Maliarik MJ, Johnson CC. The role of endotoxin and its receptors in allergic disease. *Ann Allergy Asthma Immunol* 2005; **94**: 323–32.

4 Janeway CA Jr. Approaching the asymptote? Evolution and revolution in immunology. *Cold Spring Harb Symp Quant Biol* 1989; **54** (Pt 1): 1–13.

5 Matzinger P. Tolerance, danger, and the extended family. *Annu Rev Immunol* 1994; **12**: 991–1045.

6 Beutler, B. Inferences, questions and possibilities in Toll-like receptor signalling. *Nature* 2004; **430**: 257–63.

7 Avalos AM, Busconi L, Marshak-Rothstein A. Regulation of autoreactive B cell responses to endogenous TLR ligands. *Autoimmunity* 2010; **43**: 76–83.

8 Miyake K. Innate immune sensing of pathogens and danger signals by cell surface Toll-like receptors. *Semin Immunol* 2007; **19**: 3–10.

9 Seong SY, Matzinger P. Hydrophobicity: an ancient damage-associated molecular pattern that initiates innate immune responses. *Nat Rev* 2004; **4**: 469–78.

10 Hashimoto C, Hudson KL, Anderson KV. The Toll gene of Drosophila, required for dorsal-ventral embryonic polarity, appears to encode a transmembrane protein. *Cell* 1988; **52**: 269–79.

11 Gay NJ, Keith FJ. Drosophila Toll and IL-1 receptor. *Nature* 1991; **351**: 355–6.

12 Belvin MP, Anderson KV. A conserved signaling pathway: the Drosophila toll-dorsal pathway. *Annu Rev Cell Dev Biol* 1996; **12**: 393–416.

13 Lemaitre B, Nicolas E, Michaut L, Reichhart JM, Hoffmann JA. The dorsoventral regulatory gene cassette spatzle/Toll/cactus controls the potent antifungal response in Drosophila adults. *Cell* 1996; **86**: 973–83.

14 Rutschmann S, Kilinc A, Ferrandon D. Cutting edge: the toll pathway is required for resistance to gram-positive bacterial infections in Drosophila. *J Immunol* 2002; **168**: 1542–6.

15 Beutler B, Rietschel ET. Innate immune sensing and its roots: the story of endotoxin. *Nat Rev* 2003; **3**: 169–76.

16 Medzhitov R, Preston-Hurlburt P, Janeway CA Jr. A human homologue of the Drosophila Toll protein signals activation of adaptive immunity [see comments]. *Nature* 1997; **388**: 394–7.

17 Poltorak A, He X, Smirnova I, *et al.* Defective LPS signaling in C3H/HeJ and C57BL/10ScCr mice: mutations in Tlr4 gene. *Science* 1998; **282**: 2085–8.

18 Qureshi ST, Lariviere L, Leveque G, *et al.* Endotoxin-tolerant mice have mutations in Toll-like receptor 4 (Tlr4) [see comments]. *J Exp Med* 1999; **189**: 615–25.

19 Takeda K, Kaisho T, Akira S. Toll-like receptors. *Annu Rev Immunol* 2003; **21**: 335–76.

20 Jin MS, Kim SE, Heo JY, *et al.* Crystal structure of the TLR1–TLR2 heterodimer induced by binding of a tri-acylated lipopeptide. *Cell* 2007; **130**: 1071–82.

21 Liu L, Botos I, Wang Y, *et al.* Structural basis of toll-like receptor 3 signaling with double-stranded RNA. *Science* 2008; **320**: 379–81.

22 Kang JY, Nan X, Jim MS, *et al.* Recognition of lipopeptide patterns by Toll-like receptor 2-Toll-like receptor 6 heterodimer. *Immunity* 2009; **31**: 873–84.

23 Park BS, Song DH, Kim HM, Choi BS, Lee H, Lee JO. The structural basis of lipopolysaccharide recognition by the TLR4–MD-2 complex. *Nature* 2009; **458**: 1191–5.

24 Kagan JC, Su T, Horng T, Chow A, Akira S, Medzhitov R. TRAM couples endocytosis of Toll-like receptor 4 to the induction of interferon-beta. *Nat Immunol* 2008; **9**: 361–8.

25 Iwasaki A, Medzhitov R. Toll-like receptor control of the adaptive immune responses. *Nat Immunol* 2004; **5**: 987–95.

26 Crampton SP, Voynova E, Bolland S. Innate pathways to B-cell activation and tolerance. *Ann N Y Acad Sci* 2010; **1183**: 58–68.

27 Nagai Y, Garrett KP, Ohta S, *et al.* Toll-like receptors on hematopoietic progenitor cells stimulate innate immune system replenishment. *Immunity* 2006; **24**: 801–12.

28 O'Neill LA. When signaling pathways collide: positive and negative regulation of toll-like receptor signal transduction. *Immunity* 2008; **29**: 12–20.

29 Kawai T, Akira S. TLR signaling. *Semin Immunol* 2007; **19**: 24–32.

30 Jiang Z, Georgel P, Du X, *et al*. CD14 is required for MyD88-independent LPS signaling. *Nat Immunol* 2005; **6**: 565–70.

31 Perera PY, Vogel SN, Detore GR, Haziot A, Goyert SM. CD14-dependent and CD14-independent signaling pathways in murine macrophages from normal and CD14 knockout mice stimulated with lipopolysaccharide or taxol. *J Immunol* 1997; **158**: 4422–9.

32 Hoebe K, Georgel P, Rutschmann S, *et al*. CD36 is a sensor of diacylglycerides. *Nature* 2005; **433**: 523–7.

33 Triantafilou M, Gamper FGJ, Haston RM, *et al*. Membrane sorting of toll-like receptor (TLR)-2/6 and TLR2/1 heterodimers at the cell surface determines heterotypic associations with CD36 and intracellular targeting. *J Biol Chem* 2006; **281**: 31002–11.

34 Wang M, Krauss JL, Domon H, *et al*. Microbial hijacking of complement-toll-like receptor crosstalk. *Sci Signal* 2010; **3**, ra11.

35 Jia HP, Kline JN, Penisten A, *et al*. Endotoxin responsiveness of human airway epithelia is limited by low expression of MD-2. *Am J Physiol Lung Cell Mol Physiol* 2004; **287**: L428–37.

36 Kuronuma K, Mitsuzawa H, Takeda K, *et al*. Anionic pulmonary surfactant phospholipids inhibit inflammatory responses from alveolar macrophages and U937 cells by binding the lipopolysaccharide-interacting proteins CD14 and MD-2. *J Biol Chem* 2009; **284**: 25488–500.

37 Cross AS. Endotoxin tolerance—current concepts in historical perspective. *J Endotoxin Res* 2002; **8**: 83–98.

38 Foster SL, Hargreaves DC, Medzhitov R. Gene-specific control of inflammation by TLR-induced chromatin modifications. *Nature* 2007; **447**: 972–8.

39 Liew FY, Xu D, Brint EK, O'Neill LA. Negative regulation of Toll-like receptor-mediated immune responses. *Nat Rev* 2005; **5**: 446–58.

40 Gilchrist M, Thorsson V, Li B, *et al*. Systems biology approaches identify ATF3 as a negative regulator of Toll-like receptor 4. *Nature* 2006; **441**: 173–8.

41 Ober C, Hoffjan S. Asthma genetics 2006: the long and winding road to gene discovery. *Genes Immun* 2006; **7**: 95–100.

42 Wills-Karp M, Santeliz J, Karp CL. The germless theory of allergic disease: revisiting the hygiene hypothesis. *Nat Rev* 2001; **1**: 69–75.

43 Yazdanbakhsh M, Kremsner PG, van Ree R. Allergy, parasites, and the hygiene hypothesis. *Science* 2002; **296**: 490–4.

44 Kilpelainen M, Terho EO, Helenius H, Koskenvuo M. Farm environment in childhood prevents the development of allergies. *Clin Exp Allergy* 2000; **30**: 201–8.

45 Von Ehrenstein OS, Von Mutius E, Illi S, Baumann L, Bohm O, von Kries R. Reduced risk of hay fever and asthma among children of farmers. *Clin Exp Allergy* 2000; **30**: 187–93.

46 Ernst P, Cormier Y. Relative scarcity of asthma and atopy among rural adolescents raised on a farm. *Am J Respir Crit Care Med* 2000; **161**: 1563–6.

47 Braun-Fahrlander C, *et al*. Prevalence of hay fever and allergic sensitization in farmer's children and their peers living in the same rural community. SCARPOL team. Swiss Study on Childhood Allergy and Respiratory Symptoms with Respect to Air Pollution. *Clin Exp Allergy* 1999; **29**: 28–34.

48 Braun-Fahrlander C, Gassner M, Grize L, *et al*. Environmental exposure to endotoxin and its relation to asthma in school-age children. *N Engl J Med* 2002; **347**: 869–77.

49 Gehring U, Bischof W, Fahlbusch B, Wichmann HE, Heinrich J. House dust endotoxin and allergic sensitization in children. *Am J Res Crit Care Med* 2002; **166**: 939–44.

50 von Mutius E, Braun-Fahrlander C, Shierl R, *et al*. Exposure to endotoxin or other bacterial components might protect against the development of atopy. *Clin Exp Allergy* 2000; **30**: 1230–4.

51 Riedler J, Braun-Fahrlander C, Eder W, *et al*. Exposure to farming in early life and development of asthma and allergy: a cross-sectional survey. *Lancet* 2001; **358**: 1129–33.

52 Gereda JE, Leung DY, Thatayatikom A, *et al*. Relation between house-dust endotoxin exposure, type 1 T-cell development, and allergen sensitisation in infants at high risk of asthma. *Lancet* 2000; **355**: 1680–3.

53 Bolte G, Bischof W, Borte M, *et al*. Early endotoxin exposure and atopy development in infants: results of a birth cohort study. *Clin Exp Allergy* 2003; **33**: 770–6.

54 Douwes J, van Strien R, Doekes G, *et al*. Does early indoor microbial exposure reduce the risk of asthma? The Prevention and Incidence of Asthma and Mite Allergy birth cohort study. *J Allergy Clin Immunol* 2006; **117**: 1067–73.

55 Lau S, Illi S, Platts-Hills TA, *et al*. Longitudinal study on the relationship between cat allergen and endotoxin exposure, sensitization, cat-specific IgG and development of asthma in childhood—report of the German Multicentre Allergy Study (MAS 90). *Allergy* 2005; **60**: 766–73.

56 Vercelli D. Gene–environment interactions in asthma and allergy: the end of the beginning? *Curr Opin Allergy Clin Immunol* 2010; **10**: 145–80.

57 Simpson A, Martinez FD. The role of lipopolysaccharide in the development of atopy in humans. *Clin Exp Allergy* 2010; **40**: 209–23.

58 Eder W, Klimecki W, Yu L, *et al*. Opposite effects of CD 14/-260 on serum IgE levels in children raised in different environments. *J Allergy Clin Immunol* 2005; **116**: 601–7.

59 Simpson A, John SL, Jury F, *et al*. Endotoxin exposure, CD14, and allergic disease: an interaction between genes and the environment. *Am J Res Crit Care Med* 2006; **174**: 386–92.

60 Williams LK, McPhee RA, Ownby DR, *et al*. Gene–environment interactions with CD14 C-260T and their relationship to total serum IgE levels in adults. *J Allergy Clin Immunol* 2006; **118**: 851–7.

61 Williams LK, Oliver J, Peterson EL, *et al*. Gene–environment interactions between CD14 C-260T and endotoxin exposure on Foxp3+ and Foxp3- CD4+ lymphocyte numbers and total serum IgE levels in early childhood. *Ann Allergy Asthma Immunol* 2008; **100**: 128–36.

62 Zambelli-Weiner A, Ehrlich E, Stockton ML, *et al*. Evaluation of the CD14/–260 polymorphism and house dust endotoxin exposure in the Barbados Asthma Genetics Study. *J Allergy Clin Immunol* 2005; **115**: 1203–9.

63 Eder W, Kilmecki W, Yu L, *et al*. Toll-like receptor 2 as a major gene for asthma in children of European farmers. *J Allergy Clin Immunol* 2004; **113**: 482–8.

64 Michel O, Duchateau J, Sergysels R. Effect of inhaled endotoxin on bronchial reactivity in asthmatic and normal subjects. *J Appl Physiol* 1989; **66**: 1059–64.

65 Eduard W, Douwes J, Omenaas E, Heederik D. Do farming exposures cause or prevent asthma? Results from a study of adult Norwegian farmers. *Thorax* 2004; **59**: 381–6.

66 Rylander R, Bake B, Fischer JJ, Helander IM. Pulmonary function and symptoms after inhalation of endotoxin. *Am Rev Respir Dis* 1989; **140**: 981–6.

67 Becker S, Clapp WA, Quay J, *et al*. Compartmentalization of the inflammatory response to inhaled grain dust. *Am J Res Crit Care Med* 1999; **160**: 1309–18.

68 Michel O, Kips J, Duchateau J, *et al*. Severity of asthma is related to endotoxin in house dust. *Am J Res Crit Care Med* 1996; **154**: 1641–6.

69 Tulic MK, Wale JL, Holt PG, Sly PD. Modification of the inflammatory response to allergen challenge after exposure to bacterial lipopolysaccharide. *Am J Respir Cell Mol Biol* 2000; **22**: 604–12.

70 Eisenbarth SC, Piggott DA, Huleatt JW, Visintin I, Herrick CA, Bottomly K. Lipopolysaccharide-enhanced, toll-like receptor 4-dependent T helper cell type 2 responses to inhaled antigen. *J Exp Med* 2002; **196**: 1645–51.

71 Herrick CA, Bottomly K. To respond or not to respond: T cells in allergic asthma. *Nature Rev Immunol* 2003; **3**: 1–8.

72 Dabbagh K, Dahl ME, Stepick-Biek P, Lewis DB. Toll-like receptor 4 is required for optimal development of Th2 immune responses: role of dendritic cells. *J Immunol* 2002; **168**: 4524–30.

73 Strohmeier GR, Walsh JH, Klings ES, *et al*. Lipopolysaccharide binding protein potentiates airway reactivity in a murine model of allergic asthma. *J Immunol* 2001; **166**: 2063–70.

74 Phipps S, Lam CE, Kaiko GE, *et al*. Toll/IL-1 signaling is critical for house dust mite-specific Th1 and Th2 responses. *Am J Res Crit Care Med* 2009; **179**: 883–93.

75 Hammad H, Chieppa M, Perros F, *et al*. House dust mite allergen induces asthma via Toll-like receptor 4 triggering of airway structural cells. *Nat Med* 2009; **15**: 410–16.

76 Tan AM, Chen HC, Pochard P, Eisenbarth SC, Herrick CA, Bottomly HK. TLR4 signaling in stromal cells is critical for the initiation of allergic Th2 responses to inhaled antigen. *J Immunol* 2010; **184**: 3535–44.

77 Redecke V, Hacker H, Datta SK, *et al*. Cutting edge: activation of Toll-like receptor 2 induces a Th2 immune response and promotes experimental asthma. *J Immunol* 2004; **172**: 2739–43.

78 Pulendran B, Kumar P, Cutler CW, Mohamadzadeh M, Van Dyke T, Banchereau J. Lipopolysaccharides from distinct pathogens induce different classes of immune responses *in vivo*. *J Immunol* 2001; **167**: 5067–76.

79 Broide D, Schwarze J, Tighe H, *et al*. Immunostimulatory DNA sequences inhibit IL-5, eosinophilic inflammation, and airway hyperresponsiveness in mice. *J Immunol* 1998; **161**: 7054–62.

80 Serebrisky D, Teper AA, Huang CK, *et al*. CpG oligodeoxynucleotides can reverse Th2-associated allergic airway responses and alter the B7.1/B7.2 expression in a murine model of asthma. *J Immunol* 2000; **165**: 5906–12.

81 Broide DH, Stachnick G, Castaneda D, *et al*. Systemic administration of immunostimulatory DNA sequences mediates reversible inhibition of Th2 responses in a mouse model of asthma. *J Clin Immunol* 2001; **21**: 175–82.

82 Hessel EM, Chu M, Lizcano JO, *et al*. Immunostimulatory oligonucleotides block allergic airway inflammation by inhibiting Th2 cell activation and IgE-mediated cytokine induction. *J Exp Med* 2005; **202**: 1563–73.

83 Moisan J, Camateros P, Thuraisingam T, *et al*. TLR7 ligand prevents allergen-induced airway hyperresponsiveness and eosinophilia in allergic asthma by a MYD88-dependent and MK2-independent pathway. *Am J Physiol Lung Cell Mol Physiol* 2006; **290**: L987–99.

84 Sel S, Wegmann M, Bauer S, Garn H, Alber G, Renz H. Immunomodulatory effects of viral TLR ligands on experimental asthma depend on the additive effects of IL-12 and IL-10. *J Immunol* 2007; **178**: 7805–13.

85 Xirakia C, Koltsida O, Stavropoulos A, *et al.* TLR7-triggered immune response in the lung mediates acute and long-lasting suppression of experimental asthma. *Am J Res Crit Care Med* 2010; **181**: 1207–16.

86 Trompette A, Divanovic S, Visintin A, *et al.* Allergenicity resulting from functional mimicry of a Toll-like receptor complex protein. *Nature* 2009; **457**: 585–8.

87 Maunsell K, Wraith DG, Cunnington AM. Mites and house-dust allergy in bronchial asthma. *Lancet* 1968; **1**: 1267–70.

88 Tovey ER, Chapman MD, Wells CW, Platts-Mills TA. The distribution of dust mite allergen in the houses of patients with asthma. *Am Rev Respir Dis* 1981; **124**: 630–5.

89 Heymann PW, Chapman MD, Aalberse RC, Fox JW, Platts-Mills TA. Antigenic and structural analysis of group II allergens (Der f II and Der p II) from house dust mites (Dermatophagoides spp). *J Allergy Clin Immunol* 1989; **83**: 1055–67.

90 Inohara N, Nunez G. ML—a conserved domain involved in innate immunity and lipid metabolism. *Trends Biochem Sci* 2002; **27**: 219–21.

91 Gangloff M, Gay NJ. MD-2: the Toll "gatekeeper" in endotoxin signalling. *Trends Biochem Sci* 2004; **29**: 294–300.

92 Derewenda U, Li J, Derewenda Z, *et al.* The crystal structure of a major dust mite allergen Der p 2, and its biological implications. *J Mol Biol* 2002; **318**: 189–97.

93 Kim HM, Park BS, Kim JI, *et al.* Crystal structure of the TLR4–MD-2 complex with bound endotoxin antagonist Eritoran. *Cell* 2007; **130**: 906–17.

94 Ohto U, Fukase K, Miyake K, Satow Y. Crystal structures of human MD-2 and its complex with antiendo-toxic lipid IVa. *Science* 2007; **316**: 1632–4.

95 Mueller GA, Edwards LL, Aloor JJ, *et al.* The structure of the dust mite allergen Der p 7 reveals similarities to innate immune proteins. *J Allergy Clin Immunol* 2010; **25**: 909–17.

96 Wills-Karp M, Nathan A, Page K, Karp CL. New insights into innate immune mechanisms underlying allergenicity. *Mucosal Immunol* 2009; **3**: 1041–10.

97 Guan Y, Ranoa DR, Jiang S, *et al.* Human TLRs 10 and 1 Share common mechanisms of innate immune sensing but not signaling. *J Immunol* 2010; **184**: 5094–103.

Index

Notes: Page numbers in *italics* refer to figures, those in **bold** refer to tables. *vs.* indicates a comparison or differential diagnosis. The following abbreviations have been used in subentries:

G-CSF   granulocyte colony-stimulating factor
GM-CSF   granulocyte–macrophage colony-stimulating factor
IL   interleukin
MMP   matrix metalloproteinase
NKT cells   natural killer T cells
TGF-β   transforming growth factor β
Th1 cells   T helper cells type 1
Th2 cells   T helper cells type 2
TLR   Toll-like receptor
Treg   regulatory T cells

A

A-122058 259
acidic mammalian chitinase (AMCase) 178
  epithelial cells 143, 144
acquired (adaptive) immune response
  B cells 68–9
  mast cells 91–3
  recognition 307–8
  regulation 67
activin A 238, 298
activin receptor-like kinase (ALK) family 152
AD *see* atopic dermatitis (AD)
adalimumab 226
ADAM33 244
adenosine, mast cell activation 93
adherens junctions *140*
adherens junctions (AJs) 139
adoptive transfer experiments
  IL-15 202
  Th2 cells 17
  Th17 cells 199–200
  Treg in asthma 44
adrenoceptors, β agonists *see* β₂-adrenergic agonists
AECs *see* epithelial cells
AER 001 (pitrakinra, IL-4 mutein, AEROVANT™) 22, 179–80
AEROVANT™ (IL-4 mutein, pitrakinra, AER 001) 22, 179–80

AHR *see* airway hyperresponsiveness (AHR)
AIRE (autoimmune regulator) 40
air pollution, IL-17R⁺ NKT cells 62–3
airway
  mast cells 93–4
  TGF-β effects 46–7
airway epithelial cells (AECs) *see* epithelial cells
airway fibrosis 237–41
  collagen 237
  extracellular matrix 237–8
  TGF-β 238–9
airway hyperresponsiveness (AHR) 237
  IL-17RB NKT cells 60
airway inflammation
  dendritic cells 8
  prostanoids 278–9
airway remodeling 149–51, 237, 298
  animal models 150
  beneficial effects 151
  fibroblasts 149, 151
  MMPs 152
  SD-208 153
  smooth muscle cells 149
  targets 150–1
  TGF-β 150
airway smooth muscle (ASM) 163–71, 298
  asthma pathogenesis 165–6, *167*
  chemokines 255

contractile 163
functional diversity 165, *166*
IL-5, effects of 190–1
leukotrienes **288**
mast cell infiltration 79–80, 93–4, 298
PGE₂ 276
phenotype plasticity 163–5
  cell culture 164
  maturation 164, *164*
  phenotype modulation 164
prostanoids 276–8
synthetic/proliferative 163
treatment indications 167–8
in vitro culture 163
ALK *see* activin receptor-like kinase (ALK) family 152
allele frequencies, IL-17RB polymorphisms 61–2
allergic airway disease
  cytokines 189
  Th2 cells 17
allergic airway inflammation
  IL-15 202
  IL-25 200–1
allergic asthma, TNF 226–7
allergic inflammation
  chemokines 253–5
  chronic *see* chronic allergic inflammation
  cytokines 7
  IL-10 effects 45–6

Inflammation and Allergy Drug Design, First Edition. Edited by Kenji Izuhara, Stephen T. Holgate, Marsha Wills-Karp.
© 2011 Blackwell Publishing Ltd. Published 2011 by Blackwell Publishing Ltd.